Cardiology
1994

Cardiology

1994

WILLIAM C. ROBERTS, M.D.
Executive Director
Baylor Cardiovascular Institute
Baylor University Medical Center
Dallas
Editor-in-Chief, The American Journal of Cardiology

CHARLES E. RACKLEY, M.D.
Professor of Medicine
Division of Cardiology
Department of Medicine
Georgetown University Medical Center
Washington, D.C.

DEAN T. MASON, M.D.
Physician-in-Chief, Western Heart Institute
Chairman, Department of
Cardiovascular Medicine
St. Mary's Medical Center
at Golden Gate Park, San Francisco
Editor-in-Chief, American
Heart Journal

WILLIAM W. PARMLEY, M.D.
Professor of Medicine
University of California
San Francisco, School of Medicine
Chief of Cardiology
Moffitt/Long Hospital, San Francisco
Editor-in-Chief, Journal of the
American College of Cardiology

JAMES T. WILLERSON, M.D.
Edward Randall III Professor and
Chairman
Department of Internal Medicine
University of Texas Medical School at
Houston
Chief of Medical Service
Hermann Hospital
Medical Director and Director of
Cardiology Research
The Texas Heart Institute
Houston
Editor-in-Chief, Circulation

THOMAS P. GRAHAM, JR., M.D.
Director of Pediatric Cardiology
Vanderbilt University Medical Center
Nashville

Butterworth–Heinemann
Boston London Oxford Singapore Sydney Toronto Wellington

ISBN 07506-9591-9

ISSN 0275-0066

Butterworth–Heinemann
313 Washington Street
Newton, MA 02158

10 9 8 7 6 5 4 3 2 1
Printed in the United States of America

Contents

2. Coronary Artery Disease   62

3. Acute Myocardial Infarction and Its Consequences   **180**

Preface

Cardiology 1994 is the fourteenth book to be published in this series. It contains summaries of 738 articles, all published in 1993. A total of 22 medical journals (Table I) were examined and at least one and usually many articles were summarized from each journal. The number of articles summarized by each of the six authors is listed in Table II. All of Dr. Rackley's submissions were from *The American Journal of Cardiology;* Dr. Willerson's from *Circulation;* Dr. Mason's from *The American Heart Journal;* and Dr. Parmley's from *The Journal of the American College of Cardiology.* The contributions of Dr. Graham and myself were from a variety of medical journals. The summaries from each contributor were submitted to me, organized into the various sections in each of the ten chapters, and edited.

A book of this type is made possible because of unselfish contributions from several individuals, none of whom is rewarded by authorship.

Table I. *Journals containing articles summarized in* Cardiology 1994.

1. American Heart Journal
2. American Journal of Cardiology
3. American Journal of Hypertension
4. American Journal of Medicine
5. Annals of Internal Medicine
6. Annals of Surgery
7. Annals of Thoracic Surgery
8. Archives of Internal Medicine
9. Arteriosclerosis and Thrombosis
10. British Heart Journal
11. British Medical Journal
12. Chest
13. Circulation
14. European Heart Journal
15. International Journal of Cardiology
16. Journal of the American College of Cardiology
17. Journal of American Medical Association
18. Journal of Thoracic and Cardiovascular Surgery
19. Lancet
20. Medicine
21. New England Journal of Medicine
22. Southern Medical Journal

Table II. *Contributions of the Six Authors to* Cardiology 1994.

AUTHOR	1	2	3	4	5	6	7	8	9	10	Totals
					CHAPTERS						
1) WCR	60	36	38	23	17	23	10	6	5	23	241 (32.66%)
2) CER	14	49	33	12	4	9	8	1	5	7	142 (19.24%)
3) JTW	9	37	26	9	4	3	4	1	10	7	110 (14.90%)
4) DTM	0	38	24	18	3	5	3	5	4	6	106 (14.36%)
5) WWP	1	32	22	13	2	1	5	0	9	7	92 (12.47%)
6) TPG, Jr	0	0	0	1	0	0	0	46	0	0	47 (6.37%)
Totals	84	192	143	76	30	41	30	59	33	50	738 (100%)
Figures	12	27	20	5	7	9	5	8	3	2	98
Tables	17	6	17	3	6	8	2	3	2	10	74

I am enormously grateful to Donna Robertson for typing the summaries contributed by me; to Angie Esquivel, Leslie Flatt, Azora L. Irby, and Joy Phillips also for typing many summaries; to Michelle St. Jean-Richards, Editorial Assistant, for all her work obtaining permissions, and to Barbara Murphy, Medical Editor, and Karen Oberheim, Associate Editor, for efficiently coordinating the publishing of the book in Boston.

William C. Roberts, M.D.
Editor

Cardiology
1994

Conversion of Units

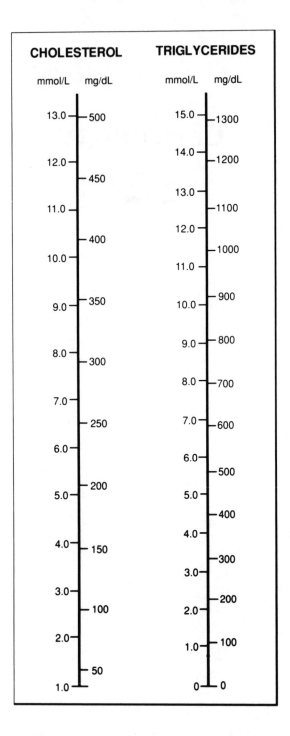

CHOLESTEROL

mmol/L	mg/dL
13.0	500
12.0	
	450
11.0	
	400
10.0	
9.0	350
8.0	
	300
7.0	
	250
6.0	
	200
5.0	
4.0	150
3.0	
	100
2.0	
	50
1.0	

TRIGLYCERIDES

mmol/L	mg/dL
15.0	1300
14.0	1200
13.0	1100
12.0	
	1000
11.0	
10.0	900
9.0	800
8.0	700
7.0	600
6.0	500
5.0	400
4.0	300
3.0	
	200
2.0	
1.0	100
0	0

Cholesterol mg/dL = mmol/L x 38.6
Triglyceride mg/dL = mmol/L x 88.5

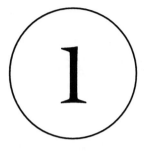

Factors Causing, Accelerating, or Preventing Coronary Arterial Atherosclerosis

---

BLOOD LIPIDS

Interesting Cardiologists in Lipids

Roberts,[1] from Dallas, Tex, examined the possible reasons why cardiologists ranked low in considering cholesterol of major importance for the development of atherosclerosis: (1) cardiologists as a group are not completely convinced of the important role of cholesterol in atherosclerosis; (2) cardiologists view cholesterol management as unexciting; (3) cardiologists avoid cholesterol management because they know that successful management requires expert knowledge of nutrition, expert knowledge of cholesterol-lowering drugs, and a change in their own lifestyles; (4) cardiologists are a bit confused by the recommendations of the lipid experts regarding whom to treat and whom not to treat with diet and lipid-lowering agents; (5) cardiologists resent being excluded from important roles in the cholesterol-lowering world; (6) cardiologists view the lipid-lowering drugs as too expensive; (7) cardiologists consider cholesterol-lowering drugs to have too many side effects with too high risk-benefit ratios; and (8) cardiologists view cholesterol management as financially unrewarding. The author concluded that because secondary prevention is in the hands of cardiologists and because cholesterol lowering has proved beneficial after atherosclerotic events, cardiologists must increase their knowledge of and use of low-fat, low-cholesterol diets and lipid-lowering agents.

Screening

The High Blood Cholesterol Education Program recommends that all adults aged ≥20 years be screened for high blood cholesterol at least once every 5 years. One of the national health objectives for the year 2000 is to increase to 75% the percentage of adults screened for high blood cholesterol within the preceding 5 years. To measure progress toward this objective, data from the Center for Disease Controls Behavioral Risk Factors Surveillance System[2] were used to examine state-specific trends in cholesterol screening from 1988 to 1991. Data were available for 258,782 persons aged ≥20 years in 47 states and the District of Columbia who participated in the Behavioral Risk Factors Surveillance System, a population-based, random-digit-dialed telephone survey. Respondents were asked whether they had ever had their cholesterol checked, and if so, the length of time that had elapsed since they last had their cholesterol checked. Persons who reported that they had been screened within the preceding 5 years were classified as having been screened for high blood cholesterol. In the 37 states that participated continuously for all 4 years in the Behavioral Risk Factor Surveillance Study from 1988 to 1991, the percentage of adults screened for high blood cholesterol increased from 51% to 64%. These findings indicate substantial increases in cholesterol screening from 1988 to 1991, representing an additional 19 million adults aged ≥20 years who have been screened for high blood cholesterol. If current trends continue, by 1994 populations of half the states will attain the national year 2000 objective for cholesterol screening.

As Predictors of Coronary Artery Disease

The increased risk of cardiovascular disease associated with higher serum cholesterol levels in middle-aged persons has been clearly established, but there have been few opportunities to examine a potential link between serum cholesterol levels measured in young men and clinically evident premature cardiovascular disease later in life. Klag and associates[3] from Baltimore, Md, and Peking, China performed a prospective study of 1,017 young men (mean age, 22 years) followed for 27 to 42 years to quantify the risk of cardiovascular disease and total mortality associated with serum cholesterol levels during early adult life. The mean serum cholesterol level at entry was 192 mg/dL (5.0 mol/L). During a median follow-up of 30.5 years, there were 125 cardiovascular-disease events, 97 of which were due to CAD (Figure 1-1, Table 1-1). The serum cholesterol level at baseline was strongly associated with the incidence of events related to coronary heart disease and cardiovascular disease, as well as to total mortality and mortality due to cardiovascular disease. The

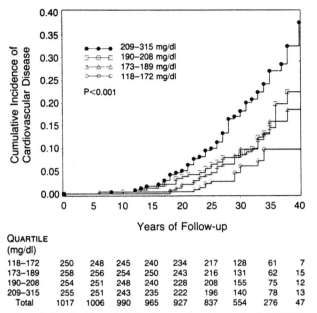

Quartile (mg/dl)								
118–172	250	248	245	240	234	217	128	61	7
173–189	258	256	254	250	243	216	131	62	15
190–208	254	251	248	240	228	208	155	75	12
209–315	255	251	243	235	222	196	140	78	13
Total	1017	1006	990	965	927	837	554	276	47

Figure 1-1. Cumulative Incidence of Cardiovascular Disease in 1,017 White Men, According to the Serum Cholesterol Level at a Median Age of 22 Years. To convert values for cholesterol to millimoles per liter, multiply by 0.02586. The numbers below the figure are the numbers of men included in the analysis at each time point. Reproduced with permission from Klag et al.[3]

risks were similar whether the events occurred before or after the age of 50. In a proportional-hazards analysis adjusted for age, body-mass index (the weight in kilograms divided by the square of the height in meters), the level of physical activity, coffee intake, change in smoking status, and the incidence of diabetes and hypertension during follow-up, a difference in the serum cholesterol level at baseline of 36 mg/dL (0.9 mol/L)—the difference between the 25th and 75th percentiles of cholesterol level in the study population at baseline—was associated with an increased risk of cardiovascular disease (relative risk, 1.72), coronary heart disease (relative risk, 2.01), and mortality due to cardiovascular disease (relative risk, 2.02). A difference in the baseline serum cholesterol level of 36 mg/dL was significantly associated with an increased risk of death before the age of 50 (relative risk, 1.64) but not with the overall risk of death (relative risk, 1.21). These findings indicate a strong association between the serum cholesterol level measured early in adult life in men and cardiovascular disease in midlife.

The association of lipoprotein levels with cardiovascular disease is less well understood in women than in men. To better characterize any relations, Bass and associates,[4] from Baltimore, Md, explored HDL and LDL cholesterol and triglyceride levels in women using data from female participants in the Lipid Research Clinics' Follow-up Study. Using a sample of 1,405 women aged 50 to 69 years, age-adjusted cardiovascular disease death rates and summary relative risk estimates by categories of lipid and lipoprotein levels were calculated. Average follow-up was 14 years. HDL cholesterol and triglyceride levels were strong predictors of cardiovascu-

Table 1-1. Relative Risk of Cardiovascular Disease Associated with a Difference in the Serum Cholesterol Level of 36 mg per Deciliter during Medical School in 1,017 White Men as a Group and According to the Age of the Men at the Time of the Event.* Reproduced with permission from Klag et al.[3]

Variable	Overall		<50 Years of Age		≥50 Years of Age	
	No. of Events	Relative Risk (95% CI)	No. of Events	Relative Risk (95% CI)	No. of Events	Relative Risk (95% CI)
Cardiovascular disease						
Crude	125	1.76 (1.46–2.12)†	37	1.93 (1.40–2.68)†	88	1.67 (1.33–2.10)†
Adjusted‡		1.72 (1.39–2.14)†		2.05 (1.36–3.08)†		1.60 (1.24–2.06)†
Coronary heart disease						
Crude	97	2.04 (1.66–2.50)†	30	2.18 (1.54–3.08)†	67	1.97 (1.53–2.52)†
Adjusted‡		2.01 (1.59–2.53)†		2.25 (1.47–3.45)†		1.92 (1.44–2.55)†
Myocardial infarction						
Crude	62	2.42 (1.90–3.08)†	20	2.44 (1.62–3.68)†	42	2.40 (1.78–3.23)†
Adjusted‡		2.22 (1.67–2.94)†		2.09 (1.25–3.47)§		2.31 (1.63–3.25)†
Angina pectoris						
Crude	49	1.56 (1.15–2.11)§	16	1.75 (1.05–2.92)¶	33	1.47 (1.02–2.14)¶
Adjusted‡		1.54 (1.10–2.17)¶		2.09 (1.15–3.80)¶		1.34 (0.88–2.04)
Cardiovascular-disease mortality						
Crude	21	2.03 (1.37–3.00)†	5	3.29 (1.53–7.06)§	16	1.74 (1.10–2.77)¶
Adjusted‡		2.02 (1.23–3.32)‖		5.63 (1.63–19.48)§		1.70 (0.97–2.98)
Total mortality						
Crude	95	1.33 (1.06–1.66)¶	32	1.49 (1.02–2.19)¶	63	1.25 (0.95–1.65)
Adjusted‡		1.21 (0.93–1.58)		1.64 (1.03–2.61)¶		1.06 (0.77–1.47)

*Cox proportional-hazards analysis was used. A total of 874 men were included in the multivariate analyses. Serum cholesterol was analyzed as a continuous variable. Relative risks are presented for a difference in the cholesterol level between the 25th and 75th percentiles of cholesterol in this study population at base line. CI denotes confidence interval.

†$P<0.001$.

‡The multivariate Cox model was adjusted for the calendar year, age at graduation, body-mass index, coffee intake, degree of physical activity, and three time-dependent covariates: a change in cigarette-smoking status during follow-up, the development of hypertension, and the development of diabetes mellitus during follow-up.

§$P<0.01$.   ¶$P<0.05$.   ‖$P = 0.005$.

lar disease death in age-adjusted and multivariate analyses. LDL and total cholesterol levels were poorer predictors of cardiovascular disease mortality. After adjustment for other cardiovascular disease risk factors, HDL levels <1.30 mmol/L (50 mg/dL) were strongly associated with cardiovascular mortality (RR = 1.74). Triglyceride levels were associated with increased cardiovascular disease mortality at levels of 2.25 to 4.49 mmol/L (200 to 399 mg/dL) (RR = 1.65) and 4.50 mmol/L (400 mg/dL) or greater (RR = 3.44). At total cholesterol levels of 5.20 mmol/L (200 mm/dL) or greater and at all levels of LDL and triglycerides, women with HDL levels of <1.30 mmol/L (<50 mg/dL) had cardiovascular disease death rates that were higher than those of women with HDL levels of 1.30 mmol/dL (50 mg/dL) or greater. Thus, HDL cholesterol and triglyceride levels are independent lipid predictors of cardiovascular disease death in women.

To evaluate the relationship between serum cholesterol level and all-cause CAD and non-CAD mortality as a function of age, Kronmal and associates,[5] from Seattle, Wash., examined data from the biennial examination from 1948 through 1980 for 5,209 men and women enrolled in the Framingham Heart Study. The authors performed an age-specific analyses by the Cox proportional-hazards regression model of survival subsequent to ages 40, 50, 60, 70, and 80 years for all subjects enrolled and alive at each of the stated ages. Complementary models were studied that used HDL cholesterol, LDL cholesterol, or total cholesterol level as predictors of survival subsequent to examination at which lipoprotein subfractions were determined (1968 through 1973). The relation between total cholesterol level and all-cause mortality was positive—that is, higher cholesterol levels were associated with higher mortality—at age 40 years, negative at age 80 years, and negligible at ages 50 to 70 years (Table 1-2). The relation with CAD mortality was significantly positive at ages 40, 50, and 60 years but attenuated with age until the relationship was positive, but not significant, at age 70 years and negative, but not significant, at age 80 years. Results for the relation between LDL cholesterol and HDL cholesterol and mortality help explain these findings. Non-CAD mortality was significantly negatively related to cholesterol level for ages 50 years and above. The negative results in the oldest age group for all-cause and CAD mortality appeared to be due to a negative relation with LDL cholesterol levels rather than the protective effect of high HDL cholesterol levels. Similar results from several modified analyses make low cholesterol level due to severe illness an unlikely explanation for the results. Physicians should be cautious about initiating cholesterol-lowering treatment in men and women above 65 to 70 years of age.

Laakso and associates,[6] from Kuopio, Finland, investigated the association of lipoprotein fractions with the future risk of CAD in patients with non-insulin-dependent diabetes. At baseline, lipoprotein fractions were determined in 313 diabetic patients with non-insulin-dependent diabetes, including 153 men and 160 women. These patients were followed for 7 years to determine their development of CAD events, including

Table 1-2. Crude Mortality Within Age Categories by Sex and Total Serum Cholesterol Interval. Reproduced with permission from Kronmal et al.[5]

		Men			Women		
Age, y	Total Serum Cholesterol Interval, mmol/L (mg/dL)	N	No. of Deaths	Deaths/100 Person-Years (±SE)	N	No. of Deaths	Deaths/100 Person-Years (±SE)
40	<5.17 (<200)	233	40	0.7±0.1	456	60	0.6±0.1
	5.17-6.18 (200-239)	343	66	0.8±0.1	393	51	0.5±0.1
	6.21-7.21 (240-279)	217	67	1.4±0.2	189	27	0.6±0.1
	≥7.24 (≥280)	114	36	1.4±0.2	71	19	1.1±0.3
50	<5.17 (<200)	291	74	1.5±0.2	337	60	1.0±0.1
	5.17-6.18 (200-239)	633	193	1.8±0.1	676	119	1.0±0.1
	6.21-7.21 (240-279)	462	163	2.1±0.2	610	107	0.9±0.1
	≥7.24 (≥280)	219	78	2.1±0.2	394	97	1.3±0.1
60	<5.17 (<200)	469	175	3.4±0.3	267	60	2.3±0.3
	5.17-6.18 (200-239)	743	270	3.3±0.2	772	185	2.1±0.2
	6.21-7.21 (240-279)	483	219	3.8±0.3	836	228	2.1±0.1
	≥7.24 (≥280)	223	97	3.6±0.4	635	188	2.2±0.2
70	<5.17 (<200)	259	115	6.4±0.6	141	46	4.6±0.7
	5.17-6.18 (200-239)	365	168	6.0±0.5	414	109	3.4±0.3
	6.21-7.21 (240-279)	208	94	5.5±0.6	463	149	3.8±0.3
	≥7.24 (≥280)	91	49	6.2±0.9	339	121	3.8±0.3
80	<5.17 (<200)	81	41	12.2±1.9	68	29	9.3±1.7
	5.17-6.18 (200-239)	87	46	12.0±1.8	147	44	6.4±1.0
	6.21-7.21 (240-279)	34	12	6.8±2.0	120	45	8.1±1.2
	≥7.24 (≥280)	10	2	4.3±3.0	75	14	3.6±1.0

CAD-associated death and myocardial infarction. Fifty-six non-insulin-dependent diabetes patients died from CAD and 25 had a nonfatal AMI during the follow-up. The non-insulin-dependent diabetes patients having these CAD events had higher levels of total and VLDL triglycerides and very LDL cholesterol and lower levels of HDL cholesterol than those without CAD events (Figure 1-2). CAD-associated deaths and all CAD events were increased 4-fold if there were low HDL cholesterol values (<0.9 mmol/L) as compared with diabetics with HDL cholesterols ≥0.9 mmol/L. High triglyceride levels (>2.3 mmol/L) were associated with a 2-fold increase in the risk of CAD events. HDL was inversely associated with CAD events and VLDL triglycerides with CAD events in non-insulin-dependent diabetes patients with low HDL cholesterol levels (≤1.12 mmol/L). Thus, these data indicate that low HDL cholesterol, high VLDL cholesterol, and high total and VLDL triglycerides are important risk factors for CAD events in patients with non-insulin-dependent diabetes mellitus.

To study the association between nonfasting serum triglyceride concentrations and mortality in women from coronary and cardiovascular disease and all causes, Stensvold and associates,[7] from Oslo, Norway, determined, at initial screening, total serum cholesterol concentration; serum triglyceride concentration; BP; height; weight; and self-reported

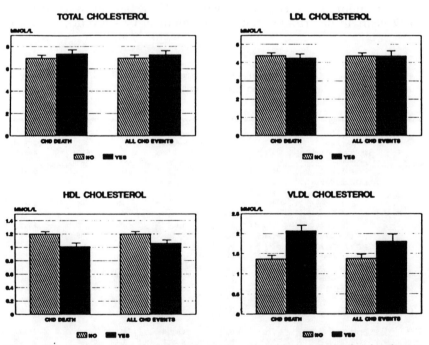

Figure 1-2. Total and lipoprotein cholesterol concentrations measured at baseline in non-insulin-dependent diabetic patients for those with CAD with and without subsequent death and serious CAD events, including CAD death or nonfatal myocardial infarction during a 7-year follow-up. LDL indicates low-density lipoprotein; HDL, high-density lipoprotein; and VLDL, very-low-density lipoprotein. Total and lipoprotein cholesterol concentrations were measured in mmol/L. The results are expressed as mean ± standard error of the mean. Reproduced with permission from Laakso et al.[6]

information about smoking habits, physical activity, and time since last meal in 25,048 men and 24,535 women aged 35 to 49 years. During subsequent follow-up, 108 women died from CAD, 238 from cardiovascular diseases, and 931 from all causes. In women, mortality increased steadily with increasing triglyceride concentration for all three causes of death. With the proportional hazards model and adjustment for age, systolic BP, total cholesterol concentration, time since last meal, and number of cigarettes per day, the relative risk between triglyceride concentrations 23.5 mmol/L and 1.5 mmol/L was 4.7 for deaths from CAD, 3.0 for deaths from cardiovascular disease, and 2.3 for total deaths in all women. A raised nonfasting concentration of triglycerides is an independent risk factor for mortality from CAD, cardiovascular disease, and any-cause mortality among middle-aged Norwegian women in contrast to what is seen in men.

Risk of Excessively Low Levels

LaRosa,[8] from Washington, DC, reviewed the cholesterol-lowering clinical studies over the past 2 decades and examined the manner in which these results should influence current public policy on cholesterol. Cholesterol lowering in both primary and secondary prevention has been clearly demonstrated to lower coronary morbidity and, in secondary prevention, to lower coronary mortality as well. Putative dangers of cholesterol lowering remain unproven. Population studies linking low cholesterol to noncoronary mortalities do not demonstrate cause-and-effect relations. In fact, based on current studies, the opposite is more likely to be the case. Neither gender nor age should automatically exclude persons from cholesterol screening. Drug intervention, however, should be used conservatively, particularly in young adults and the elderly. Drugs should be used only after diet and lifestyle interventions have failed. The evidence linking high blood cholesterol to coronary atherosclerosis and cholesterol lowering to its prevention is broad-based and definitive (Figure 1-3). Concerns about cholesterol lowering and spontaneously low cholesterols should be pursued but should not interfere with the implementation of current public policies to reduce the still heavy burden of atherosclerosis in Western society.

Lipoprotein(a)

Plasma lipoprotein(a) (Lp[a]) concentrations are associated with an increased risk of CAD in adults with familial hypercholesterolemia. Hegele and associates,[9] from Toronto, Canada, hypothesized that Lp(a) concentrations in children with familial hypercholesterolemia were higher among those with myocardial ischemia on stress thallium scans and among those with a family history of premature CAD. Twenty-nine asymptomatic heterozygotes with familial hypercholesterolemia (range: 9 to 23 years) and 7 homozygotes (range: 4 to 13 years) were evaluated with clinical assessment, lipoprotein measurement, and stress thallium scans. Compared with subjects with normal stress thallium scans, mean Lp(a) was significantly higher in homozygotes with stress thallium abnormalities and tended to be higher in heterozygotes with stress thallium abnormalities. Lp(a) tended to be higher in heterozygotes with a family history of premature CAD. The investigators concluded that Lp(a)

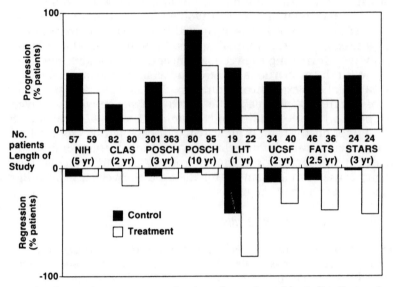

Figure 1-3. Progression versus regression in major angiographic studies. Progression of coronary atherosclerosis on angiography is less in cholesterol-treated subjects than in control subjects. Regression is better in treated patients. CLAS = Cholesterol-Lowering Atherosclerosis Study; FATS = Familial Atherosclerosis Treatment Study; LHT = Lifestyle Heart Trial; NIH = National Institutes of Health; POSCH = Program on the Surgical Control of the Hyperlipidemias; STARS = St Thomas' Atherosclerosis Regression Study; UCSF = University of California at San Francisco. Reproduced with permission from LaRosa et al.[8]

is higher in hypercholesterolemic children who have abnormal stress thallium scans. Lp(a) may be useful in assessing CAD risk in children with familial hypercholesterolemia.

Jenner and associates,[10] from Framingham, Mass, measured Lp(a) in 1,284 men and 1,394 women, mean ages 48 ± 10 years, without cardiovascular and cerebrovascular disease and not on medications known to affect lipids. Plasma Lp(a) levels were measured by an enzyme-linked immunosorbent assay. Mean plasma Lp(a) concentrations were 14 ± 7 mg/dL in men and 15 ± 17 mg/dL in women. Values of >38 mg/dL were above the 90th percentile and values of >22 mg/dL were above the 75th percentile in both men and women. There was an inverse association between plasma levels of Lp(a) and triglycerides for both sexes, but triglycerides accounted for only approximately 0.5% of the variation in Lp(a) levels. Associations of Lp(a) levels with total and LDL cholesterol levels were not significant. After controlling for age, Lp(a) values were 8% greater in postmenopausal women than in premenopausal women. Body-mass index, alcohol consumption, cigarette smoking, use of β-blockers or cholesterol-lowering medications, and the use of drugs for the treatment of diabetes and hypertension were not correlated with Lp(a) levels.

Elevated mean levels of Lp(a) have been associated with symptomatic cardiovascular diseases including AMI, other CAD syndromes, restenosis of coronary vein grafts after CABG, and family history of AMI. Schreiner and associates,[11] from Chapel Hill, NC, Houston, Tex, and

Bethesda, Md, evaluated associations of Lp(a) with arterial wall thickening in asymptomatic individuals participating in the Atherosclerosis Risk in Communities (ARIC) Study. Intima-media wall thickening in the extracranial carotid arteries was assessed noninvasively with B-mode ultrasonography; Lp(a) was measured as its total protein component. Individuals with wall thickening ≥90% of the population maximum far-wall thickness were pair matched to individuals with wall thickening <75%, by race, gender, center, 10-year age group, and time of examination. These selection criteria yielded 492 matched pairs, with 395 white pairs and 97 black pairs. The mean Lp(a) protein level for all black participants was 175 µg/mL compared with 78 µg/mL for whites. Conditional logistic regression analysis for the association of Lp(a) with case-control status yielded a statistically significant prevalence odds ratio estimate of 1.49, based on a 1-SD difference in Lp(a) protein, after adjusting for age, LDL cholesterol, HDL cholesterol, fibrinogen, hypertension, and cigarette smoking. None of these risk factors significantly altered the odds ratio, in agreement with reports that Lp(a) is unaffected by environmental influences. In addition, no differential effect of Lp(a) protein on case-control status (effect modification) was observed by race, gender, LDL cholesterol, or fibrinogen in this population. The authors concluded that Lp(a) is an independent risk factor for intima-media carotid thickening in individuals free of prevalent cardiovascular disease.

To assess prospectively the risk of AMI associated with elevated levels of Lp(a), Ridker and associates,[12] from Boston, Mass, studied a total of 14,916 male physicians aged 40 to 84 years with no prior history of AMI or stroke. The physicians provided plasma samples at baseline and were then followed up prospectively for an average period of 60.2 months. Samples from 296 physicians who subsequently developed AMI were analyzed for Lp(a) level together with paired controls, matched for smoking status and age. The distribution of Lp(a) level among cases was virtually identical to that of controls, and there was no significant difference between groups for median Lp(a) levels (103.0 mg/L v 102.5 mg/L). In analyses controlling for age and smoking status, the authors found no evidence of association between increasing level of Lp(a) and risk of AMI (relative risks from lowest to highest quintiles of Lp(a): 1.00, 0.97, 0.83, 0.88, and 1.07) or a threshold effect at any prespecified cutoff of Lp(a) level (relative risks associated with Lp[a] levels above the 25th, 50th, 75th, 90th, and 95th percentiles of the control distribution, respectively: 1.04, 1.00, 1.19, 1.00, and 1.07; all P values nonsignificant). Further adjustment for both lipid and nonlipid cardiovascular risk factors had no material impact. In this prospective study of predominantly middle-aged white men, the authors found no evidence of association between Lp(a) level and risk of future AMI. These data do not support the use of Lp(a) level as a screening tool to define cardiovascular risk among this population.

Very Low High-Density Lipoproteins

Epidemiological studies have established that concentrations of plasma HDL are inversely associated with premature atherosclerosis, but the physiological basis of this relation remains unknown. Rader and associates,[13] from Bethesda, Md, and Portland, Ore, investigated five probands with very low plasma HDL. None had clinical or biochemical findings typical of the known genetic disorders with low HDL nor had evidence of premature coronary atherosclerosis by sensitive diagnostic methods. All five probands and the son of one of them had rapid catabolism of the HDL apolipoproteins A-I and A-II. These results indicate that not all people with low HDL are necessarily at risk of premature CAD.

Oxidative Modification of Low-Density Lipoproteins

To test whether LDL from subjects with an atherogenic lipoprotein phenotype characterized by small, dense LDL (pattern B) demonstrates greater susceptibility to oxidative modification than LDL from subjects exhibiting primarily larger, more buoyant LDL particles (pattern A), Chait and associates,[14] from Seattle, Wash, and Stanford and Berkeley, Calif, compared measures of susceptibility with oxidative modification in six density subfractions of LDL isolated from pattern A and pattern B subjects. Seven male and three female pattern A subjects and five male and two female pattern B subjects, classified on the basis of peak LDL particle size, were studied. Plasma lipid and lipoprotein levels, apolipoprotein B, mean LDL particle diameter, lag phase, and rate of oxidation after initiation of oxidation by copper sulfate were measured. The lag time, a measure of resistance to oxidative modification, was inversely related to LDL density in both groups of subjects, without an independent effect of phenotype. The fraction that had the major LDL peak had a shorter lag time in pattern B than in pattern A. Pattern B subjects also demonstrated an increased rate of oxidation in fraction 1, which includes remnants of triglyceride-rich lipoproteins. The increased atherogenic risk associated with the pattern B phenotype may result in part from increased concentrations of lipoprotein subpopulations that are relatively susceptible to oxidative modification.

Nitric Oxide

Casino and associates,[15] from Bethesda, Md, investigated the role of nitric oxide in the endothelium-dependent vasodilation in patients with hypercholesterolemia by studying the effect of N^G-monomethyl-L-arginine (L-NMMA), an inhibitor of endothelial nitric oxide synthesis, on basal vascular tone and on the responses to acetylcholine, an endothelium-dependent vasodilator. Vascular responses to sodium nitroprusside, a direct smooth muscle dilator, were also studied. This study included 33 hypercholesterolemic patients (17 men from the age of 51 years with a plasma cholesterol ≥240 mg/dL) and 23 normal controls (12 men, 48 years of age, with a plasma cholesterol <210 mg/dL). The drugs were infused into the brachial artery, and the response of the forearm vasculature was measured by strain-gauge plethysmography. Basal blood flow and vascular resistance were similar in hypercholesterolemic patients and normal controls. The reduction in basal blood flow and increase in vascular resistance provoked by L-NMMA were not different between the two groups. L-NMMA markedly blunted the response to acetylcholine in normal individuals, but it did not significantly modify the response to acetylcholine in the hypercholesterolemic patients (Figure 1-4). L-NMMA did not modify the vasodilator response to sodium nitro-

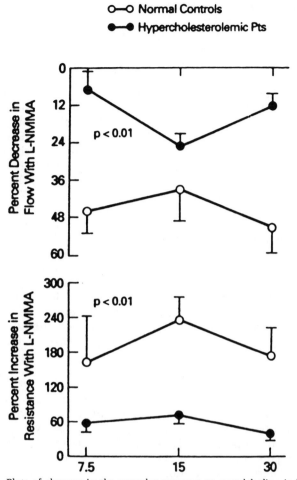

Figure 1-4. Plots of changes in the vascular response to acetylcholine induced by N^G-monomethyl-L-arginine (L-NMMA), expressed as percentage of decrease in forearm flow and percentage of increase in vascular resistance, in 10 normal controls (open circles) and 20 hypercholesterolemic patients (closed circles). Values represent mean and SEM. Reproduced with permission from Casino et al.[15]

prusside in either controls or patients. Thus, hypercholesterolemic patients have a defect in the bioactivity of nitric oxide that may help explain their impaired endothelium-dependent vascular relaxation.

Hypocholesterolemia and Apolipoprotein E Phenotype

Persons with total cholesterol levels <130 mg/dL (<3.26 mmol/L) make up <1% of a healthy population. Causes of hypocholesterolemia include a diet very low in cholesterol and saturated fat, disease, genetic factors (including low apolipoprotein B-100 [apo B-100] and the apo E allele), and drug therapy. Snyder and associates,[16] from San Francisco, Oakland, Berkeley, and San Diego, Calif, determined the causes of hypocholesterolemia in a healthy Kaiser Foundation Health Plan population. The authors conducted a dietary and health survey of 201 healthy hypocholesterolemic adults (range: 2.04 to 3.88 mmol/L [79 to 150 mg/dL]) and 200 matched control subjects with total cholesterol levels in the middle quintile of the population (range: 5.0 to 5.61 mmol/L [194 to 217 mg/dL]) who had routine health screening from 1983 through 1985. The authors did apo E phenotyping studies and lipid and apo A-1 and B-100 measurements in a subgroup of 45 hypocholesterolemic subjects (mean total cholesterol level: 3.26 mmol/L [126 mg/dL]) and in a comparison group of 49 unmatched volunteers (mean total cholesterol level: 5.04 ± 0.75 mmol/L [195 ± 29 mg/dL]). The authors found no differences in dietary intake or clinically significant medical illness between hypocholesterolemic and control subjects. In the hypocholesterolemic subgroup, an increased frequency of the apo E2 allele (ε2) and a decreased frequency of the apo E4 allele (ε4) were found; the frequencies of the ε2, ε3, and ε4 alleles were 33.3%, 63.3%, and 3.3%, respectively. The corresponding apo E allele frequencies in the comparison subgroup were 8.2%, 73.5%, and 18.4%, similar to those previously reported for the general population and significantly different from those found in the hypocholesterolemic subgroup. One hypocholesterolemic subject (a 46th patient) had a mutation in the apo B gene that resulted in the synthesis of a truncated species of apo B (apo B-46). The study indicates that hypocholesterolemia in the Kaiser Foundation Health Plan urban population is usually not caused by diet or disease. Biochemical factors, including the increased frequency of the apo E-2 phenotype and the decreased frequency of the apo E-4 phenotype, are more important.

Homozygous Familial Hypercholesterolemia

Variation in plasma-cholesterol concentration and the expression of CAD in patients with homozygous familial hypercholesterolemia (FH) is well documented, but the underlying reasons for variation are not clearly defined. Because FH is caused by mutations at the LDL gene locus, Moorjani and associates,[17] from Quebec, Canada, compared plasma-cholesterol concentrations in 21 FH homozygotes with either the >10 kb deletion (promoter region and exon 1) (11 subjects) or the exon 3 missense (trp_{66}εgly) mutation (10 subjects) of the LDL gene. Subjects with the >10 kb deletion had a higher mean plasma-cholesterol concentration than those with the exon 3 mutations (26.7 v 16.1 mmol/L), and there was no overlap in individual plasma-cholesterol concentrations between subjects in the two groups. Although the frequency of CAD was similar in the two groups, age-of-onset was earlier in subjects with the >10 kb deletion. Also, coronary deaths were more frequent and occurred at an earlier age in subjects with the >10 kb deletion. These results provided evidence that there is less variation in plasma-cholesterol concentrations among FH homozygotes when they are subdivided into groups according to LDL receptor-gene defect. Furthermore, differences in plasma-cholesterol concentrations are reflected in the severity of CAD expression.

In Twins

The extent to which serum lipid levels are affected by genetic and environmental factors remains a point of controversy. Heller and associates,[18] from University Park, Pa, and Stockholm and Umeå, Sweden, studied

Table 1-3. Mean Lipid Levels (±SD) in 302 Pairs of Twins, According to Zygosity, Rearing Status, and Sex. Reproduced with permission from Heller et al.[18]

Lipid	Monozygotic Twins Reared Apart		Monozygotic Twins Reared Together		Dizygotic Twins Reared Apart		Dizygotic Twins Reared Together	
	Men (N = 44)	Women (N = 48)	Men (N = 50)	Women (N = 84)	Men (N = 62)	Women (N = 138)	Men (N = 80)	Women (N = 98)
Total cholesterol (mg/dl)*	253.32±44.11	271.03±44.07	236.15±34.53	274.06±48.66	251.98±45.56	275.97±55.97	242.64±41.59	274.87±50.88
HDL (mg/dl)*	45.36±13.13	55.78±16.68	48.87±15.64	63.91±16.52	50.92±14.36	61.18±16.76	54.19±11.48	61.57±14.71
Apolipoprotein A-I (g/liter)	1.25±0.23	1.39±0.27	1.25±0.29	1.48±0.25	1.28±0.21	1.49±0.30	1.28±0.20	1.48±0.23
Apolipoprotein B (g/liter)	1.14±0.23	1.15±0.21	1.05±0.18	1.09±0.25	1.09±0.23	1.14±0.29	1.05±0.19	1.10±0.25
Triglycerides (mg/dl)†	158.11±71.72	138.43±50.14	145.00±87.90	150.21±92.45	153.44±77.90	136.87±75.72	144.60±79.54	138.75±64.17

*To convert values for HDL to millimoles per liter, multiply by 0.02586.   †To convert values for triglycerides to millimoles per liter, multiply by 0.01129.

302 pairs of twins (mean age, 66 years); 146 pairs had been reared apart. The authors simultaneously compared the twins on the basis of both zygosity and rearing status, which allowed joint estimation of genetic and environmental influences on serum lipid levels. Genetic influence was expressed in terms of heritability, the proportion of the population variation attributable to genetic variation (a value of 1.0 indicates that all of the population variation is attributable to genetic variation). The serum lipids and apolipoproteins measured included total cholesterol, HDL cholesterol, apolipoproteins A-1 and B, and triglycerides. Structural-equation analyses revealed substantial heritability for the serum levels of each lipid measured, ranging from 0.3 to 0.8. Comparisons of the twins reared together with those reared apart suggested that the environment of rearing had a substantial impact on the level of total cholesterol (accounting for 0.2 to 0.4 of the total variance) (Table 1-3). Sharing the same environment appeared to affect the other lipid measures much less, however, than did genetic factors and unique environmental factors not shared by twins. Comparisons of younger with older twins suggested that heritability for apolipoprotein B and triglyceride levels decreased with age. The effect of genetic factors on the serum levels of some but not all lipids appears to decrease with age. Early rearing environment appears to remain an important factor in relation to levels of total cholesterol later in life, but it has less effect on other serum lipids and apolipoproteins in the elderly.

In Depressed Men

In several clinical trials of interventions designed to lower plasma total and LDL cholesterol, reduction in CAD mortality have been offset by an unexplained rise in suicides and other violent deaths. Morgan and associates,[19] from San Diego and La Jolla, Calif, tried to find out whether depressive illness is related to low plasma-cholesterol concentrations in men aged 50 years and older. In 1985–1987, Beck depression inventories were obtained from 1,020 white men, aged 50 to 89 years, in Rancho Bernardo, Calif. Disease history and behaviors were assessed by standard questionnaires. Plasma cholesterol and weight were measured at this time, as they had been in 1972 to 1974. Among men aged 70 years and older, categorically defined depression was three times more common in those with low plasma cholesterol (<4.14 mmol/L) than in those with higher concentrations (5/31 [16%] v 22/363 [6%]). Depressive symptom scores correlated significantly and inversely with plasma-cholesterol concentrations, even after adjustment for age, health status, number of chronic illnesses, number of medications, and exercise, as well as measured weight loss and change in plasma cholesterol in the previous 13 years. The findings that low plasma cholesterol is associated with depressive symptoms in elderly men is compatible with observations that a very low total cholesterol may be related to suicide and violent death.

Effects of in Utero Growth

To see whether reduced rates of fetal growth are related to raised serum cholesterol concentrations in adult life Barker and associates,[20] from Southampton and Cambridge, United Kingdom, performed a follow-up study of men and women whose size at birth had been recorded. The subjects included in the study were 219 men and women born in a single hospital during 1939 to 1940. Men and women who had a small abdominal circumference at birth had raised serum concentrations of total and LDL cholesterol and apolipoprotein B. This was independent of the duration of gestation. Serum concentrations of total cholesterol fell by 0.25 mmol/L with each 1 inch (2.54 cm) increase in abdominal circumference. The corresponding figure for serum LDL cholesterol was 0.26 mmol/L (0.11 to 0.42) and for serum apolipoprotein B 0.04 g/L (0.02 to 0.07). Small head and chest circumferences at birth and short length were each associated with raised serum LDL cholesterol concentrations, but the trends disappeared in a simultaneous regression with abdominal circumference at birth. The association between abdominal circumference at birth and LDL cholesterol concentration was independent of social class, current body weight, cigarette smoking, and alcohol consumption. Thus, raised serum cholesterol concentrations in adult life are associated with impaired growth during late gestation, when fetal undernutrition has a disproportionate effect on liver growth. Impaired liver growth may permanently alter LDL cholesterol metabolism.

Effects of Excessive Body Weight

Denke and associates,[21] from Dallas, Tex, and Hyattsville, Md, examined the association between body weight adjusted for height as calculated by body-mass index (BMI) and serum lipid and lipoprotein levels in white men using the National Health and Nutrition Examination Survey (NHANES II). Lipid results were categorized into six different levels of BMI: (1) 21.0 kg/m^2 or lower, (2) 21.1 to 23.0 kg/m^2, (3) 23.1 to 25.0 kg/m^2, (4) 25.1 to 27.0 kg/m^2, (5) 27.1 to 30.0 kg/m^2, and (6) greater than 30.0 kg/m^2; and three age groups: (1) young men (20 through 44 years), (2) middle-aged men (45 through 59 years), and (3) older men (60 through 74 years). Using linear trend analysis, changes in BMI from categories 2 to 5 in young men were associated with a total cholesterol level 0.59 mmol/L (23 mg/dL) higher and a LDL cholesterol level 0.59 mmol/L (23 mg/dL) higher. For middle-aged men and older men, the same change in BMI was associated with smaller but still significant differences in total cholesterol levels (higher by 0.31 mmol/L [12 mg/dL] and 0.28 mmol/L [11 mg/dL], respectively) and non-HDL cholesterol levels (higher by 0.37 mmol/L [14 mg/dL] and 0.25 mmol/L [10 mg/dL], re-

Table 1-4. Adjusted* Mean Serum Lipoprotein Levels by Age and Body-Mass Index (BMI) Group for Adult White Men in the United States, 1976–1980, in NHANES II[†]. Reproduced with permission from Denke et al.[21]

Age, y	BMI Group, kg/m²	LDL Cholesterol[‡]		HDL Cholesterol[§]	
		No. of Values	mmol/L (mg/dL)	No. of Values	mmol/L (mg/dL)
20-44	≤21.0	80	2.87 (111)	254	1.22 (47)
	21.1-23.0	129	3.05 (118)	343	1.19 (46)
	23.1-25.0	146	3.47 (134)	439	1.19 (46)
	25.1-27.0	125	3.59 (139)	327	1.14 (44)
	27.1-30.0	100	3.65 (141)	295	1.06 (41)
	>30.0	64	3.78 (146)	162	1.01 (39)
45-59	≤21.0	18	3.62 (140)	46	1.16 (45)
	21.1-23.0	31	4.11 (159)	93	1.27 (49)
	23.1-25.0	69	3.98 (154)	173	1.16 (45)
	25.1-27.0	68	4.03 (156)	174	1.16 (45)
	27.1-30.0	61	4.01 (155)	147	1.11 (43)
	>30.0	44	3.70 (143)	109	0.98 (38)
60-74	≤21.0	54	3.52 (136)	149	1.42 (55)
	21.1-23.0	100	4.09 (158)	211	1.22 (47)
	23.1-25.0	112	3.65 (141)	289	1.16 (45)
	25.1-27.0	132	3.88 (150)	339	1.14 (44)
	27.1-30.0	102	3.98 (154)	291	1.14 (44)
	>30.0	80	3.59 (139)	203	1.03 (40)

*Adjusted for smoking status (present smokers vs nonsmokers), percentage of energy intake from saturated fatty acids, and dietary cholesterol intake (milligrams), as well as sample weight.
[†]From the Second National Health and Nutrition Examination Survey (NHANES II).
[‡]To convert milligrams per deciliter to millimoles per liter, multiply by 0.02586.
[§]To convert milligrams per deciliter to millimoles per liter, multiply by 0.01129.

spectively), whereas the LDL cholesterol levels were unchanged. Although advancing age may blunt the BMI-associated differences in total and LDL cholesterol levels, the BMI-associated differences in triglyceride levels (higher by 0.7 to 1.33 mmol/L [62 to 188 mg/dL]) and HDL cholesterol levels (lower by 0.18 to 0.39 mmol/L [7 to 15 mg/dL]) were of similar magnitude in all age groups. Excess body weight is associated with deleterious changes in the lipoprotein profile (Table 1-4). Higher BMI was associated at all ages with higher plasma triglyceride levels, lower HDL cholesterol levels, and higher total and non-HDL cholesterol levels. In young men, the higher total cholesterol level was reflected mainly in the LDL cholesterol level; in middle-aged and older men, in the non-HDL fraction. Programs to reduce CAD by improving lipid levels should include more emphasis on achieving and maintaining ideal body weight.

Effects of Walnuts

A previous study had shown that frequent consumption of nuts was associated with a reduced risk of CAD. To explore possible explanations for this finding, Sabaté and associates,[22] from Loma Linda, Calif, studied the effects of nut consumption on serum lipids and BP. They randomly placed 18 healthy mean on two mixed natural diets, each diet to be followed for 4 weeks. Both diets conformed to the National Cholesterol Education Program Step 1 Diet and contained identical foods and macronutrients, except that 20% of the calories of one diet (the walnut diet) were derived from walnuts (offset by lesser amounts of fatty foods, meat, and visible fat [oils, margarine, and butter]). With the reference diet, the mean serum values for total, LDL, and HDL cholesterol were, respectively, 182 ± 23, 112 ± 16, and 47 ± 11 mg/dL (4.7 ± 0.6, 2.9 ±

0.4, and 1.2 ± 0.3 mmol/L). With the walnut diet, the mean total cholesterol level was 22.4 mg/dL (0.6 mmol/L) lower than the mean level with the reference diet; the LDL and HDL cholesterol levels were, respectively, 18.2 mg/dL (0.5 mmol/L) and 2.3 mg/dL (0.06 mmol/L) lower. These lower values represented reductions of 12.4%, 16.3%, and 4.9% in the levels of total, LDL, and HDL cholesterol, respectively. The ratio of LDL cholesterol to HDL cholesterol was also lowered by the walnut diet. Mean BP values did not change during either dietary period. Incorporating moderate quantities of walnuts into the recommended cholesterol-lowering diet while maintaining the intake of total dietary fat and calories decreases serum levels of total cholesterol and favorably modifies the lipoprotein profile in normal men.

Effects of Trans Fatty Acids

Trans isomers of fatty acids, formed by the partial hydrogenation of vegetable oils to produce margarine and vegetable shortening, increase the ratio of plasma LDL to HDL cholesterol, so it is possible that they adversely influence risk of CAD. To investigate this possibility, Willett and associates,[23] from Boston, Mass, studied dietary data from participants in the Nurses' Health Study. The authors calculated intake of trans fatty acids from dietary questionnaires completed by 85,095 women without diagnosed CAD, stroke, diabetes, or hypercholesterolemia in 1980. During 8 years of follow-up, there were 431 cases of new CHD (nonfatal AMI or death from CAD). After adjustment for age and total energy intake, intake of trans isomers was directly related to risk of CAD (relative risk for highest v lowest quintile 1.50). Additional control for established CAD risk factors, multivitamin use, and intakes of saturated fat, monounsaturated fat, linoleic acid, dietary cholesterol, vitamins E or C, carotene, or fiber did not change the relative risk substantially. The association was stronger for the 69,181 women whose margarine consumption over the previous 10 years had been stable (1.67 [1.5-2.66]). Intakes of foods that are major sources of trans isomers (margarine, cookies [biscuits], cake, and white bread) were each significantly associated with higher risk of CAD. These findings support the hypothesis that consumption of partially hydrogenated vegetable oils may contribute to occurrence of CAD.

Effects of Colorectal Adenomas

To study the relation between serum lipoprotein levels and the frequency of colorectal adenomas, the benign precursors of colorectal cancer, Bayerdörffer and associates,[24] from Munich, studied 822 of 1,124 consecutive patients who underwent colonoscopy; and of the 822 studied patients, 194 had colorectal adenomas. Serum cholesterol fractions (HDL, LDL, and VLDL) and presence or absence of adenomas were examined. Univariate analysis of the total patient group showed that the HDL cholesterol level was inversely related to the frequency of colorectal adenoma (odds ratio, 0.4) and that LDL and VLDL cholesterol levels were positively associated with adenoma frequency (odds ratio, 2.3 and 1.7, respectively). Univariate analysis of the subgroup of 89 patients with high-risk adenomas showed an inverse association between such adenomas and HDL cholesterol (odds ratio, 0.4). A logistic regression analysis that included age and body-mass index showed an association between lipoprotein levels and the presence of adenomas. The relative strength (in descending order) of these associations was as follows: HDL, LDL, VLDL, and total serum cholesterol. A logistic regression analysis of patients with high-risk adenoma showed a significant association between such adenomas and the HDL cholesterol level. Patients with colorectal adenomas have lower HDL cholesterol levels and higher LDL and VLDL cholesterol levels; these lipoproteins may have prognostic significance for the development of colorectal adenomas.

Effects of Human Immunodeficiency Virus (HIV)

Patients with acquired immunodeficiency (AID) syndrome exhibit marked disturbances in lipid metabolism. Because altered lipid metabolism may affect immune processes, Shor-Posner and associates,[25] from Miami, Fla, determined in 94 asymptomatic HIV-1-infected homosexual men and 42 health seronegative control subjects, serum levels of triglycerides and cholesterol. Immune assessment included measurements of lymphocyte subpopulations (CD4), immune activation (β_2-microglobulin), natural killer cell function, and lymphocyte proliferation in response to mitogens phytohemagglutinin and pokeweed. Dietary intake was determined using a semiquantitative food-frequency questionnaire. Despite greater consumption of saturated fat and cholesterol, significantly lower levels of total, HDL, and LDL cholesterol were observed in HIV-1-seropositive men, relative to seronegative controls, with 40% of the HIV-1-infected group demonstrating hypocholesterolemia (<150 mg/dL). Low values of total, HDL, and LDL cholesterol were associated with elevated levels of β_2-microglobulin in HIV-1-seropositive men. No differences between the groups were noted for serum triglycerides. HIV-1-infected subjects did not demonstrate the significant inverse relationship between cholesterol and mitogen response observed in seronegative controls. These findings indicate that low levels of cholesterol are prevalent during the early stages of HIV-1 infection and associated with specific alterations in immune function, suggesting that hypocholesterolemia may be a useful marker of disease progression.

Effects of Premarin ± Provera

Exogenous female hormone use appears to affect cardiovascular disease risk in both premenopausal and postmenopausal women. Vaziri and associates,[26] from Framingham, Mass, and Bethesda, Md, evaluated the impact of exogenous female hormone usage on the lipid profile in 1,930 female participants in the Framingham Offspring Study. Of the 992 premenopausal subjects, 57 were current oral contraceptive users; among the 938 postmenopausal subjects, 80 were current hormone users. The influence of hormone use on lipid and lipoprotein levels was determined using multivariable linear regression models that adjusted for age, body-mass index, smoking, alcohol intake, β-blocker, and diuretic therapy. Adjusted least-squares means were calculated for each lipid and lipoprotein according to female hormone usage and menopausal status. In the premenopausal analysis, pooled oral contraceptive use was significantly related to increased levels of total cholesterol, triglycerides, HDL cholesterol, and apolipoprotein A-I (Table 1-5). Increased estrogen content was

Table 1-5. Impact of Oral Contraceptive Use on the Lipid Profile in Premenopausal Subjects: Results From Multiple Linear Regression Models.* Reproduced with permission from Vaziri et al.[26]

	Adjusted Means†		Estimate of Difference Between Users and Nonusers (95% CI)	P
	Nonusers (N = 935)	Users (N = 57)		
Total cholesterol, mmol/L (mg/dL)	4.98 (192.1)	5.33 (205.6)	0.35 (0.10–0.60) (13.5 [3.7-23.3])	.007
LDL cholesterol, mmol/L (mg/dL)	3.04 (117.4)	3.22 (124.2)	0.18 (−0.07-0.42) (6.9 [−2.6-16.3])	.16
HDL cholesterol, mmol/L (mg/dL)	1.46 (56.3)	1.59 (61.3)	0.13 (0.04-0.22) (5.1 [1.5-8.7])	.006
Total cholesterol/ HDL cholesterol, mmol/L (mg/dL)	3.64 (3.64)	3.58 (3.58)	−0.06 (−0.37-0.25) (−0.06 [−0.37-0.25])	.72
Triglycerides, mmol/L (mg/dL)	0.91 (81.0)	1.04 (96.8)	0.18 (0.04-0.31) (15.8 [3.7-27.8])	.01
VLDL cholesterol, mmol/L (mg/dL)	0.46 (17.8)	0.52 (19.9)	0.06 (−0.02-0.14) (2.2 [−1.0-5.3])	.17
Apolipoprotein A-1, μmol/L (mg/dL)	54.05 (151.8)	63.46 (178.3)	9.42 (6.13-12.71) (26.5 [17.2-35.7])	.0001
Apolipoprotein B, μmol/L (mg/dL)	1.47 (73.6)	1.60 (80.0)	0.13 (−0.01-0.26) (6.3 [−0.5-13.2])	.07

*CI indicates confidence interval; LDL, low-density lipoprotein; and VLDL, very-low-density lipoprotein.

†Adjusted for age, body mass index, current smoking, alcohol intake, β-blocking agents, and diuretics.

inversely associated with LDL cholesterol and apolipoprotein B levels, and increased progestin content was inversely related to HDL cholesterol and apolipoprotein A-I levels. Combination use of premarin and provera was significantly associated with increased apolipoprotein A-I levels; less powerful but still significant associations with increased HDL cholesterol and decreased LDL cholesterol were also observed. In this cross-sectional analysis, oral contraceptive use is associated with both favorable and unfavorable lipid alterations with respect to atherogenic risk. Among postmenopausal women, hormone replacement therapy (both premarin only and combined premarin and provera) appears to be associated with favorable effects on the lipid profile.

Effects of Atenolol v Celiprolol

Antihypertensive drugs may affect serum lipoprotein levels in mixed populations, but data in hyperlipidemic patients are scanty. Dujovne and associates[27] from Kansas City, Kan, compared atenolol v celiprolol effects on serum lipoproteins in 159 hyperlipoproteinemic hypertensive patients. This was a randomized, double-blind, parallel-group, positive-controlled multicenter trial with centralized lipoprotein laboratory and diet constancy monitoring. BP reduction and serum lipoprotein and apoprotein levels were monitored for 3 months. Both drugs reduced systolic and diastolic BP. Atenolol had greater effects than celiprolol on diastolic pressure, but effects on systolic BP were not different. Patients receiving atenolol had lower serum HDL cholesterol levels and higher LDL/HDL cholesterol ratios; patients treated with celiprolol showed no contrasting changes. These differences in lipoprotein levels between drug treatment groups were statistically significant at weeks 9 and 12 (Figure 1-5). The difference between drug treatments was also significant if the values of the 9- and 12-week visits were averaged. Patients taking atenolol had statistically significantly higher serum levels of total cholesterol, triglycerides, and apoprotein B at 9 weeks. These divergent directional changes were consistent throughout and statistically significantly different between drugs.

THERAPY OF HYPERLIPIDEMIA

Treatment Surveillance

To investigate recent trends in the percentage and characteristics of patients being treated by a physician for high blood cholesterol and to assess missed clinical opportunities to screen for high blood cholesterol, Giles and associates,[28] from Atlanta, GA, and Baltimore, Md, interviewed by telephone 154,735 adults in 37 states that participated in the Behavioral Risk Factor Surveillance System during 1988–1990 to assess trends in the percentage of patients treated for high blood cholesterol by a physician. An opportunity was considered missed if a person did not report being screened for high blood cholesterol despite seeing a physician for preventive care in the last 2 years. Between the first quarter of 1988 and the last quarter of 1990, the percentage of persons treated by a physician for high blood cholesterol increased from 7.6% to 11.7% (Table 1-6). However, because an estimated 36% of US adults need treatment for high blood cholesterol, fewer than one third of persons who need treatment are receiving it. Persons with two or more cardiac risk factors were more likely to be treated; and men, blacks, persons from lower socioeconomic groups, and persons between ages 20 and 34 were less likely to be treated. Among the 126,571 persons who had seen

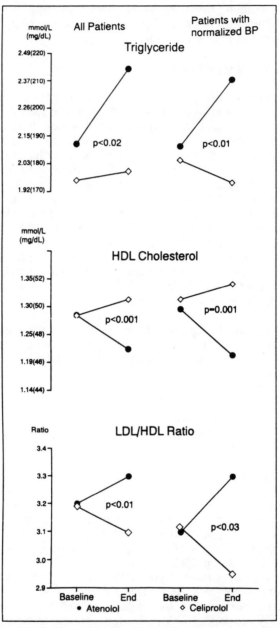

Figure 1-5. Blood lipid changes from baseline to the averaged results between weeks 9 and 12 (end) by treatment group for all patients (*left*) (atenolol = 72; celiprolol = 71) and patients with diastolic blood pressure (BP) at week 12 ≤ 90 mm Hg (*right*) (atenolol = 44; celiprolol = 32). HDL = high-density lipoprotein; LDL = low-density lipoprotein. Reproduced with permission from Dujovne et al.[27]

a physician for preventive care within the last 2 years, missed opportunities to screen for high blood cholesterol were most common among persons aged 20 through 34 years (59%) and among women who had seen obstetricians/gynecologists for preventive care (43%). Fewer than one

Table 1-6. Persons Being Treated for High Blood Cholesterol, Behavioral Risk Factor Surveillance System, 1988-1990. Reproduced with permission from Giles et al.[28]

Characteristic	No. of Persons	% Being Treated*	Adjusted† Odds Ratio (95% Confidence Interval)
Sex			
F	88 822	11.5	1.00‡
M	65 913	8.3	0.71 (0.68-0.74)
Race			
W	134 794	10.1	1.00‡
B	13 083	9.1	0.81 (0.76-0.87)
Hispanic	6858	10.4	1.12 (1.04-1.20)
Age group, y			
20-34	51 406	2.7	1.00‡
35-49	45 386	8.5	3.02 (2.86-3.19)
50-64	28 496	18.6	7.44 (7.04-7.87)
≥65	29 447	19.3	8.31 (7.78-8.88)
Education, y			
<12	25 232	12.7	1.00‡
12	52 157	9.0	1.09 (1.03-1.15)
>12	77 346	8.5	1.25 (1.18-1.32)
Cardiac risk factor score			
0-1	72 808	9.6	1.00‡
2-3	75 132	10.2	1.28 (1.22-1.33)
4-6	6795	16.3	2.27 (2.08-2.47)
Total	**154 735**	**10.0**	. . .

*Advised by a physician to reduce blood cholesterol or blood fat level.
†Adjusted for all variables presented in the table.
‡Referent.

third of persons who need treatment for high blood cholesterol as estimated by data from the Second National Health and Nutrition Examination Survey are receiving treatment. Better use of clinical opportunities to screen for high blood cholesterol could substantially accelerate the progress in identifying persons, young adults in particular, who are likely to benefit from cholesterol reduction.

Meta-analysis of Cholesterol-Lowering Trials

To investigate the level of risk of death from CAD above which cholesterol-lowering treatment produces net effects, Smith and associates,[29] from Glasgow, Leeds, and York, United Kingdom, performed meta-analysis of results of randomized controlled trials of cholesterol-lowering treatments. Published and unpublished data from all identified randomized controlled trials of cholesterol-lowering treatments with 6 months or more follow-up and with at least one death were included in the meta-analysis. In the pooled analysis, net benefit in terms of total mortality from cholesterol lowering was seen only for trials including patients at very high initial risk of CAD (odds ratio, 0.74). In a medium-risk group, there was no net effect; and in the low-risk group, there were adverse treatment effects (1.22). In a weighted regression analysis, a significant trend of increasing benefit with increasing initial risk of CAD was shown. Raised mortality from causes other than CAD was seen in trials of drug treatment (1.21) but not in trials of nondrug treatment (1.02). The authors concluded that currently evaluated cholesterol-lowering drugs seem to produce mortality benefits in only a small proportion of patients at very high risk of death from CAD.

Reducing serum cholesterol lowers the risk for CAD, but its effects on other vascular diseases are unknown. Atkins and associates,[30] from Seattle, Wash, performed a meta-analysis of randomized, controlled trials and found that 13 studies met three eligibility criteria: (1) patients randomized to intervention or control; (2) fatal or nonfatal stroke reported separately; and (3) endpoints assessed without knowledge of treatment status. For fatal stroke, the overall odds ratio associated with cholesterol-lowering interventions in 13 trials was 1.32, and the odds ratio for the 10 single-intervention trials was 1.34. Among 8 trials reporting nonfatal events, the summary odds ratio for nonfatal stroke for treated participants compared with controls was 0.9; and the odds ratio for total strokes was 0.1. Among 3 trials using clofibrate, treatment significantly increased the risk for fatal stroke but not for nonfatal stroke. Regression analysis showed no statistical association between the magnitude of cholesterol reduction and the risk for fatal stroke. Lowering serum cholesterol through modified diets or medications does not reduce stroke mortality or morbidity in middle-aged men. Clofibrate appears to increase the risk for fatal strokes, but the mechanism of this effect is unknown.

Diet

To examine the rationale for preventive nutrition intervention and the potential efficacy of nutrition-related risk-factor modification on CAD incidence, Posner and associates,[31] from Boston and Framingham, Mass, compared the cardiovascular risk and dietary profiles of Framingham men and women, aged 30 to 79 years (n = 1,798 and 1,845, respectively), with the Health People 2000: National Health Promotion and Disease Prevention Objectives for the Nation. The information was used to project the 10-year incidence of CAD with and without lowering serum cholesterol levels. Data for this report were derived from the 1984 to 1988 cycle III examinations of the Framingham offspring-spouse cohort. Estimates of the reduction in CAD risk associated with modifications in serum cholesterol levels and other CAD risk factors are projected using Framingham models. About 40% met guidelines for desirable total cholesterol levels (<5.17 mmol/L [<200 mg/dL]); 20% were hypertensive; 25% smoked; and 10% of women and 20% of men were obese. Twenty-four-hour dietary data, adjusted for estimates of usual intake, indicated that about 50% to 80% met dietary cholesterol objectives (<300 mg) and 55% to 94% met dietary sodium objectives (<3 g/d). In contrast, mean total fat intakes were high (38% of total energy); and only 6% to 9% of subjects met total fat guidelines, 9% to 14% met saturated fat guidelines, and fewer than 3% met dietary fiber guidelines. Ten-year cumulative incidence for CAD was projected to be up to 25% lower with reduction in serum cholesterol level. Risk factors lowering, emphasizing preventive nutrition measures, is an important element of health care reform, particularly strategies to reduce cardiovascular disease rates and to promote population health.

To define how much regression to the mean confounds apparent responsiveness in subgroups analyses and to test, using techniques that remove regression to the mean, whether hypercholesterolemic subjects are more likely to respond to diet, Denke and Frantz,[32] from Dallas, Tex, and Minneapolis, Minn, collected data on 812 men and women participating in the Minnesota Coronary Survey Dietary Trial who had at least two total cholesterol measurements on a high-saturated-fat diet and one cholesterol measurement on a low-saturated-fat diet. If regression toward the mean is not taken into account, dietary responsiveness in patients with mean cholesterol levels of 280 mg/dL was -25%, were as dietary responsiveness in subjects with mean serum cholesterol levels of 156 mg/dL was −5%. After regression toward the mean was taken into account, subjects with high initial serum cholesterol levels had an 18% reduction in serum cholesterol levels, and subjects with low levels had an 11% reduction. Even after regression toward the mean is accounted for, subjects with high serum cholesterol levels were significantly more diet-responsive. The efficacy of a cholesterol-lowering diet for individuals can be overestimated or underestimated if only single measurements are used to determine response. Subjects with hypercholesterolemia, even after adjustment for regression toward the mean, are more diet-responsive than subjects with lower cholesterol levels. Dietary therapy should remain the first step in the treatment of hypercholesterolemia and should also be effective in reducing cholesterol levels in the population at large.

In a randomized, single-blind, controlled trial, Singh and co-associates,[33] from Moradabad, India, assigned 621 patients to either intervention diet A (group A, 310 patients) or control diet B (group B, 311 patients) for a period of 24 weeks. Group A patients received a diet with (1) a higher percentage of calories from fruits and vegetables and complex carbohydrates; (2) a higher polyunsaturated/saturated fat ratio; and (3) a larger amount of soluble dietary fiber, antioxidant vitamins and minerals, and low saturated fat and cholesterol than group B. Group A patients also did more physical and yogic exercises than group B. Adherence to diet and exercise was obtained through questionnaires, and information obtained was quantified into a formula. After 24 weeks, the overall score of diet and exercise was significantly higher in group A than in group B. There was a significant decrease in serum total cholesterol (13%), LDL cholesterol (17%), triglycerides (19%), fasting blood glucose (20%), and BP (12/6 mm Hg) in the intervention group compared with initial levels and changes in group B. The effect of exercise on the decrease in risk factors was additive. Within group A, overall score for diet and exercise was greater in one subset of 116 patients in the intervention group that had maximal lifestyle changes. A separate analysis of data in this subgroup revealed a greater decrease in risk factors compared with risk-factor changes in the remaining 194 patients with less higher overall score, indicating that the relation of lifestyle changes with reduction in risk factors may be of causal nature. It is possible that diet and physical inactivity may be important in the development of risk factors for CAD, and lifestyle changes may reverse these risk factors within 24 weeks.

Soluble Fiber

To determine if high intake of soluble rather than insoluble fiber can further reduce plasma lipids in persons with diets already low in saturated fats and cholesterol, Jenkins and associates,[34] from Toronto, Canada, studied 43 healthy persons (mean age, 58 years) who had a mean percentage of ideal body weight of 107% and mild-to-moderate hyperlipidemia after following a National Cholesterol Education Program Step II diet for ≥2 months. Participants were assigned to each diet for 4 months separated by 2 months. Both diets aimed to provide ≤20% calories as fat, 20% as protein, and at least 60% as available carbohydrate (2.5 to 3.0 g of fiber/100 kcal) and included low-fat dairy foods and vegetable-protein products. Participants chose amounts of food. The soluble-fiber diet included barley, dried lentils, peas, beans, oat bran, and a commercial cereal with added psyllium. The insoluble-fiber diet included wheat-bran breakfast cereal, high-fiber crackers, and bread with wheat bran and gluten. All diet foods were packaged centrally and delivered weekly. Twenty-two participants received the soluble-fiber diet first. Plasma total, LDL, and HDL cholesterol and serum apolipoproteins decreased during both periods with lowest levels by week 4.

Garlic

To assess the effects of standardized garlic powder tablets on serum lipids and lipoproteins, glucose, and BP, Jain and associates,[35] from New Orleans, La, randomized 42 healthy adults (mean age, 52 years) with a serum total cholesterol level of ≥220 mg/dL with either 300 mg three times/day of standardized garlic powder in tablet form or placebo. Diets and physical activity were unchanged. This study was conducted in an outpatient, clinical research unit. The baseline serum total cholesterol level of 262 ± 34 mg/dL was reduced to 247 ± 29 mg/dL after 12 weeks of standard garlic treatment. Corresponding values for placebo were 276 ± 34 mg/dL before and 274 ± 29 mg/dL after placebo treatment. LDL cholesterol was reduced by 11% by garlic treatment and 3% by placebo. There were not significant changes in HDL cholesterol, triglycerides, serum glucose, BP, and other monitored parameters. Thus, treatment with standardized garlic 900 mg/dL produced a significantly greater reduction in serum total cholesterol and LDL cholesterol than placebo. The garlic formulation was well tolerated without any odor problems.

Warshafsky and associates,[36] from Valhalla, NY, provided a meta-analysis of reported randomized and placebo-controlled clinical trials studying the effect of garlic on total serum cholesterol in persons with total cholesterol levels >200 mg/dL (5.17 mmol/L). Patients treated with garlic consistently had a greater decrease in total cholesterol levels compared to those receiving placebo. Meta-analysis of homogeneous trials estimated a net total cholesterol decrease, attributable to garlic, of 23 mg/dL (0.59 mmol/L) (Figure 1-6). The best available evidence suggests that garlic, in an amount approximating one half to one clove per day, decreases total serum cholesterol levels by about 9%.

Linoleate-Enriched Cheese Product

To test the effect of substituting a modified-fat cheese product into the diets of hypercholesterolemic adults, Davis and associates,[37] from Davis, Calif, and Paris, France, performed a 4-month, randomized, double-blind, crossover substitution involving 26 healthy adult volunteers with total cholesterol levels ≥5.69 and ≤7.24 mmol/L. Daily substitution of 100 g of cheese (either partial skim-milk mozzarella or modified-fat

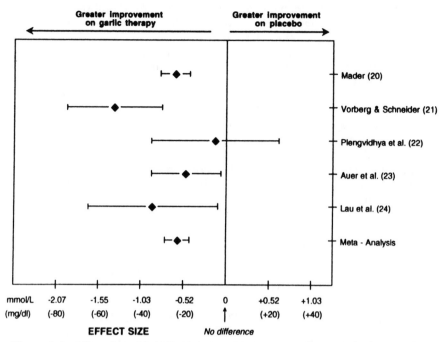

Figure 1-6. Effect sizes with 95% CIs for mean improvement during garlic therapy compared with placebo. Effect size for each trial was computed as the difference between the change of cholesterol level in the garlic and placebo groups. The pooled difference was calculated using data only from homogeneous trials. Any CI that includes zero indicates a nonsignificant result. Reproduced with permission from Warshafsky et al.[36]

[vegetable oil] mozzarella) into participants' normal diets were performed. Participants consumed an assigned cheese for 2 months, at which time they crossed over to consume the other study cheese. No differences in weight or in the amount or type of calories consumed were found during the study. No statistically significant changes in lipid values resulted from consumption of mozzarella cheese. Modified-fat cheese substitution resulted in a decreased LDL cholesterol level when compared with levels at both baseline (−0.28 mmol/L) and during consumption of the skim-milk mozzarella cheese (−0.38 mmol/L). Findings for total cholesterol were similar. HDL cholesterol, plasma triglyceride, apolipoprotein A-I and B-100 levels were unaltered. Both sexes responded similarly. Thus, a linoleate-enriched cheese product, in the absence of any other changes in diet or habits, substituted into the normal diets of hypercholesterolemic adults reduced LDL and plasma-cholesterol levels.

Psyllium

To determine the efficacy of psyllium in reducing serum cholesterol levels in patients on high- or low-fat diets, Sprecher and associates,[38] from Cincinnati, Ohio, and St. Louis, Mo, performed a double-blind, placebo-controlled, 16-week parallel trial. The study included an 8-week baseline period and an 8-week treatment period. Involved in the study were healthy men and women, aged 21 to 70 years, with total serum cholesterol levels ≥220 mg/dL (≥5.7 mmol/L). Thirty-seven participants followed a high-fat diet and 81 participants followed a low-fat diet. The participants were randomly assigned to either psyllium, 5.1 g twice a day, or placebo. Psyllium recipients in both the high- and low-fat diet groups showed small but significant decreases in total cholesterol and LDL cholesterol levels. Total cholesterol and LDL cholesterol levels decreased 5.8% and 7.2%, respectively, in psyllium recipients on high-fat diets and 4.2% and 6.4%, respectively, in psyllium recipients on low-fat diets. No significant difference was seen in LDL cholesterol response when psyllium recipients on low- and high-fat diets were compared. No significant reduction in lipid levels were observed in placebo recipients. Based on the National Cholesterol Education Program LDL cholesterol classification system, 39% of the psyllium recipients improved in LDL cholesterol classification compared with 20.3% of placebo recipients. Psyllium produces a modest but significant improvement in total cholesterol and LDL cholesterol levels in persons on either low-fat or high-fat diets and may obviate the need for typical lipid-lowering medications or may prove to be a valuable adjunct to other treatments in patients with moderately elevated LDL cholesterol levels.

High-Molecular-Weight Hydroxypropylmethylcellulose

Dressman and associates,[39] from Ann Arbor and Midland, Mich, and Athens, Greece, assessed the efficacy of a high-molecular-weight hydroxypropylmethylcellulose (K8515) as a cholesterol-lowering agent, the dose-response profile of its action, and the ability of adult subjects to tolerate its ingestion at effective doses. Efficacy was assessed in 10 normal and 12 mildly hyperlipidemic subjects in double-blind, randomized crossover trials of 1 and 2 weeks' duration, respectively. The dose-response profile was studied in 12 mildly hypercholesterolemic subjects in a nonrandomized control trial with doses given in escalating order. Tolerance was assessed by a questionnaire of adverse effects and bowel movement habits in all subjects. The authors found that 10 g of K8515 ingested in a prehydrated form three times/day with meals lowered total cholesterol levels by an average of 1.5 mmol/L (56 mg/dL) (32%) in normal subjects within 1 week (Figure 1-7). In two studies of subjects with mildly elevated cholesterol levels (with entry levels ranging from 5.4 mmol/L [207 mg/dL] to 6.7 mmol/L [260 mg/dL]), average reductions of 1.0 mmol/L (39 mg/dL) (18%) and 1.2 mmol/L (45 mg/dL) (20%) were observed within the same period. The effect was primarily due to a reduction in LDL cholesterol levels. LDL levels in normal subjects were an average of 1.1 mmol/L (42 mg/dL) (38%) lower after a week of 10 g of K8515 three times/day with meals; and in the two studies of subjects with mild hyperlipidemia, the reductions in LDL levels after 1 week were 0.9 mmol/L (37 mg/dL) (23%) and 1.05 mmol/L (40 mg/dL) (25%). Although there was a tendency for LDL cholesterol levels to decrease, this was significant only in normal subjects. Decreases in cholesterol levels were not accompanied by any rise in triglyceride levels. Dose-response studies in those with mildly elevated cholesterol levels indicated that it is possible to achieve a 15% decrease in LDL cholesterol levels within 1 week at a dose of 6.7 g three times/day, with minimal adverse effects. These results suggest a role for high-molecular-weight

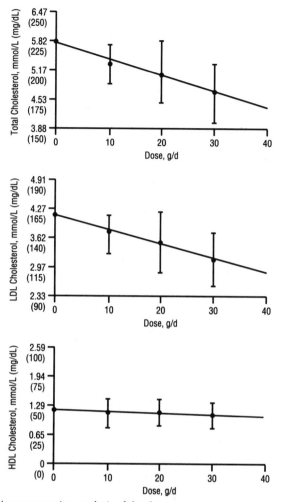

Figure 1-7. Linear regression analysis of the dose-response study results. Top, Total cholesterol levels; line of best fit is (total cholesterol) = 223 − 1.42 (daily dose of hydroxypropylmethylcellulose), R^2 = .972 (P = .014). Center, Low-density lipoprotein (LDL) cholesterol levels; line of best fit is (LDL cholesterol) = 159 − 1.27 × (daily dost of hydroxypropylmethylcellulose), R^2 = .975, P = .0124. Bottom, High-density lipoprotein (HDL) cholesterol levels; line of best fit is (HDL cholesterol) = 46 − 0.18 × (daily dose of hydroxypropylmethylcellulose), R^2 = .900, P = .0513. Error bars represent SDs. Reproduced with permission from Dressman et al.[39]

hydroxypropylmethylcellulose in the clinical treatment of mild hypercholesterolemia.

Estrogen ± Progestin

Most epidemiologic studies of cardiovascular disease in postmenopausal women suggest that estrogen-replacement therapy has a protective effect. The effects of the use of estrogen combined with progestin are less well studied. To examine the associations of hormone-replacement therapy with concentrations of plasma lipids and hemostatic factors, Nabulski and associates,[40] from multiple US Centers, studied fasting serum concentrations of glucose and insulin, and BP, in 4,958 postmenopausal women participating in a population-based investigation. Using cross-sectional data, the authors classified the women into four groups according to their use of hormone-replacement therapy: current users of estrogen alone, current users of estrogen with progestin, nonusers who had formerly used these hormones, and nonusers who had never used them. Current users had higher mean levels of HDL cholesterol, its subfractions HDL_2 and HDL_3, and apolipoprotein A-I than nonusers, and lower mean levels of LDL cholesterol, apolipoprotein B, lipoprotein(a), fibrinogen, antithrombin III, and fasting serum glucose and insulin (Table 1-7). Current users of estrogen alone had higher triglyceride, factor VII, and protein C levels than either nonusers or current users of estrogen with progestin. After making certain assumptions, the authors

Table 1-7. Unadjusted Values (Means ± SD) for Physiologic Variables, According to Use of Replacement Hormones. Reproduced with permission from Nabulski et al.[40]

VARIABLE*	CURRENT USERS		NONUSERS	
	ESTROGEN (N = 853)	ESTROGEN–PROGESTIN (N = 173)	FORMER USE (N = 813)	NO USE (N = 3119)
Total triglycerides (mg/dl)†	135±82	124±67	125±73	122±73
Cholesterol (mg/dl)‡				
LDL	123±41	124±36	142±41	142±41
HDL	68±20	69±20	58±17	57±17
HDL_3	46±11	46±12	42±11	41±11
HDL_2	22±11	22±11	17±9	16±9
Apolipoprotein (mg/dl)				
A-I	161±33	159±36	141±31	139±30
B	89±28	89±26	95±30	95±31
Lipoprotein(a) (μg/ml)	99±105	79±83	114±111	118±120
Fibrinogen (g/liter)	2.92±0.59	2.82±0.52	3.12±0.66	3.17±0.66
Factor VII (%)	134±38	123±30	126±28	125±29
Factor VIII (%)	130±35	122±30	134±41	137±42
Von Willebrand factor (%)	114±46	106±38	120±49	123±50
Antithrombin III (%)	110±21	111±23	114±23	115±22
Protein C (μg/ml)	3.45±0.63	3.29±0.61	3.29±0.67	3.28±0.62
Fasting glucose (mg/dl)§	96±9	94±8	99±11	99±11
Fasting insulin (μU/ml)¶	9.4±6.8	8.0±6.6	11.7±8.7	11.7±8.9
Blood pressure (mm Hg)				
Systolic	119±18	115±16	122±19	123±20
Diastolic	72±10	70±9	72±11	73±11

*Some data were missing for some variables.

†To convert values to millimoles per liter, multiply by 0.01129.

‡To convert values to millimoles per liter, multiply by 0.02586.

§Subjects with diabetes were excluded from this category. To convert values to millimoles per liter, multiply by 0.05551.

¶Subjects with diabetes were excluded from this category. To convert values to picomoles per liter, multiply by 7.175.

estimated that the findings, if causal, would translate into a reduction of 42% in the risk of CAD in users of hormones as compared with nonusers. Women using estrogen with progestin would have an even greater estimated benefit. A randomized trial is needed to eliminate possible selection biases in the observational study that are related to the prescription of replacement hormones. Nevertheless, hormone-replacement therapy appears to be associated with a favorable physiologic profile, which probably mediates its protective effects on CAD. The use of estrogen combined with progestin appears to be associated with a better profile than the use of estrogen alone.

Lovastatin

D'Agostino and associates,[41] from Boston, Mass, studied the efficacy and tolerability of lovastatin in 213 hypercholesterolemic patients with systemic hypertension. At baseline, standard deviation of total serum cholesterol, LDL cholesterol, HDL cholesterol, and the ratio of total serum cholesterol to HDL cholesterol were 268, 189, and 43 mg/dL and 6.6, respectively. Of the 213 hypertensive patients, only 24 were not receiving antihypertensive or related cardiac medication. Baseline mean systolic and diastolic BPs were 140 and 84 mm Hg, respectively. Within 1 month of lovastatin therapy, the observed significant reductions in total serum cholesterol, LDL cholesterol, and the ratio of total to HDL cholesterol were 19%, 27%, and 24%, respectively. HDL cholesterol was increased by 6%. Diastolic BP did not change significantly during this 1-month period. The 1-month lipid results were maintained over the full 6 months of the study. The dosage of lovastatin was 20 mg/day for the first month of therapy and could subsequently be adjusted to response, up to a maximum of 80 mg/day. Again, without changes in diastolic BP, lovastatin was generally effective in improving the serum lipids of hypercholesterolemic hypertensive patients regardless of the type of antihypertensive medications received (including diuretics and β-blockers).

A diet low in saturated fat and cholesterol is the standard initial treatment for patients with hypercholesterolemia. Little quantitative information, however, is available about the efficacy of dietary therapy in clinical practice or about the combined effect of diet and drug therapy. Hunninghake and associates,[42] from multiple US medical centers, treated 111 outpatients with an LDL cholesterol level between 160 and 200 mg/dL (4.14 and 5.17 mmol/L) at five lipid clinics with the National Cholesterol Education Program Step 2 Diet (a diet with <30% of calories derived from fat [<7% saturated, 10–15% monounsaturated, and <10% polyunsaturated] and the cholesterol intake less than 200 mg/day both alone and together). A diet high in fat and cholesterol (to provide 40% of calories as fat, with 15% saturated, 14% monounsaturated, and 8% polyunsaturated fatty acids, and a cholesterol intake of 350 to 400 mg/day) and a placebo identical in appearance to the lovastatin were used as the respective controls. Each of the 97 patients completing the study (58 men and 39 women) underwent four consecutive 9-week periods of treatment according to a randomized, balanced design: a high-fat diet–placebo period, a low-fat diet–placebo period, a high-fat diet–lovastatin period, and a low-fat diet–lovastatin period. The level of LDL cholesterol was a mean of 5% lower during the low-fat diet than during the high-fat diet (Tables 1-8 and 1-9). With lovastatin therapy as compared

Table 1-8. Lipoprotein Levels at the End of Each Intervention. Reproduced with permission from Hunninghake et al.[42]

VARIABLE*	HIGH-FAT DIET–PLACEBO	LOW-FAT DIET–PLACEBO	HIGH-FAT DIET–LOVASTATIN	LOW-FAT DIET–LOVASTATIN	P VALUE FOR DIET	P VALUE FOR DRUG
	mg/dl — mean (95% confidence interval)					
Intention-to-treat analysis, all variables						
	(N = 100)	(N = 102)	(N = 101)	(N = 102)		
Cholesterol						
Total	272	257	215	204	<0.001	<0.001
	(266–278)	(252–262)	(209–220)	(199–209)		
LDL	182	172	131	123	<0.001	<0.001
	(177–187)	(167–177)	(127–137)	(119–127)		
HDL	56.5	52.7	58.5	54.4	<0.001	<0.001
	(53.5–59.5)	(50.3–55.2)	(55.6–61.5)	(51.6–57.2)		
HDL$_2$	17.2	15.1	18.0	16.6	<0.001	0.026
	(15.4–19.0)	(13.8–16.5)	(16.2–19.8)	(14.9–18.4)		
HDL$_3$	38.7	36.6	39.9	38.0	<0.001	<0.001
	(37.0–40.3)	(35.1–38.1)	(38.6–41.3)	(36.3–39.7)		
VLDL	34.5	34.3	27.1	27.3	0.59	<0.001
	(30.3–38.6)	(30.3–38.3)	(24.9–29.4)	(24.2–30.4)		
LDL:HDL	3.40	3.42	2.38	2.39	0.73	<0.001
	(3.2–3.6)	(3.2–3.6)	(2.2–2.5)	(2.3–2.5)		
Triglycerides	146	148	121	125	0.69	<0.001
	(132–160)	(134–162)	(110–131)	(112–137)		
Apolipoproteins						
A-I	149	139	149	142	<0.001	0.25
	(142–156)	(133–144)	(143–156)	(136–148)		
A-II	50.4	49.4	51.4	48.9	0.014	0.58
	(48.5–52.3)	(47.7–51.1)	(49.4–53.5)	(46.9–50.8)		
B	143	138	111	108	0.012	<0.001
	(138–147)	(133–142)	(107–116)	(104–112)		
E	7.73	7.48	6.46	6.36	†	†
	(7.24–8.22)	(7.01–7.95)	(6.03–6.89)	(6.01–6.71)		
Lipoprotein(a)‡	15.0	17.0	17.0	17.0	0.09	0.07
	(8.0–48.3)	(8.0–43.3)	(7.5–43.0)	(7.0–42.5)		
Per-protocol analysis, principal variables						
	(N = 85)	(N = 84)	(N = 84)	(N = 82)		
Cholesterol						
Total	274	257	219	203	<0.001	<0.001
	(267–280)	(252–263)	(213–224)	(198–208)		
LDL	183	172	133	123	<0.001	<0.001
	(178–188)	(167–177)	(128–138)	(119–127)		
HDL	57.3	52.5	60.4	55.9	<0.001	<0.001
	(54.0–60.7)	(50.0–55.2)	(57.2–63.7)	(52.7–59.2)		
LDL:HDL	3.37	3.45	2.33	2.33	0.70	<0.001
	(3.20–3.54)	(3.25–3.64)	(2.18–2.48)	(2.19–2.49)		
Apolipoproteins						
A-I	151	138	153	144	<0.001	0.25
	(143–159)	(132–145)	(146–160)	(138–151)		
B	143	138	113	106	0.01	<0.001
	(138–148)	(133–143)	(108–118)	(102–111)		

*To convert values for cholesterol to millimoles per liter, multiply by 0.02586; to convert values for triglycerides to millimoles per liter, multiply by 0.01129.

†P values are not provided because of lack of fit in model.

‡Values are medians with interquartile ranges.

with placebo, the reduction was 27%. Together, the low-fat diet and lovastatin led to a mean reduction of 32% in the level of LDL cholesterol. The level of HDL cholesterol fell by 6% during the low-fat diet and rose by 4% during treatment with lovastatin. The ratio of LDL to HDL choles-

Table 1-9. Percent Change in Lipid Levels Between Interventions, According to Intention-to-Treat Analysis. Reproduced with permission from Hunninghake et al.[42]

Variable and Comparison	Cholesterol				Apolipoproteins	
	Total	LDL	HDL	LDL:HDL	A-I	B
	mean % change (95% confidence interval)					
Diet						
Low-fat diet–placebo vs. high-fat diet–placebo (n = 97)*	−5 (−7 to −2)	−5 (−8 to −2)	−5 (−7 to −3)	1 (−2 to 5)	−5 (−8 to −2)	−2 (−6 to 2)
Low-fat diet–lovastatin vs. high-fat diet–lovastatin (n = 99)	−5 (−7 to −2)	−5 (−8 to −2)	−6 (−9 to −4)	3 (−1 to 6)	−3 (−7 to 1)	−2 (−5 to 2)
Low-fat diet vs. high-fat diet (n = 99)†	−5 (−6 to −3)	−5 (−7 to −3)	−6 (−8 to −4)	2 (0 to 4)	−4 (−7 to −2)	−2 (−4 to −1)
Drug						
High-fat diet–lovastatin vs. high-fat diet–placebo (n = 97)*	−21 (−23 to −18)	−27 (−30 to −25)	5 (2 to 8)	−30 (−33 to −27)	2 (−2 to 5)	−21 (−24 to −18)
Low-fat diet–lovastatin vs. low-fat diet–placebo (n = 99)	−20 (−22 to −19)	−27 (−30 to −25)	3 (1 to 6)	−29 (−32 to −26)	3 (1 to 5)	−20 (−24 to −17)
Drug vs. placebo (n = 99)†	−20 (−22 to −19)	−27 (−29 to −25)	4 (3 to 6)	−29 (−32 to −27)	2 (0 to 5)	−21 (−23 to −18)
Diet and drug						
Low-fat diet–lovastatin vs. high-fat diet–placebo (n = 98)*	−25 (−27 to −23)	−32 (−34 to −29)	−2 (−5 to 1)	−30 (−32 to −27)	−2 (−6 to 1)	−24 (−27 to −21)
High-fat diet–lovastatin vs. low-fat diet–placebo (n = 99)*	−16 (−18 to −14)	−23 (−26 to −20)	11 (9 to 14)	−30 (−33 to −27)	8 (5 to 11)	−18 (−21 to −15)

*Simple pairwise comparison.

†Values are means of the within-patient average of the two pairwise comparisons.

terol and the level of total triglycerides were reduced by lovastatin, but not by the low-fat diet. The effects of the low-fat low-cholesterol diet and lovastatin on lipoprotein levels were independent and additive. However, the reduction in LDL cholesterol produced by the diet was small, and its benefit was possibly offset by the accompanying reduction in the level of HDL cholesterol.

The Lovastatin Study Group,[43] from multiple medical centers, reported results of treatment with lovastatin of 745 patients with severe hypercholesterolemia (mean baseline plasma cholesterol level on diet, 9.3 mmol/L [360 mg/dL]) for a median duration of 5.2 years. Their mean age at baseline was 50 years; 77% of patients had titrations of lovastatin to 80 mg/dL; and 58% took other lipid-lowering agents, usually bile acid sequestrants, concomitantly. The mean changes at 5 years in total, LDL, and HDL cholesterol were −35%, −44%, and +14%, respectively (Figure 1-8). Eighty percent of patients completed the study, 13% were unavailable for follow-up, 4% were discontinued due to adverse events unlikely to be related to lovastatin, and 3% (21) were discontinued because of drug-attributable adverse events: marked but asymptomatic increase in aminotransferase values (10 patients), gastrointestinal disturbance (3 patients), rash (2 patients), myalgia (1 patient), myopathy (2 patients), arthralgia (1 patient), insomnia (1 patient), and weight gain (1 patient). Sixteen patients died during the study, all of CAD. Of these, 14 had CAD at baseline. There were no deaths attributable to trauma, suicide, or homicide, and there were only 14 cases of cancer (v 21 expected). There was no evidence for an adverse effect on the lens. Lovastatin is a generally well-tolerated and effective drug during long-term use.

To evaluate the efficacy and safety of lovastatin in women with moderate hypercholesterolemia, Bradford and associates,[44] from the Ex-

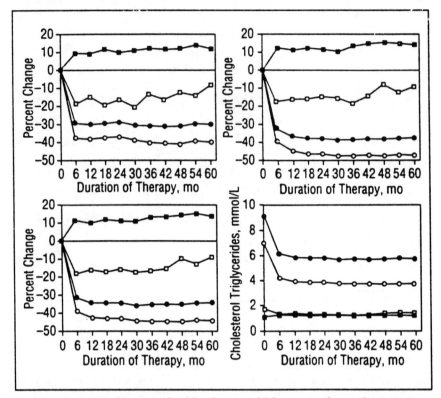

Figure 1-8. Mean changes in lipid levels (central laboratory values only) in patients completing 5 years of therapy. Closed circles indicate total cholesterol; open circles, low-density lipoprotein cholesterol; closed squares, high-density lipoprotein cholesterol; and open squares, triglycerides. Top left, Percent change, patients in the lovastatin monotherapy group (N = 133); top right, percent change, patients in the lovastatin plus concomitant therapy group (N = 213); bottom left, percent change, all patients (N = 346); and bottom right, absolute values, all patients (N = 346). To convert to milligrams per deciliter, multiple by 38.7 for cholesterol and 88 for triglycerides. Reproduced with permission from Lovastatin Study Groups I through IV.[43]

panded Clinical Evaluation of Lovastatin (EXCEL) Study, in a multicenter, double-blind, diet- and placebo-controlled trial, studied 3,390 women from the total cohort of 8,245 volunteers. Participants were randomly assigned to receive placebo or lovastatin at doses of 20 or 40 mg once daily or 20 or 40 mg twice daily for 48 weeks. Among women, lovastatin (20 to 80 mg/dL) produced sustained (12- to 48-week), dose-related changes: decreases in LDL cholesterol (24% to 40%) and triglycerides (9% to 18%) and increases in HDL cholesterol (6.7% to 8.6%) (Table 1-10). Depending on the dose, from 82% to 95% of lovastatin-treated women achieved the National Cholesterol Education Program goal of LDL cholesterol levels <4.1 mmol/L (160 mg/dL), and 40% to 87% achieved the goal of <3.4 mmol/L (130 mg/dL). Successive transaminase elevations >3 times the upper limit of normal occurred in 0.1% of women and were dose dependent above the 20-mg dose. Myopathy, defined as muscle symptoms with creatine kinase elevations >10

Table 1-10. Change From Baseline in Plasma Lipid/Lipoprotein Levels of Women.* Reproduced with permission from Bradford et al.[44]

Level	Placebo	Treatment Group			
		Lovastatin			
		20 mg Once Daily	40 mg Once Daily	20 mg Twice Daily	40 mg Twice Daily
LDL cholesterol, % *(SD)†*	+ 0.5 (10.8)	− 24.4 (11.5)	− 31.4 (12.5)	− 33.8 (12.1)	− 40.4 (12.3)
HDL cholesterol, % *(SD)†*	+ 2.3 (12.1)	+ 6.7 (11.8)	+ 7.2 (12.7)	+ 8.0 (12.1)	+ 8.6 (13.1)
Total cholesterol, % *(SD)†*	+ 1.2 (8.0)	− 16.8 (8.8)	− 21.9 (9.3)	− 23.5 (8.9)	− 28.2 (9.3)
Triglycerides‡, *median*	+ 5.7	− 9.4	− 13.6	− 14.3	− 17.9

* HDL = high-density lipoprotein; LDL = low-density lipoprotein; SD = standard deviation.
† Values are percentage change from baseline (SD). All pair-wise comparisons of lovastatin with placebo were significant ($P < 0.001$).
‡ Values are percentage change from baseline. The differences between placebo and all lovastatin treatment groups were significant ($P < 0.001$).

times the upper limit of normal, was rare and associated with the highest recommended daily dose of lovastatin (80 mg). Estrogen-replacement therapy appeared to have no effect on either the efficacy or safety profile of lovastatin. Lovastatin is highly effective and generally well tolerated as therapy for primary hypercholesterolemia in women.

Lovastatin v Pravastatin

The Lovastatin Pravastatin Study Group,[45] from Helsinki, Finland, evaluated the efficacy and safety profile of lovastatin and pravastatin across their usually recommended dose ranges (lovastatin 20 to 80 mg/day and pravastatin 10 to 40 mg/day) in a randomized, controlled, double-blind trial in 672 hypercholesterolemic patients. After a 7-week placebo and diet run-in period, patients with LDL cholesterol >160 mg/dL (4.1 mmol/L) were randomized to 20 mg/day of lovastatin or 10 mg/day of pravastatin for 6 weeks. The doses were then increased to 40 and 80 mg/day of lovastatin and 20 and 40 mg/day of pravastatin at weeks 6 and 12, respectively. Efficacy and safety evaluations were performed at weeks 6, 12, and 18. The mean percent changes from baseline in LDL cholesterol at weeks 6, 12, and 18 were −28%, −33%, and −39%, respectively, with lovastatin, and −19%, −25%, and -27%, respectively, with pravastatin. All changes were significantly different from 0, and the between-group differences were highly significant. The frequency of adverse events leading to discontinuation was low (3% with lovastatin and 2% with pravastatin), with no significant differences between groups. Across the recommended dosage ranges, lovastatin was more effective than pravastatin in reducing total and LDL cholesterol; both agents had similar safety profiles.

Pravastatin

Pitt and associates,[46] from Ann Arbor, Mich, designed a study to test the effect of pravastatin on the progression of CAD in patients with moderate hypercholesterolemia. Angiographic entry criteria included the presence of ≥1 stenosis ≥50% in a major epicardial coronary artery and certification of film quality through the core angiography laboratory. Patients qualified for randomization if after diet stabilization their LDL concentrations were ≥130 mg/dL and <190 mg/dL and triglycerides were ≤350 mg/dL. Pravastatin (40 mg) or placebo is administered once daily at bedtime. Arteriography will be repeated at the end of 3 years of treatment. The primary endpoint of the study is the change in absolute mean coronary artery diameter. During a 30-month recruitment period, 44,145 patients were screened and 408 were randomized. The most frequent reason for excluding patients during the screening and dietary lead-in periods was a low serum cholesterol level. A large proportion of patients with documented CAD have cholesterol concentrations that are considered to be normal or only modestly increased. Adherence to strict standards of quality control for digital analysis of angiograms ensures that baseline angiograms can be interpreted at the end of 3-year follow-up.

The Pravastatin Multinational Study Group for Cardiac Risk Patients[47] evaluated the use of pravastatin in 1,062 patients with hypercholesterolemia (serum total cholesterol concentrations of 5.2 to 7.8 mmol/L [200 to 300 mg/dL]) and ≥2 additional risk factors for atherosclerotic CAD. Efficacy and safety analyses were performed on the initial 26-week, randomized, double-blind, placebo-controlled period; further safety analyses were conducted on the subsequent 52 weeks, which included an additional 26-week double-blind phase permitting other lipid-lowering agents and a final 26-week open-label period. At 13 weeks, pravastatin at a dose of 20 mg once daily at bedtime significantly lowered serum LDL cholesterol 26%, total cholesterol 19%, and triglycerides 12% and significantly raised serum HDL cholesterol 7%. Efficacy of pravastatin was maintained at 26 weeks; and during this initial period, there were significantly more serious cardiovascular adverse events in the placebo group (13 events) than in the pravastatin group (1 event). Six myocardial infarctions, five cases of unstable angina, and one sudden cardiac death occurred in the placebo group, compared with none of these events in the pravastatin group. In this study, pravastatin produced beneficial effects on serum lipids and was associated with a reduction in the incidence of serious cardiovascular adverse events.

Pravastatin ± Cholestyzamine

Treatment of severe hypercholesterolemia often requires high-dose therapy with hydroxymethylglutaryl-coenzyme A reductase inhibitor alone or in combination with acid-binding resin. The Pravastatin Multicenter Study Group II[48] evaluated the efficacy and safety of pravastatin alone and in combination with cholestyramine in a randomized, double-blind, multicenter study of 311 patients for 8 weeks and in continued therapy through 24 weeks. The dose of pravastatin was 20 to 40 mg twice daily alone or 20 mg twice daily with cholestyramine, 12 g twice daily, v placebo. After 8 weeks of therapy, pravastatin in a dosage of 20 mg twice daily reduced LDL cholesterol levels by 31%; a dosage of 40 mg twice daily reduced LDL cholesterol levels by 32%. Cholestyramine combined with 40 mg of pravastatin reduced the level by 51%. Pravastatin, 40 or 80 mg daily, reduced the triglyceride level by 13% to 19%, resin alone increased the triglyceride level by 21%, and no change was seen with combined therapy. HDL cholesterol levels increased by about 5% regardless of regimen. Similar effects were seen at 24 weeks. Symptoms reported were indistinguishable among placebo and pravastatin users and were less than with cholestyramine alone or cholestyramine in combination with pravastatin. Elevations of liver enzyme levels were small in all groups, indistinguishable between resin and pravastatin, and were highest when the two drugs were combined. Plasma creatine kinase levels did not increase in any treatment group. Pravastatin treatment of hypercholesterolemia is highly effective and well tolerated alone and in combination with bile acid-binding resin and shows no tendency to increase muscle enzyme levels.

Pravastatin ± Gemfibrozil

To compare the efficacy and safety of pravastatin, gemfibrozil, combined therapy, and placebo in the treatment of hypercholesterolemia (total plasma cholesterol ≥6.0 mmol/L or in at least the 90th percentile by age and sex and triglycerides less than 4.0 mmol/L despite dietary interventions), Wiklund and associates,[49] from five medical centers in Sweden and two in Finland, randomized 290 ambulatory patients to active treatment or placebo for 12 weeks following a single-blind placebo lead-in period. Pravastatin reduced total cholesterol (26% v 15%), LDL cholesterol (34% v 17%), and apolipoprotein B (29% v 15%) more than gemfibrozil. Gemfibrozil reduced VLDL cholesterol (49% v 22%) and triglycerides (42% v 14%) and increased HDL cholesterol (15% v 6%) more than pravastatin. Pravastatin and gemfibrozil increased apolipoprotein A-I comparable (3.3% v 5.0%). The combination significantly reduced total cholesterol (29%), LDL cholesterol (37%), VLDL cholesterol (49%), and apolipoprotein B (32%) and increased HDL cholesterol (17%). The combination reduced the total cholesterol/HDL cholesterol (39%) and LDL cholesterol/HDL cholesterol (46%) ratios significantly. Adverse events and clinical laboratory abnormalities were generally mild and transient in all groups, although creatine kinase tended to be higher with combination therapy. Study drugs were withdrawn from two patients with asymptomatic creatine kinase elevations. Severe myopathy was not observed; however, the presence of subclinical musculoskeletal effects cannot be excluded. Co-administration of pravastatin and gemfibrozil combined the specific effects of the two drugs on lipoprotein concentrations and ratios. The incidence of side effects was low; severe myopathy did not occur. The combination may be useful in selected cases of combined hyperlipidemia; however, because myopathy at a low incidence or after long-term therapy cannot be excluded, the routine of combination therapy is not advisable.

Pravastatin vs Simvastatin

The efficacy and safety profile of simvastatin and pravastatin across their most commonly recommended dosage ranges were compared in a double-blind, parallel, multicenter study in 550 patients with primary hypercholesterolemia by the Simvastatin Pravastatin Study Group,[50] from Rahway, NJ. The study consisted of a 6-week placebo period followed by 18 weeks of active treatment. Patients were randomized to 10 mg of simvastatin or pravastatin once in the evening; doses were titrated at 6-week intervals to a maximum of 40 mg/day if the LDL cholesterol remained ≥130 mg/dL (3.4 mmol/L). Baseline characteristics were similar in both groups. At the end of the study with simvastatin and pravastatin, respectively, 30% and 14% continued to take the 10-mg dose and 48% and 66% were titrated to the maximal dose. After 18 weeks of treatment with simvastatin and pravastatin, the mean percent decreases from baseline were, respectively, 27% and 19% for total plasma cholesterol, 38% and 26% for LDL cholesterol, 30% and 16% for VLDL cholesterol, and 18% and 14% for triglycerides. The mean percent increase from baseline in HDL cholesterol was 15% with simvastatin compared with 12% with pravastatin. The efficacy goal of LDL cholesterol <130 mg/dL was achieved in 65% of the patients treated with simvastatin v 39% of those treated with pravastatin. There was no significant difference between groups in the frequency of drug-related adverse experiences. A standard sleep questionnaire given at baseline and after 6, 12, and 18 weeks of treatment showed no impairment of sleep with either drug. Simvastatin was significantly more effective than pravastatin in reducing total, LDL, and VLDL cholesterol and triglycerides and in increasing HDL cholesterol and had a comparable safety and tolerability profile.

Cholestyzamine

Because hypercholesterolemia is associated with impaired endothelium-dependent vasodilation, Leung and associates,[51] from Hong Kong, conducted a study to find out whether cholesterol reduction improved endothelial function in patients with hypercholesterolemia and normal coronary arteries. Twenty-five men (mean age, 51 years) with total serum cholesterol >6.2 mmol/L and angiographically normal coronary arteries had their coronary vasomotor responses to intracoronary acetylcholine and nitroglycerin assessed by computer-assisted quantitative angiography at baseline and after 6 months of cholesterol-reducing diet and cholestyramine. Between baseline and follow-up, mean total serum cholesterol level, mean LDL cholesterol level, and mean total cholesterol to HDL cholesterol ratio fell by 29%, 37%, and 29%, respectively. Acetylcholine significantly reduced the mean segment diameter at baseline (22%), but it increased the diameter at follow-up (6%), the difference between the two occasions being significant. Nitroglycerin significantly increased the mean segment diameter, both at baseline (19%) and at follow-up (19%), the difference between the two responses being not significant. At baseline, total cholesterol and LDL cholesterol did not correlate with acetylcholine response, but they did at follow-up. Impairment of endothelium-dependent (acetylcholine-induced) dilation of the epicardial coronary arteries in hypercholesterolemic patients with angiographically normal coronary arteries is thus reversible by reducing serum cholesterol. In addition, the degree of impairment of acetylcholine-induced vasomotor response is related to the cholesterol concentrations after therapy.

Cholestyramine or Colestipol v Niacin v Lovastatin v Psyllium

Veterans are frequently older, have more chronic illnesses, and take more medications than subjects volunteering for clinical trials. Because these factors may impair the effectiveness of lipid-lowering drug therapy, the effectiveness of drug therapy in veterans may differ from that measured in randomized controlled trials. In 297 patients with type IIa hyperlipidemia attending a large Veterans Administration Medical Center lipid clinic, adverse effects, compliance, and lipid and lipoprotein responses to drug therapy were prospectively monitored by Schectman and associates,[52] from Milwaukee, Wis. Bile acid sequestrants (4 packets/day) were associated with a high rate of adverse effects and had the highest drug discontinuance rate (37%) and poorest compliance (73%) of all agents. Patients aged >60 years tolerated therapy with bile acid sequestrants less well than did younger veterans. Niacin (1.5 g/day) also had a high drug discontinuance rate (27%). Lovastatin (20 mg/day) had the lowest drug discontinuance rate (2%) and the highest compliance (90%). Lovastatin also reduced LDL cholesterol the most (−22%), but niacin produced the largest increase in HDL cholesterol (14%); both niacin and lovastatin produced similar reductions in the LDL/HDL ratio. However, psyllium (10.4 q/day) reduced LDL cholesterol by only 2% and had no effect on the LDL/HDL ratio. Psyllium produced larger LDL cholesterol reductions in patients aged <60 years than in older patients. Niacin and lovastatin are effective drugs for hypercholesterolemia management in the Veterans Administration Medical Center setting. In elderly veterans, bile acid sequestrants were associated with a higher rate of adverse effects limiting compliance, and psyllium was ineffective.

Colestipol + Niacin

Blankenhorn and associates,[53] from Los Angeles, Calif, used carotid ultrasound imaging in the Cholesterol Lowering Atherosclerosis Study to determine the impact of colestipol plus niacin in altering carotid artery atherosclerosis. Seventy-eight patients had ultrasound studies at baseline, 2, and 4 years. Twenty-four patients receiving colestipol and niacin and 22 placebo patients had carotid ultrasound images at baseline, 2, and 4 years with matching cervical angiograms. Carotid ultrasound measurements were tested for treatment effects and compared with measurements of atherosclerosis in coronary and cervical angiograms. Patients treated with colestipol and niacin showed progressive reduction in carotid thickness at 2 and 4 years. Subjects treated with placebo developed increased wall thickness at the same time periods. Reduced levels of apolipoprotein B and increased levels of HDL cholesterol and apolipoprotein C-III were significant predictors of carotid wall thinning. Ultrasound-measured carotid intima-media thickness was correlated at baseline with visually read coronary angiographic stenosis and at 2 years with a computer measurement of mild carotid atherosclerosis. Thus, these data indicate that common carotid intima-media thickening may be reduced by colestipol-niacin treatment.

Gemfibrozil

To evaluate the efficacy of gemfibrozil in men with primary isolated low HDL cholesterol levels, Miller and associates,[54] from Baltimore, Md, studied 14 men with low levels of HDL cholesterol but desirable total cholesterol levels and gave them gemfibrozil in a randomized, double-blind, placebo-controlled, crossover trial. They were randomly to receive placebo and gemfibrozil each for 3 months, with a 1-month washout period between phases. Overall, gemfibrozil increased the total HDL cholesterol concentration by 9%, reduced triglyceride levels by 38%, and significantly lowered the total cholesterol/HDL cholesterol ratio. Those with fasting triglyceride levels of 1.07 mmol/L or greater had a significant elevation in the HDL cholesterol level (14.6%) and a reduction in triglyceride levels (50%) with gemfibrozil; those with fasting triglyceride levels <95 mg/dL had a smaller increase in the HDL cholesterol level (4%) and a smaller reduction in triglyceride levels (15%). There were no significant differences in the plasma levels of LDL cholesterol, HDL_2-cholesterol, apolipoproteins A-I and B, or Lp(a). HDL_3-cholesterol and apo A-II levels rose slightly. The adverse effects attributable to gemfibrozil were minimal. In men with desirable total cholesterol levels, gemfibrozil raised HDL-cholesterol and lowered triglyceride levels to a similar extent as reported for hyperlipidemic men in the Helsinki Heart Study. These lipid-altering effects were most pronounced in those with the highest fasting triglyceride levels.

In a randomized, parallel-group, multicenter clinical trial, Gotto and associates,[55] from Houston, Tex, compared a newly developed, once-daily, extended-release formulation of gemfibrozil and gemfibrozil twice daily in terms of lipid-regulating effects and toxicity. Patients were men and women with elevations of LDL cholesterol and low levels of HDL cholesterol. The trial consisted of a l-week screening period, an 8-week diet baseline period (Step One Diet), and a 24-week double-blind treatment period (extended release gemfibrozil 1,200 mg once daily v gemfibrozil 600 mg twice daily). At the end of the trial, the two treatment groups showed comparable improvements in all primary lipid factors: mean percent changes in triglyceride, HDL cholesterol, and LDL cholesterol were −32%, +10%, and −10%, respectively, for extended release (n = 325) and −36%, +11%, and −10%, respectively, for twice daily (n = 330) (Table 1-11). The 90% confidence interval for the relative difference between the treatment means fell within the equivalence bounds of ±35% for all three factors, demonstrating equivalence of efficacy. Adverse effects were reported at low rates and were similarly distributed in frequency and intensity between treatment groups; they were preponderantly mild or moderate and gastrointestinal effects were the most frequent. The once-

Table 1-11. Comparison of Efficacy: Mean Percent Changes From Baseline in Primary Factors at Six Months, With Confidence Intervals (qd: n = 325; bid: n = 330). Reproduced with permission from Gotto et al.[55]

	Mean Percent Change ±SD Gemfibrozil		90% CI for Difference of the Means*	90% CI for Relative Difference†
	QD	BID		
TG	−32 ± 25	−36 ± 22	0.9, 7.1	−19.5%, −2.6%
HDL-C	+10 ± 16	+11 ± 16	−2.6, 1.4	−23.7%, 15.7%
LDL-C	−10 ± 14	−10 ± 14	−2.2, 1.3	−12.3%, 24.0%

*Gemfibrozil qd minus gemfibrozil bid. See "Statistical Analysis."
†[(Gemfibrozil qd minus gemfibrozil bid)/gemfibrozil bid] × 100. See "Statistical Analysis."
CI = confidence interval; HDL-C = high-density lipoprotein cholesterol; LDL-C = low-density lipoprotein cholesterol; TG = triglyceride; other abbreviations as in Table I.

daily formulation of gemfibrozil may afford better control of dyslipidemia through improved compliance by patients who have this asymptomatic disease.

Beta-Carotene and/or Vitamin E

Experimental and epidemiologic evidence supports the hypotheses that oxidation of LDL appears to be important in mediating the atherogenicity of LDL. To test this hypothesis in humans, it was necessary to perform intervention studies in large populations. Reaven and associates,[56] from La Jolla, Calif, assessed the effectiveness of supplementation with β-carotene and vitamin E, used alone and in combination with each other, and with vitamin C, to protect LDL from oxidation. In phase 1, after a placebo period, 8 subjects were given β-carotene (60 mg/day) for 3 months, then β-carotene plus vitamin E (1,600 mg/day) for another 3 months, and then β-carotene plus vitamin E plus vitamin C (2 g/day) for 3 months. During phase 2, β-carotene and vitamin C were discontinued, and subjects took only vitamin E for 5 months. During each period, LDL samples were isolated, and measurements of susceptibility to oxidation were performed. β-Carotene levels in LDL increased nearly 20-fold, but LDL susceptibility to oxidation did not change. Addition of vitamin E increased LDL levels nearly 2.5-fold, and this decreased LDL oxidation 30% to 40%. During the vitamin C supplementation period, plasma levels of β-carotene and vitamin E rose, but only β-carotene increased in LDL. However, the susceptibility of LDL to oxidation in this period was not decreased further. During phase 2, when subjects took only vitamin E, LDL susceptibility to oxidation was decreased by 50% as measured by thiobarbituric acid-reactive substances, conjugated dienes, and lipid peroxide formation, as well as by macrophage degradation. Thus, long-term supplementation with large doses of vitamin E alone, but not β-carotene, conferred increased protection to LDL in vitro assays of oxidation.

Heparin-Induced Extracorporeal Low-Density Lipoprotein Precipitation

Heparin-induced extracorporeal LDL precipitation therapy was evaluated by Lane and associates,[57] from Oklahoma City, Okla, for safety and efficacy in selectively reducing LDL cholesterol levels. Weekly treatments were given to high-risk hypercholesterolemic patients (n = 33) with LDL cholesterol levels >160 mg/dL despite prior diet and drug therapy. Lipids, lipoprotein cholesterol, apolipoproteins A-I and B, and fibrinogen were measured on plasma samples before and after treatment. Mean plasma volume treated was 2.7 L and mean treatment duration was 1.7 hours. Therapy complications were infrequent and were primarily vascular access problems or hypotension. Treatment goals were >30% LDL cholesterol reduction with each treatment. In 98% of 686 extracorporeal treatments, LDL cholesterol levels were reduced 230%. Mean LDL cholesterol levels were reduced 111.0 mg/dL with a time-averaged decrease of 39% over a 25-week course. Mean HDL cholesterol was reduced only 6.2 mg/dL (15%). Total cholesterol (47% decrease) and apolipoprotein B (53% decrease) levels were also reduced. Fibrinogen decreased 58% without bleeding complications. Thus, heparin-induced extracorporeal

LDL precipitation therapy can safely and selectively remove plasma LDL cholesterol, producing consistent reductions in LDL cholesterol, total cholesterol, and apolipoprotein B levels.

DIABETES MELLITUS

Effects on Left Ventricular Mass

Sasson and associates,[58] from Toronto, Canada, tested the hypothesis that insulin resistance is an important independent contributing factor to LV mass in the healthy obese population. Study population consisted of 40 normotensive, nondiabetic, otherwise healthy obese subjects with a body-mass index >25 kg/m². LV mass was determined electrocardiographically using standard formulae. Insulin resistance was assessed using indices derived from intravenous glucose tolerance tests' insulin levels at baseline, insulin level at 90 minutes of intravenous glucose tolerance test, insulin integration over 90 minutes of an intravenous glucose tolerance test, and the rate of glucose disposal were evaluated. The insulin level at 90 minutes of the intravenous glucose tolerance test and the rate of glucose disposal, insulin integration over 90 minutes, basal insulin, and body-mass index were all correlated with LV mass by univariate analysis (Table 1-12). Thus, LV mass in the normotensive, nondiabetic obese population is strongly associated with the degree of insulin resistance and is associated hyperinsulinemia.

Table 1-12. Univariate Correlates of Left Ventricular Mass/Height (n = 40). Reproduced with permission from Sasson et al.[58]

Variable	r	P
BMI	.59	.0001
Indices of insulin resistance		
Insulin-90	.61	.0001
Insulin integration	.46	.003
Basal insulin (fasting)	.44	.005
k Value	.55	.003
Blood pressure		
Systolic	.22	.18
Diastolic	.19	.24
Age	.2	.89

BMI indicates body mass index (kg/m²); insulin-90, insulin levels at 90 minutes of Intravenous Glucose Tolerance Test (IVGTT); insulin integration, integration of insulin values over 90 minutes of IVGTT; and k value, rate of glucose disposal derived from IVGTT.

Effects on Endothelium-Dependent Vasodilation

Johnstone and associates,[59] from Boston, Mass, evaluated vascular reactivity in the forearm resistance vessels of 15 patients with insulin-dependent diabetes mellitus and 16 age-matched normal subjects. No patients had hypertension or dyslipidemia. Each subject was pretreated with aspirin to inhibit endogenous production of prostanoids. Methacholine chloride was administered through the brachial artery to assess endothelium-dependent vasodilation. Sodium nitroprusside and verapamil were infused intra-arterially to assess endothelium-independent vasodilation. Phenylephrine was administered to examine vasoconstrictor responsiveness. Forearm blood flow, as determined by venous occlusion plethysmography, and dose-response curves were estimated for each drug. Basal forearm blood flows in diabetic and normal subjects were comparable. The forearm vasodilator response to methacholine was less in diabetic than in normal subjects. At the highest dose of methacholine, the forearm blood flow increased in diabetic subjects but less than in normal subjects. The forearm blood flow responses to nitroprusside and verapamil and the forearm vasoconstrictor responses to phenylephrine were similar in diabetic and normal subjects. In the diabetic patients, endothelium-dependent vasodilation correlated inversely with serum insulin concentration but not with glucose concentration or duration of diabetes. Therefore, endothelium-dependent vasodilation is abnormal in forearm resistance vessels of patients with insulin-dependent diabetes mellitus. This abnormality might be relevant to the high prevalence of vascular disease that occurs in diabetic patients.

Effects on Left Ventricular Function

Diabetes mellitus has been reported to have controversial effects on LV function in patients with no evidence of CAD. Ferraro and associates,[60] from Naples, Italy, evaluated LV function at rest in two groups of diabetic patients, with insulin-dependent (n = 16) and non-insulin-dependent (n = 23) diabetes mellitus, with no evidence of CAD. All patients underwent an electrocardiographic stress test and first-pass and equilibrium radionuclide angiography at rest and during supine exercise. Data in each group of diabetic patients were compared with data obtained from age- and sex-matched normal subjects. In both groups of diabetic patients, plasma catecholamine levels were significantly greater than in control subjects. Ejection fraction at rest and during exercise did not differ between each group of diabetic patients and their respective control group. In patients with insulin-dependent diabetes, peak ejection rate was significantly greater than in control subjects; similarly, peak filling rate was significantly greater than in controls. Cardiac output and systemic vascular resistances did not differ between patients with insulin-dependent diabetes and control subjects. In contrast, patients with non-insulin-dependent diabetes had significantly reduced cardiac output, compared with that of control subjects, and increased systemic vascular resistances. Peak filling rate in patients with non-insulin-dependent diabetes was also significantly reduced compared with that of control subjects. Thus, LV function at rest is preserved in patients with insulin-dependent diabetes, but both systolic and diastolic LV function are compromised in those with non-insulin-dependent diabetes despite increased catecholamine levels.

MISCELLANEOUS TOPICS

Birth Weight and Head Circumference

To determine how fetal growth is related to death from cardiovascular disease in adult life, Barker and associates,[61] from Southhampton, United Kingdom, performed a follow-up study of men born during 1907 to 1924 whose birth weights, head circumferences, and other body measurements were recorded at birth. Of the 1,586 men studied, mortality ratios for cardiovascular disease fell from 119 in men who weighed 5.5 pounds (2,495 g) or less at birth to 74 in men who weighed more than 8.5 pounds (3,856 g). This fall was significant for premature cardiovascular deaths up to 65 years of age. Mortality ratios also fell with increasing head circumference and increasing ponderal index (weight/length^3). These findings showed that reduced fetal growth is followed by increased mortality from cardiovascular disease.

Early Growth

To determine whether the link suggested between growth in utero and during infancy and death from cardiovascular disease in men is also present in women, Osmond and associates,[62] from Southampton, United Kingdom, performed a follow-up study of men and women whose birth weight and weight at 1 year of age had been recorded. A total of 5,585 women and 10,141 men born during 1911 to 1930 were studied. Among women and men, death rates from cardiovascular disease fell progressively between the low and high birth weight groups. Cardiovascular deaths in men but not in women were also strongly related to weight at 1 year, falling progressively between the low and high weight groups. The highest cardiovascular death rates were among those with below average birth weight but above average weight at 1 year. In men, the highest rates were among those with below average birth weight and below average weight at 1 year. Thus, relations between cardiovascular disease and birth weight are similar in men and women. In men, cardiovascular disease is also related to weight gain in infancy.

Body Height

Hebert and associates,[63] from Boston, Mass, evaluated 22,071 male physicians and a population homogeneous for high educational attainment and socioeconomic status in adulthood to determine whether there is an association between height and risk of CAD. The study population was comprised of participants in the Physicians' Health Study, randomized, double-blind, placebo-controlled trial of low-dose aspirin and β-carotene in the primary prevention of cardiovascular disease and cancer among US male physicians aged 40 to 84 years. Participants were classified into five height categories at study entry from the shortest to the tallest and were followed for an average of 60 months to determine whether myocardial infarction, stroke, and/or death occurred from CAD. Men in the tallest (≥73 in) compared with the shortest (≤67 in) height category had a 35% lower risk of myocardial infarction after adjusting for all other known cardiovascular risk factors (Figure 1-9). For every

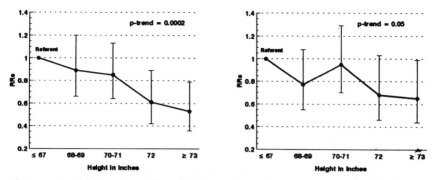

Figure 1-9. Relative risks (RR) and 95% confidence intervals for myocardial infarction (fatal and nonfatal events) by height categories are shown. Left panel is control for age in years, aspirin assignment, and β-carotene assignment. In the right panel, there is a control for age, aspirin assignment, β-carotene assignment, body-mass index, smoking, history of hypertension, diabetes, history of elevated cholesterol, history of angina pectoris, parental history of myocardial infarction prior to age 60, alcohol use, and exercise frequency at least weekly. The relationship between height and risk of myocardial infarction is demonstrated in the figure. Reproduced with permission from Hebert et al.[63]

inch of added height, there was an approximately 2% to 3% decline in the risk of myocardial infarction. Men in the tallest height bracket compared with those in the shortest height bracket had only small and nonsignificant decreases in the risk of stroke and cardiovascular death. However, the number of events for stroke and cardiovascular death were far fewer than for myocardial infarction; thus, the confidence intervals were wide. These data indicate that height is inversely correlated with the risk of myocardial infarction in male physicians in the United States.

Body Weight, Obesity, and Weight Loss

To investigate the nature of the relation between body weight and all-cause mortality, Lee and associates,[64] from Boston, Mass, and Stanford, Calif, performed a prospective cohort study, following up men from 1962 or 1966 (1962/1966) through 1988. The men were Harvard University alumni with a mean age of 47 years in 1962/1966; they were without self-reported, physician-diagnosed CAD, stroke, or cancer; and they completed questionnaires on weight, height, cigarette smoking habit, and physical activity (n = 19,297). The authors calculated body-mass index (weight in kilograms divided by the square of height in meters) using self-reported measures. In multivariate analysis adjusting for age, cigarette smoking habit, and physical activity, they found a J-shaped relation between body-mass index and mortality. Relative risks of dying for men with a body-mass index of <22.5, 22.5 to <23.5, 23.5 to <24.5, 24.5 to <26.0, and 26.0 or greater were 1.00 (referent), 0.99, 0.95, 1.01, and 1.18, respectively. Among current smokers, the relation between body-mass index and mortality was U-shaped, with lowest risk of death at a body-mass index of 23.5 to <24.5. During early follow-up (1962/1966 through 1974), the authors also observed a U-shaped curve, this time with lowest mortality risk at a body-mass index of 24.5 to <26.0. To minimize confounding by cigarette smoking and bias from antecedent disease and early mortality, they conducted analysis only among never smokers and omitted the first 5 years of follow-up (510 deaths). The corresponding relative risk from this analysis, adjusted for age and physical activity, were 1.00, 1.23, 0.90 to 1.06, 1.27, and 1.67, respectively. Therefore, in these prospective data, body weight and mortality were directly related. After accounting for confounding by cigarette smoking and bias resulting from illness-related weight loss or inappropriate control for the biologic effects of obesity, the authors found no evidence of excess mortality among lean men. Indeed, lowest mortality was observed among men weighing, on average, 20% below the US average for men of comparable age and height.

To test the hypothesis that both body-mass index (expressed as the ratio of weight in kilograms per height in meters squared) and the ratio of waist circumference to hip circumference are positively associated with mortality risk in older women, Folsom and associates,[65] from Minneapolis, Minn, and Miami, Fla, studied a random sample of 41,837 Iowa women aged 55 to 69 years prospectively with a 5-year follow-up period. The main outcome measure was total mortality (1,504 deaths). Body-mass index, an index of relative weight, was associated with mortality in a J-shaped fashion: rates were elevated in the leanest as well as in the most obese women. In contrast, waist/hip circumference ratio was strongly and positively associated with mortality in dose-response manner. Adjusted for age, body-mass index, smoking, education level, marital status, estrogen use, and alcohol use, a 0.15-unit increase in waist/hip circumference ratio (eg, a 15-cm [6-in] increase in waist measurement in a woman with 100-cm [40-in] hips) was associated with a 60% greater relative risk of death. The observed associations were not explained to any great degree by bias from weight loss prior to baseline or higher early deaths among lean participants. Waist/hip circumference ratio is a better marker than body-mass index of risk of death in older women. Waist/hip circumference ratio should be measured as part of routine surveillance and risk monitoring in medical practice.

Alpert and associates,[66] from Mobile, Ala, measured heart rate and BP and performed echocardiography in 39 patients whose actual body weight was greater than twice their ideal body weight to identify factors influencing LV systolic function in morbidly obese patients and to assess the effect of weight loss on LV systolic function. Patients were studied before and after weight loss induced by gastroplasty. The study cohort was 133% overweight before weight loss and 39% overweight at the nadir of weight loss. Before weight loss, LV fractional shortening varied inversely with LV internal dimension in diastole (an indirect index of preload), LV end-systolic wall stress, and systolic BP. The weight loss induced change in LV fractional shortening varied directly with pre-weight loss LV internal dimension in diastole, LV end-systolic wall stress, and systolic BP, and inversely with the pre-weight loss LV fractional shortening. The weight loss-induced change in LV fractional shortening varied inversely with the weight loss-induced changes in LV end-systolic stress, and systolic BP. In patients with reduced LV fractional shortening, weight loss produced a significant increase in LV fractional shortening that was accompanied by a significant decrease in LV internal dimension in diastole, LV end-systolic stress, and systolic BP. The results suggest that LV loading conditions have an important role in determining LV systolic function in morbidly obese patients. Improvement in LV systolic function in these patients is closely related to weight loss-induced alterations in LV loading conditions.

In a supplement to the October 1, 1993, issue of *The Annals of Internal Medicine*, a symposium was published[67] (sponsored by the NIH Nutrition Coordinating Committee and the NIH Office of Medical Applications of Research). The symposium, an excellent one on voluntary weight loss and control, contains 26 articles.

Baldness

To examine the relation between male pattern baldness and the risk of AMI in men under the age of 55 years, Lesko and associates,[68] from Brooklyn, Mass, performed a hospital-based, case-control study of 665 men admitted to a hospital for a first nonfatal AMI; control group were 772 men admitted to the same hospitals with noncardiac diagnoses. Extent of baldness was assessed using the 12-point modified Hamilton Baldness Scale; other information was obtained by personal interview. Among the controls, the prevalence of any baldness was 34%, and the prevalence of baldness involving the vertex scalp was 23%. After allowing for age, the relative risk estimate for frontal baldness compared with no hair loss was 0.9 and for baldness involving the vertex scalp it was 1.4. Risk of AMI increased as the degree of vertex baldness increased; for severe vertex baldness the relative risk was 3.4. The relation between vertex baldness and AMI was consistent within strata defined by age and other risk factors for CAD. These data support the hypothesis that male pattern baldness involving the vertex scalp is associated with CAD in men under the age of 55 years.

Dental Disease

To investigate a reported association between dental disease and risk of CAD, DeStefano and associates,[69] from Marshfield, Wis, and Atlanta, Ga, analyzed prospectively 9,760 subjects who participated in a health examination survey in the early 1970s and were followed up to 1987. The subjects with periodontitis had a 25% increased risk of CAD relative to those with minimal periodontal disease. Poor oral hygiene, determined by the extent of dental debris and calculus, was also associated with an increased incidence of CAD. In men <50 years at baseline, periodontal disease was a stronger risk factor for CAD; men with periodontitis had a relative risk of 1.7. Both periodontal disease and poor oral hygiene showed stronger associations with total mortality than with CAD. Thus, dental disease is associated with an increased risk of CAD, particularly in young men. Whether this is a casual association is unclear. Dental health may be a more general indicator of personal hygiene and possibly health care practices.

Number of Pregnancies

Whether increasing parity or gravidity is a risk factor for CAD has been debated, but the question remains unresolved. Ness and associates,[70] from multiple US medical centers, tested the association between the number of pregnancies and a variety of cardiovascular endpoints in two groups of women who had completed childbearing. One group comprised 2,357 women who were followed for 28 years through the Framingham Heart Study, and the other comprised 2,533 women who were followed for at least 12 years through the first National Health and Nutrition Examination Survey National Epidemiologic Follow-up Study (NHEFS). The rates of CAD were higher among multigravid women than among women who had never been pregnant, in both the Framingham Heart Study and the NHEFS, but in both studies, the higher rates were statistically significant only in women with six or more pregnancies. For the women in the Framingham Study, the rate ratio adjusted for age and educational level in the group with six or more pregnancies (as compared with women who had never been pregnant) was 1.6. For the women in the NHEFS, the same adjusted rate ratio was 1.5. Adjustments for other known cardiovascular risk factors, including weight, did not markedly alter this risk. The rate of total CAD was also significantly higher among multigravid women in the Framingham Study than in the women who had never been pregnant. In two prospective American studies, having six or more pregnancies was associated with a small but consistent increase in the risk of CAD and cardiovascular disease.

Plasma Fibrinogen

Iso and associates,[71] from two Japanese and two US medical centers, used data from 1,020 Japanese men and women in a 1989 to 1991 Akita, Japan, population and from >15,000 men and women from the 1986 to 1989 Atherosclerosis Risk in Communities (ARIC) Study. To examine further the correlates of plasma fibrinogen level, subsamples of nonsmoking Akita Japanese and Minneapolis Caucasians were also studied separately in 1990. Compared with the Japanese in the Akita study, Caucasians and African Americans in ARIC had a 23 to 40 mg/dL higher age-adjusted fibrinogen level for men and a 25 to 67 mg/dL higher level for women (Figure 1-10). In the subsample, the mean plasma fibrinogen value was 288 mg/dL in Caucasian men and 248 mg/dL in Japanese men. Women showed a similar racial difference: 300 mg/dL in Caucasians and 257 mg/dL in Japanese. There were weak but positive correlations of plasma fibrinogen with age and body-mass index and weak inverse correlations with alcohol intake, HDL cholesterol, and triglycerides in most of the sex-race groups. For women, plasma fibrinogen was positively associated with menopause and inversely associated with the use of hormone-replacement therapy. Total fish intake was inversely associated with plasma fibrinogen in all sex-race groups, and the association was statistically significant for Caucasian men. After controlling for these correlates, the Japanese-Caucasian difference in mean fibrinogen value was smaller but was not eliminated: mean difference of 23 mg/dL for men and 41 mg/dL for women. These results confirm and extend the preliminary finding that plasma fibrinogen level is higher in American than in Japanese populations. This may contribute to the higher rate of CAD mortality in the United States than in Japan.

Fibrinolytic Activity

Fibrinolytic activity (FA) was measured by Meade and associates,[72] from London, United Kingdom, by dilute blood clot lysis time at entry to the Northwick Park Heart Study in 1,382 white men, aged 40 to 64 years, of

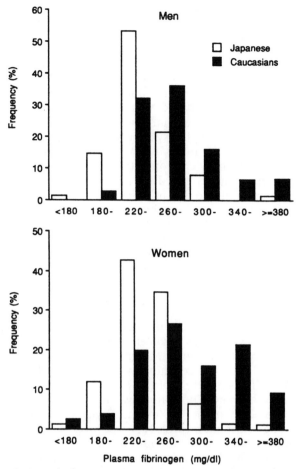

Figure 1-10. Sex-specific frequency distributions of plasma fibrinogen concentrations in nonsmoking Akita Japanese and Minneapolis Caucasians aged 47 to 69 years (1990). Reproduced with permission from Iso et al.[71]

whom 179 subsequently had episodes of myocardial ischemia during a mean follow-up period of 16.1 years. There was a significant interaction between age and low FA with respect to CAD: a difference of one standard deviation in FA was associated with a difference of about 40% in ischemic heart disease risk in those aged 40 to 54 at entry. The FA association remained after adjusting for plasma fibrinogen. High fibrinogen concentrations were also associated with CAD, as was high factor VII activity with fatal events. Low FA in younger men may exert a long-term influence by impairing the removal of fibrin deposits that contribute to atherogenesis. Low FA appears to be a leading determinant of CAD in younger men, and methods of enhancing fibrinolytic activity, whether by lifestyle changes or pharmacologically, should be considered.

Plasma Renin Activity

An earlier prospective study reported an association between high levels of plasma renin activity (as measured by the renin-sodium profile) and the incidence of AMI in patients with systemic hypertension. Mead and associates,[73] from London, United Kingdom, investigated the relation between plasma renin and CAD in their local population. The study included 803 white men, aged 40 to 64 years, selected from industrial workers in London. Plasma renin activity and established risk factors for CAD were measured at entry, which was between 1972 and 1978. Ascertainment of the primary clinical endpoints of fatal or nonfatal AMI and sudden death from coronary causes was carried out until the end of 1991. In an analysis of the 86 first coronary events, the authors found an independent relation between higher systolic BP and coronary endpoints (relative risk per 1 SD increase in BP, 1.47) but no relation between plasma renin activity and coronary endpoints (relative risk per 1 SD increase in the level of plasma renin activity, 1.04). In the 242 men who had hypertension of a degree similar to that of the subjects in the earlier prospective study of the renin profile, and in whom 44 of the 86 coronary events occurred, the relative risk of those in the highest as compared with the lowest third for plasma renin activity was 1.26. The results suggest that there is no association between plasma renin activity and AMI or sudden death from coronary causes, at least in normotensive men.

Alcohol Consumption

Most studies suggest that alcohol use decreases the risk of CAD in men. This association, however, has not been well established in women. Garg and associates,[74] from Hyattsville, Md, investigated the relation between alcohol use and CAD incidence among women aged 45 to 74 years in the Epidemiologic Follow-up Study of the First National Health and Nutrition Examination Survey. The cohort was free of heart disease at baseline. During the follow-up period (mean, 13 years), 884 CAD cases were identified through hospital records, reported hospital stays, or death certificates. Women reporting any amount of alcohol use had about a 20% decrease in risk of CAD incidence compared with abstainers. Using a Cox regression model to adjust for known cardiovascular risk factors, this relative risk of CAD remained essentially unchanged. The greatest reduction in the risk of CAD (36% to 39%) was among women who consumed about half to two drinks per day compared with abstainers. This study of a nationally representative sample with a mean follow-up of 13 years and a substantial number of CAD cases suggests that moderate alcohol use decreases the risk of CAD. However, the risk and benefits of moderate alcohol consumption need to be viewed within a broader perspective, especially because the potentially harmful effects of alcohol have been well documented.

Single Electrocardiogram

Sutherland and associates,[75] from Charleston, SC, determined the predictive ability of a single ECG tracing in predicting mortality among white and black men in the Charleston Heart Study. In 1960, baseline tracings of men aged 35 to 74 in the Charleston Heart Study were coded. Tracings were categorized as being normal or having minor or major abnormalities (Table 1-13). The 30-year vital status was ascertained and the association between ECG findings and coronary and all-cause mortality evaluated. The proportion of black men with major abnormalities

Table 1-13. Specific ECG Abnormalities by Race. Reproduced with permission from Sutherland et al.[75]

	White Men (n=584)	Black Men (n=307)	High Socioeconomic Status Black Men (n=102)
Major abnormalities			
ST depression (4-1)	2 (0.3%)	1 (0.3%)	0 (0%)
STJ depression (4-2)	2 (0.3%)	2 (0.7%)	0 (0%)
T-wave negative (5-1)	1 (0.2%)	2 (0.7%)	0 (0%)
T-wave negative (5-2)	10 (1.7%)	23 (7.5%)	4 (3.9%)
Left bundle branch block (7-1)	0 (0%)	0 (0%)	0 (0%)
Right bundle branch block (7-2)	0 (0%)	0 (0%)	0 (0%)
Intraventricular block (7-4)	0 (0%)	0 (0%)	0 (0%)
Premature beats (8-1)	30 (5.1%)	25 (8.1%)	1 (1.0%)
Atrial fibrillation/flutter (8-3)	0 (0%)	0 (0%)	0 (0%)
Minor abnormalities			
Q duration (1-3)	2 (0.3%)	0 (0%)	1 (1.0%)
ST sloping (4-3)	3 (0.5%)	6 (2.0%)	0 (0%)
T flat/negative (5-3)	49 (8.4%)	55 (17.8%)	10 (9.8%)
PR interval (6-3)	1 (0.2%)	2 (0.7%)	2 (2.0%)
Low QRS amplitude (9-1)	20 (3.4%)	1 (0.3%)	1 (1.0%)
High-amplitude R waves (3-1)	2 (0.3%)	9 (2.9%)	7 (6.9%)
Left-axis QRS deviation (2-1)	31 (5.3%)	22 (7.1%)	2 (2.0%)
Right-axis QRS deviation (2-2)	5 (0.9%)	0 (0%)	0 (0%)
Clinical findings			
Left-axis deviation	45 (7.7%)	30 (9.8%)	3 (2.9%)
Early repolarization	66 (11.3%)	100 (32.7%)	59 (57.8%)
Nonspecific T waves and/or ST-segment changes	48 (8.2%)	90 (29.4%)	21 (20.6%)
Left ventricular hypertrophy	5 (0.9%)	30 (9.8%)	2 (2.0%)

at the 1960 baseline examination was almost twice that of white men. Rate of all-cause mortality increased with severity of abnormalities for white and black men. The absolute excess risk for black men with major abnormalities was 23 per 1,000 person-years and for white men, 12.8. The excess risk for coronary mortality was 7.3 for white men and 6.5 for black men. These data confirm earlier associations derived from studies of white populations and extend the observations to black men. The magnitude of the relative risk for mortality was different for white and black men. After controlling for traditional coronary disease risk factors, white men with major abnormalities on the ECG were 2.7 times more likely to die of CAD compared with black men who were 1.95 times more likely to die of CAD (Figure 1-11).

Physical Activity and Fitness

Recent trends toward increasing physical activity, stopping cigarette smoking, and avoiding obesity may increase longevity. Paffenbarger and associates,[76] from Boston, Mass, analyzed changes in the lifestyles of Harvard alumni and the associations of these changes with mortality. Men who

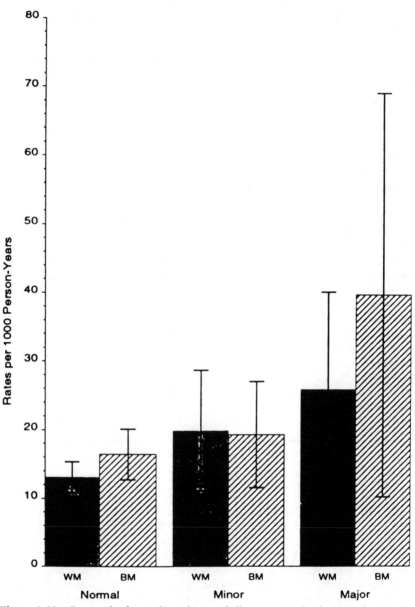

Figure 1-11. Bar graph of age-adjusted rates of all-cause mortality by ECG abnormality. WM indicates white men and BM, black men. Reproduced with permission from Sutherland et al.[75]

were 45 to 84 years of age in 1977 and who had reported no life-threatening disease on questionnaires completed in 1962 or 1966 and again in 1977 were classified according to changes in lifestyle characteristics between the first and second questionnaires. The authors analyzed changes in their level of physical activity, cigarette smoking, BP, and body weight, and the relation of these factors to mortality between 1977 and 1985. Of the 10,269 men, 476 died during this period (which totaled 90,650 man-years of observation). Beginning moderately vigorous sports activity (at an intensity of 4.5 or more metabolic equivalents) was associated with a 23% lower risk of death than not taking up moderately vigorous sports. Quitting cigarette smoking was associated with a 41% lower risk than continuing smoking, but with a 23% higher risk than constant nonsmoking. Men with recently diagnosed hypertension had a lower risk of death than those with long-term hypertension, as did men with consistently normal BP. Maintenance of lean body mass was associated with a lower mortality rate than long-term, recent, or previous obesity. The associations between changes in lifestyle and mortality were independent and were largely undiminished by age. These findings on death from CAD mirrored those on death from all causes. Beginning moderately vigorous sports activity, quitting cigarette smoking, maintaining normal BP, and avoiding obesity were separately associated with lower rates of death from all causes and from CAD among middle-aged and older men.

Despite many studies suggesting that poor physical fitness is an independent risk factor for death from cardiovascular causes, the matter has remained controversial. Sandvik and associates,[77] from Oslo, Norway, studied this question in a 16-year follow-up investigation of Norwegian men that began in 1972. The study included 1,960 healthy men, aged 40 to 59 years (84% of those invited to participate). Conventional coronary risk factors and physical fitness were assessed at baseline, with physical fitness measured as the total work performed on a bicycle ergometer during a system-limited exercise-tolerance test. After an average follow-up time of 16 years, 271 men had died, 53% of them from CAD. The relative risk of death from any cause in fitness quartile 4 (highest) as compared with quartile 1 (lowest) was 0.5 after adjustment for age, smoking status, serum lipids, BP, resting heart rate, vital capacity, body-mass index, level of physical activity, and glucose tolerance. Total mortality was similar among the subjects in fitness quartiles 1, 2, and 3 when the data were adjusted for these same variables. The adjusted relative risk of death from cardiovascular causes in fitness quartile 4 as compared with quartile 1 was 0.4. The corresponding relative risks for quartiles 3 and 2 (as compared with quartile 1) were 0.5 and 0.6, respectively. Physical fitness appears to be a graded, independent, long-term predictor of mortality from cardiovascular causes in healthy, middle-aged men. A high level of fitness was also associated with lower mortality from any cause.

CAD is newly diagnosed in approximately 1.5 million persons each year and accounts for an estimated $47 billion in direct and indirect health care costs. A report in the Morbidity and Mortality Weekly Report of September 10, 1993,[78] summarized information about the potential efficacy and cost-effectiveness of physical activity promotion as a strategy for preventing CAD. A review of 43 epidemiologic studies in 1987 concluded that moderate to vigorous physical activity reduced risk of CAD. Two thirds of the studies documented a substantially inverse relation between physical activity and risk for CAD. Additionally, the risk for CAD increased nearly 2-fold for persons who were physically inactive, a level comparable to the relative risks associated with increased systolic BP, cigarette smoking, and elevated serum cholesterol. A subsequent meta-analysis and results from other longitudinal studies supported the role of physical inactivity as a strong and independent risk factor for CAD. Based on a national survey in 1985, 56% of men and 61% of women in the United States either never or irregularly engaged in physical activity. Specifically, 25% of men and 30% of women reported no leisure-time physical activity during the preceding month, and an additional 31% of men and women reported irregular physical activity. Of the 36% of men and 31% of women who were regularly active during leisure time, 8% of the men and 7% of the women reported participating in vigorous and intense activity. An estimate of the population-attributable risk for CAD mortality associated with physical inactivity among a selected group of men from 1977 through 1985 was 14%. In comparison, the risk for systemic hypertension was 20%; for cigarette smoking, 13%; and for a positive family history of premature parental death, 20%. A total of 205,254 deaths associated with CAD were attributed to never or irregularly engaging in physical activity—a number in excess of estimates for smoking, obesity, and hypertension but similar to the estimates for elevated serum cholesterol.

Based on 1989 mortality estimates for CAD, the extrapolated cost of physical inactivity is $5.7 billion; among other risk factors for CAD, only elevated serum cholesterol (≥200 µg/dL) has a higher estimated cost (Table 1-14). A cost-effectiveness analysis to estimate the health and economic implications of a physical activity program in preventing CAD was conducted using a model of two hypothetical cohorts (one physically active and the other inactive) of 1,000 men aged 35 years. This analysis was based on a 30-year period to observe differences in the occurrence of CAD events, life expectancy, and quality-adjusted life expectancy. Physical activity was associated with 78 fewer CAD events and 1,138 quality-adjusted life-years gained during the 30-year period. For each quality-adjusted life-year gained, the direct cost was $1,395, and the total cost was $11,313—amounts similar to the cost savings of other CAD intervention strategies (Table 1-15).

Vaitkevicius and associates,[79] from Baltimore, Md, measured coronary arterial pressure and augmentation index using applanation tonometry and aortic pulse wave velocity in 146 male and female volunteers, aged 21 to 96 years, from the Baltimore Longitudinal Study of Aging. Volunteers were rigorously screened to exclude clinical and occult cardiovascular disease. Aerobic capacity was determined in all individuals by measurement of maximal oxygen consumption during treadmill exercise. In this healthy, largely sedentary cohort, the arterial stiffness indices of carotid arterial pressure and augmentation index and

Table 1-14. Population-Attributable Risk of Coronary Heart Disease (CHD) Deaths and Estimated Societal Costs, by Selected Risk Factors—United States.* From Morbidity and Mortality Weekly Report.[78]

Risk factor	Attributable risk (%)[†] (n=593,111)	Estimated cost (billions)[§]
Physical inactivity	34.6	$5.7
Obesity	32.1	$5.3
Smoking	25.0	$4.1
Hypertension	28.9	$4.7
Elevated serum cholesterol (≥200 µg/dL)	42.7	$7.0

*Source: *Reference 8.*
[†]Percentages cannot be summed because they are calculated independently for each risk factor.
[§]Costs include hospital, physician, and nursing services; medicines; and lost productivity.

Table 1-15. Selected Risk Factors for Coronary Heart Disease, by Prevalence, Population-Attributable Risk, and Cost-Effectiveness—United States. From Morbidity and Mortality Weekly Report.[78]

Risk factor	Prevalence (%)	Attributable risk (%)*	Cost effectiveness
Physical inactivity	58.0	34.6	$11,313 per QALY[†]
Hypertension	18.0	28.9	$25,000 per QALY[§]
Smoking	25.5	25.0	$21,947 total lifetime benefits of quitting[¶]
Obesity	23.0	32.1	NA**
Elevated serum cholesterol (≥200 µg/dL)	37.0	42.7	$28,000 per QALY[††]

*Percentages cannot be summed because they are calculated independently for each risk factor.
[†]Quality-adjusted life-years.
[§]Source: *Reference 9.*
[¶]Source: *Reference 10.*
**Not available.
[††]Source: *Reference 11.*

aortic pulse wave velocity increased almost 5-fold and 2-fold, respectively, as patients aged, including both men and women. This occurred in spite of only a 14% increase in systolic BP. In endurance-trained male athletes, aged 54 to 75 years, the arterial stiffness indexes were significantly reduced compared with their sedentary aged peers, despite similar blood pressures (Figure 1-12). Thus, in normotensive, rigorously screened volunteers in whom systolic BP increases an average of only 14% between ages 20 and 90 years, there are still important age-associated increases in arterial stiffness. Higher physical condition status is associated with reduced arterial stiffness both within the predominantly sedentary population and in endurance-trained older men. These findings suggest that interventions to improve exercise conditioning may reduce stiffening of arteries that normally accompany the aging process.

Cigarette Smoking

Cigarette smoking is the single most preventable cause of premature death in the United States. An estimated 390,000 smoking-attributable deaths in the US occurred in 1985, and more than 434,000 deaths occurred in 1988; in 1988, an estimated 1,198,887 years of potential life lost (YPLL) before age 65 were attributed to smoking. To estimate the national impact of cigarette smoking on mortality and YPLL, calculations were performed using the Smoking-Attributable Mortality, Morbidity, and Economic Cost (SAMMEC) software. A report in the Morbidity and Mortality Weekly Report analyzed the results[80] (Table 1-16).

To compare diet, nutrient intakes, and biochemical measure between smokers and nonsmokers, Margetts and Jackson,[81] from Southampton, United Kingdom, undertook dietary assessment in 2,197 subjects aged 16 to 64 years. The data was collected in a cross-sectional survey conducted in 1986 and 1987. Of the 2,197 subjects, 1,842 were considered to have kept a record typical of their usual dietary intake and had given data on smoking, and the results were analyzed: 1,224 nonsmokers (631 men), 359 light smokers (166 men), and 259 heavy smokers (153 men). Smokers ate more white bread, sugar, cooked meat dishes, butter, and

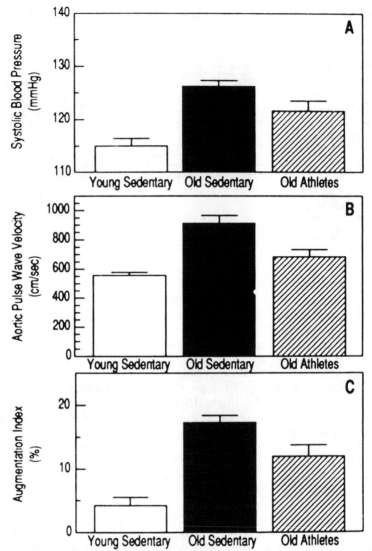

Figure 1-12. Bar graphs of systolic blood pressure, augmentation index, and aortic pulse wave velocity are shown and compared among young and old sedentary and older athletic men using analysis of variance methods. The values shown are means ± standard errors of mean. In panel A, systolic blood pressure assessment demonstrate that older control patients differ from younger control patients. In panel B, older controls differ from younger controls and older athletes in their aortic pulse wave velocity; and in panel C, older sedentary patients differ from younger sedentary patients and older athletes. Reproduced with permission from Vaitkevicius, et al.[79]

whole milk and less wholemeal bread, high-fiber breakfast cereals, fruit, and carrots. Smokers had lower intakes of polyunsaturated fat, protein, carbohydrate, fiber, iron, carotene, and ascorbic acid. Adjusting for other covariates did not substantially alter the pattern of intakes. At the same dietary intake of carotenoids, smokers were more likely to have lower circulating serum β-carotene concentrations than nonsmokers. The diet

Table 1-16. Relative Risks* (RRs) for Death Attributed to Smoking and Smoking-Attributable Mortality (SAM) for Current and Former Smokers, by Disease Category and Sex—United States, 1990. From Morbidity and Mortality Weekly Report.[80]

Disease Category (ICD-9 Code)†	Male RR Current Smokers	Male RR Former Smokers	SAM	Female RR Current Smokers	Female RR Former Smokers	SAM	Total SAM
Adult diseases (persons aged ≥35 y)							
Neoplasms							
Lip, oral cavity, pharynx (140-149)	27.5	8.8	5033	5.6	2.9	1442	6475
Esophagus (150)	7.6	5.8	5668	10.3	3.2	1616	7284
Pancreas (157)	2.1	1.1	2667	2.3	1.8	3447	6114
Larynx (161)	10.5	5.2	2379	17.8	11.9	611	2990
Trachea, lung, bronchus (162)	22.4	9.4	81 179	11.9	4.7	35 741	116 920
Cervix uteri (180)	...‡	...	...	2.1	1.9	1294	1294
Urinary bladder (188)	2.9	1.9	3046	2.6	1.9	980	4026
Kidney, other urinary (189)	3.0	2.0	2866	1.4	1.2	353	3219
Cardiovascular diseases							
Hypertension (401-404)	1.9	1.3	3299	1.7	1.2	2151	5450
Ischemic heart disease (410-414)							
Persons aged 35-64 y	2.8	1.8	26 431	3.0	1.4	7701	34 132
Persons aged ≥65 y	1.6	1.3	38 918	1.6	1.3	25 871	64 789
Other heart diseases (390-398, 415-417, 420-429)	1.9	1.3	23 295	1.7	1.2	12 019	35 314
Cerebrovascular diseases (430-438)							
Persons aged 35-64 y	3.7	1.4	4557	4.8	1.4	4114	8671
Persons aged ≥65 y	1.9	1.3	10 421	1.5	1.0	4189	14 610
Atherosclerosis (440)	4.1	2.3	3737	3.0	1.3	2675	6412
Aortic aneurysm (441)	4.1	2.3	5913	3.0	1.3	1382	7295
Other arterial disease (442-448)	4.1	2.3	2032	3.0	1.3	1115	3147
Respiratory diseases							
Pneumonia and influenza (480-487)	2.0	1.6	11 292	2.2	1.4	7881	19 173
Bronchitis, emphysema (491-492)	9.7	8.8	9324	10.5	7.0	5541	14 865
Chronic airway obstruction (496)	9.7	8.8	30 385	10.5	7.0	18 597	48 982
Other respiratory diseases (010-012, 493)	2.0	1.6	787	2.2	1.4	668	1455
Pediatric diseases (persons aged <1 y)							
Short gestation, low birth weight (765)	1.8		285	1.8		222	507
Respiratory distress syndrome (769)	1.8		219	1.8		141	360
Other respiratory conditions of newborn (770)	1.8		214	1.8		160	374
Sudden infant death syndrome (798)	1.5		288	1.5		182	470
Burn deaths§			863			499	1362
Environmental tobacco smoke deaths‖			1055			1945	3000
Total			276 153			142 537	418 690

*Relative to never smokers.
†ICD-9 indicates *International Classification of Diseases, Ninth Revision.*
‡Ellipses indicate not applicable.
§Data from the National Fire Protection Association, 1993.
‖Deaths among nonsmokers from lung cancer attributable to environmental tobacco smoke (Environmental Protection Agency, 1992).

and nutrient intakes and circulating levels of nutrients of smokers were different from those of nonsmokers. Smokers were more likely to have an imbalance between the dietary intake of antioxidant nutrients and the metabolic demand for antioxidant protection. This imbalance is likely to make smokers more susceptible to oxidative damage. Smokers are at increased risk of chronic disease because their diets are different and because smoking creates an altered pattern of demand for specific nutrients. The diets of smokers not only fail to meet the usual requirements for specific nutrients to satisfy the altered pattern of demand but are likely to exacerbate the damage caused by smoking.

To examine the temporal relation between stopping smoking and total mortality rates among middle-aged women, Kawachi and associates,[82] from Boston, Mass, performed a prospective cohort study with 12 years of follow-up involving 117,001 female registered nurses, aged 30 to 55 years, who were free of manifest CAD, stroke, and cancer, in 1976. A total of 2,847 deaths (933 among never smokers, 1,115 among current smokers) occurred during 1.37 million person-years of follow-up. The multivariate relative risks for total mortality compared with never smokers were 1.87 for current smokers and 1.29 for former smokers. Participants who started smoking before the age of 15 years had the highest risks for total mortality (multivariate relative risk, 3.15), cardiovascular disease mortality (relative risk, 9.94), and deaths from external causes of injury (relative risk, 5.39). Compared with continuing smokers, former smokers had a 24% reduction in risk for cardiovascular disease mortality within 2 years of quitting. The excess risks for total mortality and both cardiovascular disease and total cancer mortality among former smokers approached the level of that for never smokers after 10 to 14 years of abstinence. The health benefits of cessation were clearly present regardless of the age at starting and daily number of cigarettes smoked. The risk of cigarette smoking on total mortality among former smokers decreased nearly to that of never smokers 10 to 14 years after cessation.

To identify and quantify the major external (nongenetic) factors that contribute to death in the US, McGinnis and Foege,[83] from Washington, DC, and Atlanta, Ga, identified articles published between 1977 and 1993 through MEDLINE searches, reference citations, and expert consultation. Government reports and compilations of vital statistics and surveillance data were also obtained. Data used were those for which specific methodological assumptions were stated. A table quantifying the contributions of leading factors was constructed using actual counts, generally accepted estimates, and calculated estimates that were developed by summing various individual estimates and correcting to avoid double counting (Table 1-17). For the factors of greatest complexity and uncertainty (diet and activity patterns and toxic agents), a conservative approach was taken by choosing the lower boundaries of the various estimates. The most prominent contributors to mortality in the US in 1990 were tobacco (an estimated 400,000 deaths), diet and activity patterns (300,000), alcohol (100,000), microbial agents (90,000), toxic agents (60,000), firearms (35,000), sexual behavior (30,000), motor vehicles (25,000), and illicit use of drugs (20,000). Socioeconomic status and access to medical care are also important contributors but difficult to quan-

Table 1-17. Actual Causes of Death in the United States in 1990. Reproduced with permission from McGinnis et al.[83]

| | Deaths | |
Cause	Estimated No.*	Percentage of Total Deaths
Tobacco	400 000	19
Diet/activity patterns	300 000	14
Alcohol	100 000	5
Microbial agents	90 000	4
Toxic agents	60 000	3
Firearms	35 000	2
Sexual behavior	30 000	1
Motor vehicles	25 000	1
Illicit use of drugs	20 000	<1
Total	**1 060 000**	50

*Composite approximation drawn from studies that use different approaches to derive estimates, ranging from actual counts (eg, firearms) to population attributable risk calculations (eg, tobacco). Numbers over 100 000 rounded to the nearest 100 000; over 50 000, rounded to the nearest 10 000; below 50 000, rounded to the nearest 5000.

tify independent of the other factors cited. Because the studies reviewed used different approaches to derive estimates, the stated numbers should be viewed as first approximations. Approximately half of all deaths that occurred in 1990 could be attributed to the factors identified. Although no attempt was made to further quantify the impact of these factors on morbidity and quality of life, the public health burden they impose is considerable and offers guidance for shaping health policy priorities.

Smoking has both acute and chronic adverse effects in patients with CAD. Quillen and associates,[84] from Iowa City, Iowa, evaluated the potential effects of cigarette smoking on proximal and distal epicardial conduit and coronary resistance vessels. Twenty-four long-term smokers were studied during cardiac catheterization after vasoactive medications had been discontinued. The effect of smoking one cigarette 10 to 15 mm long on proximal and distal conduit vessel segments was assessed before and immediately after smoking and at 5, 15, and 30 minutes after smoking (n = 8). Coronary flow velocity was measured in a nonobstructed artery with a 3F intraocoronary Doppler catheter before and 5 minutes after smoking. Eight patients were studied without smoking to control for spontaneous changes in conduit arterial diameter and resistance vessel tone. The average diameter of proximal coronary artery segments decreased from 2.56 mm to 2.41 mm 5 minutes after smoking. Distal coronary diameter decreased from 1.51 to 1.39 mm. Marked focal vasoconstriction after smoking was observed in two patients. Coronary diameter returned to baseline by 30 minutes after smoking. There was no change in vessel diameter in control patients. Despite a significant increase in the rate/pressure product, coronary flow velocity decreased by 7% and coronary vascular resistance increased by 21% 5 minutes after smoking. There was no change in these variables in the control subjects. These authors concluded that smoking causes immediate constriction of proximal and distal epicardial coronary arteries and increased coronary resistance vessel tone despite an increase in myocardial oxygen demand. These acute coronary hemodynamic effects may contribute to the adverse acute consequences of cigarette smoking.

References

1. Roberts WC: Getting cardiologists interested in lipids. Am J Cardiol 1993 (Sep 15);72:744–745.
2. State-specific changes in cholesterol screening—behavioral risk factors surveillance system, 1988–1991. MMWR 1993 (Sep 3);42/34:663–668.
3. Klag MJ, Ford DE, Mead LA, et al: Serum cholesterol in young men and subsequent cardiovascular disease. N Engl J Med 1993 (Feb 4);328:313–318.
4. Bass KM, Newschaffer CJ, Klag MJ, et al: Plasma lipoprotein levels as predictors of cardiovascular disease in women. Arch Intern Med 1993 (Oct 11);153:2209–2216.
5. Kronmal RA, Cain KC, Ye Z, et al: Total serum cholesterol levels and mortality risk as a function of age. Arch Intern Med 1993 (May 10);153:1065–1073.
6. Laakso M, Lehto S, Penttilälä K: Lipids and lipoproteins predicting coronary heart disease mortality and morbidity in patients with non-insulin-dependent diabetes. Circulation 1993 (Oct);88[part 1]:1421–1430.

7. Stensvold E, Tverdal A, Urdal P, et al: Nonfasting serum triglyceride concentration and mortality from coronary heart disease and any cause in middle-aged Norwegian women. Br Med J 1993 (Nov 20);307:1318–1322.

8. LaRosa JC: Cholesterol lowering, low cholesterol, and mortality. Am J Cardiol 1993 (Oct 1);72:776–786 (Abstract #3).

9. Hegele RA, Connelly PW, Cullen-Dean G, et al: Elevated plasma lipoprotein(a) associated with abnormal stress thallium scans in children with family hypercholesterolemia. Am J Cardiol 1993 (Aug 15);72:402–406.

10. Jenner JL, Ordovas JM, Lamon-Fava S, et al: Effects of age, sex, and menopausal status on plasma lipoprotein(a) level (The Framingham Offspring Study). Circulation 1993 (April);87:1135–1141.

11. Schreiner PJ, Morrisett JD, Sharrett AR, et al: Lipoprotein(a) as a risk factor for preclinical atherosclerosis. Arteriosclerosis and Thrombosis 1993 (June);13:826–833.

12. Ridker PM, Hennekens CH, Stampfer MJ: A prospective study of lipoprotein(a) and the risk of myocardial infarction. JAMA 1993 (Nov 10);270:2195–2199.

13. Rader DJ, Lkewaki K, Duverger N, et al: Very low high-density lipoproteins without coronary atherosclerosis. Lancet 1993 (Dec 11);342:1455–1458.

14. Chait A, Brazg RL, Tribble DL, et al: Susceptibility of small, dense, low-density lipoproteins to oxidative modification in subjects with the atherogenic lipoprotein phenotype, pattern B. Am J Med 1993 (April);94:350–356.

15. Casino PR, Kilcoyne CM, Quyyumi AA, et al: The role of nitric oxide in endothelium-dependent vasodilation of hypercholesterolemic patients. Circulation 1993 (Dec);88:2541–2547.

16. Snyder SM, Terdiman JF, Caan B, et al: Relation of apolipoprotein E phenotypes to hypocholesterolemia. Am J Med 1993 (Nov);95:480–488.

17. Moorjani S, Roy M, Torres A, et al: Mutations of low-density-lipoprotein-cholesterol-receptor gene, variation in plasma cholesterol, and expression of coronary artery disease in homozygous familial hypercholesterolemia. Lancet 1993 (May 22);341:1303–1306.

18. Heller DA, Faire U, Pedersen NL, et al: Genetic and environmental influences on serum lipid levels in twins. N Engl J Med 1993 (April 22);328:1150–1156.

19. Morgan RE, Palinkas LA, Barrett-Connor EL, Wingard DL: Plasma cholesterol and depressive symptoms in older men. Lancet 1993 (Jan 1993);341:75–79.

20. Barker DJP, Martyn CN, Osmond C, et al: Growth in utero and serum cholesterol concentrations in adult life. Br Med J 1993 (Dec 11);307:1524–1527.

21. Denke MA, Sempos CT, Grundy SM: Effect of excess body weight on blood cholesterol levels in white American men. Arch Intern Med 1993 (May 10);153:1093–1103).

22. Sabaté J, Fraser GE, Burke K, et al: Effects of walnuts on serum lipid levels and blood pressure in normal men. N Engl J Med 1993 (March 4);328:603–607.

23. Willett WC, Stampfer MJ, Manson JE, et al: Intake of *trans* fatty acids and risk of coronary artery disease among women. Lancet 1993 (March 6);341:581–585.

24. Bayerdörffer E, Mannes GA, Richter WO, et al: Decreased high-density lipoprotein cholesterol and increased low-density cholesterol levels in patients with colorectal adenomas. Ann Intern Med 1993 (April 1);118:481–487.

25. Shor-Posner G, Basit A, Lu Y, et al: Effects of HIV infection on serum levels of cholesterol and triglycerides. Am J Med 1993 (May);94:515–523.

26. Vaziri SM, Evans JC, Larson MG, et al: The impact of female hormone usage on the lipid profiles (The Framingham Offspring Study). Arch Intern Med 1993 (Oct 11);153:2202–2206.

27. Dujovne CA, Eff J, Ferraro L, et al: Comparative effects of atenolol versus celiprolol on serum lipids and blood pressure in hyperlipidemic and hypertensive subjects. Am J Cardiol 1993 (Nov 15);72:1131–1136.

28. Giles WH, Anda RF, Jones DH, et al: Recent trends in the identification and treatment of high blood cholesterol by physicians. JAMA 1993 (March 3);269:1133–1138.

29. Smith GD, Song F, Sheldon TA: Cholesterol lowering and mortality. Br Med J 1993 (May 22);306:1367–1373.

30. Atkins D, Psaty BM, Koepsell TD, et al: Cholesterol reduction and the risk of stroke in men. Ann Intern Med 1993 (July 15);119:136–145.

31. Posner BM, Cupples LA, Gagnon D, et al: Rational and potential efficacy of preventive nutrition in heart disease. Arch Intern Med 1993 (July 12);153:1549–1556.

32. Denke MA, Frantz ID: Response to a cholesterol-lowering diet. Am J Med 1993 (June);94:626–631.

33. Singh RB, Singh NK, Rastogi SS, et al: Effects of diet and lifestyle changes on atherosclerotic risk factors after 24 weeks on the Indian Diet Heart Study. Am J Cardiol 1993 (June 1);71:1283–1288.

34. Jenkins DJ, Wolever TM, Rao AV, et al: Lipid lowering by soluble fiber in low-fat, low-cholesterol diets. N Engl J Med 1993 (July 1);329:21–26.

35. Jain AK, Vargas R, Gotzkowsky S, et al: Can garlic reduce levels on serum lipids? Am J Med 1993 (June);94:632–635.

36. Warshafsky S, Kamer RS, Sivak SL: Effect of garlic on total serum cholesterol. Ann Intern Med 1993 (Oct 1);119:599–605.

37. Davis PA, Planton J-F, Gershwin ME, et al: A linoleate-enriched cheese product reduces low-density lipoprotein in moderately hypercholesterolemic adults. Ann Intern Med 1993 (Oct 1);119:555–559.

38. Sprecher DL, Harris BV, Goldberg AC, et al: Efficacy of psyllium in reducing serum cholesterol levels in hypercholesterolemic patients on high- or low-fat diets. Ann Intern Med 1993 (Oct 1);119:545–554.

39. Dressman JB, Adair CH, Barnett JL, et al: The cholesterol-lowering affect of high-molecular-weight hydroxypropylmethylcellulose. Arch Intern Med 1993 (June 14);153:1345–1353.

40. Nabulski AA, Folsom AR, White A, et al: Association of hormone-replacement therapy with various cardiovascular risk factors in postmenopausal women. N Engl J Med 1993 (April 15);328:1069–1075.

41. D'Agostino RB, Kannel WB, Stepanians MN, et al: Efficacy and tolerability of lovastatin in hypercholesterolemia in patients with systemic hypertension. Am J Cardiol 1993 (Jan 1);71:82–87.

42. Hunninghake DB, Stein EA, Dujovne CA, et al: The efficacy of intensive dietary therapy alone or combined with lovastatin in outpatients with hypercholesterolemia. N Engl J Med 1993 (April 29);328:1213–1219.

43. Lovastatin Study Groups I through IV: Lovastatin 5-year safety and efficacy study. Arch Intern Med 1993 (May 10);153:1079–1087.

44. Bradford RH, Downton M, Chremos AN, et al: Efficacy and tolerability of lovastatin in women with moderate hypercholesterolemia. Ann Intern Med 1993 (June 1);118:850–855.

45. Lovastatin Pravastatin Study Group: A multicenter comparative trial of lovastatin and pravastatin in the treatment of hypercholesterolemia. Am J Cardio 1993 (April 1);71:810–815.

46. Pitt B, Ellis SG, Mancini GBJ, et al (for the PLAC I Investigators): Design and Recruitment in the United States of a multicenter quantitative angiographic trial of pravastatin to limit atherosclerosis in the coronary arteries (PLAC I). Am J Cardiol 1993 (July 1);72:31–35.

47. Pravastatin Multinational Study Group for Cardiac Risk Patients: Effects of pravastatin in patients with serum total cholesterol levels from 5.2 to 7.8 mmol/L (200 to 300 mg/dL) plus two additional atherosclerotic risk factors. Am J Cardiol 1993 (Nov 1);72:1031–1037.

48. Pravastatin Multicenter Study Group II: Comparative efficacy and safety of pravastatin and cholestyramine alone and combined for hypercholesterolemia. Arch Intern Med 1993 (June 14);153:1321–1329.

49. Wiklund O, Angelin B, Bergman M, et al: Pravastatin and gemfibrozil alone and in combination for the treatment of hyper-cholesterolemia. Am J Med 1993 (Jan 1993);94:13–20.

50. Simvastatin Pravastatin Study Group: Comparison of the efficacy, safety and tolerability of simvastatin and pravastatin for hypercholesterolemia. Am J Cardiol 1993 (June 15);71:1408–1414.

51. Leung W-H, Lau C-P, Wong C-K: Beneficial effect of cholesterol-lowering therapy on coronary endothelium-dependent relaxation in hypercholesterolemic patients. Lancet 1993 (June 12);341:1496–1500.

52. Schectman G, Hiatt J, Hartz A: Evaluation of the effectiveness of lipid-lowering therapy (bile acid sequestrants, niacin, psyllium and lovastatin) for treating hypercholesterolemia in veterans. Am J Cardiol 1993 (April 1);71:759–765.

53. Blankenhorn DH, Selzer RH, Crawford DW, et al: Beneficial effects of colestipol-niacin therapy on the common carotid artery. Two- and four-year reduction of intima-media thickness measured by ultrasound. Circulation 1993 (July);88:20–28.

54. Miller M, Bachorik PS, McCrindle BW, et al: Effect of gemfibrozil in men with primary isolated low high-density lipoprotein cholesterol. Am J Med 1993 (Jan);94:7–12.

55. Gotto AM Jr, Breen WJ, Corder CN, et al (for the Lopid SR Work Group I): Once-daily extended-release gemfibrozil in patients with dyslipidemia. Am J Cardiol 1993 (May 1);71:1057–1063.

56. Reaven PD, Khouw A, Beltz WF, et al: Effect of dietary antioxidant combinations in humans. Arteriosclerosis and Thrombosis 1993 (April);13:590–600.

57. Lane DM, McConathy WJ, Laughlin LO, et al: Weekly treatment of diet/drug-resistant hypercholesterolemia with the heparin-induced extracorporeal low-density lipoprotein precipitation (HELP) system by selective plasma low-density lipoprotein removal. Am J Cardiol 1993 (April 1);71:816–822.

58. Sasson Z, Rasooly Y, Bhesania T, et al: Insulin resistance is an important determinant of left ventricular mass in the obese. Circulation 1993 (Oct);88[part 1]:1431–1436.

59. Johnstone MT, Creager SJ, Scales KM, et al: Impaired endothelium-dependent vasodilation in patients with insulin-dependent diabetes mellitus. Circulation 1993 (Dec);88:2510–2516.

60. Ferraro S, Perrone-Filardi P, Maddalena G, et al: Comparison of left ventricular function in insulin- and non-insulin-dependent diabetes mellitus. Am J Cardiol 1993 (Feb 15);71:409–414.

61. Barker DJP, Osmond C, Simmonds SJ, et al: The relation of small head circumference and thinness at birth to death from cardiovascular disease in adult life. Br Med J 1993 (Feb 13);306:422–426.

62. Osmond C, Barker DJ, Winter PD, et al: Early growth and death from cardiovascular disease in women. Br Med J 1993 (Dec 11);307:1519–1524.

63. Hebert PR, Rich-Edwards JW, Manson JE, et al: Height and incidence of cardiovascular disease in male physicians. Circulation 1993 (Oct);88[part 1]:1437–1443.

64. Lee I-M, Manson JE, Hennekens CH, et al: Relation of body weight and all-cause mortality. JAMA 1993 (Dec 15);270:2823–2828.

65. Folsom AR, Kaye SA, Sellers TA, et al: Body fat distribution and 5-year risk of death in older women. JAMA 1993 (Jan 27);269:483–487.

66. Alpert MA, Terry BE, Lambert CR, et al: Factors influencing left ventricular systolic function in nonhypertensive morbidly obese patients, and effect of weight loss induced by gastroplasty. Am J Cardiol 1993 (March 15);71:733–737.

67. NIH Nutrition Coordinating Committee and NIH Office of Medical Applications of Research: Methods for voluntary weight loss and control, Danford D, Fletcher SW (eds). Ann Intern Med 1993 (Oct suppl).

68. Lesko SM, Rosenberg L, Shapiro S: Relation of baldness to acute myocardial infarction in men. JAMA 1993 (Feb 24);269:998–1003.

69. DeStefano F, Anda RF, Kahn HS, et al: Dental disease and risk of coronary artery disease and mortality. Br Med J 1993 (March 13);306:688–692.

70. Ness RB, Harris T, Cobb J, et al: Number of pregnancies and the subsequent risk of cardiovascular disease. N Engl J Med 1993 (May 27);328: 1528–1533.

71. Iso H, Folsom AR, Sato S, et al: Plasma fibrinogen and its correlates in Japanese and U.S. population samples. Arteriosclerosis and Thrombosis 1993 (June);13:783–790.

72. Meade TW, Ruddock V, Stirling Y, et al: Fibrinolytic activity, clotting factors, and long-term incidence of coronary artery disease in the Northwick Park Heart Study. Lancet 1993 (Oct 30);342:1076–1079.

73. Meade TW, Cooper JA, Peart WS: Plasma renin activity and coronary artery disease. N Engl J Med 1993 (Aug 26);329:616–619.

74. Garg R, Wagener DK, Madans JH: Alcohol consumption and risk of ischemic heart disease in women. Arch Intern Med 1993 (May 24);153:1211–1216.

75. Sutherland SE, Gazes PC, Keil JE, et al: Electrocardiographic abnormalities and 30-year mortality among white and black men of the Charleston Heart Study. Circulation 1993 (Dec);88:2685–2692.

76. Paffenbarger RS, Hyde RT, Wing AL, et al: The association of changes in physical-activity level and other lifestyle characteristics with mortality among men. N Engl J Med 1993 (Feb 25);328:538–545.

77. Sandvik L, Erikssen J, Thaulow E, et al: Physical fitness as a predictor of mortality among healthy, middle-aged norwegian men. N Engl J Med 1993 (Feb 25);328:533–537.

78. Public health focus: Physical activity and the prevention of coronary heart disease. MMWR 1993 (Sep 10);42:669–672.

79. Vaitkevicius PV, Fleg JL, Engel JH, et al: Effects of age and aerobic capacity on arterial stiffness in healthy adults. Circulation 1993 (Oct);88[part 1]:1456–1462.

80. Cigarette smoking-attributable mortality and years of potential life lost–United States, 1990. MMWR 1993;42:645–649.

81. Margetts BM, Jackson AA: Interactions between people's diet and their smoking habits. Br Med J 1993 (Nov 27);307:1381–1384.

82. Kawachi I, Colditz GA, Stampfer MJ, et al: Smoking cessation in relation to total mortality rates in women. Ann Intern Med 1993 (Nov 15);119: 992–1000.

83. McGinnis JM, Foege WH. Actual causes of death in the United States. JAMA 1993 (Nov 10);270:2207–2212.

84. Quillen JE, Rossen JD, Oskarsson HJ, et al: Acute effect of cigarette smoking on the coronary circulation: Constriction of epicardial and resistance vessels. J Am Coll Cardiol 1993 (Sep);22:642–647.

2

Coronary Artery Disease

Trends in Nonfatal Disease

Although CAD mortality has been decreasing, little is known about trends in morbidity from CAD. DeStefano and associates,[1] from Atlanta, evaluated trends in nonfatal CAD in the United States from 1980 to 1989. They analyzed data from the National Health Interview Survey, an ongoing survey of representative samples of the civilian, noninstitutionalized population of the United States. Survey respondents were determined to have CAD if they reported ever having an AMI, angina pectoris, or CAD. Incidence was defined as initial onset of a CAD condition during the year preceding the interview date. About 6 million people were estimated to be living with CAD (Table 2-1). The age-standardized prevalence was relatively constant at about 25 per 1000. Among white men, however, prevalence increased significantly over the 10-year period. Among men aged 75 to 84 years, prevalence increased from 100 per 1000 in 1980 to 179 per 1000 in 1989. Among men and women aged 45 to 54 years, prevalence decreased. Overall, the incidence rate of nonfatal CAD was relatively flat (at about 3 per 1000 per year after 1983). Among white women, the incidence rate increased from 1.4 to 2.8 per 1000; and by the end of the decade, it nearly equaled the incidence rate among white men. Overall, the burden of nonfatal CAD remained fairly constant during the 1980s. The trends, however, were not uniform in all population groups. The apparent increasing incidence among women deserves continued monitoring. An encouraging trend is the decreasing prevalence in the younger age groups.

Table 2-1. Estimated Number of People Living with Coronary Heart Disease and Age-Standardized Prevalence, by Year, United States, 1980 through 1989. Reproduced with permission from DeStefano et al.[1]

Year	No. of People, Millions	Prevalence per 1000 Population (95% Confidence Limits)
1980	4.72	21.6 (18.9, 24.3)
1981	5.02	22.4 (20.3, 24.5)
1982	5.06	22.2 (19.7, 24.7)
1983	5.90	25.5 (23.2, 27.8)
1984	6.07	25.9 (23.6, 28.2)
1985	5.80	24.4 (22.1, 26.7)
1986	6.09	25.2 (22.6, 27.9)
1987	6.10	24.8 (22.6, 26.9)
1988	6.26	25.2 (22.9, 27.5)
1989	5.75	22.7 (20.4, 25.0)

In Women

To determine the effects of female gender on long-term survival and subsequent CAD events in a population developing first clinical manifestations of CAD, Orencia and associates,[2] from Rochester, Minn, did a follow-up on all Rochester residents first diagnosed with either angina pectoris or AMI/sudden unexpected death between Jan 1, 1960, and Dec 31, 1979. Patients with angina pectoris were followed up through 1982 for survival and time to initial AMI/cardiac death. Patients with AMI were followed up through 1982 for survival and time to recurrent AMI/cardiac death. Angina pectoris was the initial diagnosis for 529 women and 504 men. AMI or sudden unexpected death was the initial diagnosis for 611 women and 997 men. The average age of patients diagnosed with angina pectoris was 67 years for women and 60 years for men. The average age of patients diagnosed with AMI/sudden unexpected death was 72 years for women and 62 years for men. Women presenting with angina pectoris survived significantly longer and had a lower incidence of subsequent AMI/cardiac death compared with men of similar age. When rates of AMI and sudden unexpected death were combined to assess all cardiac endpoints with objective criteria ("hard" endpoints), women presenting with AMI/sudden unexpected death had survival rates and risk of subsequent AMI/coronary death that were similar to men of the same age. When survival following AMI was analyzed separately, survival also did not vary by gender. In this population, women with angina pectoris as an initial diagnosis, but not those with AMI or sudden unexpected death, have longer survival and lower risk of subsequent AMI/cardiac death than do men with the same presentation and of a similar age.

After age 40 years, CAD is the leading cause of death in both women and men, yet in women the factors associated with, or leading to, CAD have been less extensively studied. Solymoss and associates,[3] from Montreal, Canada, examined the strength of association of a number of risk factors to CAD in groups of women <60 years of age with (n = 108) and without (n = 66) angiographically documented significant narrowing of coronary arteries. In univariate analyses, there were significant differences between control subjects and patients with regard to age and total lipids and apolipoproteins measured. The relative frequency of cigarette smoking and diabetes was higher and that of estrogen replacement therapy lower in patients with CAD than in control subjects. In multivariate analysis, the following factors were independently associated with CAD: total cholesterol to HDL cholesterol, lipoprotein(a), estrogen replacement, age, and smoking. The nonadjusted odds ratio of CAD, based on combined tercile values of lipoprotein(a) serum level and total cholesterol to HDL cholesterol ratio, was very low when both values were within the first tercile, but very high when both were in the third tercile. In conclusion, the serum lipoprotein(a) level and the total cholesterol to HDL cholesterol ratio were the risk factors most closely associated to CAD in women, and the determination of lipoprotein(a) should complement the measurement of classic lipids in the screening and the diagnostic workup of the disease. (Kuhn and Rackley,[4] from Washington, DC, provide a fine review of CAD in women.)

Composition of Plaques in Women v Men

Composition of atherosclerotic plaques has been described in various subsets of patients with fatal CAD and after coronary bypass operations, but no reports have investigated the composition of coronary plaque or saphenous vein grafts according to gender. Mautner and associates,[5] from Bethesda, Md, studied a total of 979, 5-mm segments of native coronary arteries and 842, 5-mm segments of saphenous vein grafts by a computerized planimetric technique in 11 women and 11 men who were matched for survival after the bypass operation. Comparison of the plaque components revealed that atherosclerotic plaques in women, compared with those in men, contained significantly more cellular fibrous tissue, both in native coronary arteries (mean, 38% v 4%) and in saphenous vein grafts (mean, 70% v 36%) (Figure 2-1). In contrast, the proportion of dense fibrous tissue was significantly less in the atherosclerotic plaques of women than in those of men, both in native coronary arteries (mean, 50% v 85%) and in saphenous vein grafts (mean, 25% v 57%). Therefore, cellular fibrous tissue is often found at an early stage of plaque development, and dense fibrous tissue is a major component in later stages. Thus, the plaque composition of the native coronary arteries and saphenous venous conduits differed in men and women, with the plaques of the women appearing younger than those of the men.

Effects of Race on Management

To compare racial differences in clinical presentation, natural history, and access to medical care and procedures among emergency-department patients with acute chest pain, Johnson and associates,[6] from Boston, Mass, and Cincinnati, Ohio, prospectively studied 3,031 patients, aged 30 years or older, who came to the emergency department with acute chest pain from 1984 to 1986. African Americans tended to have slightly, but not al-

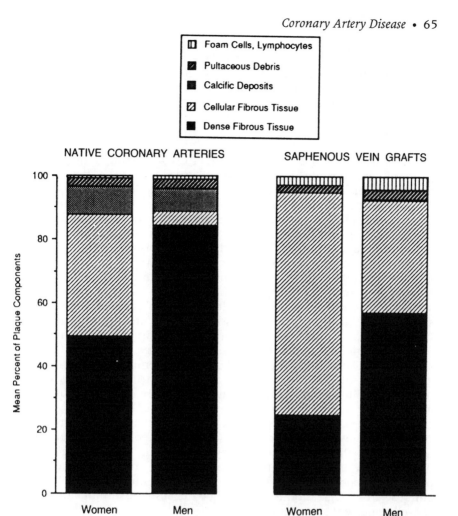

Figure 2-1. Graph comparing the mean composition of the plaques in the native coronary arteries and saphenous vein grafts of women and men. The plaques in women had a higher percentage of cellular fibrous tissue than did those in men. This difference was observed in the saphenous vein grafts and was even more pronounced in the native coronary arteries. In both men and women, calcific deposits were found mainly in native coronary arteries. Reproduced with permission from Mautner et al.[5]

ways significantly, lower rates of AMI, acute CAD, and major complications, after adjusting for presenting symptoms and signs; the adjusted odds ratios for African Americans were as follows: 0.77 for AMI, 0.75 for CAD, and 0.79 for death or major complications. Clinical factors classically associated with AMI were equally predictive in African Americans and whites. After adjustments were made for multiple clinical factors, a lower proportion of African Americans were admitted to the hospital (odds ratio, 0.69) and, once admitted, were somewhat less likely to be triaged to the coronary care unit (odds ratio, 0.81). In adjusted analyses, African Americans were as likely to undergo cardiac catheterization as whites (odds ratio, 0.86) but were less likely to undergo CABG once severity of CAD was included in the analysis (odds ratio, 0.24). African Americans and whites had a similar presentation and natural history of AMI and, after adjusting for probability of clinical events, similar access to most medical care and cardiac procedures. However, the rate of CABG was much lower among African Americans than among whites.

Coronary Progression

Previous studies of the natural history of CAD generally relied on estimates of percent stenosis derived from visual assessment of the coronary angiogram. In a study of 26 patients, Stone and associates,[7] from Boston, Mass, performed serial quantitative angiography 3 years apart to determine changes in both absolute measurements of the luminal diameter and relative percent stenosis. Initially, the mean minimal diameter of 74 coronary obstructions was 1.9 mm, the mean "normal" reference diameter was 3.1 mm, and the mean percent stenosis was 37%. At follow-up, there was a mild reduction of 0.1 mm in the minimal diameter and an increase in percent stenosis to 39%. The average diameter of 85 arterial segments without a focal obstruction either initially or at follow-up showed mild but significant progression. Using a minimal change of 0.3 mm in arterial diameter as a categoric variable, progression occurred in 26% of 74 arterial segments, no significant change in 65%, and regression in 9% (Figure 2-2). The only significant determinant of disease progression was the initial severity of disease. Obstructed arteries with a larger initial minimal diameter and presumably milder disease progressed more rapidly than did those with a smaller diameter. There was no effect of age on the rate of progression. Although overall there was a correlation between the direction and magnitude of change in minimal diameter and those in percent stenosis, changes in percent stenosis can be misleading, because the minimal and adjacent normal diameters may progress independently at different rates. The outcome variable of an atherosclerosis regression trial should be the absolute minimal diameter, as well as percent stenosis.

Waters and associates,[8] from Winston-Salem, NC, and Montreal, Canada, evaluated the angiographic progression of coronary atherosclerosis in 335 patients who underwent repeat coronary arteriography after a 2-year interval as part of a clinical trial. Progression was defined as an increase in diameter stenosis by ≥15% of at least one coronary lesion, and it was seen in 141 (42%) of the patients. Coronary lesions were measured quantitatively from comparable end diastolic frames selected by a radiologist viewing each pair of films together. During a mean follow-up of 44 ± 10 months after the second arteriogram, cardiac death occurred in 19 patients (6%), cardiac death or nonfatal AMI occurred in 40 patients (12%), and 90 patients (27%) underwent CABG. Of the 19 cardiac deaths, 16 were in patients who demonstrated progression of their CAD, a relative risk of 7.3. The relative risk of cardiac death or nonfatal AMI for those with progression of coronary disease was 2.3 and of any cardiac event 1.7. A stepwise multivariate Cox regression model of time to event was used to assess the relative contribution of progression as a predictor of coronary events. Low LVEF, progression of lesion severity, and hypertension were identified as predictors of cardiac death. Angina and the number of diseased vessels were the strongest predictors

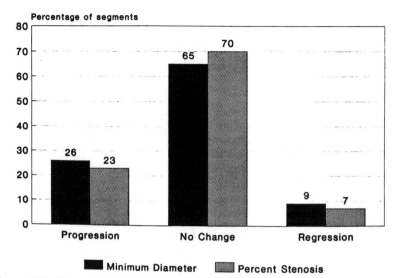

Figure 2-2. Natural history of coronary obstructions as expressed by minimal diameter and percent stenosis over 3.0 ± 0.6 year (n = 74 atherosclerotic obstructions). Reproduced with permission from Stone et al.[7]

of future revascularization. Thus, coronary progression is a strong, independent predictor of future coronary events, especially cardiac death (Figure 2-3).

The International Nifedipine Trial on Antiatherosclerotic Therapy (INTACT) provided the database for this study. Jost and associates,[9] from Rotterdam, The Netherlands, and Hannover, Germany, prospectively analyzed the quantitative association of progression of CAD with anatomic site and diameter. Data from 348 patients were evaluated 3 years apart and analyzed quantitatively. Results showed that decreases in the minimal diameter of preexisting stenoses were largest in segments that were greater than 3 mm in diameter. Similarly these changes were greater in a proximal position and in the right coronary artery as compared to a distal position. The number of new stenoses per segment was lowest in segments that were less than 2 mm in diameter and in a distal position, and was highest in segments of the right coronary artery. Thus, they concluded that progression of CAD occurs most frequently in coronary segments that are greater than 2 mm in diameter in a proximal or mid-artery position and in the right coronary artery. One limitation of the study is that only patients with moderate CAD were initially included in this trial. Therefore overall progression of CAD may be underestimated in this group of patients.

Relation of Coronary Diameter to Body Surface Area

Coronary artery dilation has been described as an early effect of atherosclerosis. No noninvasive technique has been available to measure coro-

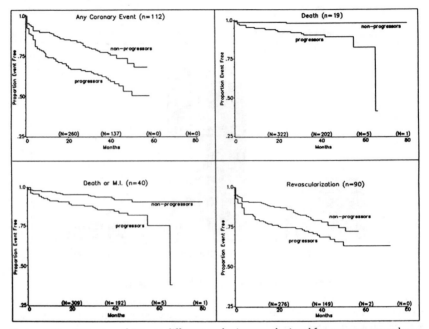

Figure 2-3. Estimates of time to different endpoints are depicted for progressors and non-progressors. For any coronary event (upper left), cardiac death (upper right), and the combined endpoint of cardiac death or nonfatal myocardial infarction (MI) (bottom left), the differences between groups are highly significant (p < 0.001). For revascularization (bottom right), the difference is less marked but still statistically significant (p = 0.014). Reproduced with permission from Waters et al.[8]

nary size. In this study by Guerra and associates,[10] from Miami Beach, Fla, coronary diameters were measured in 100 asymptomatic individuals (89 men and 11 women; mean age, 40 ± 6 years) by means of ultrafast computed tomography with 3 mm thick electrocardiographic gated scans. Individuals without evidence of coronary calcium were studied. The diameter of the LM and right coronary arteries were measured. Total coronary diameter was determined, and univariate analysis was performed with respect to total, HDL, and LDL cholesterol; mean BP; age; body surface area; and triglycerides. Mean LM was 4.23 ± 0.85 mm and mean right coronary artery was 3.06 ± 1.08 mm. Total coronary diameter increased with body surface area. No other variable showed any significant effect on total coronary diameter in this group without evidence of atherosclerosis.

Dilating Capacity in Runners

Haskell and associates,[11] from Stanford, Calif, studied 11 male volunteers who had participated in ultradistance running during the past 2 years and 11 physically inactive men referred for arteriography but without visible CAD to determine whether ultradistance running alters coronary artery size and dilating capacity in humans. The subjects were aged 39 to

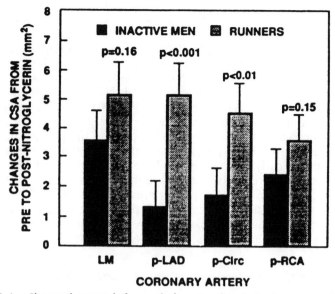

Figure 2-4. Changes between before and after nitroglycerin in the cross-sectional area (CSA) (mm²) for the left main (LM) and proximal left anterior descending (p-LAD), circumflex (p-Circ), and right (p-RCA) coronary arteries in physically inactive men and ultradistance runners are shown. Reproduced with permission from Haskell et al.[11]

66 years. The internal diameter of the proximal segments of each major epicardial coronary artery was measured before and after nitroglycerin administration using a computer-based quantitative arteriographic analysis system. Before nitroglycerin, the sum of the cross-sectional areas for the proximal right, LAD, and circumflex arteries was not different for the runners and inactive men. However, the increase in the sum of the cross-sectional areas for the proximal right, LAD, and circumflex arteries in response to nitroglycerin was greater for the runners (Figure 2-4). LV mass index, but not LV mass, was significantly greater for the runners. Among the runners, dilating capacity was positively correlated with aerobic capacity and negatively related to adiposity, resting heart rate, and plasma lipoprotein concentrations. Thus, well-trained, middle-aged endurance runners demonstrate significantly greater dilating capacity of their epicardial coronary arteries in response to nitroglycerin as compared to inactive men.

Compensatory Dilatation

Necropsy examinations and epicardial ultrasound studies have suggested that atherosclerotic coronary arteries undergo compensatory enlargement. This increase in vessel size may be an important mechanism for maintaining myocardial blood flow. It also is of fundamental importance in the angiographic study of coronary disease progression and regression. Hermiller and associates,[12] from Durham, NC, designed a study to determine, using intracoronary ultrasound, whether coronary arteries undergo adaptive expansion in vivo. Forty-four consecutive patients were studied and 80 intravascular ultrasound images were analyzed. Internal elastic laminal area, a measure of overall vessel size, increased as plaque area expanded. When the left main, LAD, and right coronary arteries were examined individually, there continued to be as great or greater positive correlation between internal elastic lamina and plaque area, implying that each of the vessels and all in aggregate underwent adaptive enlargement. When only those vessels with <30% area stenosis were examined, internal elastic lamina correlated well with plaque area, and for each 1 mm^2 increase in plaque area, internal elastic lamina increased 2.7 mm^2. This suggests that arterial enlargement may overcompensate for early atherosclerotic lesions. As a result, there was no relation between percent area stenosis and lumen area for <30% stenosis, but with greater stenoses, lumen area significantly declined. These human in vivo results validate the hypothesis that individual coronary arteries undergo adaptive enlargement that maintains or augments lumen area during the early stages of atherosclerosis.

Coronary Arterial Ectasia in Abdominal Aortic Disease

Coronary artery ectasia is the saccular or fusiform dilatation of a coronary artery. Coronary artery ectasia is found in 1.2% to 4.9% of patients at autopsy or during angiographic studies, with a similar prevalence of coronary artery ectasia found in patients with atherosclerotic peripheral vascular disease. Abdominal aortic aneurysm and coronary artery ectasia are similar in pathogenesis and histology. In an investigation by Stajduhar and associates,[13] from Tacoma, Wash, and Washington, DC, to determine whether coronary artery ectasia occurs more frequently in patients with abdominal aortic aneurysm than in occlusive forms of atherosclerotic peripheral vascular disease, examination of coronary angiograms was performed in patients who underwent cardiac catheterization and vascular reconstruction for abdominal aortic aneurysm or occlusive atherosclerotic peripheral vascular disease of the lower extremities. Of 72 patients with abdominal aortic aneurysm, 15 had coronary artery ectasia (21%) compared with only 2 of 69 patients with atherosclerotic peripheral vascular disease (3%). Coronary artery ectasia was predominantly discrete, located in the left coronary system, and associated with significant coronary atherosclerosis. Coronary artery ectasia may be more prevalent in patients with abdominal aortic aneurysm resulting from a similar pathogenetic process.

Effects of Mental Stress

Jiang and associates,[14] from Durham, NC, studied 46 patients with documented CAD to examine the relation of cardiovascular reactivity to mental stress and cardiac vagal activity. Cardiac vagal activity was measured by means of frequency-domain analysis of heart rate variability with 48-hour out-of-hospital Holter monitoring. The amplitude of the high frequency component of heart rate variability is considered to be an index of cardiac vagal activity. Cardiovascular reactivity was measured in the laboratory during a three-minute public speaking task. Results revealed (1) that the amplitude of the high-frequency component was significantly higher during sleep than during waking and (2) that compared to subjects with low diastolic BP reactivity, those who displayed high diastolic BP reactivity exhibited a significantly lower amplitude of the high-frequency component. These results indicate that decreased cardiac vagal activity may contribute to the exaggerated diastolic BP reactivity to mental stress in patients with CAD.

To determine the effects of anger on coronary vasoconstriction, Boltwood and associates,[15] from Stanford, Calif, studied 12 patients with symptomatic myocardial ischemia during cardiac catheterization. During catheterization, the patients were asked to recall a recent event that had produced anger. One narrowed and two non-narrowed arterial segments were selected using predetermined criteria. Patients also completed various self-report measurements upon entering the catheterization laboratory before any procedures, after completion of the clinical angiogram and after the anger recall stressor. There was a significant increase in subject reports of anger and arousal during the anger stressor. There were no significant changes in heart rate, systolic or diastolic BP, or heart rate × systolic BP product during the anger stressor. A total of 27 arterial segments (9 narrowed and 18 non-narrowed) were selected and analyzed using quantitative angiographic techniques. Repeated-measures analysis of variance found no significant group differences with regard to changes in arterial diameter between conditions or among segments. Reported anger was significantly correlated with a decrease in both mean and minimal diameter changes in narrowed arteries. Vasoconstriction only occurred with high levels of anger. There were no significant correlations between anger report and diameter change in non-narrowed arteries. Thus, anger may produce coronary vasoconstriction in previously narrowed coronary arteries.

Depression and Ventricular Tachycardia

Carney and associates,[16] from St. Louis, Mo, studied 103 patients who were found to have significant CAD by coronary angiography. The patients were given a standardized psychiatric interview plus 24-hour Holter monitoring to determine if depressed patients with CAD had a higher prevalence of VT than nondepressed patients with CAD. Twenty-one patients (20%) met the criteria for either major or minor depression. There were no significant differences between depressed and nondepressed patients with CAD in severity of CAD or in ventricular function. Five (23.8%) of the depressed patients and 3 (3.7%) of the non-depressed patients had episodes of VT during 24 hours of Holter monitoring. This difference remained significant even after controlling for relevant covariates. These authors concluded that there is a higher prevalence of VT among patients with CAD and depression than among those CAD patients without depression.

Exercise-Induced QRS Prolongation

Michaelides and associates,[17] from Columbus, Ohio, investigated the effect of myocardial ischemia on the QRS duration in patients with CAD, because acute myocardial ischemia decreases conduction velocity through the ischemic myocardium and may produce QRS prolongation on the surface electrocardiogram. One hundred fifty patients who underwent cardiac catheterization and exercise radionuclide ventriculography within 1 month of each other were studied. Forty patients had normal coronary arteries and 110 had CAD. QRS duration decreased with exercise in patients with normal coronary arteries (−3.0 msec), but increased in patients with CAD; exercise-induced QRS prolongation was directly related to the number of diseased vessels (4.8, 7.8, and 13 ms in patients with one-, two-, and three-vessel CAD, respectively). Likewise, QRS duration decreased with exercise in patients without exercise-induced segmental contraction abnormalities (−1.8 msec) but increased in patients with segmental contraction abnormalities (6.7, 14, and 21 ms in patients with one-, two-, and three-segmental contraction abnormalities, respectively). Exercise-induced QRS prolongation was better related to the number of segmental contraction abnormalities than to the number of diseased vessels. It was concluded that exercise produces QRS prolongation in patients with CAD in direct relation to the number of diseased vessels and to exercise-induced segmental contraction abnormalities. This QRS prolongation was more closely related to the number of exercise-induced segmental contraction abnormalities than to the number of diseased vessels. Thus, exercise-induced QRS prolongation in patients with CAD may be a marker of exercise-induced myocardial ischemia.

Effects of Weight Lifting

Featherstone and associates,[18] from Davis, Calif, assessed the safety of and physiologic responses to maximal repetition, dynamic, resistive weight lifting at 40%, 60%, 80%, and 100% of maximal voluntary contraction compared with aerobic exercise using a maximal treadmill exercise test. Twelve men with CAD exercised to fatigue at four stations (overhead press, biceps curl, quadriceps extension, and supine press). The electrocardiogram was monitored continuously. Heart rate and systolic and diastolic BP were measured at rest and during peak exercise. No symptoms or electrocardiographic evidence of ischemia occurred with weight lifting, but 5 of 12 patients had ischemic ST-segment depression with the treadmill. No significant ectopy occurred with either activity. Mean peak heart rates with all lifts were less than with the treadmill. Peak systolic BP was similar, but peak diastolic BP was greater with all lifts, except 100% maximal contraction biceps curl and quadriceps extension, than with the treadmill. Peak rate BP product was greater with the treadmill than with all lifts. Diastolic time interval from the electrocardiograph was shorter with the treadmill than with all lifts. Diastolic pressure-time index was greater with all lifts than with the treadmill. The ratio of the diastolic pressure-time index to rate pressure product, an indirect estimate of the balance between myocardial oxygen supply and demand, was greater for all lifts than for the treadmill. Thus, estimated myocardial oxygen supply-to-demand balance appears more favorable with maximal repetition weight lifting than with maximal treadmill exercise.

Endothelium-Dependent Dilation

Collins and associates,[19] from London, England, studied the responses of normal human coronary arteries in seven patients (six women and one man; mean age, 51 ± 11 years) to acetylcholine, an endothelium-dependent vasodilator and isosorbide dinitrate, an endothelium-independent vasodilator, before and after the administration of reduced free human hemoglobin. Hemoglobin 10^{-5} M infusion had no effect on coronary artery diameter. Acetylcholine and isosorbide dinitrate were infused into the coronary artery and diameter changes were assessed by quantitative angiography. Acetylcholine (10^{-7} M) increased LAD diameter. Hemoglobin, at concentrations of 10^{-6} M and 10^{-5} M, reversed the vasodilator effect causing constriction of the coronary artery. Isosorbide dinitrate in the presence of hemoglobin caused dilatation of the coronary artery in all cases. Therefore, reduced free hemoglobin is an inhibitor of acetylcholine's vasodilator effects, presumably as a result of hemoglobin's inhibition of nitric oxide (Figure 2-5).

Low doses of acetylcholine induce "endothelium-dependent" dilatation in normal coronary arteries and constriction of diseased vessels. Arbustini and associates,[20] from Pavia, Italy, investigated morphologic changes induced by perfusion of normal and diseased coronary arteries with low and high doses of acetylcholine. Vessels were excised from a series of beating hearts explanted at transplantation for idiopathic dilated cardiomyopathy and CAD. Coronary arteries from other explanted hearts, perfused with saline solution under similar conditions were taken as controls. Samples were studied using conventional histopathologic and immunohistochemical methods. Coronary arteries were grouped according to presence or absence of histologically detectable structural modifications of any type and extent. Low doses of acetylcholine induced changes in all but one structurally diseased coronary artery, whereas no change was induced in any but one histologically normal coronary artery. High doses of acetylcholine induced contraction changes in both normal and diseased vessels. Changes observed in the

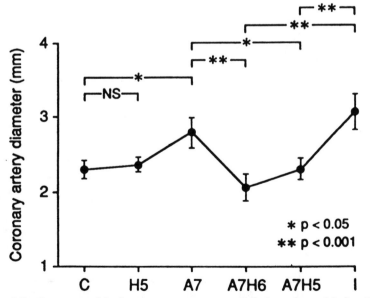

Figure 2-5. Responses of the human coronary artery to infusions of acetylcholine (A) in concentrations of 10^{-7} M and two concentrations of hemoglobin: 10^{-6} M and 10^{-5} M infused with acetylcholine. After the infusions, marked dilation is induced by isosorbide dinitrate (I). Hemoglobin infusion prevented the vasodilator effect of acetylcholine as shown in the figure. Reproduced with permission from Collins et al.[19]

wall of the contracted vessels were (1) endothelial cell contraction with protruding nuclei and detachment of their intercellular junctions with exposure of subjacent collagen to flow, (2) contraction of plaque smooth muscle cells, and (3) formation of cushions protruding into vessel lumens causing blunt microchannels. Contraction in both intimal and plaque cells occurred even in diseased vessel segments with intimal denudation. These effects seemed to be dose-dependent in structurally normal vessels because low doses of acetylcholine did not produce any morphologically detectable changes in histologically normal coronary arteries, and low doses of acetylcholine induced similar reactions in vessels affected by both atherosclerosis and subintimal fibrocellular thickening.

Egashira and associates,[21] from Fukuoka, Japan, determined if endothelium-dependent dilation of the coronary arteries was altered with aging in 18 patients, aged 23 to 70 years, with atypical chest pain with angiographically normal coronary arteries and no obvious risk factors for CAD. An endothelium-dependent vasodilator, acetylcholine (1, 3, 10, and 30 µg/min) and an endothelium-independent vasodilator, papaverine (10 mg), were injected into the left coronary artery. The large coronary diameter was assessed by arteriography, and the increase in coronary blood flow was measured using the intracoronary Doppler catheter technique. Acetylcholine increased coronary blood flow in a dose-dependent manner with no changes in arterial pressure and heart rate. The maximum increase in coronary blood flow produced by acetylcholine varied among patients, but it was highly correlated with aging (Figure 2-6). The percent increase in blood flow response to acetylcholine to the response to papaverine also correlated with aging. The slope of the

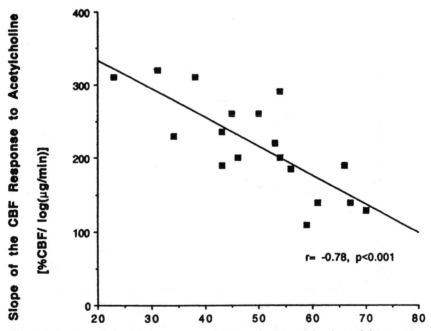

Figure 2-6. The relationship between age (horizontal axis) and the slope of the coronary blood flow response to acetylcholine (vertical axis). Reproduced with permission from Egashira et al.[21]

coronary blood flow response to acetylcholine correlated significantly with aging. The results of this study demonstrate that endothelium-dependent dilation of coronary arteries associated with acetylcholine administration is decreased with aging in humans.

Nitric Oxide Synthesis

Lefroy and associates,[22] from London, England, used N^G-monomethyl-L-arginine (L-NMMA), an inhibitor of nitric oxide synthesis, to determine the effects of inhibition of nitric oxide synthesis in the human coronary circulation. Twelve patients (mean age, 52 ± 2 years) with normal epicardial coronary arteries were studied. The ECG, systemic BP, and coronary venous oxygen saturation, an index of coronary blood flow, were monitored continuously. Coronary artery diameter was measured by quantitative arteriography. L-NMMA was given as intracoronary infusions at 2 Ml/min through a diagnostic arteriography catheter. In two patients, low doses of L-NMMA were infused into a nondominant right coronary artery. There was no evidence of ischemia in these patients who were not included in the final analysis. In the remaining ten patients, higher doses of L-NMMA (4, 10, and 25 µmol/min, each for five minutes) were infused into the left coronary artery. In six patients, incremental doses of acetylcholine were infused at 1, 10, and 100 µmol/min, each for three minutes before and after the L-NMMA infusion. Sodium nitroprusside, a nitric oxide donor, was infused at the end of the study. No patient developed myocardial ischemia. Heart rate and systemic BP remained unchanged throughout the infusions. L-NMMA at 25 µmol/min compared with the control saline infusion caused a significant reduction in distal but not proximal LAD diameter and a fall in coronary venous oxygen saturation. Sodium nitroprusside dilated the proximal and distal LAD and increased the coronary venous oxygen saturation. Acetylcholine caused significant dilatation of the distal but not proximal LAD and a significant increase in coronary venous oxygen saturation. After L-NMMA, acetylcholine-induced dilatation of the distal LAD was abolished (Figure 2–7). Therefore, inhibition of nitric oxide synthesis in human coronary circulation causes a decrease in basal distal LAD diameter and basal coronary blood flow indicating that there is a small basal release of nitric oxide in the distal epicardial coronary arteries and resistive vessels. Distal epicardial coronary artery dilatation in response to acetylcholine is nitric oxide dependent, but coronary resistive vessel dilatation does not appear to be nitric oxide dependent.

Chlamydia Pneumoniae

Linnanmäki and associates,[23] from Helsinki, Finland, investigated whether Chlamydia pneumoniae species-specific immune complexes are present in patients with chronic CAD. The presence of Chlamydia-specific circulating immune complexes was studied in 46 patients with chronic CAD and in control subjects. Chlamydial lipopolysaccharide-containing immune complexes were detected with the antigen-specific capture method, and they were present in 41% of patients and 15% of control subjects. The presence of C. pneumoniae antibodies in circulating immune complexes was studied by testing the specificity of antibodies derived from isolated and dissociated immune complexes by micro-

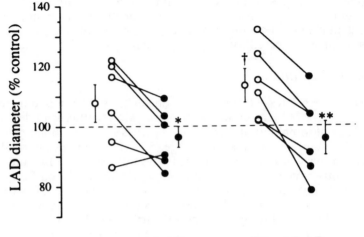

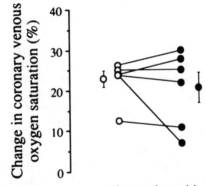

Figure 2-7. The effects of intracoronary infusion of acetylcholine (100 nmol/min) on proximal and distal LAD coronary artery diameters and coronary venous oxygen saturation before (O) and after (•) LNMMA infusion in six patients. Individual patient responses are shown with a mean ± SEM. †P < 0.05 compared with control saline infusion. *P < 0.05, **P < 0.01 compared with before LNMMA infusion. Reproduced with permission from Lefroy et al.[22]

immunofluorescence testing and immunoblotting. The C. pneumoniae indexes based on the relative amount of immune complex-derived antibodies and free antibodies were significantly higher among patients compared with control subjects. Immune complex bound antibodies showed specificity for 98-kd and 42-kd proteins of C. pneumoniae. Therefore, these results suggest that many patients with chronic CAD have a chronic C. pneumoniae infection in which chlamydial components have easy access to the circulation to form immune complexes with preexisting antibodies. These findings provide evidence for associated chronic C. pneumoniae infection in patients with CAD.

Sealing Arterial Puncture Sites

Arterial bleeding after cardiac catheterization sometimes prolongs hospital stay. Smaller catheters have helped to alleviate this problem somewhat. To shorten compression time further, a biodegradable collagen plug was developed that enhances the formation of fibrin and the subsequent formation of a clot at the puncture site immediately after a diagnostic or interventional procedure. Ernst and associates,[24] from Nieuwegein, The Netherlands, reported an international registry using this device. Two hundred fifty-two patients admitted for routine coronary angiography or PTCA to four large hospitals received this device immediately after the procedure. Hemostasis was achieved with the collagen plug in 87% of patients after a mean compression time of 4.8 minutes. The time to hemostasis was independent of the heparin load. A total of 54 hematomas (21%) were reported and all but 2 resolved without additional treatment. Two patients had a severe hematoma requiring blood transfusion, and two patients required surgery to repair a pseudoaneurysm. No severe late complications were noted during a 4 week follow-up. These authors concluded that a collagen plug appears to be a safe device to achieve hemostasis at an arterial puncture site, independent of anticoagulation. This device looks promising, although a controlled study will be required to assess its safety and efficacy.

DETECTION

By Family History

It has been suggested that a family history positive for CAD increases the risk of CAD. Castro-Beiras and associates,[25] from La Coruña, Spain, studied this association to determine the degree of risk, the independence of this association, and the presence of interaction of a family history of CAD with the major known risk factors in a low incidence area. One hundred and six hospital cases (85 men and 21 women) of CAD and 106 hospital controls individually matched with each case for sex, age, and place of residence (rural-urban) were studied. From every participant, information was collected on personal and family history of cardiovascular disease and risk factors; height, weight, lipid profile, and BP were measured, and an electrocardiogram was recorded. Conditional logistic regression was used in the analysis. The observed odds ratio of patients suffering from CAD among those with, compared to those without, a positive family history of CAD was 4.95 after adjusting for the major known risk factors in each individual and their families (no interaction term remained in the model). The results support the hypothesis that a family history of CAD, acting through mechanisms other than known risk factors or their familial aggregation, is an independent risk factor for CAD even in a low incidence area. No interaction effect was observed between family history and the presence of the three major risk factors of CAD. This finding should help to identify individuals at greater risk of CAD.

By Low Levels of High-Density Lipoprotein

French and associates,[26] from Auckland, New Zealand, compared the prevalence of risk factors for atherosclerosis in 488 consecutive patients undergoing cardiac catheterization for the investigation of chest pain with that in 868 subjects from a population sample. The presence and severity of angiographic CAD (defined as mean diameter stenosis >50%), total and HDL cholesterol, triglycerides, history of systemic hypertension, smoking, diabetes mellitus, family history, and drug therapy were assessed. Low HDL cholesterol (<0.9 mmol/L [35 mg/dL]) was more prevalent in patients with CAD than in the population sample in both men and women. There were no differences in total cholesterol levels between these two groups. Total/HDL cholesterol ratios were significantly greater in patients with CAD. History of systemic hypertension was more prevalent in both men and women with CAD than in the population sample. The prevalence of other risk factors was not significantly different between the two groups. In patients with CAD, the severity of disease was inversely correlated with levels of HDL cholesterol in both men and women, and positively correlated with total cholesterol in men aged <55 years. Low HDL cholesterol was more frequent when total cholesterol was ≤5.2 mmol/L (200 mg/dL) than when it was >5.2 mmol/L (200 mg/dL). Men and women with angiographic CAD are more likely to have low HDL cholesterol levels and history of hypertension than is an age-matched population sample.

By Aortic Plaque

Fazio and associates,[27] from San Francisco, Calif, tested the hypothesis that atherosclerotic plaque in the thoracic aorta detected by transesophageal echocardiography might be a marker for CAD. Sixty-one patients who had previously undergone coronary angiography underwent transesophageal echocardiography. The indications for angiography were angina in 26, valvular heart disease in 17, a positive noninvasive evaluation for ischemia without angina in 6, post-AMI in 5, familial hypercholesterolemia in 4, coronary cameral fistula in 1, atrial myxoma in 1, and suspected aortic dissection in 1. Forty-one of the 61 patients had obstructive CAD with at least >70% stenosis in one artery. In 37 of the 41 patients, atherosclerotic plaque was detected in the thoracic aorta. Twenty of the 61 patients had normal coronary angiography. In 2 of these 20 patients, plaque was detected by transesophageal echocardiography in the thoracic aorta. In this small series, therefore, the presence of aortic plaque on transesophageal echocardiography had a sensitivity of 90% and a specificity of 90% in angiographically proved obstructive CAD. A positive predictive value of aortic plaque for obstructive CAD was 95%, and the negative predictive value was 82%.

By Peripheral Atherosclerosis

Because the excess mortality rate associated with an ankle-brachial BP index (ABPI) <0.9 was only partly explained by an excess cardiovascular mortality, Ögren and associates,[28] from Malmö, Sweden, investigated 439 men, aged 68 years, who were part of a prospective population study in Malmö, Sweden, and performed an examination on each of them that included ABPI, carotid-artery ultrasonography, and 24-hour ambulatory electrocardiographic monitoring. Cause-specific mortality and incidence of AMI during 8 years of follow-up was compared with men with and without signs of arteriosclerotic disease. Of 60 men with an ABPI of 0.9, twenty (33%) had angina pectoris or previous AMI; 11 (18%) had silent ST-segment depression (≥1 mm); 3 (5%) had a history of stroke; and 17 (28%) had symptom-free carotid stenosis (>30% reduction of the cross-sectional diameter). Total mortality rate in men with no signs of arteriosclerotic disease was 19.6 per 1000 person-years and cardiac event rate (fatal and nonfatal AMI and death from chronic CAD 2.1; 1.2 to 3.9, respectively), whereas no independent association with total mortality was found.

After Major Vascular Surgery

Major vascular surgery is associated with a high incidence of cardiac ischemic complications. By means of continuous perioperative electrocardiographic recording, Landesberg and associates,[29] from Jerusalem, Israel, studied 151 consecutive patients undergoing major vascular surgery to find out the characteristics of any myocardial ischemia and the relation to outcome. Thirteen patients had postoperative cardiac events (six AMIs, two unstable angina, and five CHF). There were 342 perioperative ischemic episodes shown by ST-segment depression; 164 (48%) occurred postoperatively. Postoperative ischemic episodes were significantly longer than episodes before or during operations (3.2 v 1.7 and 1.5 min/hour monitored). Both Detsky's cardiac risk index and long-duration (>2 hour) preoperative ischemia were predictive of postoperative cardiac complications. However, long-duration ST-segment depression preceded most (84.6%) postoperative cardiac events, including AMIs, and no cardiac event was preceded by ST-segment elevation. Five of the six postoperative AMIs were non-Q-wave infarctions. These authors concluded that long-duration subendocardial ischemia, rather than acute coronary artery occlusion, may bring about postoperative myocardial injury and complications.

The relative prognostic value of widely accessible resting two-dimensional echocardiographic ventricular function data has not been compared with recognized clinical and scintigraphic risk markers in patients who are unable to exercise before major nonvascular surgery. In this report by Takase and associates,[30] from St. Louis, Mo, 53 consecutive patients, aged 67 ± 13 years, undergoing preoperative evaluation (intra-abdominal 23%, orthopedic 30%, thoracic 9%, and other 38%) for known or suspected CAD were followed up to evaluate the prognostic value of these studies for the perioperative cardiac events (cardiac death [n = 4], myocardial infarction [n = 2], unstable angina [n = 3], and pulmonary edema [n = 8]) that occurred in 13 of the 53 patients (25%). Dipyridamole thallium-201 myocardial redistribution defects occurred in 15 patients (28%). Resting echocardiographic LV dysfunction was present in 21 patients (40%). Multivariate analysis of clinical, echocardiographic, and scintigraphic risk predictors revealed that cardiac events were not predicted by clinical variables, including Goldman class or score. Cardiac events were independently predicted only by the presence of significant LV dysfunction on resting two-dimensional echocardiography and dipyridamole thallium-201 defect redistribution. A dipyridamole-induced reversible thallium-201 perfusion defect was predictive of subsequent cardiac death or myocardial infarction, whereas LV dysfunction on resting echocardiography was predictive of perioperative pulmonary edema. It was concluded that stress thallium-201 perfusion imaging and resting two-dimensional echocardiography provide independent prognostic information in patients undergoing major nonvascular surgery who are at significant risk for ischemic cardiac events and who are unable to perform standard exercise stress tests. Clinical risk indexes were not predictive of cardiac events in these patients when analyzed in combination with noninvasive risk assessment.

By Occult Pseudoxanthoma Elasticum

Pseudoxanthoma elasticum is an inherited disorder of connective tissue that is associated with numerous systemic manifestations, including premature CAD. The typical patient presents with yellow macules or papules that can become confluent to form plaques and, in severe cases, redundant folds of skin. Cutaneous lesions have been likened to "plucked chickens skin." In patients whose skin is mildly affected, the condition may be difficult to recognize. Ocular complications occasionally occur without the characteristic skin lesions. Lebwohl and associates,[31] from New York, described four patients, aged 27, 32, 39, and 59 years, who presented with premature cardiovascular disease and were found to have angioid streaks and histologic evidence of pseudoxanthoma elasticum, despite the absence of characteristic skin lesions. The authors suggested that a diagnosis of pseudoxanthoma elasticum be considered in any patient presenting with signs of accelerated atherosclerosis at an early age in the absence of known risk factors. Additionally, the authors suggested that arterial grafts should not be used for CABG in patients with pseudoxanthoma elasticum because of possible calcific deposits in the internal elastic laminae.

Electrocardiogram

Gorgels and associates,[32] from Maastricht, The Netherlands, studied the value of the electrocardiogram recorded during chest pain for identifying high-risk patients with three-vessel or left main stem CAD. The number of leads with abnormal ST segments, the amount of ST-segment deviation, and specific combinations of leads with abnormal ST segments were correlated with the number of coronary arteries with proximal narrowing of >70%. Electrocardiograms recorded during chest pain were compared with one from a symptom free episode. In this retrospective analysis, 113 consecutive patients were included. One-vessel CAD was present in 47 patients, two-vessel CAD in 22, three-vessel CAD in 24, and left main CAD in 20. Stratification was performed according to the presence of an old myocardial infarction. The number of leads with ST-segment deviations and the amount of ST-segment deviation in the electrocardiogram obtained during chest pain at rest showed a positive correlation with the number of diseased coronary arteries. These findings were more marked when the absolute shifts from baseline were considered, because ST-segment abnormalities could be present also in the electrocardiogram obtained during the symptom free episode. Left main and three-vessel CAD showed a frequent combination of leads with abnormal ST segments: ST-segment depression in leads I, II, and V_4-V_6, and ST-segment elevation in lead aVR. The negative predictive and positive accuracy of this pattern were 78% and 62%, respectively. When the total amount of ST-segment changes was >12 mm, the positive predictive accuracy for three-vessel or left main stem CAD increased to 86%. The findings show that the electrocardiogram during chest pain at rest is of great value in diagnosing the number of diseased coronary arteries in patients with rest angina.

To determine which computer ST criteria are superior for predicting patterns and severity of CAD during exercise testing, Ribisl and associates,[33] from Long Beach, Calif, studied 230 male veterans who had both coronary angiography and a treadmill exercise test. Significant differences in computer-scored ST criteria were observed among patients with progressively increasing disease severity. Three-vessel/left main CAD produced responses significantly different from one- and two-vessel disease or those with <70% occlusion. Discriminant function analysis revealed that horizontal or downsloping ST depression measured at the J junction during exercise or recovery, or both, was the most powerful predictor of severe disease. With use of a cut point of 0.075 mV ST depression, horizontal, or downsloping ST depression alone yielded a sensitivity of 50% and specificity of 71% for prediction of severe disease; the only additional variable that added significantly to the prediction was exercise capacity, which improved sensitivity to 57% with no change in specificity. Measurements of ST amplitude at the J junction and at 60 ms after the J point without slope considered and other scores, including the Treadmill Exercise Score, ST Integral, and ST/heart rate index, had a lower but comparable predictive accuracy when compared with horizontal or downsloping ST depression. Prediction of CAD severity can be achieved using computerized electrocardiographic measurements obtained during exercise testing. The most powerful marker for severe CAD is the amount of horizontal or downsloping ST-segment depression during exercise or recovery, or both, a measurement that simulates the traditional visual approach.

Gallik and associates,[34] from Houston, Tex, studied 12 patients with exercise-induced ST-segment elevation without prior AMI, electrocardiographic evidence of LV hypertrophy, or LBBB who underwent thallium-201 tomography immediately after exercise and four hours later. Coronary angiography and left ventriculography were performed within an average of eight days of exercise testing. Five patients had repeat exercise thallium-201 tomography after medical therapy or revascularization. All patients had large, reversible perfusion defects (average defect size, 34%), with 11 of 12 patients having a ≥25% stress perfusion defect. In 10 patients with atherosclerotic CAD, the average stenosis of the involved vessel was 93%. The electrocardiographic leads with ST-segment elevation predicted the site of reversible hypoperfusion. Two patients had extensive, reversible anterior hypoperfusion due to exercise-induced spasm of minimally stenosed LAD coronary arteries. Follow-up exercise testing in 5 patients showed abolition of reversible hypoperfusion and ST changes after medical therapy or revascularization. In patients without prior AMI, exercise-induced ST-segment elevation signifies extensive, reversible hypoperfusion than can be abolished by revascularization in patients with critical coronary stenoses and by medical therapy in those with coronary vasospasm.

Holter Monitoring

To determine if Holter monitoring can predict cardiac risk in patients when the exercise test is nondiagnostic, Raby and associates,[35] from Boston, Mass, monitored a total of 90 eligible patients for 24 hours after their exercise test without alterations in baseline medications. Prospective follow-up was obtained, and events were confirmed by investigators unaware of subjects' clinical data. Nineteen patients (21%) had a total of 71 episodes of ST depression, all of which were asymptomatic. During a mean follow-up of 719 days, there were 10 patients with adverse events: 3 with cardiac deaths, 3 with nonfatal AMIs, and 4 with admissions for unstable angina. Of the 10 adverse events, 9 occurred in the group of 19 with ST depression detected by Holter. The sensitivity of ST depression was 90%, the specificity 88%, the predictive positive value 47%, and the predictive negative value 99%. In a multivariate Cox proportional-hazards model that controlled for prior history of CAD, hypercholesterolemia, and all exercise test variables, the presence of ST depression detected by Holter was the only independent predictor of outcome. In patients with nondiagnostic exercise tests, ST depression detected by Holter monitoring identified those with an increased risk of adverse cardiac events. The absence of ST depression detected by Holter was a useful predictor of low risk.

Coronary Angiography

To determine the appropriateness of coronary angiography in New York State, Bernstein and associates,[36] from multiple US medical centers, studied a random sample of 1,335 patients undergoing coronary angiography in New York State in 1990 at 15 randomly selected hospitals. Approximately 76% of coronary angiographys were rated appropriate; 20% were rated uncertain; and 4% were rated inappropriate. Inappropriate use did not vary significantly between the elderly (ie, patients aged ≥65 years) and nonelderly, 4.7% and 3.9%, respectively. Although the rate of inappropriate use varied from 0% to 9% among hospitals, the difference was not significant. Rates of appropriateness did not vary by hospital location (upstate v downstate), volume (fewer than 750 procedures annually or at least 750 procedures annually), teaching status, or whether revascularization was available at the hospital where angiography was performed. Although coronary angiography was used for few inappropriate indications in New York State, many procedures were performed for uncertain indications in which the benefit and risk were approximately equal or unknown.

Dobutamine Stress Echocardiography

Poldermans and associates,[37] from Rotterdam, The Netherlands, determined the predictive value of dobutamine stress echocardiography for perioperative cardiac events in patients scheduled for elective major noncardiac vascular surgery. Patients unable to exercise had a dobutamine stress test before surgery. One hundred thirty-six patients (mean age, 68 years) received incremental dobutamine infusions from 10 to 40 μg/kg/min continued with atropine, if necessary, to achieve 85% of the age-predicted maximal HR without symptoms or signs of myocardial ischemia. Echocardiographic images were evaluated by two observers blinded to the clinical data of the patients. Technically adequate images were obtained in 134 of 136 patients. One major complication occurred, ventricular fibrillation, and three tests were discontinued because of side effects. Data from 131 patients were analyzed with univariate and multivariate analyses. The dobutamine stress test was positive with new or worsened wall motion abnormalities in 35 of 131 patients. In the postoperative period, 5 patients died of AMI, 9 patients had unstable angina, and 1 patient developed pulmonary edema. All patients with cardiac complications, 15 patients in total, had abnormal dobutamine stress tests (Table 2-2). No cardiac events occurred in patients with negative tests. Five patients with a technically inadequate or prematurely stopped test were operated on without complications. By multivariate analysis, only age >70 years and new wall motion abnormalities during the dobutamine test were significant predictors of perioperative cardiac events. Therefore, dobutamine stress echocardiography is a feasible, safe, and useful method for identifying patients at high or low risk of perioperative cardiac events. The test provides additional information beyond that provided by clinical variables for patients who are scheduled for major noncardiac vascular surgery. Some patients with abnormal wall motion responses to dobutamine did not develop cardiac events; thus, the sensitivity of the information provided in this study is high, but the specificity is less certain.

The problems of population referral bias in the calculation of specificity in diagnostic testing for CAD have been previously described. Previous studies investigating the sensitivity and specificity of dobutamine stress echocardiography have been subject to pretest and posttest referral biases, largely as a result of the requirement for coronary arteriography. This study by Bach and associates,[38] from Ann Arbor, Mich, determines the normalcy rate for dobutamine stress echocardiography by examining a population at statistically low risk for CAD. The probability of signifi-

Table 2-2. Clinical Data on Patients with Perioperative Cardiac Events. Reproduced with permission from Poldermans et al.[37]

Patient	Age (years)	Preoperative clinical data							DSE				Perioperative event	Time after surgery (days)
		HTN	DM	Smoking	AP	MI	Detsky	ECG	Med.	NWMA	CHP	ST		
1	70	−	−	+	−	+	10	Inf. MI	−	+	+	+	Fatal MI	3
2	76	−	−	−	−	+	10	Ant. MI	−	+	−	+	Fatal MI	5
3	76	−	−	+	+	+	15	Ant. MI	−	+	−	−	Fatal MI	5
4	62	+	+	−	−	−	0	Normal	+	+	−	+	Fatal MI	3
5	85	−	−	−	−	+	10	Ant. MI	−	+	−	−	Fatal MI	7
6	83	+	−	+	−	−	5	RBBB	+	+	−	+	UAP	1
7	50	+	+	−	+	+	10	LVH	+	+	+	+	UAP	1
8	72	−	+	−	+	+	25	Inf. MI	+	+	−	−	UAP	1
9	76	−	−	+	+	+	15	Inf. MI	+	+	+	+	UAP	1
10	76	−	−	+	−	−	15	Normal	−	+	−	−	UAP	1
11	73	+	−	−	+	−	15	Normal	−	+	−	−	UAP	5
12	77	+	−	−	+	−	15	Inf. MI	+	+	−	−	UAP	1
13	51	−	−	−	+	+	35	Inf. MI	+	+	+	+	UAP	2
14	72	−	−	+	+	+	25	Ant. MI	+	+	−	+	UAP	3
15	66	+	−	+	−	+	5	Normal	+	+	−	−	Pulmonary edema	2

DSE, dobutamine stress echocardiography; HTN, hypertension; DM, diabetes mellitus; AP, history of angina pectoris; MI, myocardial infarction; Detsky, Detsky's score; Med., antianginal medication; NWMA, new or worsened wall motion abnormality; CHP, chest pain during stress echo; ST, ST changes >1 mm during stress echocardiography; −, negative; +, positive; inf., inferior; ant., anterior; RBBB, right bundle branch block; LVH, left ventricular hypertrophy; UAP, unstable angina pectoris.

cant CAD was determined for 828 consecutive patients referred for dobutamine stress echocardiography and groups were identified with <10% and <5% probability of disease. Four of 72 patients (5.6%) with a normal baseline echocardiogram and a probability of CAD of <10%, and 3 of 38 patients (7.9%) with a probability of <5% were found to have an abnormal dobutamine stress echocardiogram, yielding normalcy rates of 94% and 92%, respectively. The area of abnormality involved the posterior circulation in 3 of 4 patients (75%). This study demonstrates that dobutamine stress echocardiography has a normalcy rate of 92% to 94% and is an accurate test for excluding the presence of significant CAD.

A number of stress tests have emerged using pharmacologic agents. Dobutamine stress has been combined with both echo and perfusion techniques. Marwick and associates,[39] from Brussels, Belgium, examined the efficacy of these two techniques in patients with CAD. Two hundred seventeen patients without previous infarction were studied with dobutamine stress echocardiography and technetium-99m methoxy isobutyl nitrile (sestamibi) single-photon emission computed tomography at the time of diagnostic coronary angiography. The presence of coronary stenoses of greater than 50% diameter were compared with the presence of rest or stress-induced abnormalities of perfusion and regional function. Significant CAD was found in 142 patients; 75% were identified by dobutamine echocardiography and 76% by perfusion imaging. In 75 patients without significant disease, the specificity of dobutamine echocardiography was 83% compared with 67% for scintigraphy. Echocardiographic sensitivity was lower in patients unable to complete the test because of side effects. Selective use of scintigraphy in the 31 patients with a negative submaximal stress echo led to a sensitivity of 80% for this combination. Patients with left ventricular hypertrophy accounted for most of the difference in specificity between echo and scintigraphy (94% v 59%). These authors concluded that dobutamine stress echo and perfusion scintigraphy have equivalent results. In patients with left ventricular hypertrophy, echo appears to be the test of choice. Selective use of sestamibi scintigraphy in patients with a negative submaximal echo stress test enhances the accuracy of stress echocardiography.

Mertes and associates,[40] used dobutamine stress echocardiography for the evaluation of CAD in 1,118 consecutive patients. Dobutamine stress testing was performed for evaluation of chest pain, risk assessment before noncardiac surgery, after recent AMI, or as part of ongoing research protocols. Maximal dose of dobutamine used was increased from 30 to 50 μg/kg/min and atropine was used in 420 (37%) of the patients. There were no deaths, AMIs, or episodes of sustained VT as a result of dobutamine stress testing. The major reasons for test termination were achievement of target heart rate in 52%, maximum dose given in 23%, and angina pectoris in 13%. The test was discontinued in 3% of patients because of noncardiac side effects, including nausea, anxiety, headache, tremor, and urgency. In the patients who developed angina, sublingual nitroglycerin, a short-acting β-blocker, or both types of medications relieved angina. The most common arrhythmias in response to dobutamine were frequent VPCs in 15% and frequent atrial premature complexes in 8% of the patients. Forty patients developed nonsustained VT with dobutamine administration. No patient had symptoms associated with tachycardia. This study demonstrates that dobutamine stress echocardiography is relatively safe and may be performed using supplemental atropine and a high dose dobutamine infusion. Symptomatic ischemia was effectively treated with test termination, sublingual nitroglycerin, or short-acting β-blockers.

In 66 patients with suspected CAD, exercise electrocardiography, exercise echocardiography, dobutamine stress echocardiography, single-photon emission computed tomography using methoxy-isobutyl-isonitrile and coronary angiography were performed by Hoffmann and associates,[41] from Aachen, Germany, to compare methods for detecting CAD. CAD was defined as 70% luminal area stenosis in at least one coronary artery at coronary angiography. Significant CAD was present in 50 patients. Exercise echocardiography, dobutamine stress echocardiography, and computed tomography had a significantly higher sensitivity compared with exercise electrocardiography. There were no significant differences in sensitivity between exercise echocardiography, dobutamine stress echocardiography, and computed tomography. Specificity of computed tomography was lowest (71%), whereas exercise electrocardiography, exercise echocardiography, and dobutamine echocardiography had higher specificities (93%, 87%, and 81%, respectively). Significance, however, was not achieved. Differences in overall accuracy between exercise echocardiography, dobutamine stress echocardiography, and computed tomography were not significant. Comparison with accuracy of exercise electrocardiography was significant. In one-vessel CAD, exercise electrocardiography had a lower sensitivity than exercise and dobutamine echocardiography and computed tomography. Regarding the 24 patients with false-negative exercise electrocardiography results, 67% had positive exercise echocardiographic findings, 71% positive dobutamine echocardiographic results, and 84% positive computed tomography results. Thus, exercise echocardiography and dobutamine stress echocardiography are markedly superior in sensitivity to exercise electrocardiography, especially in one-vessel CAD and represent a useful alternative to myocardial emission computed tomography.

To compare the value of dobutamine and dipyridamole stress echocardiography with exercise stress testing for the diagnosis of CAD, Previtali and associates,[42] from Pavia, Italy, studied 80 patients with chest pain of suspected myocardial ischemic origin (57 with CAD and 23 without significant CAD) who underwent dobutamine stress echocardiography, dipyridamole echocardiography, and bicycle exercise electrocardiography after discontinuation of antianginal treatment. Dobutamine echocardiography and exercise testing revealed a higher overall sensitivity than dipyridamole echocardiography (79% v 60%; 77% v 60%, respectively); this finding was due to a higher dobutamine and exercise sensitivity in one-vessel CAD, whereas sensitivity of the three tests was similar in multivessel CAD. Dobutamine and dipyridamole showed a higher specificity than exercise (83% v 43%; 96% v 43%, respectively). Diagnostic accuracy of dobutamine echocardiography was higher than that of exercise, whereas the difference with dipyridamole was not significant. In the tests that yielded positive results, double product during exercise was significantly higher than that during dobutamine and dipyridamole echocardiography. No major complications occurred during the tests, but adverse effects were more frequent during dobutamine testing. Thus, dobutamine echocardiography may be superior to dipyridamole echocardiography and exercise electrocardiography for the diagnosis of CAD.

Intravascular Ultrasonic Imaging

Intracoronary ultrasound provides a unique in vivo look at coronary artery lesions. In 65 patients, Hodgson and associates,[43] from Cleveland, Ohio, compared diagnostic ultrasound imaging with angiography to evaluate lumen, total vessel, and plaque areas and to classify plaques as soft, fibrous, calcific, mixed, or concentric subintimal thickening. Compared with patients with stable angina, patients with unstable angina had more soft lesions (74% v 41%) fewer calcified and mixed plaques (25% v 59%) and fewer intralesional calcium deposits (16% v 45%). Ultrasound was more sensitive than angiography for identifying unstable lesions (74% v 40%). The morphologic plaque calcification by ultrasound had only minimal relationship to established angiographic morphology characteristics. As more information is collected with this technique, it is possible that a knowledge of plaque composition and lumen dimension will help in selecting specific treatment strategies for individual patients and may relate to long-term clinical success with different interventions.

Hermiller and associates,[44] from Durham, NC, obtained selective, coronary arteriographic, catheter-based, intravascular ultrasound images to determine the presence and extent of angiographically undetected or underestimated LM coronary arterial narrowing in patients receiving coronary interventional therapy. Coronary arteriograms were determined to be either normal or abnormal by visual inspection. Abnormal arteriograms were digitized and quantitated using a semiautomated edge-detection algorithm. Thirty-eight patients receiving percutaneous treatment of stenoses in the left coronary artery system were studied. Optimal LM coronary angiograms were obtained in two views, and intravascular ultrasound images were obtained after the coronary interventional procedure. Intravascular ultrasound detected plaque in 24 of 27 angiographically normal LM arteries (89%), and narrowing was observed in 11 of 11 angiographically abnormal LM arteries (100%) (Figure 2-8). Of 38 patients, 8 had >40% area stenosis by intravascular ultrasound. In patients

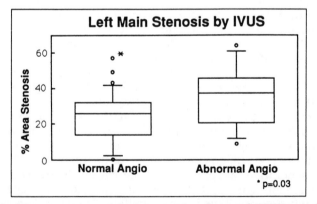

Figure 2-8. Percent area stenosis by intravascular ultrasound (IVUS) was significantly less in normal than abnormal angiographic (Angio) group. This figure depicts data in box plot. *Upper and lower edges of box* represent 75th and 25th percentiles, respectively, and *middle line*, the median. *Upper and lower bars* represent 90th and 10th percentiles, respectively, and *points* above or below 90th and 10th percentiles are plotted. Reproduced with permission from Hermiller et al.[44]

with angiographic CAD, there was no correlation between quantitative angiographic and ultrasound percent area stenosis. The median plaque area was not different between angiographically normal and abnormal patients. The median percent area stenosis in arteriographically normal subjects was less than that in abnormal ones. Unrecognized left main disease is widespread and often underestimated in patients with normal LM angiograms undergoing interventional procedures. Plaque area is similar for angiographically normal and insignificantly abnormal arteries. This study suggests that intravascular ultrasound overcomes the limitations of silhouette imaging.

This study by Dupouy and associates,[45] from Creteil, France, was performed to evaluate the accuracy of intravascular ultrasound for the assessment of coronary artery vasomotion and endothelial function in patients with atherosclerosis. Twenty patients with luminal irregularities on the coronary angiogram and a high cholesterol level (287 ± 19 mg/dL) (group 1) and six patients with angiographically smooth arteries and a minimally elevated cholesterol level (197 ± 12 mg/dL) (group 2) were studied. A 4.3 French mechanical intravascular ultrasound probe was placed into the proximal segment of the coronary artery. The ultrasound images were recorded on videotape and were then digitized allowing the measurement of the lumen area and then the calculation of a mean intimal thickness index. Endothelial function was studied during sympathetic stimulation by cold pressor test and, after increasing coronary blood flow, by intracoronary papaverine administration; a 1 mg bolus of nitrate was then administered into the coronary artery. Patients in group 1 had a higher mean intimal thickness (1.52 ± 0.64 mm) than those in group 2 (0.18 ± 0.08 mm). In response to sympathetic stimulation, a vasoconstricting effect occurred in group 1 (9.5 ± 1.3 mm^2 v 11 ± 1.2 mm^2 at baseline), and a vasodilating action was observed in the control group (12 ± 2.1 mm^2 v 10 ± 1.8 mm^2 at baseline). After papaverine infusion, a trend toward a vasoconstricting effect was observed in response to increased flow in group 1 that was not observed in group 2. Nitrate infusion induced a significant vasodilating effect in both groups. In conclusion, intravascular ultrasound may be considered a useful tool to assess endothelial function of large coronary arteries and to obtain the precise relation between wall thickness and the vasomotor response.

Thallium-201 Emission Tomography

In an investigation by Maublant and associates,[46] from Clermont-Ferrand, France, exercise thallium-201 single-photon emission computed tomography images were compared prospectively with four-hour redistribution images, with four-hour reinjection images, and with images obtained at rest on a separate day in 37 patients with documented CAD. Exercise images were abnormal in 35 patients (95%). On the basis of an improvement in thallium-201 distribution between exercise and nonexercise images, overall sensitivity for the detection of CAD was significantly higher with reinjection at four hours or with a rest injection on a separate day than with redistribution imaging (84%, 83%, and 70%, respectively). Reinjection and rest injection were positive more frequently in patients with a wall-motion abnormality (76% and 80%, respectively, v 64% at redistribution). Among the 11 patients who had no evidence of redistribution at four hours, 5 (45%) demonstrated ischemia with reinjection, and 5 demonstrated ischemia in the separate rest study; a total of 7 patients showed improvement either at reinjection or rest. Among these, 86% had a wall-motion abnormality associated with stenosis of >90%; in the other 30 patients, these two conditions were observed concomitantly in only 43%. This study demonstrates that the thallium-201 four-hour postexercise reinjection technique is as sensitive as the two-day rest/exercise method for the detection of CAD and provides additional information when severe stenosis is associated with a wall-motion abnormality.

Iskandrian and associates,[47] from Philadelphia, Pa, examined the ability of single photon emission computed tomographic imaging with thallium-201 during adenosine-induced coronary hyperemia to detect high-risk patients with LM or three-vessel CAD. There were 339 patients: 102 with either LM or three-vessel CAD (group 1) and 237 with no CAD, one-, or two-vessel disease (group 2). By means of univariate analysis, several variables were found to differ between groups 1 and 2: Q-wave myocardial infarction (35% v 25%), ST segment depression (35% v 19%), age (67 ± 9 v 62 ± 10 years), resting systolic BP (142 ± 22 v 135 ± 20 mm Hg), abnormal thallium images (95% v 74%), multivessel thallium abnormality (76% v 39%), extent of thallium abnormality (24% ± 11% v 19% ± 13%), and increased lung thallium uptake (39% v 15%). According to stepwise discriminant analysis, only three variables were predictors of high risk: multivessel thallium abnormality, increased lung thallium uptake, and ST depression. On the basis of these variables, patients were divided into three groups with different prevalence rates for LM and three-vessel CAD: 63% in 68 patients, 30% in 137 patients, and 13% in 137 patients. Thus, adenosine-thallium imaging permits stratification of patients into different risk groups; 20% of patients have a high, 40% an intermediate, and 40% a low prevalence of LM or three-vessel CAD.

Patients with left bundle branch block on the electrocardiogram frequently have artifactual reversible septal perfusion defects with exercise thallium-201 scintigraphy. O'Keefe and associates,[48] from Kansas City, Mo, evaluated adenosine thallium scintigraphy as an attractive alternative in these patients. One hundred seventy three consecutive patients with left bundle branch block were evaluated with either exercise thallium scintigraphy or adenosine thallium scintigraphy. Follow-up cardiac catheterization was performed in 31 of the 56 patients in the exercise group and 42 of the 117 patients in the adenosine thallium group. The overall predictive accuracy was 93% in the adenosine thallium group and 68% in the exercise thallium group. The specificity was 42% with exercise thallium and 82% with adenosine thallium scintigraphy. These authors concluded that adenosine thallium imaging was superior to exercise thallium imaging in the detection of CAD in patients with left bundle branch block. Adenosine thallium appears to obviate septal artifacts thereby improving the specificity in the left anterior descending and right coronary arteries. It also was safe in patients with left bundle branch block. This retrospective study would need to be more carefully evaluated in a prospective manner. It should also be noted that these studies were based on tomographic thallium imaging and may not be generalized to planar thallium scintigraphy.

To assess the prevalence and functional significance of ischemic ambulatory electrocardiographic responses, Klein and associates,[49] from New York and Los Angeles, Calif, prospectively performed ambulatory electrocardiographic monitoring in 244 patients (mean age, 61 ± 10 years) referred for stress redistribution thallium-201 myocardial perfusion scintigraphy. The prevalence of ST-segment depression during ambulatory electrocardiography was 33% among patients with positive exercise electrocardiograms, but prevalence varied in selected patient subgroups. Among three groups with CAD, the group with ambulatory electrocardiographic ischemia (group 1) had a greater frequency of ischemic thallium responses, a greater median number of reversible thallium defects, and a greater summed thallium reversibility score than did the group with positive exercise electrocardiograms but negative ambulatory electrocardiographic responses (group 2) or that with negative exercise and ambulatory electrocardiographic responses (group 3). Exercise ST depression in group 1 versus group 2 was significantly greater, occurred at a lower heart rate threshold, and lasted longer after exercise. Notably, one third of group 1 patients also manifested evidence of transient ischemic dilation of the left ventricle after exercise, a sign of severe ischemia. However, although functionally less sick than group 1 patients, 66% of group 2 patients and 50% of group 3 patients still had an ischemic thallium response, which was sometimes severe. Thus transient ischemia during ambulatory electrocardiographic monitoring identifies a functionally sicker cohort of patients with CAD and occurs in approximately one third of CAD patients with positive results of exercise tests. A negative ambulatory electrocardiographic response, however, does not exclude functionally significant disease among CAD patients. These results imply that caution should be applied in the interpretation of a negative ambulatory electrocardiographic response for the purpose of patient risk stratification.

Some patients are unable to undergo either exercise or vasodilator pharmacologic stress testing. Hays and associates,[50] from Houston, Tex, assessed the feasibility, safety, and accuracy of a high-dose dobutamine infusion in conjunction with thallium-201 computed tomography in 144 patients. Dobutamine was administered intravenously at incremental doses up to 40 µg/kg/min with increasing doses at three minute intervals. After one minute at the maximal dose, 3 mCi of thallium-201 was injected, and the infusion continued for an additional two minutes. Dobutamine significantly increased the heart rate from 75 to 120 and systolic pressure from 136 to 148. Seventy-five percent of patients experienced side effects during the infusion, but 74% tolerated a dobutamine dose of 40 µg/kg/min and 97% a dose of 30µg/kg/min. The most common side effects were chest pain, palpitation, flushing, headache, and dyspnea. The sensitivity of dobutamine tomography was 86% in patients who underwent coronary angiography; 84% on those with single vessel CAD, 82% on those with double-vessel CAD, and 100% on those with triple-vessel CAD. Seventy-eight percent of arteries with severe stenosis were identified with dobutamine tomography. The specificity was 90% for patients and 86% for individual vessels. These authors concluded that a high-dose dobutamine infusion in conjunction with thallium tomography is well tolerated and a good method for diagnosing CAD in patients who cannot exercise or undergo a vasodilator pharmacologic stress test. A limitation of this study was the need to visually assess both regional wall motion and myocardial perfusion.

Matzer and associates,[51] from Los Angeles, Calif, examined the relation between the quantitative myocardial perfusion defect severity of exercise thallium-201 single-photon emission computed tomography and the quantitative degree of coronary stenosis in 18 patients with one-vessel disease (≥50% diameter stenosis). A total of 26 vessels were analyzed. Thallium-201 quantitative defect severity score was derived by summing the number of pixels in a coronary territory in which counts fell below the normal mean and multiplied by the number of standard deviations by which they fell below the normal mean. The thallium-201 defect severity score was significantly related to the maximal percent luminal diameter narrowing, percent area narrowing, absolute stenotic area, and absolute stenotic diameter. As expected, the strongest relation between thallium-201 defect severity and quantitative angiographic indexes was in the low and high ranges of coronary stenosis, with more variability and lower correlation coefficients. This observation is likely to be due to the complex flow characteristics across stenotic lesions. The findings suggest that in a select population, thallium-201 defect severity is potentially useful for noninvasive characterization of the functional severity of coronary artery stenosis and may complement coronary angiography in predicting functionally significant stenosis.

Dilsizian and associates,[52] from Bethesda, Md, determined whether stress-redistribution-reinjection and rest-redistribution imaging provide the same information regarding myocardial viability. Both stress-redistribution-reinjection and rest-redistribution thallium single-photon emission computed tomographic imaging were performed in 41 patients with chronic stable CAD with quantitative analyses of regional thallium activity. Thallium reinjection was performed immediately after the three- to four-hour redistribution images were completed. Of the 155 myocardial regions with perfusion defects on the stress images, 91 (59%) were irreversible on conventional three- to four-hour redistribution images. When the outcomes of these irreversible regions were assessed after reinjection and compared with rest-redistribution images, there was a concordance of data regarding myocardial viability in 72 of the 91 (79%) irreversible defects. Of the 41 patients, 20 also underwent positron emission tomography at rest with [18F]fluorodeoxyglucose and [15O]water. In these patients, stress-redistribution-reinjection and rest-redistribution imaging provided concordant information regarding myocardial viability in 427 (72%) of 594 myocardial regions and discordance in 167 regions. However, when discordant regions, 149 of 167 (89%) demonstrated only mild to moderate reduction in thallium activity and positron emission tomography verified 98% of these regions to be metabolically active and viable. Therefore, when the severity of thallium activity is considered within irreversible thallium defects, the concordance between stress-redistribution-reinjection and rest-redistribution imaging regarding myocardial viability increased to 94% (Figure 2-9). These data indicate that one of two imaging modalities, either stress-redistribution-reinjection or rest-redistribution imaging may be used for identifying viable myocardium. When there is no contraindication to stress testing, stress-redistribution reinjection imaging provides a more comprehensive assessment of the extent and severity of CAD by demonstrating regional myocardial ischemia without jeopardizing information regarding myocardial viability.

Transesophageal pacing echocardiography is a new diagnostic technique that uses simultaneous graded transesophageal LA pacing and biplane transesophageal echocardiography for the detection of pacing-

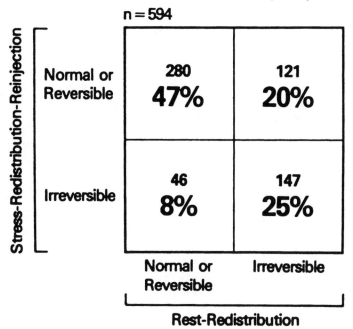

Figure 2-9. Concordance and discordance between stress-redistribution-reinjection and rest-redistribution images in the 20 patients who underwent positron emission tomographic studies. Five myocardial regions of interest were drawn on the transaxial tomograms from the five sets of thallium images, and thallium activities were then computed within each region. Thallium defects were classified as normal/reversible or irreversible. Reproduced with permission from Dilsizian et al.[52]

induced wall motion abnormalities. In a prospective study by Norris and associates,[53] from San Antonio, Tex, 30 patients underwent biplane transesophageal pacing echocardiography, dipyridamole thallium-201 single-photon emission computed tomography, and coronary arteriography. The sensitivity (86% v 95%), specificity (89% v 56%), positive predictive value (95% v 73%), and negative predictive value (83% v 83%) of biplane transesophageal pacing echocardiography and thallium-201 single-photon emission computed tomography in identifying patients with significant CAD was similar. In the 90 vascular territories analyzed, the agreement between biplane transesophageal pacing echocardiography and thallium-201 single-photon emission computed tomography for presence or absence of significant disease was 71%. Analysis of the three major vascular territories demonstrated that each imaging modality had a high sensitivity and specificity in the LAD and right coronary artery segments. However, the two techniques demonstrated poor sensitivity in the segmental distribution of the LC. It was concluded that biplane transesophageal pacing echocardiography compared favorably with thallium-201 single-photon emission computed tomography in terms of safety and accuracy for detecting significant CAD. Accordingly, biplane transesophageal pacing echocardiography may be a suitable alternative for those patients with nondiagnostic thallium-201 single-photon emission computed tomography studies and in those with contraindications to adenosine or dipyridamole.

Manning and associates,[54] from Boston, Mass, developed a magnetic resonance angiographic technique that allows the acquisition of complete images of coronary flow within a single-breath hold. By this method, the feasibility of noninvasive magnetic resonance coronary angiography was evaluated in 25 subjects, including 19 healthy adult volunteers and 6 patients after diagnostic coronary angiography. Noninvasive magnetic resonance coronary angiography was performed with a fat-suppressed ECG-gated gradient-echo sequence with a k-space segmentation. Overlapping transverse sections were initially used to image coronary flow, with oblique images obtained after identification of proximal anatomy. The left main coronary artery was seen in 24 subjects (96%) with a mean diameter of 4.8 mm and an average length of 10 mm. The LAD was visualized in 100% of subjects with a mean proximal diameter of 3.6 mm. The LC coronary artery was visualized in 76% of subjects and the right coronary artery in 100% of subjects (Figure 2-10). Quantitative angiography of normal proximal segments demonstrated a good correlation with magnetic resonance determined lumen diameters. Occluded arteries in patients with CAD displayed an absence of flow signal distal to the occlusion, whereas vessels with significant angiographic stenoses demonstrated signal loss corresponding to the area of the stenosis with visualization of the more distal vessel. These data suggest that breath-held magnetic resonance coronary angiography allows visualization of the major epicardial coronary arteries. With further development, this may become a noninvasive means for the evaluation of patients with known or suspected CAD in the future.

Magnetic Resonance Imaging

The ability to assess the patency of coronary arteries to noninvasive means would represent an important advance. Manning and associates,[55] from Boston, Mass, developed a magnetic resonance imaging (MRI) coronary angiographic technique that permits the display of areas of abnormal coronary blood flow. They compared this method with conventional contrast angiography for the identification of coronary-artery stenoses. MRI coronary angiography was performed with an electrocardiographically gated sequence in 39 subjects, aged 33 to 84 years, who were scheduled for elective cardiac catheterization with coronary angiography. Sequential overlapping transverse and oblique sections were acquired during periods of breath-holding and were displayed as cine loops for analysis. MRI and conventional angiographic data were compared in a blinded manner. The four major epicardial coronary arteries were classified by MRI coronary angiography as being normal (or having only minimal irregularities) or as having disease that was moderately severe to severe. The sensitivity and specificity of MRI coronary angiography, as compared with conventional angiography, for correctly identifying individual vessels with ≥50% angiographic stenoses were 90% and 92%, respectively. The corresponding positive and negative predictive values were 0.85 and 0.95, respectively. The sensitivity and specificity of the technique were 100% and 100%, respectively, for the left coronary artery. MRI coronary angiography provides a new approach to evaluating the patency of coronary arteries. These preliminary data suggest that this technique may provide a noninvasive means of evaluating patients with known or suspected CAD. At its current stage of development, this proce-

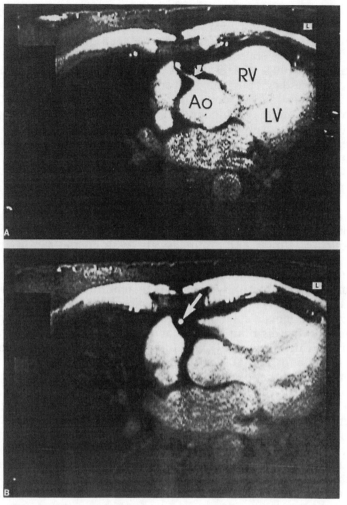

Figure 2-10. Magnetic resonance coronary angiographic images are shown using a breath-hold technique and the acquisition of transverse magnetic resonance sections 5 mm thick in a healthy volunteer (panel A) at the level of the proximal right coronary artery (white arrow). Panel B demonstrates subsequent transverse sections of the right coronary artery at a more inferior level (white arrow). LV = left ventricular cavity; RV = right ventricular cavity; Ao = aortic root. Reproduced with permission from Manning et al.[54]

dure may be most helpful for excluding clinically important stenoses in patients referred for diagnostic contract angiography.

Cine MRI has the capability of evaluating wall motion. Van Rugge and associates,[56] from Leiden, The Netherlands, evaluated the clinical usefulness of cine MRI during dobutamine stress for the detection of CAD in 45 patients with chest pain who were admitted for coronary arteriography. Dobutamine was administered to a maximal dose of 20 µg/kg/min. MRI images were obtained both at rest and during peak dobutamine stress. The test was positive if any new or worsening wall-motion abnormality developed. Dobutamine electrocardiography was also performed outside the magnetic environment, and all patients performed symptom-limited exercise electrocardiography. Significant CAD (>50% diameter stenosis) was present in 37 patients. During peak dobutamine stress, wall motion changes developed or worsened in 30 patients, giving an overall sensitivity for the detection of CAD of 81% and a specificity of 100%. Corresponding data was 51% and 63% for dobutamine electrocardiography and 70% and 63% for exercise electrocardiography. The sensitivity of dobutamine MRI for the detection of CAD in patients with single, double, and triple vessel disease was 75%, 80%, and 100%, respectively. These authors concluded that dobutamine MRI is a reasonable non-exercise-dependent method for the assessment of myocardial ischemia in patients with CAD.

Ultrafast Computed Tomography

Coronary artery calcium is a marker of atherosclerosis in asymptomatic patients. Ultrafast computed tomography can detect and quantify coronary calcium, simply and noninvasively, with greater sensitivity than can other techniques. Janowitz and associates,[57] from Miami Beach, Fla, measured and compared the prevalence and extent of coronary calcium in a large population of asymptomatic men and women. Coronary calcium studies were performed in an asymptomatic population of 1,396 male and 502 female subjects (aged 14 to 88 years). The prevalence of calcium and the distribution of total calcium scores (which reflect the amount of calcium present) were determined and compared for men and women at 5- and 10-year intervals. The prevalence of calcium in women was half that of men, until the age of 60 years when the difference diminished. The mean total calcium score distributions of men between the ages of 40 and 69 years were virtually identical to those of women between the ages of 50 and 79. The quantitative data obtained by ultrafast computed tomography showed very close agreement with autopsy studies of coronary calcium (Figure 2-11). Ultrafast computed tomography is a sensitive technique to measure coronary calcium in both men and women. The differences in prevalence and extent of coronary calcium appear to be parallel to those observed in the clinical incidence of CAD in men and women. Ultrafast computed tomography may have a greater impact on the treatment of women than of men, because it can be used to provide objective evidence of.coronary atherosclerosis.

Infrared Thermography

Lawson and associates,[58] from Stony Brook, NY, used infrared thermography to measure and map precordial skin temperature in 60 patients undergoing elective coronary angiography; 9 patients were normal and 51 had CAD. Thermograms were graded by quartile area (zero to 4 plus) and magnitude of thermal asymmetry (recorded as degrees Celsius). The presence, mean area, and degree of thermal asymmetry were significantly greater in patients with CAD. Twenty-two patients subsequently underwent successful revascularization with PTCA with a highly significant decrease in the presence, magnitude, and degree of thermal asymmetry. The results demonstrate that CAD is associated with precordial thermal asymmetry. The area and magnitude of thermal asymmetry is greater in patients with CAD than in control subjects without angiographically significant CAD. Successful revascularization changed the

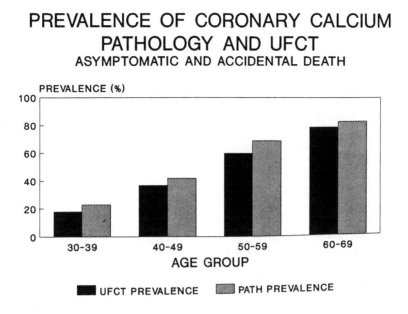

PREVALENCE OF CORONARY CALCIUM PATHOLOGY AND UFCT
ASYMPTOMATIC AND ACCIDENTAL DEATH

Figure 2-11. Comparison of prevalence of coronary calcium from this study with autopsy prevalence of calcium from published data of International Atherosclerosis Project. Autopsy study is from 361 subjects with accidental deaths. Ultrafast computed tomographic (UFCT) data were adjusted to reflect 2:1 male:female ratio in autopsy study. Reproduced with permission from Janowitz et al.[57]

asymmetric precordial pattern to a more symmetric one. Infrared thermography is a promising technique for the detection of CAD before and after revascularization.

PROGNOSIS INDICES

Exercise Testing

To develop prediction rules from clinical and exercise test data identifying patients at high and low risk for cardiovascular events among a group of male veterans, Morrow and associates,[59] from Long Beach, Calif, studied 3,609 men referred to their Veterans Affairs Medical Center for exercise testing between 1984 and 1990. Of the 3,609 patients, 2,546 remained evaluatable after exclusion of those who underwent subsequent cardiac catheterization, those with significant CAD, and those who had previous CABG. During a mean follow-up period of 2.8 years, 119 cardiovascular deaths and 44 nonfatal AMIs occurred in 2,546 patients. The Cox proportional-hazards model showed the following characteristics to be statistically independent predictors of time until cardiovascular death: history of CHF or digoxin use, exercise-induced ST depression, change in systolic BP during exercise, and exercise capacity. Using a simple score based on one item of clinical information (history of

CHF or digoxin use) and 31 exercise test responses (ST depression, exercise capacity, and change in systolic BP), 77% of patients were categorized as low risk (annual cardiac mortality rate, <2%), 18% as moderate risk (annual cardiac mortality rate, 7%), and 6% as high risk (annual cardiac mortality rate, 15%) (hazard ratio, 10). This model has not yet been validated. Variables available from the usual noninvasive workup of patients with known or suspected CAD can be used to predict future risk for cardiovascular death.

Morris and associates,[60] from Long Beach and Palo Alto, Calif, developed a population-specific prediction rule based on clinical and exercise test data that would estimate the risk of cardiovascular death in patients selected for cardiac catheterization. Prospective data and follow-up information were obtained from patients who underwent cardiac catheterization soon after clinical assessment and exercise testing. Males (n = 588) referred for evaluation of CAD from 1984 to 1990 were selected after exclusion of patients with significant valvular heart disease and patients with prior cardiac surgery. Half had a prior myocardial infarction and half complained of typical angina pectoris. All patients performed a treadmill test and were selected for clinical reasons to undergo coronary angiography within 3 months. Over a mean follow-up period of 2.5 years (± 1.4 years), there were 39 cardiovascular deaths and 45 nonfatal myocardial infarctions. The Cox proportional-hazards model demonstrated the following characteristics to be statistically independent predictors of time until cardiovascular death: history of CHF (hazard ratio, 4), ST depression on the resting electrocardiogram (hazard ratio, 3), and a drop in systolic BP below the resting value during exercise (hazard ratio, 5). Exercise-induced ST depression was not associated with either death or nonfatal myocardial infarction. A simple score based on one item of clinical information (history of CHF), a resting electrocardiogram finding (ST depression), and an exercise test response (exertional hypotension) stratified these patients for 4 years after testing from 75% with a low risk (annual cardiac mortality rate, 1%), 17% with a moderate risk (annual mortality rate, 7%), and 1% with a high risk (annual cardiac mortality rate, 12%) (hazard ratio, 20). It was concluded that the variables available from the usual noninvasive workup of patients with known or suspected CAD enable prediction of risk of cardiovascular death. Three quarters of those usually undergoing cardiac catheterization can be identified by simple noninvasive variables as being at such low risk that invasive intervention is unlikely to improve prognosis.

Stress Echocardiography

To examine the value of transient regional asynergy on dobutamine stress echocardiography as a noninvasive predictor of future cardiac events, Mazeika and associates,[61] from London, England, studied 51 symptomatic patients with suspected CAD using an incremental regimen of 5, 10, 15, and 20 µg/kg/min. Pretest likelihood of CAD was 80% before and 83% after exercise electrocardiography using probability analysis based on age, sex, and symptoms. Two-dimensional images were analyzed with reference to an 11-segment model and gave good interrater agreement. During 24 months of follow-up, 23 patients had events (1 AMI, 9 unstable angina, 10 CABG, and 3 PTCA) and 28 were event free. Age, proportion with baseline asynergy, and both pretest echocardiographic EF and its response to dobutamine were similar in these two groups. Transient asynergy was seen in 17 of 23 patients (74%) with events and 8 of 28 patients (29%) without events; 5 of 6 patients with involvement of three segments had events. AMI or unstable angina occurred in 8 of 25 (32%) with a positive stress echocardiogram and 2 of 26 (8%) with a negative stress echocardiogram. Both exercise duration and time to diagnostic ST-segment shift were shorter in those with inducible asynergy. These data suggest that patients with probable CAD and a positive dobutamine echocardiogram are at higher risk of an adverse outcome. Dobutamine echocardiography may aid selection for coronary angiography and prognostic revascularization, particularly in patients unable to exercise.

Stress echocardiography is useful in diagnosing myocardial ischemia in patients with significant CAD. Krivokapich and associates,[62] from Los Angeles, Calif, examined the correlation between the results of exercise stress echocardiography and cardiac event rates within 12 months after testing in patients referred for evaluation of possible myocardial ischemia. Cardiac events, defined as AMI, CABG, PTCA, or death, were tabulated for 360 patients with ≥12 months of follow-up, or a cardiac event within 12 months of follow-up, or both. Wall motion abnormalities at rest were present in 60% of patients. A positive stress echocardiogram, defined as the development of new or worsened wall-motion abnormalities, was obtained in 18% of patients (65 of 360), and ≥1 cardiac event during follow-up was present in 14%. A cardiac event occurred in 34% of patients (22 of 65) with a positive stress echocardiogram and in 9% (27 of 295) with a negative one. AMIs occurred in 9% of patients with a positive stress echocardiogram compared with 2% with a negative test. An insufficient exercise capacity to reliably exclude ischemia was present in 63% of patients (17 of 27) with a cardiac event despite a negative stress echocardiogram. The predictive value of the stress echocardiographic results was enhanced by combining these results with the electrocardiographic results. In summary, a positive stress echocardiogram was associated with a three-fold increased incidence of any cardiac event and a four-fold increased incidence of AMI within 12 months of follow-up compared with a negative stress echocardiogram. Thus, stress echocardiography is a useful prognosticator of future events in patients with CAD.

Thallium-201 Exercise Testing

Travin and associates,[63] from Boston, Mass, reviewed 268 patients to determine the exercise workload, the electrocardiographic and thallium-201 image parameters that are most closely associated with a poor prognosis from ischemic heart disease. Only patients with unequivocal thallium-201 redistribution were selected. A multivariate analysis was performed to find the variables that were most strongly associated with the outcomes of coronary revascularization, AMI, and cardiac death during a follow-up period of 25 ± 19 months. Patients who underwent early elective revascularization had poorer exercise tolerance and more thallium image abnormalities than those with no events. In the remaining patients, myocardial infarction was most closely related to the extent and severity of thallium ischemia, whereas cardiac death was associated with abnormal thallium lung uptake and an inability to exercise to 9.6 MET. Thus, unlike AMI, cardiac death is best predicted by variables that reflect poor LV function rather than those that indicate ischemia.

UNSTABLE ANGINA PECTORIS

New Clinical Classification

The diagnosis of unstable angina encompasses a broad spectrum of patients with myocardial ischemia, varying widely in cause, prognosis, and responsiveness to therapy. Ahmed and associates,[64] from Boston, proposed a new clinical classification on unstable angina based on the following two components: the severity and the clinical setting in which unstable angina develops. The hypothesis that this clinical classification correlates with the underlying coronary artery anatomy was tested. In 238 consecutive patients, an unstable angina score ranging from 2 to 6 was determined by adding the scores for severity (1 = unstable angina without pain at rest; 2 = pain at rest >48 hours before angiography; and 3 = pain at rest ≤48 hours before angiographic evaluation) and the clinical setting of unstable angina (1 = unstable angina secondary to a noncardiac condition; 2 = primary unstable angina; and 3 = early postinfarction unstable angina). Fifty concurrently studied consecutive patients with stable angina were assigned a score of 0. Patients with unstable angina averaged 63 years of age, and 165 (69%) were men. Pain at rest occurred in 202 of 238 patients (85%), and angiography was performed ≤48 hours in 139 of these patients (69%). Among patients with unstable angina, 5 (2%) had secondary unstable angina, 143 (60%) had primary unstable angina, and 90 (38%) had postinfarction unstable angina (Figure 2-12). Multivariable regression analysis identified the unstable

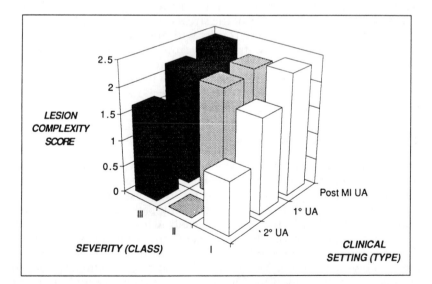

Figure 2-12. Lesion complexity. Lesion complexity (0 = no obstruction; 1 = simple stenosis; 2 = complex stenosis; 3 = thrombus; and 4 = total occlusion) is related to severity and timing of last episode of pain at rest (class I = unstable angina without pain at rest; class II = pain at rest > 48 hours before angiography; and class III = pain at rest ≤ 48 hours before angiographic evaluation), and clinical circumstances of presentation (ie, type of unstable angina). Post MI UA = postinfarction angina; 1° UA = primary unstable angina; 2° UA = secondary unstable angina. Reproduced with permission from Ahmed et al.[64]

angina score as the most important predictor of intracoronary thrombus and lesion complexity in the ischemia related artery. The new clinical classification of unstable angina correlates with the underlying angiographic anatomy and may thus aid in decisions regarding diagnostic procedures and provide a useful basis for comparing the response to therapy among patients with unstable angina.

Silent Myocardial Ischemia

Serneri and associates,[65] from Florence, Italy, studied [³H]norepinephrine kinetics in patients with active unstable angina compared with patients with inactive unstable angina, stable effort angina, and control. Silent myocardial ischemia was evaluated by three 24-hour Holter monitoring periods on alternate days and [³H]norepinephrine kinetics were assessed under normal conditions and following the cold pressor test. Simultaneously, catecholamine concentrations were measured in the aortic, coronary sinus, and peripheral venous blood. Different from the other groups, the majority of silent ischemic episodes in patients with unstable angina occurred without increase in heart rate. These patients had a positive coronary sinus-aorta norepinephrine gradient, both at rest and following the cold pressor test. [³H]Norepinephrine kinetics demonstrated an increased selective cardiac spillover at rest and during the cold pressor test. Reduced cardiac [³H]norepinephrine extraction was also found. There was a significant relation between the number of ischemic events or the overall duration of silent ischemia and norepinephrine spillover, both at rest and following cold application. Therefore, during the acute phase of unstable angina, a disorder in cardiac norepinephrine metabolism occurs (Figure 2-13) resulting in a reflex cardiac sympathetic overactivity that probably contributes to the development of silent myocardial ischemia.

Smooth-Muscle Cells and Fibroblast Growth Factors

Flugelman and associates,[66] from Bethesda, Md, determined whether additional mechanisms play a role in the transformation of stable angina to unstable angina in addition to plaque rupture and thrombosis. The histological findings of atherectomy specimens from 34 patients with unstable angina were compared with those of 24 patients with postangioplasty restenosis and 10 patients with stable angina. The expression of acidic and basic fibroblast growth factor was examined. Specimens from patients with unstable angina resembled those from patients with postangioplasty restenosis as regards smooth-muscle cell abundance and differed from those from patients with stable angina. Thrombus and/or hemorrhage occurred in 34% of patients with unstable angina compared with 8% of restenosis lesions and none in the patients with stable angina. Active lesions consisting of thrombus, hemorrhage, and abundant and disorganized smooth-muscle cells in the presence of loose connective tissue were observed in 56% of the unstable angina patients and in 50% of the restenosis patients but in none of the stable angina patients. The expression of acidic and basic fibroblast growth factor was detected in 80% to 100% of lesions from patients with unstable angina and restenosis specimens but in only one of five stable angina patients. Thus, microscopic evidence of thrombosis and plaque rupture was found in one third

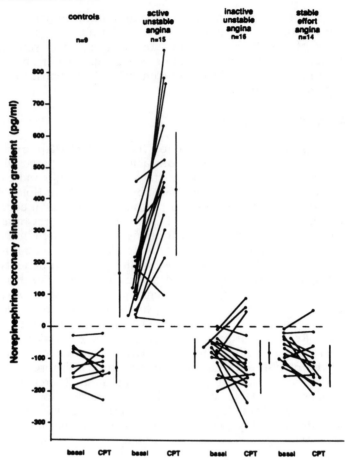

Figure 2-13. Graph of norepinephrine coronary sinus-aorta gradient both at rest and after cold pressor test (CPT) in controls and in the three groups of anginal patients (p < 0.001 among the groups both at rest and after CPT). Bars indicate SD. Reproduced with permission from Serneri et al.[65]

of unstable angina patients, perhaps because this was a selected group of patients who had no angiographic evidence of intracoronary thrombus. The lesions of the patients with unstable angina resembled those of restenosis patients regardless of smooth muscle cell abundance, lesion activity, and the expression of fibroblast growth factor.

Neutrophil and Monocyte Adhesion

Mazzone and associates[67] studied 39 patients who underwent diagnostic coronary arteriography to assess whether upregulation of granulocyte and monocyte CDllb/CD18 receptors take place during the passage of blood through the coronary tree of patients with clinical manifestations of CAD. Group 1 patients (15) had a clinical diagnosis of unstable angina; group 2 (14 patients) had stable angina; and group 3 (10 patients) had atypical chest pain. Sampling from the coronary sinus and aorta were obtained before coronary arteriography. Cell surface receptors were detected by immunofluorescence evaluated by flow cytofluorimetry using monoclonal antibodies tagged with fluorescent markers. Leukocytes were stained in unseparated blood to avoid in vitro manipulation that could cause phagocytosis. Group 1 and 2 patients had significant CAD >50% coronary narrowing in at least one major coronary artery, whereas group 3 patients had normal coronary arteries. In group 1, granulocytes and monocytes showed a significantly higher expression of the CDllb/CD18 adhesion receptor in the coronary sinus than in the aorta, whereas no differences in CDllb/CD18 expression were seen in groups 2 and 3. Patients with unstable angina have an increased expression of granulocytes and monocyte CDllb/CD18 adhesion receptors indicating that an inflammatory reaction takes place within the coronary system. Activation of these leukocytes may induce coronary vasoconstriction, promote thrombosis, and activate platelets; thus, these alterations may play a role in the development of acute coronary heart disease syndromes.

STABLE ANGINA PECTORIS

Effects of Eating

One of the well recognized characteristics of angina has been the worsening of exercise tolerance after eating a meal. Previous studies have been contradictory in evaluating the mechanism of this phenomenon. Colles and associates,[68] from Montreal, Canada, determined the effect of a standardized meal on ischemic threshold and exercise capacity in 20 patients with stable angina, exercise-induced ischemia, and reversible exercise-induced perfusion defects. One test was performed in the fasting state and the other 30 minutes after a 1,000 calorie meal. In the postprandial state, exercise time to ischemia was reduced by 20%, time to angina by 15%, and exercise tolerance by 9%. The rate pressure products at the end points of these exercise tests were not significantly different in the fasting and postprandial test. Quantitative 99mTc-sestamibi ischemia score was also unchanged. Thus they concluded that a reduced time to ischemia, time to angina, and exercise tolerance, occurred because of a more rapid increase in myocardial demand with exercise and not due to vasoconstriction. The extent and severity of the exercise-induced ischemia was unchanged. The clinical implication of this study is that all patients with angina should be cautioned about vigorous exercise after meals.

Wall Motion

Amanullah and associates,[69] from Stockholm, Sweden, assessed myocardial perfusion and regional wall motion during adenosine-induced coronary vasodilation in 40 patients with angina pectoris by technetium-99m sestamibi single-photon emission computed tomography and simultaneous two-dimensional echocardiography. Adenosine was infused intravenously at a dose of 140 µg/kg body weight per minute for six minutes, and technetium-99m sestamibi was injected at three minutes. Adenosine caused a significant decrease in systolic and diastolic BP and a significant increase in heart rate BP product. Adverse effects were mild and transient and no patient required aminophylline. Completely or partially reversible defects on computed tomography were present in 28 patients, a fixed defect was seen in 4 patients, and no defect was seen in 8 patients. Two-dimensional echocardiography revealed a new or worsening wall-motion abnormality in 21 patients, a fixed abnormality in 4 patients, and no abnormality in 15. Transient perfusion defects were associated with transient wall-motion abnormalities in 71% of cases. The overall sensitivity, specificity, and predictive accuracy of adenosine echocardiography in detecting significant CAD (>50% diameter stenosis) were 74%, 100%, and 78%, respectively; those of adenosine computed tomography were 94%, 100%, and 95%, respectively. Thus, adenosine technetium-99m sestamibi computed tomography has a higher sensitivity and predictive accuracy than adenosine echocardiography, suggesting that adenosine-induced perfusion defects are not always associated with wall-motion abnormality. Although the principal underlying mechanism of myocardial ischemia during adenosine infusion is a "coronary steal" phenomenon, the ischemia is also due to an enhanced myocardial oxygen demand, as indicated by an increased rate-pressure product.

Collateral-Dependent Myocardium

Vanoverschelde and associates,[70] from Bearse, Belgium, and Limburg, The Netherlands, determined mechanisms responsible for chronic regional LV dysfunction in patients with angina and noninfarcted collateral-dependent myocardium. Twenty-six patients with angina were studied, including 19 men (mean age, 60 years) with chronic occlusion of a major coronary artery but without previous AMI. Positron emission tomography was performed to measure absolute regional myocardial blood flow with ^{13}N-ammonia at rest (n = 26) and after intravenous dipyridamole (n = 11). The kinetics of ^{18}F-deoxyglucose and ^{11}C-acetate were measured to calculate the rate of exogenous glucose uptake and regional oxidative metabolism in 15 individuals. Global and regional LV function were calculated by contrast ventriculography at baseline (n = 26) and after revascularization (n = 12). Transmural myocardial biopsies from the collateral-dependent areas were obtained in 7 patients during CABG and analyzed by optical and electron microscopy. The patients were separated into groups with and without dysfunction of the collateral-dependent segments. In patients with normal wall motion (n = 9), regional myocardial blood flow, oxidative metabolism, and glucose uptake were similar among collateral-dependent and remote segments. However, in patients with regional dysfunction (n = 17), collateral-dependent segments had lower myocardial blood flow and higher glucose uptake compared with remote segments. Myocardial blood flow was similar among collateral-dependent segments of patients with and without segmental dysfunction. After intravenous dipyridamole, collateral-dependent myocardial blood flow increased in three patients with normal wall motion, but there were lesser increases in patients with regional dysfunction. There was a significant inverse correlation between wall motion abnormality and collateral flow reserve. Analysis of the tissue samples obtained at the time of the surgery showed structural changes in dysfunctional, collateral-dependent areas, including cellular swelling, loss of myofibrillar content, and accumulation of glycogen. However, regional wall motion improved in the patients studied before and after revascularization. Therefore, in a subgroup of patients with noninfarcted collateral-dependent LV segments, insufficiently developed collaterals do not provide adequate flow reserve. Despite nearly normal resting flow and oxygen consumption, these collateral-dependent segments exhibit depressed wall motion and marked ultrastructural alterations. These alterations presumably result from repeated episodes of ischemia and may represent the flow, metabolic, and morphologic correlates of myocardial "hibernation."

Effects of Serotonin

Tousoulis and associates,[71] from the Hammersmith Hospital in London, England, studied the effects of intracoronary infusion of serotonin on 38 coronary stenoses of different morphologies in 11 patients with stable angina and 4 with variant angina. While receiving the maximal infused concentration of serotonin, 100% of complicated stenoses and 50% of concentric stenoses constricted by ≥20%. The magnitude of constriction was greater at eccentric sites than concentric sites and greater in complicated stenoses than eccentric stenoses. At complicated stenoses, the constriction was greater than at the adjacent reference segment. The constriction at the stenosis was also greater for irregular or complicated lesions than for smooth lesions in both patients with stable and those with variant angina. Thus, the magnitude of the vasoconstrictor response to serotonin at the site of an atheromatous coronary plaque depends on the morphological characteristics of the plaque and is more closely related to irregular contour than stenosis severity or length. This relation suggests that variations in receptor type or density or in the smooth-muscle cell response to stimulation may determine the response to locally released serotonin in patients with CAD.

SILENT MYOCARDIAL ISCHEMIA

Silent ischemia is common in patients with coronary artery disease. In previous studies, the presence of silent ischemia has always seemed to worsen the outlook, particularly in patients with high-risk CAD. Quyyumi and associates,[72] from Bethesda, Md, evaluated the incidence and prognostic significance of ischemia detected by ambulatory monitoring in low-risk medically managed patients with CAD. They prospectively studied the significance of ST-segment changes during daily activities in 116 asymptomatic or mildly symptomatic low-risk patients with native CAD. Patients excluded from this group included those with LM CAD, three-vessel CAD, and LV dysfunction at rest, three-vessel CAD and inducible ischemia during exercise, and two-vessel CAD with LV dysfunction and inducible ischemia. Thirty-nine percent of patients had transient episodes of ST-segment depression during 48-hour electrocardiographic monitoring. Eighty-two percent of these episodes were silent. There were eight cardiac events overall, and nine patients underwent elective revascularization. Seven of the eight acute events occurred in patients without silent ischemia during monitoring. They concluded that in patients categorized as low risk on the basis of cardiac catheterization and stress testing results, silent myocardial ischemia during daily life was not uncommon, but its presence did not predict future coronary events. This study suggests that there is no value in doing ambulatory monitoring in patients with low-risk CAD.

Andrews and associates,[73] from Boston, Mass, determined whether episodes of ambulatory myocardial ischemia are caused by increases in myocardial oxygen demand or may be due to episodic coronary vasoconstriction in patients with stable CAD. Mean minute heart rate activity during ambulatory ECG monitoring was determined for 50 patients treated with propranolol, diltiazem, nifedipine, or placebo in a randomized, double-blind, crossover trial. Periods of heart rate increases of varying magnitudes and durations identified throughout a 48-hour ECG monitoring period and the number of these periods associated with an ischemic episode were determined. The circadian variation of ischemic episodes characterized by the presence or absence of an increase in heart rate were analyzed. Eighty-one percent of ischemic episodes were preceded by an increase in heart rate ≥5 beats per minute. The likelihood of developing ischemia associated with a heart rate increase was proportional to the magnitude and duration of the heart rate increase and the baseline heart rate before the increase occurred. The likelihood of developing ischemia ranged from 4% when heart rate increased <10 beats per minute and lasted <10 minutes to 60% when the heart rate increased ≥20 beats per minute and lasted ≥40 minutes. Propranolol therapy significantly reduced the magnitude and duration of heart rate increase compared with placebo, diltiazem, or nifedipine. Ischemic episodes associated with a heart rate increase displayed a daytime peak, whereas ischemia occurring without a heart rate increase occurred evenly throughout the day. Propranolol reduced the proportion of heart rate-related ischemic episodes and increased the proportion of non-heart rate-related episodes compared with placebo (Figure 2-14).

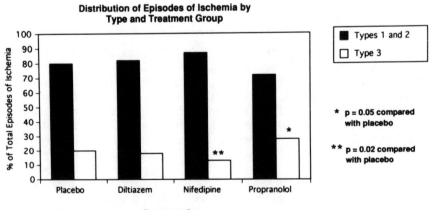

Figure 2-14. The distribution of ischemic episodes by type and treatment group. The treatment group is plotted on the horizontal axis with the percentage of each type of ischemic episode plotted on the vertical axis. Compared with placebo therapy, propranolol was associated with more episodes of myocardial ischemia and nifedipine with fewer episodes of ischemia. Reproduced with permission from Andrews et al.[73]

Nifedipine exerted the opposite effect. Multivariate analysis indicated that the probability of developing ischemia was strongly associated with heart rate variables and was unaffected by time of day. Thus, most episodes of ambulatory ischemia are associated with a preceding period of increased heart rate and the likelihood of developing myocardial ischemia may be predicted by heart rate variables. A minority of ischemic episodes are not associated with preceding periods of increased heart rate and may be caused by episodic coronary vasoconstriction.

A total of 389 patients with angiographically determined CAD, who exhibited a complete absence of angina pectoris in the presence of reproducible myocardial ischemia, were studied by Droste and associates,[74] from Bad Krozingen, Germany, in a follow-up investigation. After an initial coronary angiogram, anti-ischemic medication was prescribed as treatment. After a mean follow-up time of 5 years, patients were sent a questionnaire that assessed any new development of angina pectoris pain and cardiac events. In 48 of these patients, a second angiogram was recorded after a mean period of 4 years. Asymptomatic patients had a worse prognosis than an age-adjusted normal population. After 5 and 10 years, 9% and 26% of the patients, respectively, had died; nonfatal cardiac events (AMI, CABG, or PTCA) occurred after 5 and 10 years in 19% and 46%, respectively. A large number of initially asymptomatic patients developed angina pectoris pain over the follow-up period (34% after 5 years and 58% after 10 years). Novel angina pectoris pain often preceded cardiac events by months to years. Multivariate analysis indicated that vessel disease and degree of ischemia (defined by ST-segment depression free exercise tolerance) proved to have independent predictive value with respect to mortality rate. Newly developed angina pectoris was associated with an increase in objective signs of myocardial ischemia and a progression in coronary stenosis. The results indicate that patients who originally had myocardial ischemia with a marked absence of pain can develop angina pectoris over the course of years and that newly developed pain often precedes cardiac events.

The differences between diabetic and nondiabetic patients with silent myocardial ischemia were investigated by Hikita and associates,[75] from Saitama, Japan. Based on the results of previous exercise testing, a total of 110 patients (15 diabetic and 95 nondiabetic) with exercise-induced myocardial ischemia were divided into the following three groups: 15 diabetics with silent myocardial ischemia, 49 nondiabetics with silent myocardial ischemia, and 46 nondiabetics with anginal symptoms. All patients underwent treadmill exercise testing and 24-hour ambulatory electrocardiographic recording. Before and during exercise, blood samples from the antecubital vein were obtained to determine the plasma β-endorphin levels, and the pain threshold of each patient was measured with the electrical skin stimulation test. Furthermore, with regard to the ambulatory electrocardiographic recording, the mean of the standard deviations of all normal sinus RR intervals during successive five-minute recording periods over 24 hours was analyzed and considered as an index of the autonomic function. The plasma β-endorphin level during exercise was significantly greater in nondiabetic patients with silent ischemia than in diabetic ones. The SD mean was significantly less in the diabetic group than in the two nondiabetic ones. The findings suggest that the role of β endorphin in diabetic patients with silent myocardial ischemia may be less significant than in nondiabetic ones; therefore, a diabetic neuropathy that affects the autonomic pain fibers that innervate the heart may be involved in the mechanism of silent myocardial ischemia in diabetics.

Data concerning the natural history of asymptomatic CAD has been limited to epidemiologic rather than angiographic studies, thus leading to uncertainty as to whether warning symptoms and signs will identify subjects with silent myocardial ischemia before morbid events. To address this issue, Thaulow and associates,[76] from Oslo, Norway, followed prospectively 50 apparently healthy men with angiographically proven CAD and asymptomatic exercise-induced ST depression in the Oslo Ischemia Study. Fourteen men died. The initial presenting clinical event in these 14 men was chest pain in 4 (30%) (but in only one case was it recognized as typical angina), silent AMI in 5 (35%), and sudden death in 5 (35%). Thirty-six men survived, with 19 developing symptoms. Overall, chest pain was the first clinical event in 22 of the total of 33 men with symptoms (66%), whereas AMI occurred in 6 (18%) and sudden death in 5 (16%). Although chest pain occurred in 22 men, it was clinically diagnosed as typical angina pectoris in only 6. These observations suggest that there is an absence of clear-cut ischemic symptoms in many asymptomatic patients before morbid events.

To determine the clinical significance of silent and symptomatic myocardial ischemia detected by noninvasive testing in stable postcoronary patients, Moss and associates,[77] for the Multicenter Myocardial Ischemia Research Group, from multiple US medical centers, studied 936 patients (76% male; mean age, 58 years) who were clinically stable 1 to 6 months after hospitalization for AMI or unstable angina. The interventions included noninvasive testing involving rest, ambulatory, and exercise electrocardiograms and stress thallium-201 scintigraphy. Cox regression analysis was used to evaluate the risk (hazard ratio) of first recurrent primary events (cardiac death, nonfatal infarction, or unstable angina) or restricted events (cardiac death or nonfatal infarction) associated with ischemic noninvasive test results. ST-segment depression on the rest electrocardiogram was the only noninvasive test variable that identified a significantly increased risk for first recurrent primary events (hazard ratio): rest electrocardiogram ST depression (1.5); ambulatory electrocardiogram ST depression (0.9); exercise electrocardiogram ST depression (1.1); and stress thallium-201 reversible defects (1.3). Test results were similar for first recurrent restricted events, and in patients with and without angina. Significantly increased risk was noted when exercise-induced ST depression occurred in patients who also had reduced exercise duration (3.4) or when reversible thallium-201 defects occurred in patients who also had increased lung uptake (2.8). Each high-risk subset made up less than 3% of the population and contained less than 6% of patients with first primary events. Detection of silent or symptomatic myocardial ischemia by noninvasive testing in stable patients 1 to 6 months after an acute coronary event is not useful in identifying patients at increased risk for subsequent coronary events.

Variant, Spastic, or Microvascular Angina Pectoris

Sugiishi and Takatsu,[78] from Aichi, Japan, evaluated the relationship between cigarette smoking and coronary artery spasm by studying 175 patients with angiographically determined coronary artery spasm but no coronary artery luminal diameter narrowing from atherosclerosis exceeding 25%. The control group of patients comprised 176 patients with completely normal coronary arteries and a negative response to ergonovine maleate. The adjusted odds ratio and 95% confidence interval for smoking as a risk factor for vasospasm was 2.4 and 1.5 to 3.8, respectively. The adjusted odds ratio for total, LDL, and HDL cholesterol; triglycerides; diabetes mellitus; and body-mass index calculated by multivariate logistic regression analysis were not statistically significant. Thus, smoking appears to be an important risk factor for vasospastic angina in patients without significant coronary artery narrowing.

Patients with syndrome X have been found to have an abnormal coronary blood flow reserve. The physical performance during exercise, however, has been incompletely investigated. Cardiopulmonary exercise testing is a reliable noninvasive method to provide indexes of lung, heart, circulation, and muscle functions. In an investigation by Montorsi and associates,[79] from Milan, Italy, cardiopulmonary exercise testing was performed twice a day (8 AM and 4 PM) on two separate occasions 2 months apart, in 15 patients (10 women) with syndrome X and in age- and sex-matched normal individuals. Time and oxygen consumption at peak exercise, at ventilatory anaerobic and electrocardiographic thresholds, as well as norepinephrine plasma concentrations at each work load and at peak exercise in both tests were obtained. In syndrome X in both evaluations, the 4 PM performance was characterized by an earlier onset of both ventilatory anaerobic and electrocardiographic thresholds, despite lower values of oxygen consumption and double product, and by a greater peak ST-segment depression, despite similar total exercise time, oxygen consumption, and double product. No difference between tests was found in the norepinephrine response to exercise. Normal individuals showed reproducible cardiopulmonary exercise testing and hormonal responses in the two tests. Thus, these data suggest a circadian variation of coronary vascular response to exercise in patients with syndrome X, leading to a lower ischemic threshold early in the afternoon. The parallel earlier onset of the ventilatory anaerobic threshold reflects a concomitant abnormal muscular blood flow response (ie, vasoconstriction of working muscle arteries), suggesting a link between coronary and peripheral circulations.

Romeo and associates,[80] from Rome, Italy, evaluated the clinical course of 30 patients diagnosed with syndrome X (angina pectoris, positive exercise test, and normal coronary arteries) during a 5-year follow-up. Patients were divided at the control examination into two groups according to the median value of the heart rate/blood pressure product variation from rest to the first stage of a modified Bruce protocol, as follows: group 1, ≤1,050 and group 2, >1,050 mm Hg × beats/min. All patients were followed at 6-month intervals during a mean follow-up of 60 months. During follow-up, chest pain was unchanged in 20 patients, decreased in severity and frequency in 9, and disappeared in 1 in group 2; three patients in group 1 had prolonged episodes of anginal chest pain that needed hospitalization. In group 2, seven patients developed systemic hypertension, 4 had a progression of exercise-induced left bundle branch block to constant left bundle branch block, and 4 continued to develop rate-dependent block during exercise, but at a reduced heart rate. In the latter 8 patients, LVEF at rest during follow-up decreased significantly from 61% to 51%. Therefore, during follow-up, patients in group 1 remained clinically stable or improved, whereas it was possible to identify two subgroups among those in group 2: a subgroup who became clearly hypertensive, and a subgroup who had a progressive reduction in LV function and a progression of intraventricular conduction disturbances. In conclusion, syndrome X comprises patients with possible myocardial ischemia, borderline hypertension, and early stage cardiomyopathy.

Calcium antagonists are now considered the agents of choice for the treatment of vasospastic angina. Most of the early studies were carried out with short acting agents. Chahine and associates,[81] from Miami, Fla, evaluated amlodipine as a once-a-day agent in the management of patients with vasospastic angina. Fifty-two patients with well-documented vasospastic angina underwent a single-blind placebo run-in period. They were then randomized in a double-blind protocol to receive either 10 mg of amlodipine or placebo every morning for 4 weeks. The rate of anginal episode per week was significantly decreased with amlodipine treatment compared with placebo (5 v 15). Peripheral edema was the only major adverse event seen in the amlodipine treated patients. These authors concluded that amlodipine is efficacious and safe in the treatment of vasospastic angina. As a once-daily drug, it would appear to have efficacy similar to the other calcium entry blockers.

Egashira and associates,[82] from Fukuoka, Japan, attempted to determine whether endothelium-dependent vasodilatation of the coronary vasculature was impaired in patients with syndrome X or microvascular angina, that is, patients with chest pains resembling angina and positive exercise tests but normal coronary angiograms and no coronary-artery spasm. The authors infused the endothelium-dependent vasodilator acetylcholine and the endothelium-independent vasodilators papaverine and isosorbide dinitrate into the left coronary artery of nine patients and ten control subjects. The diameter of the LAD coronary artery was assessed by quantitative angiography, and changes in coronary blood flow were estimated with the use of an intracoronary Doppler catheter. Acetylcholine, given in doses of 1, 3, 10, and 30 µg/min, increased coronary blood flow in a dose-dependent manner in both groups. However, the mean acetylcholine-induced increases in coronary blood flow were significantly less in the patients than in the controls. The changes in coronary blood flow in response to 2 mg of isosorbide dinitrate and 10 mg of papaverine did not differ significantly between the patients and controls. The administration of papaverine resulted in myocardial lactate production in the patients but not in the controls. The three lower doses of acetylcholine caused a similar degree of dilatation of the LAD coronary artery in the two groups, and the highest dose caused a similar degree of constriction in the two groups. Isosorbide dinitrate and papaverine caused a similar degree of dilatation in both groups. These findings suggest that endothelium-dependent dilatation of the resistance coronary arteries is defective in patients with anginal chest pain and normal coronary arteries, which may contribute to the altered regulation of myocardial perfusion in these patients.

Chauhan and associates,[83] from Cambridge, United Kingdom, assessed the effect of clinical presentation on functional prognosis in patients with coronary syndrome X. Eighty-two patients with syndrome X presenting with unstable angina and stable angina were prospectively followed up with a questionnaire to examine their functional state. Forty-one patients with syndrome X had unstable angina, and 41 patients with syndrome X had stable angina. Syndrome X was defined as typical anginal chest pain, a positive exercise test, and normal coronary angiogram. The mean follow-up time was 36 (range, 20 to 51) months for the unstable angina group and 35 (range, 19 to 51) months for the stable angina group. No patient was lost to follow-up in either group. At follow-up, 28 patients in the unstable angina group were pain free compared with 15 patients in the stable angina group. Seven patients in the unstable angina group had further hospital admissions with chest pain after the cardiac catheterization compared with 12 patients in the stable angina group. Seven patients in the unstable angina group believed that they had heart disease compared with 27 in the stable angina group. Twenty-six patients in the unstable angina group but only 8 patients in the stable angina group were unlimited in their physical activity. Twelve patients in the unstable angina group compared with 27 patients in the stable angina group were unable to work normally because of chest pain. The mean duration of symptoms before cardiac catheterization was 7.9 months in the unstable angina group and 13.4 months in the stable angina group. Ten patients in the unstable angina group and 24 patients in the stable angina group still attended hospital outpatient clinics because of chest pain. Sixteen patients in the unstable angina group and 29 patients in the stable angina group were still taking regular antianginal medications. In conclusion, patients with syndrome X who present with unstable angina have a significantly better functional prognosis than those presenting with symptoms of stable angina. This may reflect differences in underlying pathophysiological mechanisms.

Tousoulis and associates,[84] from London, England, evaluated the relationship between LV function and exercise capacity in patients with syndrome X. Thirty-seven patients (9 men and 28 women) who had angina with normal coronary arteries and a positive exercise test had evaluation of LV function and exercise duration. LV hypercontractility (EF >80%) was observed in 12 patients; 25 patients had normal LV contraction. The time to 1 mm ST depression on exercise testing was significantly earlier in the patients with hypercontractility. Similarly, the magnitude of ST-segment depression at peak exercise was significantly greater in this group as was the mean time for ST-segment depression to normalize. These authors concluded that approximately one third of patients with syndrome X have LV hypercontractility, which is associated with the development of ST depression at a lower heart rate and work load during exercise.

DIET, EXERCISE, AND DRUGS FOR MYOCARDIAL ISCHEMIA

Physical Activity

To compare the cardiovascular risk of exercise in the morning and afternoon in patients with established heart disease, Murray and associates,[85] from Winston-Salem, NC, performed supervised, submaximal exercise (one hour, three times/week) performed either in the morning (7:30 AM) or the afternoon (3 PM). Documented cardiac events that occurred while patients were exercising in the rehabilitation programs were the main outcome. There were five cardiac events in 168,111 patient-hours of exercise in the morning, with an incidence of 3.0 ± 1.3 events per 100,000 patient-hours. There were two events during the 84,491 patient-hours in the afternoon, with an incidence of 2.4 ± 1.5 events per 100,000 patient-hours (not significant). The risk ratio of cardiac events during exercise in the morning compared with the afternoon was 1.27. In patients with CAD, the incidence of cardiac events is low during regular, submaximal exercise whether performed in the morning or the afternoon.

Cardiac rehabilitation and exercise training improve prognosis following major cardiac events partly by improving atherosclerotic risk factors, including plasma lipids. Limited data are available to define predictors of lipid improvements following aggressive nonpharmacologic therapy with cardiac rehabilitation. Lavie and Milani,[86] from New Orleans, La, studied 237 consecutive patients from two institutions who were enrolled in outpatient phase 2 cardiac rehabilitation and exercise programs. By univariable and multivariable analyses, we assessed the impact of numerous clinical variables, including indexes of obesity, age, gender, lipid concentrations, exercise capacity, and psychological factors, on improvements in plasma lipid values with cardiac rehabilitation. Atherosclerotic risk factors improved following cardiac rehabilitation, including levels of LDL cholesterol (-4%), HDL cholesterol (7%), and triglycerides (-13%); body-mass index (2%); percentage of body fat (-5%); and exercise capacity (26%) (Table 2-3). By both univariable and multivariable analyses, corresponding dyslipidemic baseline values were the strongest predictors of improvements in levels of LDL cholesterol, HDL cholesterol, and triglycerides. By multivariable analyses, reductions in body-mass index and older age were strong independent predictors of reduction in triglyceride values following cardiac rehabilitation. However, low-baseline triglyceride values were independently associated with improvements in both LDL and HDL cholesterol levels. Using a

Table 2-3. Improvements in Coronary Risk Factors Following Cardiac Rehabilitation (N=237). Reproduced with permission from Lavie et al.[86]

Variable*	Cardiac Rehabilitation		% Change	P
	Before, Mean±SD	After, Mean±SD		
Total cholesterol, mmol/L (mg/dL)	5.40±1.06 (209±41)	5.28±0.96 (204±37)	−2	<.03
Triglycerides, mmol/L (mg/dL)	1.89±1.02 (167±90)	1.64±0.81 (145±72)	−13	<.0001
HDL-C, mmol/L (mg/dL)	0.98±0.28 (37.9±10.9)	1.05±0.29 (40.7±11.1)	7	<.0001
LDL-C, mmol/L (mg/dL)	3.6±0.96 (139±37)	3.47±0.83 (134±32)	−4	<.05
LDL-C/HDL-C	3.9±1.3	3.5±1.2	−10	<.0001
Body mass index, kg/m²	27.3±4.2	26.8±4.1	−2	<.0001
Body fat. %	24.2±6.3	22.9±6.2	−5	<.0001
Exercise capacity, METs	7.2±2.9	9.1±3.4	26	<.0001

*HDL-C indicates high-density lipoprotein cholesterol; LDL-C, low-density lipoprotein cholesterol: and, METs. metabolic equivalents.

model incorporating 13 clinical variables, improvements in lipid values with cardiac rehabilitation were only modestly predictable with the variables assessed, accounting for only 30% to 40% of the improvements in lipid values. These authors concluded (1) that atherosclerotic risk factors markedly improved following cardiac rehabilitation and exercise training, (2) that improvements in lipid values are modestly predictable, and (3) that those patients with the worst baseline lipid values had the most improvements in lipid values following cardiac rehabilitation. Patients with combined hyperlipidemia and low levels of HDL cholesterol are likely to require drug treatment.

Regular physical exercise has been identified as having a protective effect in patients with CAD. Hambrecht and associates,[87] from Heidelberg, Germany, studied the effects of different levels of leisure-time physical activity on cardiorespiratory fitness and progression of coronary atherosclerotic lesions in unselected patients with CAD. Patients were prospectively randomized either to an intervention group (n = 29) participating in regular physical exercise or to a control group (n = 33) receiving usual care. Energy expenditure in leisure-time physical activity was estimated from standardized questionnaires and from participation in group exercise sessions. After 12 months, repeat coronary angiography was performed and coronary lesions were measured by digital imaging processing. At one year, patients in the intervention group achieved an increase in oxygen uptake at a ventilatory threshold of 7% and peak exercise of 14%, whereas a significant decrease was observed in patients in the control group. To achieve a significant improvement in cardiovascular fitness, about 1,400 kcal per week had to be expended in the form of leisure-time physical activity. The mean energy expenditure in the intervention group was 1,876 kcal per week and in the control group, 1,187 kcal per week. In the intervention group, regression of CAD was noted in 8 patients (28%), progression of disease in 3 (10%), and no change in coronary morphology in 18 (62%). By contrast, CAD progressed at a significantly faster rate in patients in the control group (progression in 45%, no change in 49%, and regression in 6%). When the two groups were combined, the lowest level of leisure-time physical activity was noted in patients with progression of disease as opposed to patients with no change or regression of disease. These authors concluded that a regular leisure-time physical activity program can improve cardiorespiratory fitness and has a favorable effect on the course of coronary artery lesions.

Aspirin v Heparin

Théroux and associates,[88] from Montreal, Canada, evaluated the relative efficacy of aspirin and antithrombotic therapy with heparin in patients with unstable angina. Aspirin (325 mg given twice a day) or heparin (5000 units intravenous bolus followed by an infusion titrated to prolong the partial thromboplastin time appropriately) were compared in a double-blind randomized trial of 484 patients in two cohorts enrolled sequentially. The study was initiated at admission to the hospital at a mean of 8 ± 8 hours after the last episode of pain. The endpoints were assessed 6 ± 3 days later, when a decision for long-term management had been made. AMI occurred in 2 of the 240 patients (0.8%) randomized to heparin and in 9 (4%) of the 244 randomized to aspirin, an odds ratio of

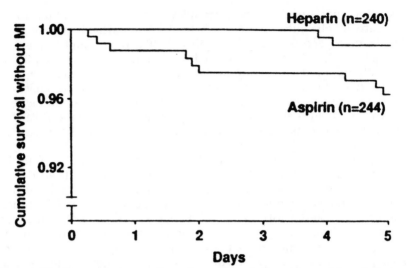

Figure 2-15. The survival curves for patients randomized to either aspirin or heparin as shown. A Cox regression logistic analysis was used to correct the baseline differences between the two groups. The differences between the two survival curves is statistically significant (p = 0.035). MI indicates myocardial infarction. Reproduced with permission from Théroux et al.[88]

0.22 and a risk difference of 3% with heparin (Figure 2-15). Survival curves with a Cox logistic regression analysis showed that the improvement in survival without AMI with heparin was independent of other clinical characteristics. Thus, this study documents that heparin prevents AMI better than aspirin during the acute phase of unstable angina.

Lovastatin

To assess the effects of lipid-lowering therapy with lovastatin on coronary angiographic findings in patients with CAD and to compare the findings with those of two lipid-lowering angiographic trials using similar endpoints, Blankenhorn and associates,[89] from the MARS Research Group, performed a randomized, double-blind, placebo-controlled, multicenter coronary angiographic trial involving 270 patients aged 37 to 67 years with total cholesterol levels ranging from 190 to 297 mg/dL (4.92 to 7.64 mmol/L) and angiographically defined CAD. All patients received a cholesterol-lowering diet and either lovastatin, 80 mg/day, or placebo. Lovastatin lowered total cholesterol level by 32%, LDL cholesterol by 38%, and the apolipoprotein B by 26% and raised the HDL cholesterol by 8.5%. Average percent diameter stenosis increased 2.2% in placebo recipients and 1.6% in lovastatin recipients (Figure 2-16). For narrowing 50% or greater, average percent diameter stenosis increased 0.9% in placebo recipients and decreased 4.1% in lovastatin recipients. The mean global change score was +0.9 (indicating progression) in the placebo group and +0.4 in the lovastatin group; 13 placebo recipients and 28 lovastatin recipients had global change scores indicating regression. Thus, treatment with lovastatin plus diet slows the rate of progression and increases the frequency of regression of coronary arterial narrowings (by

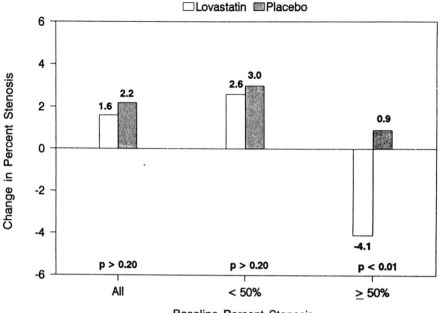

Figure 2-16. Average change in percent diameter stenosis as determined by quantitative coronary angiography. After adjusting for the percent diameter stenosis at baseline, analysis of covariance was carried out for all lesions (114 patients in the lovastatin group, 106 in the placebo group), small lesions (<50% stenosis) at baseline (112 patients in the lovastatin group, 105 in the placebo group), and large lesions (≥50% stenosis) at baseline (77 patients in the lovastatin group, 79 in the placebo group). Reproduced with permission from Blankenhorn et al.[89]

global change score), especially in more severe narrowings (by quantitative angiography). This is the third lipid-lowering trial to show a benefit using the global change score, an endpoint predictive of clinical coronary events (Table 2-4).

Differences between two of these trials, using quantitative coronary angiographic endpoints, may have theoretical bearing on the mechanisms by which lipid-lowering therapy operates at the level of the arterial wall.

Isosorbide Mononitrate

Chrysant and associates,[90] from Kenilworth, NJ, evaluated the efficacy and safety of extended-release isosorbide mononitrate tablets in patients with stable effort angina. In a double-blind study, 313 patients with stable effort-induced angina were randomized to receive placebo or extended-release isosorbide mononitrate: 30, 60, 120, or 240 mg once daily in the morning. Serial exercise testing was performed using the standard Bruce treadmill protocol on days 1, 7, 14, 28, and 42 immediately before morning drug administration and 4 and 12 hours after administration. After initial dosing, all groups that received extended-release isosorbide mononitrate had significant increases in mean total exercise time of approximately 30 to 50 seconds in relation to placebo 4 and 12 hours after

Table 2-4. Comparison of Results from the Cholesterol Lowering Atherosclerosis Study, the Program on the Surgical Control of the Hyperlipidemias Study, and the Monitored Atherosclerosis Regression Study.* Reproduced with permission from Blankenhorn et al.[89]

Trial	Baseline			Percentage Change from Baseline					GCS†
	Patients	Total Cholesterol	LDL	Total Cholesterol	LDL	Triglyceride	HDL	Apo A-I	
	n	*mmol/l.(mg/dl.)*		←		*%*		→	
CLAS (2 years)									
Niacin and colestipol	80	6.36 (246)	4.42 (171)	−26	−43	−22	+37	+19	+0.3
Placebo	82	6.28 (243)	4.37 (169)	−4	−5	−5	+2	+2	+0.8
POSCH (3 years)									
Bypass surgery	363	6.52 (252)	4.62 (179)	−28	−42	+12	+5	NA	+0.3
Control	333	6.52 (252)	4.58 (177)	−5	−7	+4	−1	NA	+0.5
MARS (2 years)									
Lovastatin	123	5.97 (231)	3.90 (151)	−32	−45	−21	+8	+3	+0.4
Placebo	123	5.95 (230)	3.98 (154)	−1	−2	+6	+1	+2	+0.9

*CLAS = Cholesterol Lowering Atherosclerosis Study
GCS = global change score
HDL = high-density lipoprotein
LDL = low-density lipoprotein
MARS = Monitored Atherosclerosis Regression Study
POSCH = Program on the Surgical Control of the Hyperlipidemias

† A positive score indicates progression of disease. In each trial, the average global change score was significantly smaller for the treated group ($P < 0.01$).

administration. On day 42, mean changes from baseline in total exercise time of patients who received 120 mg or 240 mg of extended-release isosorbide mononitrate exceeded placebo by approximately 50 to 60 seconds 4 hours after dosing and by 30 to 35 seconds 12 hours after dosing. No significant difference was detected between responses to extended release isosorbide mononitrate and placebo 24 hours after administration. Thus, there was neither significant activity nor demonstrable rebound of effort-induced angina at the end of the dosing interval. Transient headache was the most prevalent adverse experience. Extended release isosorbide mononitrate (120 mg and 240 mg administered orally once daily) significantly prolonged exercise time to development of moderate effort-induced angina 4 and 12 hours after dosing during long-term therapy, without development of nitrate tolerance. The drug was well tolerated, and no zero-hour rebound of effort-induced angina was observed.

Intranasal Propranolol

A new intranasal spray formulation of propranolol was developed to provide β-adrenergic blocking medication on an immediate basis to patients with angina pectoris. The effects of this spray or placebo were assessed by Landau and associates,[91] from New York, NY, in 16 patients with effort-induced angina in a blinded, randomized, crossover design study that compared placebo with intranasal propranolol spray (5 mg/puff) 15 minutes before exercise on a treadmill. One week later, each patient, acting as his/her own control, received the alternative treatment and repeated exercise. Mean plasma propranolol level with active therapy was 20 ng/mL. Patients with active spray demonstrated a significant increase in total exercise time than patients taking placebo (530 v 460 seconds), an increase in the time to 1 mm ST-segment depression on the electrocardiogram (384 v 327 seconds) and an increase in time to onset of angina (452 v 363 seconds). There was a blunting of maximal exercise heart rate with active therapy compared with placebo (120 v 133 beats/min), blunting of maximal exercise systolic BP (185 v 194 mm Hg), and blunting of peak double product, with more modest effects on resting heart rate. Propranolol spray is an effective approach for providing immediate β blockade and improving exercise tolerance in patients with angina pectoris.

Propranolol or Nifedipine or Diltiazem

Anti-ischemic therapy has reduced ambulatory ischemia and anginal symptoms and has improved exercise performance in patients with stable CAD. It is uncertain whether the pharmacologic response to each of these ischemic manifestations is the same for each patient. Borzak and associates,[92] from Boston, Mass, studied 50 patients in the angina and silent ischemia study who had all of these manifestations of ischemia. Patients were maximally treated with either propranolol, sustained release diltiazem, nifedipine, or placebo each for 2 week periods in a double-blind crossover fashion. With placebo, there was no correlation among the frequency of ischemic episodes by ambulatory ECG monitoring, exercise time to 1 mm ST-segment depression, or frequency of anginal episodes. Furthermore, for a given patient the efficacy of each active medication in reducing ambulatory ischemia was not correlated with response in anginal symptoms or exercise test performance. Within each of these clinical measures, efficacy of one drug was more strongly correlated with efficacy of another drug. These authors concluded that the different measures of ischemia, such as ambulatory ischemia on ECG monitoring, exercise performance on exercise test, and anginal symptoms are independent. Thus efficacy for each clinical endpoint must be assessed separately when considering response to drug treatment.

Nifedipine

Coronary vasomotion is influenced by a variety of factors, including atherosclerosis and diurnal variations in alpha-adrenergic tone. The effect of such factors on the coronary response to vasodilator drugs is unknown. To determine whether there is a diurnal variation to the response of coronary arteries to nifedipine and whether this response is altered by atherosclerosis, Raby and associates,[93] from Boston, Mass, studied 11 patients with smooth coronary arteries (6 in the morning and 5 in the afternoon), and 12 patients with irregular coronary arteries (6 in the morning and 6 in the afternoon). Changes in coronary blood flow and the vasomotor response of an epicardial coronary artery were measured before and after a 2 mg intracoronary infusion of nifedipine. There were no appreciable differences in epicardial vessel dilator response or coronary blood flow in the morning and afternoon among patients with smooth coronary arteries. By contrast, patients with irregular coronary arteries had a significantly diminished dilator response in the afternoon, without an appreciable change in coronary blood flow. It was postulated that normal coronary arteries maintain basal tone throughout the day. By contrast, atherosclerotic coronary arteries cannot do the same, increasing tone in the morning in response to catecholamines. When catecholamine levels drop in the afternoon, basal tone decreases in atherosclerotic vessels, and the dilator response to nifedipine is blunted. This observation may have an important impact on the expected benefits and timing of vasodilator therapy in CAD patients.

Nifedipine or Diltiazem or Nitroglycerin

Because it has recently been shown that ischemia in collateral-dependent myocardium may develop at a very variable threshold in angina patients, the aim of this study by Pupita and associates,[94] from Ancona, Italy, was to assess whether nifedipine and diltiazem can increase blood flow to collateralized myocardium. Nine patients with complete coronary occlusion filled by collaterals, with no other coronary stenosis, normal LV function, and reproducibly positive exercise tests were studied. They underwent exercise tests off therapy and after acute randomized administration of nifedipine (10 mg sublingually), diltiazem (120 mg orally), and nitroglycerin (0.5 mg sublingually), which is known to increase blood flow to collateralized myocardium. Following nifedipine, time to 1 mm ST-segment depression increased significantly (from 430 ± 176 to 576 ± 205 seconds), and heart rate and rate-pressure product remained unchanged. Similarly, diltiazem significantly increased time to ischemic threshold from baseline to 638 ± 125 seconds but did not change heart rate and rate-pressure product at 1 mm ST-segment depression. Submaximal rate-pressure products were significantly lowered by both nifedipine and diltiazem. Nitroglycerin not only significantly improved time to ischemic threshold but also increased heart rate and rate-pressure product; submaximal rate-pressure products were unchanged after nitroglycerin. Thus, it was concluded that in patients with chronic coronary occlusion and collateral circulation, nifedipine and diltiazem increase exercise duration; this effect is achieved through reduction of myocardial oxygen consumption rather than by increasing blood flow to collateral-dependent myocardium.

Low Molecular Weight Heparin

Collateral vessels provide an important function in maintaining viability of ischemic myocardium. Quyyumi and associates,[95] from Bethesda, Md, did a pilot study to determine whether exercise and low molecular weight heparin therapy with dalteparin sodium (Fragmin) would improve collateral function to ischemic myocardium in patients with CAD. Twenty-three patients with stable CAD were randomized to receive either subcutaneous dalteparin sodium (10,000 international units) or placebo for a 4-week period. Patients received daily subcutaneous injections of 10,000 international units for weeks 1 and 2 and 5,000 international units for weeks 3 and 4. During the first two weeks, patients were exercised to ischemia three times a day. At baseline and 4 weeks after treatment, treadmill exercise testing, exercise radionuclide ventriculography, and 48-hour ambulatory ST-segment monitoring were performed. Eight of 10 dalteparin sodium-treated patients compared with 4 of 13 placebo-treated patients had an increase in rate-pressure product at the onset of 1 mm of ST-segment depression. The duration of exercise to ischemia increased in all patients treated with low molecular weight heparin and in 62% of placebo-treated patients. The number and duration of episodes of ST-segment depression during ambulatory monitoring decreased by 30% and 35%, respectively, in the dalteparin sodium group but were unchanged in the placebo group. The decrease in LVEF with exercise was lower in 80% of dalteparin sodium-treated patients compared with 54% of placebo-treated patients. These authors concluded that this study provides interesting preliminary evidence suggesting that exercise and low molecular weight heparin therapy with dalteparin sodium lessened myocardial ischemia, presumably by enhancing collateral function. This conclusion is based on the fact that the combination of ischemia and heparin has previously been demonstrated to enhance collateral growth.

Melandri and associates,[96] from Bologna, Italy, examined the therapeutic efficacy of a low molecular weight heparin (Parnaparin) in patients with stable angina pectoris. In a double-blind, randomized, placebo-controlled trial, 29 patients with stable exercise-induced angina pectoris and angiographically proven CAD received a single daily subcutaneous injection of Parnaparin or placebo as well as aspirin and conventional antianginal medication over 3 months. Those patients randomized to Parnaparin showed a significant decrease in their fibrinogen level and improvement in the time to 1 mm ST-segment depression and the peak ST-segment depression. Canadian Cardiovascular Society class for angina pectoris was also improved by Parnaparin. Parnaparin did not affect ADP and collagen-induced platelet aggregation, but thrombin-induced aggregation was markedly reduced. The bleeding time was slightly prolonged, but this was not associated with any significant bleeding. Therefore, in patients with stable angina, low molecular weight heparin, such as Parnaparin, in addition to aspirin and conventional antianginal medication may help protect the patient with stable angina.

Hirudin

Zoldhelyi and associates,[97] from Rochester, Minn, evaluated the half-life, effect on anticoagulant variables, and safety of a new acting antithrombin, hirudin, in patients with CAD. Thirty-eight men and 1 woman with angiographic evidence of CAD were evaluated in a single-blind ascending-dosage study with a 6-hour intravenous infusion of recombinant hirudin or matching placebo. The median terminal half-life for hirudin was 2.7, 2.3, 2.9, 3.1, and 2.0 hours for the 0.02, 0.05, 0.1, 0.2, and 0.3 mg/kg/hour infusions. The prolongation in clotting as measured by the partial thromboplastin time desired was achieved in 62% to 77% of the patients within 30 minutes of starting the infusions and was directly related to dose. Plasma levels of hirudin and the activated coagulation time (ACT) in seconds correlated well, but there was considerable overlap between baseline ACT and ACT at plasma hirudin concentrations less than 1000 ng/mL. Prothrombin times were significantly prolonged only at a dosage of ≥0.05 mg/kg/hour. All variables returned to baseline values between 8 and 18 hours after the infusion. Bleeding times were not significantly prolonged. There were no obvious side effects resulting from the infusion of hirudin. No antibodies to hirudin were detected 2 weeks after the infusion. Thus, recombinant hirudin has a terminal half-life and life of 2 to 3 hours, and the activated partial thromboplastin time correlates well with plasma levels of hirudin and allows close titration over a wide range of anticoagulation. A 6 hour infusion of hirudin is well tolerated and appears to be safe in a predominantly male group of patients with stable CAD.

Hirudin v Heparin

In a study by van den Bos and associates,[98] from Rotterdam, The Netherlands, the effects of recombinant hirudin, a direct thrombin inhibitor, were evaluated in 113 patients with stable angina undergoing PTCA. Prior to PTCA, 20 mg of the recombinant hirudin was administered as a bolus followed by a continuous infusion or 10,000 units of heparin administered as a bolus and continued at a rate of 12 international units kg/hour for 24 hours. Infusions were adjusted to activated partial thromboplastin time levels. ST segments were monitored for 24 hours and angiograms were analyzed with quantitative techniques. In 74 of the hirudin treated patients and 39 of the heparin treated patients, 132 lesions were dilated. Myocardial infarction and/or emergency CABG occurred in 1 hirudin treated patient compared with 4 heparin treated patients. At 24 hours, complete perfusion was present in 91% of heparin and 100% of hirudin treated patients. Significant ST-segment displacement was found in 11% of heparin versus 4% of hirudin treated patients. Bleeding occurred only at puncture sites in 4 hirudin treated patients. Quantitative coronary arteriography did not reveal significant differences between the groups. Activated partial thromboplastin times were more often in the target range and more stable in the hirudin treated patients. Thus, these data indicate that hirudin may be safely administered to patients undergoing elective PTCA for stable angina and has at least as favorable an anticoagulant profile as heparin.

Hirulog

Selective thrombin inhibitors are a new class of antithrombotic drugs that, unlike heparin, can effectively inhibit clot-bound thrombin and escape neutralization by activated platelets. Hirulog is a 20 amino acid hirudin-based synthetic peptide that has shown promise in experimental models of thrombosis. Little information is available about the effects of hirulog in patients with CAD. Cannon and associates,[99] from Boston, Mass, randomized 45 patients undergoing cardiac catheterization, who were taking aspirin, to receive either (1) hirulog, 0.05 mg/kg intravenous bolus followed by 0.2 mg/kg/hour intravenous infusion until the end of the catheterization; (2) hirulog, 0.15 mg/kg intravenous bolus followed by 0.6 mg/kg/hour intravenous infusion; or (3) heparin, 5,000 units intravenous bolus. Serial activated partial thromboplastin time, prothrombin time, activated clotting time and fibrinopeptide A were measured. Hirulog produced a dose-dependent prolongation of all coagulation parameters; the 0.6 mg/kg/hour dose prolonged the activated partial thromboplastin time to 218% of baseline after 2 minutes and 248% of baseline after 15 minutes. The half-life of the effect on activated partial thromboplastin time was 40 minutes. The hirulog blood level correlated well with the activated partial thromboplastin time, prothrombin time, and activated clotting time. Both doses of hirulog potently suppressed the generation of fibrinopeptide A. There were no major hemorrhagic, thrombotic, or allergic complications in patients treated with hirulog or heparin. Thus, hirulog, a direct thrombin inhibitor, provides a predictable level of anticoagulation and appears to have a potent yet well-tolerated anticoagulant profile in patients with CAD.

Lidón and associates,[100] from Montreal, Canada, studied 55 patients with unstable angina to determine the efficacy of the new antithrombin, hirulog. Hirulog was given in an acute dose escalating study with each dose given for 30 minutes in 15 patients. Hirulog prolonged the activated partial thromboplastin time and fibrinopeptide A inhibition. Hirulog plasma levels correlated closely with the dose infused. A second protocol was performed to determine whether the anticoagulant and antithrombotic effects of the drug were sustained during a 72-hour infusion and whether such treatment prevented the complications of unstable angina. At the highest dose of hirulog infused (1 mg/kg/hour), failure to relieve symptoms of unstable angina occurred in only 1 of 21 patients. Fibrinopeptide A plasma levels decreased consistently at the highest infusion dose of hirulog. No deaths, myocardial infarctions, or bleeding complications occurred. Thus, these data suggest that hirulog infusions in patients with unstable angina quickly and reproducibly provide stable, dose-dependent anticoagulant and antithrombotic effects with a favorable clinical efficacy profile.

In an open-label pilot study of 20 patients with unstable angina (Braunwald class I–IIIB), Sharma and associates,[101] from Boston, Mass, administered hirulog as a continuous intravenous infusion for 5 days in a dose of 0.2 mg/kg/hour to produce an activated partial thromboplastin time of approximately 200% of control. The primary endpoints of the study were: death, development of a transmural AMI, and intractable angina needing interventions such as an intra-aortic balloon pump insertion, PTCA, and CABG. The secondary endpoints were the presence of an intracoronary thrombus detected on angiography and hemorrhagic complications during therapy. There was no death or transmural infarction in this study cohort; however, one patient developed intractable angina. Intracoronary thrombus was documented in two patients. Infusion of hirulog resulted in a steady prolongation of the activated partial thromboplastin time without any hemorrhagic or other adverse effect. Hirulog appears to be an effective antithrombotic agent that is well tolerated and may have advantages over heparin in the management of patients with unstable angina.

Amiodarone

In an investigation by Meyer and Amann,[102] from Zurich, Switzerland, 63 patients with stable angina (New York Heart Association class III) and a positive stress test despite triple therapy were randomized to a double-blind protocol, receiving either placebo or amiodarone in a dose of 600 mg/day for 10 days, followed by 400 mg/day for an additional 10 days, and then by 200 mg/day over a total period of 2 months. Comparable bicycle exercise times were observed at baseline in the amiodarone group (6.0 + 1.6 minutes) and in the placebo group (6.0 ± 1.8 minutes). With amiodarone, there was an increase in exercise duration (6.7 ± 2.2

minutes v 6.3 ± 2.2 minutes at 1 month and 7.5 ± 2.1 minutes v 6.2 ± 1.7 minutes at 2 months). Also, the amiodarone group had a significant decrease in the double product when compared with the placebo group at 1 month (14,134 ± 3,316 v 17,570 ± 4,092 mm Hg/min) and at 2 months (14,022 ± 3,303 v 17,298 ± 4,872 mm Hg/min). The degree of ST-segment depression at peak exercise was also significantly reduced. Combination therapy of amiodarone with conventional antianginal therapy is well tolerated and results in a significant improvement in exercise capacity and a mild reduction of symptoms in patients who have continued, limiting angina pectoris with conventional triple therapy.

REVASCULARIZATION PROCEDURE—GENERAL

Effects of Cost-Containment Policies

Lower rates of use of resources have been reported for the treatment of hospitalized patients covered by Medicaid than for privately insured patients. Cost-containment policies may exacerbate such differences in the use of hospital resources. Langa and Sussman,[103] from Chicago, Ill, studied patients with CAD who received care at nonfederal hospitals in California in 1983 (the year a Medicaid cost-containment program was implemented), in 1985, or in 1988. Within this sample of patients, the authors compared the rates of CABG or PTCA among patients covered by Medicaid, patients with private insurance covering fee-for-service care, and patients enrolled in a health maintenance organization (HMO). The study samples were made up of 49,167 patients in 1983, 47,809 in 1985, and 44,631 in 1988. The frequency of CABG or PTCA increased in all three insurance groups from 1983 to 1988, but it increased much faster in the fee-for-service and HMO groups than in the Medicaid group (Figure 2-17). Patients with private fee-for-service insurance were 1.66 times as likely as Medicaid patients to undergo CABG or PTCA in 1983, 2.01 times as likely in 1985, and 2.33 times as likely in 1988. Patients enrolled in HMOs were 0.96 times as likely as Medicaid patients to undergo CABG or PTCA in 1983, 1.23 times as likely in 1985, and 1.53 times as likely in 1988. Thus, the frequency of CABG or PTCA in California in 1983 was nearly twice as high for patients with private fee-for-service insurance as for patients enrolled in HMOs or for Medicaid recipients. The implementation that year of stringent cost-control measures by Medicaid may explain the slower increase in the frequency of CABG or PTCA over 5 years among Medicaid recipients as compared with patients in the fee-for-service and HMO groups. Different incentives for fee-for-service and HMO practice may explain the lower frequency of CABG or PTCA among patients enrolled in HMOs, although the rates of increase for these two groups were about the same from 1983 to 1988.

Differences in Usages by Race

To assess whether rates of coronary revascularization procedures differ between blacks and whites after PTCA is performed and to assess the relationship of these rates to hospital characteristics, Azanian and asso-

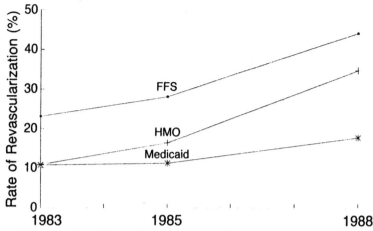

Figure 2-17. Unadjusted rates of coronary revascularization among patients covered by Medicaid, free-for-service insurance (FFS), or an HMO who had principal diagnoses indicating ischemic heart disease and received care at California hospitals in 1983, 1985, or 1988. Revascularization procedures included both coronary-artery by-pass grafting and coronary angioplasty. Reproduced with permission from Langa et al.[103]

ciates,[104] from Boston, Mass, performed a retrospective cohort study using 1987 and 1988 data on hospital claims and characteristics from the Health Care Financing Administration. One thousand four hundred twenty-nine acute care hospitals providing PTCA in the United States were examined. The patient study included a national sample of 27,485 Medicare Part A enrollees, aged 65 to 74 years, who underwent inpatient PTCA for CAD in 1987. White men and women were significantly more likely than black men and women, respectively, to receive a revascularization procedure after PTCA (57% and 50% v 40% and 43%). The adjusted odds of receiving a revascularization procedure after PTCA were 78% higher for whites than blacks. Statistically significant racial differences in the adjusted odds of receiving a revascularization procedure were present in all types of hospitals except rural hospitals, and these differences did not vary significantly by any of the four hospital characteristics. Among Medicare enrollees, whites are more likely than blacks to receive revascularization procedures after PTCA. Racial differences of similar magnitude occur in all types of hospitals. These differences may reflect overuse in whites or underuse in blacks, but they are unlikely to reflect access to cardiologists or hospitals that perform revascularization procedures. Potential explanations include unmeasured clinical or socioeconomic factors, different patient preferences, and racial bias at the hospitals performing PTCA.

Previous studies have found racial differences in the use of invasive cardiovascular procedures, which may be due in part to the greater financial incentives to perform such procedures in white patients. In Department of Veterans Affairs hospitals, direct financial incentives affecting use of the procedures are minimized for both patients and physicians. Whittle and associates,[105] from Pittsburgh, Pa, retrospectively analyzed the use of cardiovascular procedures among black and white male veterans discharged from Veterans Affairs hospitals with primary diagnoses of cardiovascular disease or chest pain during fiscal years 1987 through 1991. They used coded discharge data to determine whether PTCA or CABG was performed during or immediately after such admissions. Logistic-regression analysis was used to adjust for the primary discharge diagnosis, the presence of coexisting conditions, age, marital status, type of eligibility to receive care at Veterans Affairs hospitals, geographic region, and whether the hospital was equipped to perform CABG. Primary diagnosis was classified as AMI, unstable angina, angina, chronic ischemia, chest pain, or "other" cardiovascular diagnosis. After adjusting for all the potential confounders, they found that white veterans were more likely than black veterans to undergo PTCA (1.38), angioplasty (1.50), and CABG (2.22). Even when financial incentives are absent, whites are more likely than blacks to undergo invasive cardiac procedures.

Angioplasty v Bypass For Angina

The Randomized Intervention Treatment of Angina (RITA) trial[106] compares the long-term effects of PTCA and CABG in patients with one, two, or three significantly narrowed coronary arteries in whom equivalent revascularization was deemed achievable by either procedure. The first report is for a mean 2.5 years follow-up on the 1,001 patients randomized. Fifty-nine percent had grade 3 or 4 angina, 59% had experienced angina at rest, and 55% had two or more diseased coronary arteries. The intended procedure was done in 98% of patients. In 97% of CABG patients, all intended arteries were grafted. Dilatation of all treatment arteries was attempted in 87% of PTCA patients with an angiographic success rate per vessel of 87% (90% excluding occluded vessels). There have been 34 deaths (18 CABG, 16 PTCA), and the predefined combined primary event of death or definite AMI shows no evidence of a treatment difference (43 CABG, 50 PTCA; relative risk 0.88) (Table 2-5; Figure 2-18). Four percent of PTCA patients required emergency CABG

Table 2-5. Deaths, Myocardial Infarctions, and New Interventions During a Median 2 Year Follow-Up Since Randomization. Reproduced with permission from RITA et al.[106]

Event	CABG (n=501)	PTCA (n=510)
Death		
All causes	18	16
Pre-hospital discharge	6	4
Other cardiac death	4	4
Non-cardiac	8	8
*Non-fatal myocardial infarction**		
Definite	20	33
Silent	6	1
Patients with primary endpoint		
(death or myocardial infarction)	43	50
Subsequent interventions		
CABG	4	96
PTCA	16	93
Coronary arteriography	39	159

*Each patient is included only once; 3 patients (2 CABG, 1 PTCA) each had two infarcts. Also 1 patient in CABG group had a non-fatal infarction and died subsequently.

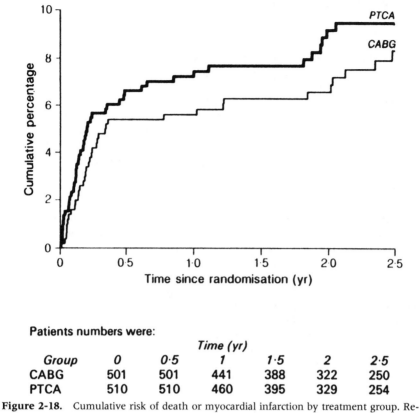

Patients numbers were:

			Time (yr)			
Group	0	0·5	1	1·5	2	2·5
CABG	501	501	441	388	322	250
PTCA	510	510	460	395	329	254

Figure 2-18. Cumulative risk of death or myocardial infarction by treatment group. Reproduced with permission from RITA.[106]

before discharge, and a further 15% had CABG during follow-up. Within 2 years of randomization, 38% and 11% of the PTCA and CABG groups, respectively, required revascularization procedure(s) or had a primary event, and repeat coronary arteriography during follow-up was 4 times more common in PTCA than in CABG patients (31% v 7%). The prevalence of angina during follow-up was higher in the PTCA group (eg, 32% v 11% at 6 months), but this difference became less marked after 2 years (31% v 22%). Anti-anginal drugs were prescribed more frequently for PTCA patients. At 1 month, CABG patients were less physically active, with greater coronary related unemployment and lower mean exercise times, than PTCA patients. Thereafter, employment status, breathlessness, and physical activity improved, with no significant differences between the two treatment groups. At 1 year, mean exercise times had increased by 3 minutes for both groups. These interim findings indicate that recovery after CABG, the more invasive procedure, takes longer than after PTCA. However, CABG leads to less risk of angina and fewer additional diagnostic and therapeutic interventions in the first 2 years than PTCA. So far, there is no significant difference in risk of death or AMI, and follow-up continues to at least 5 years.

Angioplasty v Bypass For Multivessel Narrowing

There is uncertainty regarding the selection between CABG and PTCA in many patients with CAD, especially in those with two-vessel disease. Randomized trials provide the best possible and most detailed data comparing therapy in these patients, and clinical data bases may be used to provide a current perspective. Weintraub and associates,[107] from Atlanta, Ga, compared the long-term outcome of patients with two-vessel CAD undergoing CABG or PTCA at Emory University hospitals in the years 1984 and 1985. Data on all patients with two-vessel disease diagnosed at Emory University who underwent elective PTCA or CABG in the years 1984 and 1985 were compared. Categoric variables were analyzed by chi-square and continuous variables by unpaired t test. Survival was determined by the Kaplan-Meier method and differences in survival by the Mantel Cox method. Determinants of survival were determined by Cox model analysis. There were 415 PTCA patients and 454 CABG patients. Surgical patients were older and had more frequent systemic hypertension, diabetes mellitus, prior AMI, severe angina, and CHF and more significant narrowing in the LAD coronary artery, totally occluded vessels, and LV dysfunction than did PTCA patients. Complete revascularization was achieved more often in surgical patients. There was no difference in Q-wave AMI in the hospital. No PTCA patient died compared with 1.1% of surgical patients. Five-year survival was 93% in PTCA patients and 89% in surgical patients, but there was no difference in risk-adjusted survival. Additional revascularization procedures were much more frequent in the angioplasty group (43% at 5 years) than in the surgical group (7%). Most additional procedures after PTCA were in patients with restenosis.

Patients with multivessel CAD and LV dysfunction represent a high-risk subgroup in whom CABG has been shown to improve survival compared with that of medically treated patients. The comparative benefits and risks of PTCA and CABG in this subgroup of patients are unclear. O'Keefe and associates,[108] from Kansas City, Mo, retrospectively analyzed 100 consecutive patients treated with CABG compared with a matched, concurrent cohort of 100 treated with multivessel PTCA. Early results favored PTCA; a hospital stay of 12.8 days was noted in the bypass group compared with 4.3 days in the PTCA group. In-hospital mortality rates were similar in the bypass (5%) and PTCA (3%) groups. Stroke was observed significantly more often in the CABG group (7% v 0%). However, late follow-up favored CABG patients; repeat revascularization procedures and late AMI occurred more frequently during follow-up in the PTCA group. During 5-year follow-up, superior relief from disabling angina (99% v 89%) and a trend toward improved survival (76% v 67%) were observed in the CABG group as compared with the PTCA group. Multivariate correlates of late mortality included age and incomplete revascularization but not mode of revascularization. Thus, in patients with multivessel CAD and LV dysfunction, early results favor PTCA, and late follow-up favors CABG. However, late survival was similar in both groups of patients who were completely revascularized.

The relative role of PTCA and CABG in patients with multivessel CAD is being evaluated. Rodriguez and associates,[109] from Boston, Mass, randomized 127 patients with multivessel disease and lesions suitable for either form of therapy, CABG (n = 64) or PTCA (n = 63). The characteristics of the two groups were the same. There were no differences in in-hospital deaths, frequency of periprocedure myocardial infarction, or need for emergency revascularization between the two groups. At 1-year follow-up, there were no differences in mortality or in the incidence of myocardial infarction between the groups. However, patients treated with CABG were more frequently free of angina, reinterventions, and combined cardiac events than were patients treated with coronary angioplasty (83.5% v 63.7%). In-hospital cost and cumulative cost at 1-year follow-up were greater for the CABG group than for the PTCA group. These authors concluded that the results of these techniques were relatively similar. At 1-year follow-up, however, patients in the CABG group were more frequently free from angina, reinterventions, and combined events than patients in the PTCA group.

Angioplasty v Bypass For Acute Coronary Occlusion

Although PTCA is successful in more than 90% of patients after acute coronary occlusion, overall mortality remains approximately 10% with higher subgroup mortality (ie, occlusion of the LAD coronary artery, multivessel CAD, age >70 years, cardiogenic shock) and early recovery of regional wall motion is marginal. Allen and associates,[110] from six medical centers in Europe and the United States, studied 156 consecutive patients with acute coronary occlusion documented by angiography, and they all underwent surgical revascularization with controlled reperfusion using controlled amino acid-enriched blood cardioplegic solution on total vented bypass. Ventricular wall motion was studied by echocardiography or multiple-gated acquisition scan on postoperative days five to seven and scored independently (0 = normal, 1 = mild hypokinesia, 2 = severe hypokinesia, 3 = akinesia, and 4 = dyskinesia). Results were compared with results in 1,203 patients with acute coronary occlusion treated by angioplasty in five reported medical series. Surgically treated patients were revascularized at longer ischemic intervals (6.3 v 3.9 hours) and had a greater incidence of left anterior descending occlusion (61% v 43%), multivessel disease (42% v 22%), and cardiogenic shock (41% v 10%), with 12 patients undergoing cardiopulmonary resuscitation in route to the operating room. Surgical results were superior in all categories, with overall mortality reduced from 8.7% after angioplasty to 3.9% after coronary bypass. All surgical deaths occurred in patients with preoperative cardiogenic shock. Regional wall motion recovered significantly (score <2) in 131 of 150 (87%) surgically treated patients with an average score of 0.9 ± 0.8 (normal to mild hypokinesia) despite longer ischemic times.

Rehospitalization After Angioplasty v Bypass

Lubitz and associates,[111] from Baltimore, Md, studied the rehospitalization experience of Medicare beneficiaries undergoing CABG or PTCA in 1986 and 1987 by following 53,715 patients who underwent CABG and 28,817 patients who underwent PTCA for 1 year using Medicare hospital claims data. The 1-year rehospitalization rate after CABG and PTCA was 629 and 863 per 1,000, respectively, compared with a rate of 607 for the Medicare patient population in general. About 45% of rehospitalizations after CABG and two thirds after PTCA were in categories determined by

Table 2-6. Related Event Groups* for Rehospitalization After Bypass and Coronary Angioplasty. Reproduced with permission from Lubitz et al.[111]

Event Groups	Percentage of All Related Event Rehospitalizations for Index Stays With:	
	Bypass	Angioplasty
Total	100.0	100.0
Cardiac procedures	14.1	57.1
Cardiac catheterization without revascularization	10.3	21.1
Subsequent angioplasty	2.7	25.0
Subsequent bypass surgery	1.1	11.0
Other related events	86.0	42.9
Cardiac-related groups	63.5	37.5
(1) Angina, acute myocardial infarction and other acute and subacute ischemic heart disease	17.7	23.1
Acute myocardial infarction	3.6	3.4
(2) Cardiac dysrhythmias	14.0	5.4
(3) Heart failure	23.9	7.7
(4) Other cardiac events	7.9	1.3
Infections†	8.2	1.2
Noncardiac vascular and other miscellaneous events	14.3	4.2

*The International Classification of Diseases—9th Revision—Clinical Modification codes for each event group are in reference 8.
†Most stays with principal diagnosis indicating infection were counted as a related event only if the stay occurred within 30 or 60 days of the procedure.

an expert panel to be possibly related to the original procedure (Table 2-6). After PTCA, there were 61 discharges per 1,000 for CABG and 140 discharges per 1,000 for a repeat PTCA. Rehospitalization rates for CABG after PTCA were significantly lower for female and black patients who underwent PTCA. The volume of rehospitalization after revascularizations makes it an important outcome measure. Medicare administrative records provide a unique source of information on rehospitalizations and make possible the monitoring of broad trends in the frequency and outcomes of coronary revascularization. The lower rates of CABG after PTCA for black and female patients are in line with other studies and bear further investigation.

PERCUTANEOUS TRANSLUMINAL CORONARY ANGIOPLASTY

Appropriateness of Use in New York

To determine the appropriateness of use of PTCA in New York State, Hilborne and associates,[112] from multiple US medical centers, retrospectively examined a random of 1,306 patients undergoing PTCA in New York State in 1990 at 15 randomly selected hospitals in that state. Most patients received PTCA for chronic stable angina, unstable angina, and in the post-AMI period (up to 3 weeks). Fifty-eight percent of PTCAs were rated appropriate; 38%, uncertain; and 4%, inappropriate. The inappropriate rate varied by hospital from 1% to 9%; the uncertain rate, from 26% to 50%; and the combined inappropriate and uncertain rate, from 29% to 57%. There was no difference in appropriateness when the institutions were grouped by volume (fewer than 300 procedures annually or at least 300 procedures annually), location (upstate v downstate), or by teaching status. Few PTCAs were performed for inappropriate indications in New York State. However, the large number of procedures performed for indications that were rated uncertain as to their net benefit requires further study and justification at both clinical and policy levels.

Prophylactic v Standby Cardiopulmonary Support

When patients at increased procedural risk undergo PTCA, several studies have suggested that prophylactic use of cardiopulmonary support might be helpful in maintaining stability of the patient. High-risk factors include dilatation of the LM coronary artery, poor left ventricular EF, and dilatation of the only patent coronary artery. Teirstein and associates,[113] from La Jolla, Calif, reported data from a national registry of 23 centers using cardiopulmonary support to compare the risks and benefits of prophylactic cardiopulmonary support versus standby cardiopulmonary support for patients undergoing high-risk PTCA. This retrospective study included 389 patients in the prophylactic group and 180 in the standby group. The groups were comparable regarding baseline characteristics except that left ventricular EF was lower in the prophylactic group. In the standby group, 13 of the 180 patients had irreversible hemodynamic compromise during angioplasty. Emergency institution of cardiopulmonary support was successfully initiated in 12 of the 13 patients in less than five minutes. Procedural success was 89% for the prophylactic and 84% for the standby group. Major complications did not differ between the groups. In patients with an EF less than 20%, procedural morbidity was significantly higher in the prophylactic group (41% v 9.4%), but procedural mortality was higher in the standby group (4.8% v 19%). These authors concluded that patients in the standby and prophylactic cardiopulmonary support groups had comparable success and major complication rates, but procedural morbidity was higher in the prophylactic group. Thus, for most patients standby cardiopulmonary support was preferable to prophylactic support during high-risk angioplasty. However, patients with extremely depressed left ventricular function (EF <20%) may benefit from prophylactic cardiopulmonary support.

Gradients Across Narrowings

In an investigation by Lamm and associates,[114] from Göteborg, Sweden, and Rotterdam, The Netherlands, a fiberoptic pressure sensor mounted on an 0.018-inch guidewire was used to measure the transstenotic pressure gradient in 30 patients undergoing PTCA with lesions considered suitable for quantitative coronary angiographic assessment. The aim of the study was to correlate pressure gradients with parameters obtained with quantitative coronary angiography. After intracoronary injection of 125 µg of nitroglycerin, multiple angiographic views were taken of the lesion. The pressure guide fiberoptic sensor was then positioned distal to the stenosis, and the pressure gradients were recorded before and after PTCA. There was a significant correlation between mean pressure gradients and percent diameter stenosis, absolute stenosis diameter, percent area stenosis, and absolute stenosis area. The closest relationship was found with stenotic flow reserve, which is an integrated parameter calculated from quantitative coronary angiography. With a measured gradient of >15 mm Hg, the sensitivity was 94% and the specificity 96% to predict a stenotic flow reserve <3.5. In conclusion, a statistically significant relation could be found between stenosis pressure gradients and angiographic parameters in this study, with lesions without complicated morphology. The independent information obtained by pressure gradient measurement may be of particular value in intermediately severe lesions or in stenoses where the angiographic assessment otherwise is difficult.

The functional significance of a coronary stenosis can be assessed by measuring the translesional pressure gradient. De Bruyne and associates,[115] from Aalst, Belgium, studied 34 patients in the setting of PTCA to evaluate the clinical relevance of the pressure gradient measurements by means of a PTCA balloon catheter. Both before and after PTCA, the mean pressure gradient across the stenosis was measured by means of a newly developed, 0.015-inch pressure-monitoring guidewire, first with only the wire across the stenosis (ΔP_w, considered as the actual gradient) and second with the deflated balloon catheter advanced over the wire in the stenosis (ΔP_b). Pressure gradients were correlated with quantitative coronary angiography of the stenotic segment. Before PTCA, mean ΔP_b was larger than ΔP_w. After PTCA, ΔP_b remained systematically higher than ΔP_w despite a significant reduction of percent area stenosis from 84% to 46% and an increase in minimal obstruction area from 0.98 to 3.49 mm^2. A significant correlation was found between ΔP_w and percent area stenosis, with a marked increase after percent area stenosis reached 80%. The correlation between ΔP_b and percent area stenosis was weaker, the scatter of the data was larger, and the inflection point of the curve was shifted toward less severe degrees of stenosis severity. The relation between the percent overestimation produced by the presence of the PTCA balloon catheter and either ΔP_w or the ratio between catheter and obstruction cross-sectional area suggested that in intermediate lesions and post-PTCA segments, the overestimation was poorly predictable. Thus, the presence of a PTCA catheter through a coronary stenosis causes a systematic and unpredictable overestimation of the actual pressure gradient. Even after PTCA, the pressure gradient measured with the balloon catheter does not reflect the hemodynamic significance of the dilated segment.

Measuring Collateral Flow

Collateral blood vessels are important for salvage of myocardium at risk in acute myocardial infarction. Piek and associates,[116] from Amsterdam, The Netherlands, designed a study to evaluate a new method for assessing coronary collateral flow and resistance. Angiography and flow velocity measurements of the contralateral coronary artery were performed in 38 patients undergoing coronary angioplasty for one-vessel disease. Angiography of the contralateral artery during balloon inflation revealed the presence of collateral vessels in 26 of the 38 patients (recruitable collateral vessels in 19). Fast Fourier transform spectral analysis demonstrated a significant transient increase of flow velocity during brief coronary occlusion in 15 patients with collateral vessels. Furthermore, electrocardiographic signs of ischemia were less in those 15 patients with collateral vessels. These authors concluded that the beneficial effect of collateral vessels during brief coronary occlusion is exerted by a significant increase of flow in the contralateral artery in combination with a reduced resistance in the collateral vascular bed. This method is capable of evaluating collateral vessels in terms of both flow and resistance.

In Women

Kelsey and associates,[117] from Richmond, Va, used the 1985–1986 PTCA National Heart, Lung, and Blood Institute's Registry to determine whether compared with men, women have a worse clinical outcome after PTCA. Data were collected from 16 centers, and the initial results were reported for 2,136 patients, including 546 women. Four-year follow-up status was available on 95% of the cohort. Although women were on average of 5 years older than males and had more cardiovascular risk factors and more severe angina, their CAD as determined by angiography was not more extensive. Angiographic success on a per-lesion basis was similar for women and men after PTCA (89% and 88%, respectively), and the clinical success rates were also the same, approximately 79% in both groups. However, women had more initial complications (29% v 20%) and a higher procedural mortality rate (3% v 0.3%). For patients surviving the initial procedure, four-year survival was similar for men and women. At 4 years, women had slightly fewer events, including AMIs, repeat PTCA, and/or CABG. Despite the higher proportion of women reporting the presence of angina and medication use at 4 years after PTCA, the proportion reporting improvement in symptomatic status was similar to men. Therefore, women undergoing PTCA have a higher procedural mortality risk than men, but otherwise, the success rate and long-term prognosis after PTCA are excellent.

To compare in-hospital mortality among women and men undergoing PTCA and determine whether mortality differences have changed recently, Bell and associates,[118] from Rochester, Minn, studied a consecutive series of 3,557 patients (27% women) who underwent 4,071 PTCA procedures. Two cohorts were analyzed: patients treated between 1979 and 1987 (n = 1,970) and those treated between 1988 and 1990 (n = 2,101). Women were older than men and more had class III or IV angina, unstable angina, angina at rest, cardiac failure, and diabetes mellitus, hypertension, and hypercholesterolemia. The PTCA was successful in 85% of women and 86% of men with an in-hospital mortality rate of 4.2% and 2.7%, respectively (P = .005). No significant change in mortality occurred in men between the early (2.2%) and late (3.1%) eras in contrast to a significant increase among women, 2.9% to 5.4% (P = .04). Periprocedural mortalities for women and men between 1979 and 1987 were 1.0% and 1.2% (P = not significant) and between 1988 and 1990 were 2.9% and 1.4% (P = .02), respectively. The multivariate odds ratio of in-hospital mortality for women versus men was 1.5, although six other baseline variables were more powerful predictors of in-hospital mortality. Accounting for body surface area resulted in no significant association between gender and in-hospital mortality. Periprocedural mortality was not independently associated with gender. In-hospital mortality among women has increased in recent years, but their higher mortality compared with men is related more to the severity of their underlying disease rather than gender alone.

In Mild Angina

To analyze the clinical and anatomic findings of patients undergoing PTCA for mild angina and determine the short- and long-term outcome, Berger and associates,[119] from Rochester, Minn, performed a retrospective data bank analysis of 3,729 patients who underwent PTCA at the Mayo Clinic between July 31, 1980 and Jan 30, 1991. Of these patients, 217 (6%) had stable Canadian Heart Association class I or II angina at the time of the procedure and constitute the study population. Patients were followed for a median of 37 months after the procedure. The mean age of patients was 60 years; 82% were men. Prior AMI occurred in 22% of patients. Multivessel disease was present in 68% of patients, and mean LVEF was 65%. PTCA was clinically successful in 196 patients (90%); 271 of 318 lesions (85%) were successfully dilated. There were no in-hospital deaths. CABG was performed during hospitalization in 12 patients (6%), and AMI occurred in 3 (1%); CABG or AMI occurred in 13 patients (6%). During follow-up of the 196 successfully treated patients, there were 9 deaths (5%), 16 patients (7%) developed AMI, 30 patients (15%) underwent CABG, and 36 patients (17%) developed severe angina. The probability of having any of these adverse cardiac events after 6-year follow-up was 39%; an additional 24% of patients developed recurrent mild angina during follow-up. These authors concluded that mild stable angina was an infrequent indication for PTCA at the Mayo Clinic. Although PTCA was successful in most patients with mild angina and complications were infrequent, most patients developed recurrent mild angina or had an adverse cardiac event during 6-year follow-up.

With Depressed Left Ventricular Function

Holmes and associates,[120] from Rochester, Minn, Pittsburgh, Pa, Providence, RI, Washington, DC, and Atlanta, Ga, characterized the outcome of PTCA in patients with decreased LV function and contrasted it with the results in patients with normal LV function. In the 1985–1986 National Heart, Lung, and Blood Institute's PTCA Registry of 1,802 patients undergoing PTCA, 244 patients (14%) had an LVEF of ≤45% (mean, 40 ± 7%). These patients had a greater incidence of prior AMI, longer and more complicated history of manifestations of CAD, and more extensive CAD than patients with well-preserved function. Eighty-eight percent and 91% of patients with the reduced and normal LV function, respectively, had successful PTCA of at least one coronary artery lesion. Patients with decreased LVEF had a decreased frequency of successful dilation of all lesions in which PTCA was attempted, 76% as compared with 84%, respectively. There were no differences in in-hospital complications. Death occurred in 0.8% and 0.7%, nonfatal AMIs in 5%, and emergency CABG was performed in 5% and 3% of the patients in the two groups, respectively. Patients were followed for a mean of 4 years. During this time interval, patients with decreased LVEFs had a reduced

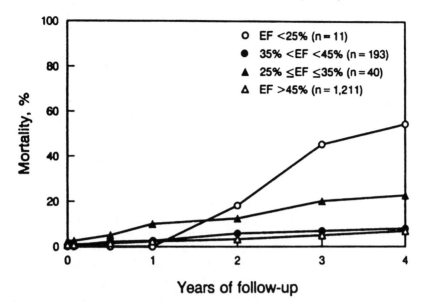

Figure 2-19. The 4-year mortality plotted by LVEF for the patients studied. Reproduced with permission from Holmes et al.[120]

survival rate compared with patients with normal LVEFs (Figure 2-19). Eighty-seven percent of the patients with mean LVEFs of 40% remained alive, and 77% were alive and had not experienced AMIs or required CABG. Thus, PTCA is effective in selected patients with depressed LVEFs. The initial outcome is good, but there is a reduced success for ideal dilation of stenosed coronary arteries and during follow-up; patients with reduced LVEFs had a reduced survival.

Effects on Blood Flow Velocity

The ability to evaluate physiology across plaques has been elusive in the past. Thallium studies after stress have provided helpful information but have been limited by a lack of quantitative measurements or observations restricted to specific arteries. Coronary velocity using Doppler measurements from intracoronary catheters has the ability to provide direct information on the physiology of stenoses before and after cardiac interventions. Ofili and associates,[121] from St. Louis, Mo, examined such measurements using a 12-MHz Doppler guidewire to measure flow velocity in proximal and distal coronary arteries utilizing fast Fourier spectral analysis. Measurements were made in normal arteries and compared to those in significantly stenosed arteries. Normal arteries had significantly higher peak diastolic velocity (64 ± 26 cm/s) and higher coronary vasodilator reserve (2.3 ± 0.8) versus stenotic arteries (41 ± 26 cm/s and 1.6 ± 0.7). There was higher flow in the first third and first half of the coronary cycle in the normal arteries. After PTCA, there was a greater increase in distal velocities in the arteries so treated. This normalization of Doppler derived flow velocity variable may prove useful as an additional endpoint measurement in interventional cases where the angiographic findings may be questionable. It should be pointed out, however, that because this is Doppler based technology, optimal placement of the transducer parallel to the blood flow is necessary to detect accurate peak velocities. This may be difficult in torturous arterial segments. Similarly, turbulence near lesions may affect the higher velocity signals.

For Long Narrowings

Balloon PTCA of long coronary artery narrowings has been associated with a lower rate of acute success and a higher rate of acute complications and restenosis than that observed for short narrowings. Angioplasty catheters with longer length balloons (30 and 40 mm) are now available, and the objective of a study by Tenaglia and associates,[122] from Durham, NC, was to determine the acute and long-term success for patients with long coronary artery narrowings treated with these longer balloons. All patients with long narrowings (≥10 mm) treated with long balloons at one institution over a 1-year period were identified, and acute and long-term outcomes were carefully documented. Procedural success (residual stenosis ≤50%) was 97%. Abrupt closure occurred in 6% and major dissection in 11% of narrowings. Clinical success (procedural success without in-hospital death, CABG, or AMI) was achieved in 90% of patients. Repeat catheterization was performed in 61 patients, and restenosis was found in 50% to 55%, depending on the definition used. The treatment of long coronary artery narrowings using angioplasty catheters with longer balloons leads to high rates of acute success. However, there is a high rate of restenosis. New interventional devices for long lesions should be compared with long balloons in a randomized controlled trial.

In Significant Left Main Narrowing

In an investigation by Nanto and associates,[123] from Osaka, Japan, to test the feasibility of synchronized retroperfusion as a support device of PTCA for high-risk patients, ten patients with LM trunk or near-LM trunk obstruction underwent PTCA with synchronized retroperfusion. An 8.5 F retroperfusion catheter was inserted from the antecubital vein into the coronary sinus. Arterial blood was supplied through the catheter into the myocardium with a retroperfusion pump during the diastolic phase by means of electrocardiographic triggering. In all patients, the narrowings were successfully dilated and an improvement of >20% in the luminal diameter stenosis was achieved; however, narrowing of >50% (58%) remained in one patient. In all patients, systemic hemodynamics were maintained for >30 seconds during balloon inflation. In seven patients, a 60-second balloon inflation was possible without any collapse of systemic hemodynamics. To test the protective effect of synchronized retroperfusion on myocardial ischemia and impairment of systemic hemodynamics, balloon inflation without synchronized retroperfusion was performed in eight patients after successful dilatation. The duration for balloon inflation with synchronized retroperfusion (71 ± 30 seconds) was significantly longer than that without synchronized retroperfusion (56 ± 30 seconds). The decrease in systolic aortic pressure, the increase in pulmonary diastolic pressure, and ST-T segment elevation in the precordial electrocardiogram during balloon inflation with synchronized retroperfusion were less than those during balloon inflation without synchronized retroperfusion. After PTCA, angina was not provoked by exercise stress testing in any of the ten patients. It was concluded that synchronized retroperfusion is a beneficial support device of PTCA for high-risk patients.

Hirulog

Topol and associates[124] determined the protective effect of a new specific thrombin inhibitor, hirulog, in 291 patients undergoing elective PTCA who were pretreated with 325 mg of aspirin and who were enrolled in sequential groups of intravenously administered hirulog instead of heparin. The hirulog infusion was maintained for 4 hours; and the primary endpoint was abrupt vessel closure within 24 hours of initiation of the procedure. Activated clotting times and activated partial thromboplastin times were monitored serially. Abrupt vessel closure occurred in 18 patients (6%). By intention to treat analysis, the abrupt closure event rate was 11% in patients receiving lowest infusion rate of hirulog and 4% in patients receiving the higher infusion rates of hirulog. There was no significant bleeding except for one patient in group 1, who received a two-unit transfusion. A strong dose-response curve of both activated clotting times and partial thromboplastin times was noted. No thrombotic closure occurred in a small number of patients with activated clotting times >300 seconds. Thus, these data indicate for the first time that it is possible to perform PTCA with an anticoagulant other than heparin in aspirin-pretreated patients. The use of the specific thrombin inhibitor, hirulog, is associated with the rapid onset, dose-dependent anticoagulant effect, minimal bleeding complications, and a rate of abrupt vessel closure of 4%.

Of Septal Perforators

Critical stenosis of a large septal perforator artery can cause significant myocardial ischemia. Because septal perforators are generally not accessible for bypass grafting, PTCA offers an excellent alternative for revascularization of these vessels. In an investigation carried out by Vemuri and associates,[125] from Philadelphia, Pa, the short-term outcome and long-term clinical follow-up following PTCA of the septal perforator was evaluated retrospectively in 21 patients. Fourteen of the 21 (66%) had previous myocardial infarction, 9 of 21 (43%) had previous CABG, 10 of 21 (48%) had previous PTCA, and 6 of 21 (28%) had CHF. Additional PTCA of ≥1 vessel was undertaken in all patients. Primary success of PTCA of the septal perforator was achieved in 20 of 21 patients (95%). The mean stenosis was improved from 98 ± 10% to 18 ± 12%. No acute closure, AMI, or emergency CABG was observed or needed during hospital stay. At long-term follow-up (18 ± 9 months), event-free survival was 95%. No cardiac death occurred. In 86% of cases, there was significant improvement in anginal class at 2 years. Five of the 6 patients with CHF showed marked improvement in functional class at 2 years. It was concluded that PTCA of the large septal perforator artery is technically feasible, with a high success rate, and does not increase the rate of acute complications of the procedure. Along with PTCA of other arteries, it provides long-term relief of angina in a majority of symptomatic patients with complex multivessel disease. Revascularization of large septal perforator arteries may provide an additional approach for more complete revascularization in multivessel PTCA.

For Left-Sided Narrowing With Totally Occluded Right Coronary Artery

Buffet and associates,[126] from Vandoeuvre les Nancy, France, compared the acute and long-term results of PTCA of the left coronary artery in 106 patients (group 1) with chronic occlusion of the right coronary artery with those of 106 patients matched for sex (92 male) and age (56 years) undergoing left PTCA with a normal right coronary artery (group 2). Before the procedure, group 1 had more unstable angina, more frequent prior AMI, and a lower LVEF. Acute results were not different in the two groups with respect to primary success and complications. At 6 months, 79 patients in group 1 and 71 patients in group 2 had reangiography; the rate of restenosis was 35% in group 1 and 42% in group 2. In both groups, LVEF increased significantly in patients without restenosis. In group 1, improvement was significant only for patients without collaterals to the occluded right coronary artery. At long-term follow-up, group 1 had higher rates of elective coronary surgery (19% v 9%), nonfatal AMI (6% v 3%), persistent angina (36% v 15%), and a trend toward a lower 4-year survival (93% v 97%). In patients with chronic occlusion of the right coronary artery, left PTCA can be performed with a low complication rate and provides a significant improvement in LVEF at 6 months in the absence of restenosis. However, at long-term follow-up, these patients have a significantly greater rate of elective CABG, death, and persistent angina.

In Saphenous Vein Bypass Grafts

Distal coronary embolization is thought to be increased in the PTCA of coronary bypass vein grafts. Liu and associates,[127] from Atlanta, Ga, performed 155 procedures of PTCA involving single vein graft dilatation. Distal coronary embolization was defined as an elevation of creatine phosphokinase greater than twice the pre-PTCA value and positive MB fraction. Twenty procedures were found to have embolism by this definition. Forty pre-PTCA angiograms were randomly selected from the remaining procedures and analyzed as a control group. Eight angiographic features were evaluated as possible risk factors for distal coronary embolization, that is, diffusely diseased vein graft, presence of thrombus, ulcerated lesion surface, marked eccentricity, large plaque volume, lesion angulation, abrupt proximal face, and ectasia. A diffusely diseased vein graft, presence of thrombus, irregular or ulcerated lesion surface, large plaque volume, and marked eccentricity were found to be important predictors by univariate analysis. A diffusely diseased vein graft and a large plaque volume were found to be important independent predictors by multivariate analysis. The presence of thrombus and an irregular or ulcerated lesion surface frequently coexist with a diffusely diseased vein graft. These authors concluded that a diffusely diseased vein graft and a large plaque volume are important independent predictors of distal embolization, and thrombus and an ulcerated lesion surface are also important.

Platelet Activation

Gasperetti and associates,[128] from Charlottesville, Va, studied 25 patients referred for PTCA of the LAD or circumflex coronary arteries. They hypothesized that PTCA in humans is associated with activation of platelets to specific platelet agonists and that this activation may be differently modified by different angiographic contrast agents. All patients were pretreated with aspirin and received heparin. Blood samples for assessment of platelet aggregation to serotonin, ADP, epinephrine, and collagen were obtained from the coronary sinus before contrast injection, after initial diagnostic contrast injection, and after three balloon inflations. Patients were randomized to receive iopamidol, diatrizoate, or ioxaglate. Contrast agents alone were not associated with altered platelet aggregation. However, PTCA was consistently associated with increased platelet aggregation to serotonin but not to ADP, epinephrine, or collagen. These effects were similar with the three contrast agents studied except that the use of iopamidol was associated with increased platelet responsiveness to all concentrations of ADP after PTCA. Therefore, PTCA in humans is associated with increased platelet aggregation in blood drawn from the coronary sinus. This effect is seen primarily when serotonin is used as an agonist.

Response to Acetylcholine Afterwards

Alterations in coronary artery responsiveness to a variety of agents, including acetylcholine, have been assumed to reflect changes in endothelial function. El-Tamimi and associates,[129] from Gainesville, Fla, and London, England, evaluated the response of coronary arteries to the intracoronary administration of acetylcholine eight days after successful coronary angioplasty. All eight patients showed a dose-dependent constriction in response to acetylcholine and experienced chest pain and ST-segment changes. Intracoronary nitroglycerin relieved the effects of acetylcholine. The coronary segments distal to the dilated site, but not at the dilated site, were hyperreactive to acetylcholine. They concluded that balloon angioplasty is accompanied by a profound alteration of distal coronary artery vessels. This may explain the positive response to exercise testing frequently observed one week after successful coronary angioplasty in the absence of restenosis.

Response to Serotonin Afterwards

McFadden and associates,[130] from Lille, France, examined by quantitative coronary arteriography the response of dilated and control coronary segments to intracoronary infusions of graded doses of serotonin, an endothelium-dependent vasoactive agent, and to intracoronary injection of isosorbide dinitrate, an endothelium-independent smooth muscle dilator in 15 patients who had undergone a single PTCA procedure and who had no clinical features of variant angina. Dose-dependent constriction to serotonin occurred at all measured sites. The mean ± SEM diameter reductions expressed as percent reduction in baseline diameter observed at proximal and distal control sites in the dilated and nondilated vessels, respectively, at the highest dose of serotonin were similar. The degree of constriction in distal segments was significantly greater than that in proximal segments. Thus, in dilated and nondilated vessels, serotonin causes significantly more constriction in distal than in proximal segments. In arteries undergoing PTCA, the vessel segments that had been subjected to PTCA had constrictor responses to serotonin that was more marked than in adjacent proximal control sites and equivalent to those in the distal vessel segments. This enhanced constrictor response could be related to changes in endothelial function after regeneration or to hyperreactivity of smooth muscle cells at the PTCA site.

Intracoronary Electrocardiogram

Progressive decrease in chest pain and surface electrocardiographic changes are commonly observed during successive balloon inflations in PTCA, which suggests a decrease in myocardial ischemic response. To assess this hypothesis, Koning and associates,[131] from Rouen, France, continuously recorded intracoronary electrocardiograms during four balloon inflations; each of the inflations was maintained to a minimum of 120 seconds in 19 patients who had significant stenosis in the LAD and normal LV function. Three successive QRS-T complexes were analyzed on surface and intracoronary electrocardiograms for measurements of ST-segment elevation 60 milliseconds after the J point. Surface electrocardiographic changes were compared with intracoronary electrocardiographic changes. On intracoronary electrocardiogram, ST area (in square millimeters) and T-wave amplitude (in millimeters) were also computed. Chest pain was noted as present or absent during each successive balloon inflation. Ability of intracoronary electrocardiogram to detect myocardial ischemia, which was defined as ST-segment elevation >1 mm during balloon inflations 1 to 4, as 89%, 89%, 84%, and 74%, respectively, and was higher than that of surface electrocardiogram, which was 68%, 63%, 68%, and 58%, respectively. On intracoronary electrocardiogram, when compared with the first balloon inflation, a significantly smaller increase in ST-segment elevation was noted during each subsequent balloon inflation, whereas a significantly smaller increase in ST area and T-wave amplitude was noted only during balloon inflation 4. The number of patients who experienced chest pain decreased from 15 to 13, 10 and 6 from the first to the fourth balloon inflation. This report demonstrates a progressive decrease in myocardial ischemic response during successive and prolonged balloon occlusions. The underlying mechanism of such an improvement, including collateral recruitment and/or metabolic adaptation process, requires clarification.

Late Outcome for Single and Multivessel Narrowing

The first PTCA was performed in Zurich, Switzerland, on Sep 16, 1977, by Dr. Andreas Gruentzig. King and Schlumpf,[132] from Atlanta, Ga, and Zurich, reported the long-term follow-up of all patients treated by Dr. Gruentzig in Zurich. Between 1977 and 1980, all 169 patients had been completely followed up for 10 years. One hundred thirty-three of the 169 patients underwent successful angioplasty with a 10-year survival rate of 89.5%. The survival rate was 95% among patients with single-vessel disease, and 81% among those with multivessel disease. Angiographic restenosis was present in 31% at 6 months. Late restenosis between 6 months and 10 years occurred in 8 patients. Additionally, progression of disease in undilated segments occurred in 31 patients. The patients with single-vessel disease were less likely to have bypass surgery and were more likely to be angina free at the 10-year follow-up than were patients with multivessel disease (79% v 67%). These authors concluded that this earliest angioplasty experience was also the first to demonstrate a difference in outcome between patients with single-vessel and multivessel disease. Although PTCA is now performed in more complex patient subsets, the long-term outcome of these earliest PTCA patients should be applicable to similar patients today.

The early and late outcome of patients who underwent multivessel PTCA in a one-stage procedure were described, and the predictors for clinical event and new revascularization procedure were identified by Le Feuvre and associates,[133] from Montreal, Canada. Of 1,937 patients treated by PTCA between 1981 and 1986, 203 (10%) had multivessel PTCA in a one-step procedure. A follow-up extending to 71 months was obtained in 195 patients (96%). Primary success was achieved in 91% of 494 attempted sites and complete revascularization in 65% of 203 patients. There were no in-hospital deaths. Acute complications occurred in 13 patients (6%), including non-Q-wave and Q-wave infarction and urgent CABG. Before PTCA, 126 patients were in class III or IV of the Canadian Cardiovascular Society classification; at follow-up, 84% were angina-free or in class I. Death occurred in 14 patients and nonfatal AMI in 18. Angiographic restenosis was diagnosed in 37% of dilated lesions in 96 patients. A repeat revascularization procedure for restenosis or progression of disease, or both, was needed in 92 symptomatic patients (47%). The survival rate at 7 years without the need for surgery or PTCA was 53%, and cardiac survival without AMI was 86% (Figure 2-20). The

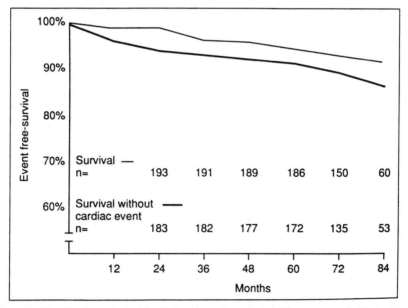

Figure 2-20. Total survival with all deaths, and survival without myocardial infarction and cardiac death in patients with multivessel angioplasty. Reproduced with permission from Le Feuvre et al.[133]

only independent predictor of cardiac death was EF. The rate of restenosis per patient was primarily determined by the number of segments dilated, whereas progression of disease was related to the number of nonsignificant coronary artery stenoses (<50%) at baseline. Thus, multivessel PTCA is a safe and effective therapeutic procedure in selected patients with multivessel disease. The long-term benefits are only limited by the high rate of restenosis in dilated segments and by progression of disease in initially nonsignificant coronary artery lesions.

Determinants of Dissection

Angiographic evidence of coronary dissection after PTCA is found in 25% to 30% of cases. Although patients are usually asymptomatic, in a small percentage, PTCA-induced coronary dissection results in luminal impairment and ischemic complications. The present study by Sharma and associates,[134] from New York, NY, was undertaken to identify factors responsible for a predisposition to coronary dissection after PTCA and to determine whether major (spiral and/or obstructive) and minor dissections share the same underlying risk factors. Clinical records and angiograms from 363 patients with 489 lesions were retrospectively graded for the presence and severity of dissection and complications. Both major and minor angiographic dissections were noted in 30%, and in 8.8% they were major. On multivariate analysis, the most significant correlates of any dissection included a balloon-to-artery ratio >1.1, calcification, presence of other lesions in the angioplasty vessel, and lesion length. However, in a multivariate model there were no variables that could predict whether a dissection would be major or minor. Only the mean total number of inflations was significantly different, but this was likely the result rather than the cause of dissection. Thus, a number of variables can predict the occurrence of angiographic coronary dissection after PTCA. Major dissections constitute a small fraction of the total number but are difficult to predict differentially.

Intra-aortic Balloon Pumping Afterwards

Kern and associates,[135] from St. Louis, Mo, and Washington, DC, measured coronary blood flow velocity with Doppler-tipped angioplasty guidewires in 15 patients who received intra-aortic balloon pumping for the usual clinical indications. Intra-aortic balloon pumping increased diastolic blood pressure 83% ± 35%. In nine patients before PTCA, peak diastolic coronary flow velocity beyond the coronary stenosis with mean diameter narrowing of 95% ± 7% was 5 ± 10 cm/s, and it was not changed by intra-aortic balloon pumping. However, after PTCA, the improved coronary luminal diameter narrowing to 18% ± 12% in 12 patients was associated with increased distal diastolic flow velocity signal and peak diastolic and mean velocities, which were further augmented by intra-aortic balloon pumping. Intra-aortic balloon pumping did not significantly increase distal systolic velocity integral or peak systolic velocity. These data indicate the lack of significant improvement in coronary blood flow velocity beyond critical coronary stenoses with intra-aortic balloon pumping and the restoration and augmentation in proximal and distal coronary blood flow velocities after reduction in critical coronary artery stenosis by PTCA.

Subcutaneous Heparin Afterwards

Abrupt closure of a coronary artery after successful angioplasty remains a problem for the interventionalist. Many laboratories continue to administer heparin intravenously for 12 to 24 hours in an attempt to alleviate this problem. But prolonged heparin therapy delays sheath removal and may lead to groin and vascular complications, and, thus, prolong the hospital stay. To test the hypothesis that subcutaneous heparin was as efficacious as intravenous heparin in preventing acute closure while reducing the vascular complications associated with extended sheath placement, Fail and associates,[136] from Philadelphia, Pa, prospectively randomized 151 patients to two groups. The intravenous group, 77 patients, received continuous intravenous heparin at 1,000 units/hour for 12 to 18 hours; the subcutaneous group, 74 patients, received 12,500 units subcutaneously every 12 hours for three doses after sheath removal 2 to 3 hours after angioplasty. The activated clotting time immediately after the angioplasty was 401 ± 108 seconds in the subcutaneous group, as compared with 368 ± 67 seconds in the intravenous group. Patients receiving subcutaneous heparin continued to show adequate anticoagulation, with a partial thromboplastin time of 85 ± 21 seconds obtained approximately 12 hours after the procedure. The partial thromboplastin time at discharge was statistically greater in the subcutaneous group at 49 ± 21 seconds versus 36 ± 13 seconds in the intravenous group. Abrupt occlusion was similar in both groups, but the hematomas and bleeding/oozing in the intravenous group was significantly higher when compared with that of the subcutaneous group, 16 versus 6 and 26 versus 7, respectively. The subcutaneous administration of heparin provides an alternative management strategy after angioplasty. It achieves adequate and extended anticoagulation, exhibiting a similar incidence of abrupt occlusion as compared with the intravenous administration, while decreasing hematoma and hemorrhagic complications because of early sheath removal.

Acute Ischemia Afterwards

The major cause of morbidity and mortality associated with PTCA is acute closure. Scott and associates,[137] from Atlanta, Ga, compared the clinical outcome of two groups of patients who experienced acute closure during PTCA. One group was treated during a period when intracoronary stents, laser balloons, and perfusion balloons were available for treatment of acute closure (group 2). These results were compared with the clinical outcome in a group of similar patients who were treated for acute closure during a period that immediately preceded the availability of these devices (group 1). One hundred sixty-six patients had acute closure in group 1, whereas 156 patients experienced acute closure in group 2. Baseline clinical characteristics were similar for both groups. There was no difference in EF, number of vessels diseased, degree of stenosis, or number of vessels attempted between the two groups. Patients in group 2 had more balloon inflations and longer balloon inflation times when compared with patients in group 1. Of the 156 patients in group 2, 47% were treated with either an intracoronary stent, laser balloon, or perfusion balloon. Group 2 patients had fewer Q-wave AMIs. In addition, peak creatine phosphokinase levels and mean residual stenosis were also lower in group 2 patients. There was also less CABG during the same admission in group 2 patients. These data suggest that there has been a recent improvement in the clinical outcome of patients with acute closure. This improvement may be related to a more aggressive use of prolonged inflation with standard balloons, in addition to the use of intracoronary stents, laser balloons, and perfusion balloons.

Coronary dissection is a major cause of abrupt arterial closure after PTCA but may also be associated with no discernable event. Deciding which dissections should receive further treatment is often a dilemma if the artery remains patent. Bell and associates,[138] from Rochester, Minn, examined predictors of major ischemic complications after coronary dissections. Fifty-eight patients with coronary dissections, but a patent artery at the completion of the PTCA procedure, subsequently had in-hospital abrupt arterial closure, AMI, emergency CABG, or died; they were matched to 58 control subjects with dissection but no event. Analysis of each angiogram was performed with the examiner unaware of the patient's history. Baseline angiographic and clinical characteristics of cases and controls were similar except for an excess of current smokers among the cases. Residual luminal diameter at the dissection site was 1.2 mm versus 1.6 mm with relative stenosis of 59% versus 43%, respectively. Dissections among cases were longer than among controls (11 mm v 7 mm). No significant difference was found in dissection morphology using two classification schemes or in final Thrombolysis in Myocardial Infarction study flow grade. Transient occlusion during the procedure, however, occurred in 47% of cases versus 5% of controls. Transient occlusion, residual percent stenosis ≥70%, and dissections ≥6 mm were independently predictive of major ischemic events.

Tschoepe and associates,[139] from Duesseldorf, Germany, investigated whether platelet activation is related to clinical outcome during the 24 hours immediately after elective PTCA. In 102 patients with high grade coronary stenosis admitted for elective PTCA, preprocedural platelet activation was characterized by flow cytometric measurement of the proteins CD62, CD63, and thrombospondin expressed on the platelet surface membrane. The prevalence of acute ischemic events during the 24 hours immediately after the procedure was related to the pre-PTCA platelet activation status. Fifty-six patients were classified as "nonactivated," whereas 46 patients showed an increased percentage of activated platelets and were classified as "activated." Two patients developed acute occlusion (2%) and four patients developed high grade restenosis (4%) as confirmed by repeat coronary angiography. All events occurred in patients classified as "activated." No patient received β-blockers, which were associated with lower expression of platelet membrane activation markers. In the nonactivated patient group, no clinical events were found. Thus, an analysis of platelet membrane activation markers may help to predict an increased risk of acute ischemic events after PTCA.

Major, adverse cardiac events (death, AMI, CABG, and reintervention) occur in 4% to 7% of all patients undergoing PTCA. Hermans and associates,[140] from Rotterdam, The Netherlands, examined prospectively collected clinical data and angiographic quantitative and qualitative lesion morphologic assessment and procedural factors to determine whether the occurrence of these events could be predicted. Of 1,442 patients undergoing PTCA for native primary CAD in two European multicenter trials, 69 had major, adverse cardiac procedural or in-hospital complications after ≥1 balloon inflation and were randomly matched with patients who completed an uncomplicated in-hospital course after successful PTCA. No quantitative angiographic variable was associated with major adverse cardiac events in univariate and multivariate analyses. Univariate analysis showed that major adverse cardiac events were associated with the following preprocedural variables: (1) unstable angina, (2) type C lesion, (3) lesion location at a bend >45°, and (4) stenosis located in the middle segment of the artery dilated; and with the following postprocedural variable: angiographically visible dissection. Multivariate logistic analysis was performed to identify variables independently correlated with the occurrence of major adverse cardiac events. The preprocedural multivariate model entered unstable angina, lesions located at a bend >45°, and stenosis located in the middle portion of the artery dilated. If all variables were included, then angiographically visible dissection, unstable angina, and lesions located at a bend >45° were independent predictors of major adverse cardiac events.

Acute occlusion after PTCA is a serious complication of coronary angioplasty. Van der Linden and associates,[141] from Leiden, The Netherlands, evaluated the potential benefit of prolonged dilation with an autoperfusion balloon catheter. Of 1,123 patients who underwent angioplasty, 83 had a refractory acute occlusion. Thirty-five patients were treated with extended dilation (17 ± 6 hours). Angiographically successful redilation with a mean residual percent diameter stenosis of 13.5% was achieved in 68% of 34 patients. Five patients underwent CABG. Three patients who were poor surgical candidates died. There was one new Q-wave AMI and one death that occurred during extended dilation. Overall success defined as angiographic success and freedom from major events was obtained in 57% of patients. Of the variables studied, only multilesion dilation was significantly associated with an unfavorable outcome. During a mean follow-up period of 14 months, two patients underwent repeat angioplasty, one sustained an infarction, and three underwent elective bypass surgery. These authors concluded that approximately half of the patients undergoing initial PTCA, who had a refractory occlusion, could be reverted to a successful procedure by prolonged dilation with an autoperfusion balloon catheter.

Restenosis

The role of supine bicycle stress echocardiography for detecting restenosis after PTCA was evaluated by Hecht and associates,[142] from Daly City, Calif, in 80 patients, 41 with single-vessel and 39 with multivessel PTCA. Total revascularization was performed in 54 patients, and partial revascularization in 26 patients. Restenosis was angiographically demonstrated in 60 patients (75%) and in 72 vessels (56%) 6 months after PTCA. The results for detecting restenosis were: (1) supine bicycle stress echocardiography versus exercise electrocardiographic sensitivity, 87% versus 55%; (2) specificity, 95% versus 79%; and (3) accuracy, 89% versus 61%. Supine bicycle stress echocardiography was 83% sensitive, 95% specific, and 88% accurate for restenosis detection in specific vessels with comparable results for single-vessel versus multivessel PTCA and total versus partial revascularization. These authors concluded that supine bicycle stress echocardiography is an excellent tool for identifying restenosis after PTCA.

Weintraub and associates,[143] from Atlanta, Ga, determined the clinical events in patients with restenosis or continued patency following PTCA in a total of 3,363 patients undergoing angiographic restudy 4 months to 1 year after PTCA compared with 3,858 patients not undergoing angiographic restudy. In the restudy population, 1,570 had restenosis and 1,793 had patent arteries at all sites dilated. The restenosis patients were older and had more systematic hypertension, more diabetes, more severe angina, and more multivessel CAD with more severe stenoses and less satisfactory original results. At restudy, in patients without restenosis, 39% had angina versus 71% in patients with restenosis. There were few deaths in the first 6 months in both groups. At 6 years, the survival rate was 0.95 without restenosis and 0.93 with restenosis. At 6 months and 6 years, freedom from AMI was 0.97 and 0.88 without restenosis and 0.93 and 0.85 with restenosis. Multivariate analysis demonstrated that restenosis after PTCA was an independent correlate of AMI but not mortality. At 6 months and 6 years, freedom from the need for CABG was 0.99 and 0.94 without restenosis and 0.91 and 0.78 with restenosis. At 6 months and 6 years, freedom from the need for repeat PTCA was 0.96 and 0.76 without restenosis and 0.44 and 0.20 with restenosis. The highest event rates were noted in the patients with restenosis with recurrent chest pain. Thus, patients with restenosis are more likely to have recurrent angina and an increased risk of AMI.

No medical therapy has been shown to reduce the rate of restenosis following PTCA. Gapinski and associates,[144] from Milwaukee, Wis, examined the existing evidence for the use of omega-3 fatty acids in this capacity with the tool of meta-analysis. A computerized search and a bibliographic review of published articles were performed. Abstracts were identified through journals, *Index Medicus*, and an unpublished listing of recent requests for fish oil for experimental use. All English-language randomized clinical trials with available reports were included in the analysis. The quality, design differences, and outcomes were evaluated for each study. For four studies that used angiography to define coronary restenosis, the absolute difference in restenosis rates between treatment and control groups was 13.9%. Furthermore, regression analysis revealed a positive linear relation between the dose of omega-3 fatty acids used and the absolute difference in restenosis rates. When three studies that used stress testing as a means of determining restenosis rates were added to the four studies that used angiography, the risk difference was 5.1%. Restenosis after PTCA is reduced by supplemental fish oils, and the extent of the observed benefit may be dependent on the dose of omega-3 fatty acids used (Figure 2-21).

Bauters and associates,[145] from Lille, France, tested by quantitative coronary angiography the angiographic probability of restenosis when repeat PTCA was performed at a site where restenosis had occurred after two previous PTCA procedures. Among 99 consecutive patients who underwent a third PTCA procedure, 96 had successful procedures. Uncomplicated failure (residual stenosis ≥50%) occurred in 3 patients. No major complications occurred. Follow-up PTCA was routinely advised. It was performed in 83 patients (86%) with successful procedures. Restenosis occurred in 32 patients (39%). An interval of <3 months between the second and third angioplasty was strongly associated with the occurrence of further restenosis after a third procedure. Thus, the angiographic probability of further restenosis after three successive PTCA

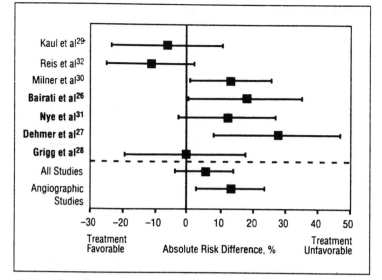

Figure 2-21. The differences in the percentage of restenosis between the treatment and control groups and 95% confidence intervals are given for the individual and pooled studies. The studies in bold print used angiography to determine the restenosis rates. The bottom estimates are pooled results. Reproduced with permission from Gapinski et al.[144]

procedures at the same site is similar to that reported after a first PTCA. Patients who undergo a third PTCA within three months of a previous procedure at the same site have a much higher risk of subsequent restenosis.

Rensing and associates,[146] for the CARPORT Study Group, used quantitative coronary angiography on 666 successfully dilated lesions at PTCA and at 6-month follow-up to attempt to determine whether a lesion characteristic would predict the risk of restenosis. Multivariate linear regression analysis was performed to obtain variables with an independent contribution to the prediction of the absolute change in minimal luminal diameter. Diabetes mellitus, duration of angina <2.3 months, gain in minimal luminal diameter at PTCA, pre-PTCA minimal luminal diameter, lesion length ≥6.8 mm, and thrombus after PTCA were independently predictive of change in minimal luminal diameter. Overall prediction of the model was poor, but percentage correct classification for a predicted change between -0.1 and -0.4 mm was approximately 10%. Lesions showing no change or regression and lesions showing large progression were more easily predictable. Thus, renarrowing after successful PTCA as determined with contrast angiography is a process that cannot be accurately predicted by simple clinical, morphological, and lesion characteristics.

Serruys and associates,[147] in a multicenter trial, evaluated the potential protective effect of ketanserin, a serotonin S_2 receptor antagonist that inhibits platelet activation and vasoconstriction induced by serotonin, and the mitogenic effect of serotonin on vascular smooth-muscle cells. A randomized, double-blind, placebo-controlled trial was performed to assess the effects of ketanserin in restenosis prevention after PTCA. Patients received either ketanserin as a loading dose of 40 mg one hour before

PTCA followed by a maintenance dose of 40 mg twice a day for 6 months or matched placebo. All patients received aspirin for 6 months. Coronary angiograms before PTCA, after PTCA, and at 6 months were analyzed by quantitative coronary arteriography. Six hundred fifty-eight patients were entered in the intention-to-treat analysis. Primary clinical endpoint was reached by 92 patients (28%) in the ketanserin group and 104 patients (32%) in the placebo group. Quantitative coronary arteriography after PTCA and at follow-up was available in 592 patients. There was no difference in mean luminal diameter between post-PTCA and follow-up angiograms in the ketanserin-treated and placebo-treated patients. Thus, ketanserin, at the dose administered in this trial, failed to reduce the loss in minimal lumen diameter during follow-up after PTCA and did not significantly improve the clinical outcome.

In a study by Marie and associates,[148] from Nancy, France, the usefulness of exercise single-photon emission computed tomography-thallium for detecting asymptomatic restenosis was assessed prospectively in 62 patients with angina before PTCA, who underwent ≤6-month reangiography and exercise single-photon emission computed tomography-thallium imaging. Among patients with restenosis, 9 had recurrence of angina, but 8 did not. These two subgroups had equivalent percentages of restenosis (71% ± 1.7% v 64% ± 16%) and extent of reversible thallium defects (2.8 ± 1.7 v 4.1 ± 2.6), and both subgroups had poorer hemodynamic responses to exercise compared with patients without restenosis. Exercise testing detected fewer patients with restenosis compared with exercise single-photon emission computed tomography-thallium imaging, especially among asymptomatic patients (25% v 100%). Asymptomatic restenosis occurs frequently, induces an amount of stress ischemia equivalent to that of symptomatic restenosis, and is efficiently detected by exercise single-photon emission computed tomography-thallium with rest reinjection but not by exercise testing.

To determine the results of PTCA for a first restenosis, the clinical, anatomic, and procedural data of 400 consecutive patients were compared with the data of 507 consecutive patients undergoing a first PTCA in a study by Piessens and associates,[149] from Leuven, Belgium. After PTCA for restenosis, emergency redilatation had to be performed in only 0.7% of the patients versus 3.1% of the control group; nevertheless, the major in-hospital event (death, AMI, emergency CABG, and cerebrovascular accident) rate for patients was only slightly lower (3.3% v 4.2%). During the 6-month follow-up period, there were no cardiac deaths and only two AMIs in the study group, but recurrent ischemia was more frequent (37% v 31%) and resulted in considerably more elective CABG (16% v 2.6%). In the study group, stepwise discriminant analysis revealed four variables significantly related to the occurrence of a second restenosis: time interval between first and second PTCA, male gender, severity of angina, and complexity of the restenotic lesions. However, their individual predictive power was low. It was concluded that, compared with PTCA for primary lesions, PTCA for restenosis was associated with fewer periprocedural complications and, after 6-month follow-up, serious cardiac events were almost nonexistent, but recurrent ischemia was more frequent.

Weintraub and associates,[150] from Atlanta, Ga, determined whether in patients with two sites dilated by PTCA, the sites undergo restenosis independently. Although restenosis remains a critical limitation after

PTCA, there is little information separating site and patient-dependent determinants of restenosis. In particular, if patients with two sites dilated have restenosis at zero or two sites more frequently and at one site less frequently than expected by random chance, then patient-related factors may be important in the restenosis process. The source of data was the clinical data base at Emory University. Patients who had previous CABG or PTCA and those who underwent PTCA in the setting of AMI were excluded. In all, 515 patients with two sites dilated undergoing angiographic restudy at 4 months to 1 year after PTCA formed the study population. Site 1 was the first site dilated. At site 1, 224 of 515 sites (45%) were restenotic, and at site 2, 193 (33%) were restenotic. Multiple clinical and angiographic variables were analyzed as possible correlates of restenosis. The most powerful univariate and multivariate correlate of restenosis at either site 1 or 2 was the behavior of the other site. If site 2 was patent, then site 1 was restenotic 28% of the time compared with 69% if site 2 was restenotic. If site 1 was patent, site 2 was restenotic 20% of the time compared with 60% if site 1 was restenotic. This relation was stronger if the 2 sites were in the same coronary artery. Thus, patients cluster with either zero or two sites restenosed. The data support the importance of patient factors that may not have been identified as part of the cause of restenosis after PTCA.

To determine the usefulness of dobutamine stress echocardiography for detecting restenosis after PTCA, Heinle and associates,[151] from Durham, NC, compared the results of coronary arteriography and dobutamine stress echocardiography in 103 patients 6 months after PTCA. The dobutamine stress echocardiograms were obtained on the same day as the coronary arteriograms, which were analyzed by both quantitative and visual estimates of luminal narrowing. The angiographic restenosis rate was 44% by quantitative and 31% by visual estimates of stenosis. Dobutamine stress echocardiography was abnormal in 38% of previously dilated regions with restenosis and normal in 79% of previously dilated regions without restenosis by quantitative coronary angiography. Dobutamine stress echocardiography was concordant in 69% of 16 patients with multivessel CAD compared with 40% of 41 patients with one-vessel CAD. By quantitative coronary angiography, 64% of patients with significant disease in the LAD were identified by dobutamine stress echocardiography compared with 12% and 24% of patients with narrowing in the LC and RC, respectively. Concordance was seen in 79% of patients with baseline wall-motion abnormalities compared with 54% of patients without baseline wall-motion abnormalities. Dobutamine stress echocardiography has a low sensitivity but high specificity for detecting restenosis after coronary angioplasty, which may be explained in part by the high prevalence of one-vessel disease in this patient population. The variables associated with significantly higher degrees of concordance were the presence of LAD disease, multivessel disease, and baseline wall-motion abnormalities.

Restenosis Differences After Angioplasty, Stenting and Atherectomy

Restenosis following interventional coronary techniques continues to be a major issue. Kuntz and associates,[152] from Boston, Mass, developed a quantitative model that explains late (6-month) lumen narrowing as

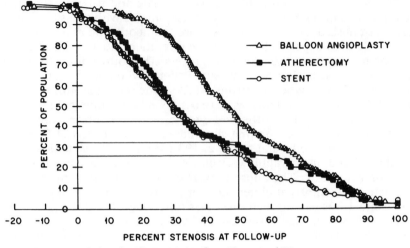

Figure 2-22. Reproduced with permission from Kuntz et al.[152]

the difference between the immediate gain and the subsequent normally distributed late loss in lumen diameter. In 524 consecutive lesions, lumen diameter was measured immediately before and after coronary intervention, which included stenting (102), directional atherectomy (134), and conventional balloon angioplasty. Four hundred seventy-five underwent follow-up angiography 3 to 6 months later. According to the model developed, three indexes of restenosis (late lumen diameter, late percent stenosis, and binary restenosis) depended solely on the immediate lumen diameter after the procedure and the immediate residual percent stenosis, but not on the specific intervention used. The late loss in lumen diameter varied directly with the immediate gain provided by the intervention and the "loss index" (a measure that corrects for differences in immediate gain) and was uniform among all three interventions. They concluded that it was the immediate result and not the procedure used that determined late outcome after coronary intervention. Figure 2-22 outlines the cumulative distribution of follow-up percent stenoses among the three interventions. As illustrated, there was a smaller mean lumen diameter in the segments treated by conventional angioplasty compared with atherectomy or stenting. The better results with the latter two techniques, however, were not due to reduced late loss but due to a larger earlier gain.

CORONARY ATHERECTOMY

A number of new devices have emerged for use by the interventional cardiologist. Stertzer and associates,[153] from Daly City, Calif, reported a consecutive series of 242 patients having 302 coronary rotational ablation procedures. Of the lesions, 7.5% were classified as American College of Cardiology/American Heart Association type A and 92.5% as either type B or type C. Procedural success was achieved in 284 or 94% of the procedures and in 95.4% of the 346 lesions. Five procedures were unsuccessful. A major cardiac event occurred in 4.3% of cases with 3% of these directly due to the ablation procedure. Six patients had a Q-wave myocardial infarction, and 2 additional patients had a Q-wave infarction and required emergency surgery. There were no procedural deaths in this initial series. Follow-up for a mean time of 9 months showed that 95.6% were alive and free of myocardial infarction. An overall estimated restenosis rate was 37%. These data suggest that this device is a reasonable candidate for use by the interventional cardiologist. This study, however, was not randomized or compared with other techniques. Subsequent to this report, the device was removed from the market for a short period of time to correct some mechanical problems and has now been returned to the marketplace.

Repeat angiography has been used as a standard technique for evaluating the results of interventional procedures on coronary lesions. Intracoronary ultrasound is a new technique that may provide direct and different kinds of information. Suarez de Lezo and associates,[154] from Cordoba, Spain, evaluated intracoronary ultrasound in 52 patients who were treated by atherectomy using ultrasound guidance. They also obtained quantitative histologic morphometric information from the specimens and follow-up echo angiographic evaluations an average of 6 months later. In correlating the echo pictures with the histology, they noted that echogenic plaques had a higher collagen and calcium content, whereas echolucent plaques had an increased level of fibrin, nuclei, and lipids. Ultrasound plaque reduction after atherectomy was greater in the echolucent as compared with the echogenic plaques as correlated with the weight of the resected material. At follow-up, an average of 6 months later, 13 of 22 patients had angiographic and ultrasound evidence of restenosis. The incidence of restenosis was higher in patients with echolucent (100%) than in echogenic (33%) plaques. These investigators also noted that there was a higher proportion of nuclear content in the resected material of patients who developed restenosis after atherectomy. One limitation of this study is that the study group predominated with patients who had unstable angina. They may have had more complex and active lesions than patients with stable CAD. It is also clear that the division into echolucent and echodense lesions is quite subjective and therefore might vary between investigators. Nevertheless it is clear that ultrasound guidance of directional atherectomy is helpful and may be predictive in the future of those plaques that are best treated with this technique.

Neointimal proliferation leading to restenosis frequently develops after PTCA. This process is associated with a change in vascular smooth-muscle cells from a contractile (quiescent) phenotype to a synthetic or proliferating (activated) one. Simons and associates,[155] from Boston, Mass, investigated whether the presence of activated smooth-muscle cells in coronary plaques at the time of coronary atherectomy predispose patients to subsequent restenosis. The authors used in situ hybridization to study the expression of messenger RNA in coronary-atherectomy specimens from 20 patients. Plaque material was hybridized with a probe for the B isoform of human nonmuscle myosin heavy chain, a major nonmuscle myosin isoform in activated, but not quiescent, smooth-muscle cells. Angiographic follow-up data were obtained a mean of 174 ± 54

days after atherectomy in 16 of the 20 patients, and the extent of recurrent luminal narrowing was analyzed quantitatively. The presence of restenosis was assessed by exercise thallium scintigraphy in the other 4 patients. Atherectomy specimens from 10 of the 20 patients showed hybridization with the probe, defined as the clustering of more than 20 silver grains per cell nucleus in more than 10 nuclei in five high-power fields (×250); specimens from the other 10 patients showed no such hybridization. At follow-up, restenosis had developed in 8 of the 10 patients with positive hybridization results but was absent in 9 of the 10 patients with negative results. The degree of late loss in luminal diameter was significantly higher in patients with positive hybridization results than in those with negative results (ratio of late loss to immediate gain after atherectomy, 0.8 ± 0.3 v 0.4 ± 0.3). The authors concluded that the expression of the B isoform of nonmuscle myosin heavy chain is increased in some coronary atherosclerotic plaques and that this increase in expression identifies a group of lesions at high risk for restenosis after atherectomy.

Although encouraging initial results have been demonstrated after directional atherectomy, the mechanisms and predictors of late lumen loss and restenosis after this procedure have not been evaluated. To examine these issues, Popma and associates,[156] from Washington, DC, obtained clinical and angiographic follow-up in 262 and 212 of 274 patients undergoing successful directional coronary atherectomy. Symptom recurrence developed in 87 patients (33%) and angiographic restenosis was found in 93 patients (44%). Restenosis was highest in restenotic lesions in saphenous vein grafts and lowest in new-onset lesions in the LAD and LC coronary arteries. Residual lumen diameter immediately after atherectomy was smaller in restenotic lesions and in lesions 210 mm in length. Late lumen loss was associated with the minimal lumen diameter immediately after atherectomy, saphenous vein graft lesion location, and male gender. Restenotic lesions, narrowings ≥10 mm in length, saphenous vein graft lesion location, and male gender were independent predictors for restenosis. It is concluded that restenosis after directional atherectomy is related both to factors resulting in a suboptimal initial result and to factors contributing to excessive late lumen loss. These results may have implications for lesion selection in patients undergoing directional coronary atherectomy.

Although intimal hyperplasia is a frequent occurrence after arterial interventional procedures, the overall frequency and significance of intimal hyperplasia in primary coronary lesions has not been previously addressed. Miller and associates,[157] from Boston, Mass, examined the incidence of intimal hyperplasia using standard light microscopy in specimens obtained from native coronary arteries of patients undergoing directional coronary atherectomy. The associated clinical history, angiographic results, and clinical outcomes were also tabulated. Intimal hyperplasia was identified in 51 of 55 patients (93%) treated with directional coronary atherectomy for restenosis after a prior intervention. These restenosis lesions had less acute gain in lumen diameter after directional coronary atherectomy, had a smaller late lumen diameter, had more severe late stenosis, and tended to have more restenosis defined as late stenosis 250% (restenosis rate 40% for prior restenosis v 26% for primary lesions). Surprisingly, however, intimal hyperplasia was also identified in 45 of 102 (44%) primary stenoses. Primary lesions with intimal hyperplasia were more likely to occur in younger patients and in the LAD artery than were either primary lesions without intimal hyperplasia or prior restenosis lesions. There were otherwise no differences in the baseline characteristics, angiographic findings, or clinical outcome or primary lesions with or without intimal hyperplasia. The event free survival (72% at 12 months) was similar in all three groups. Thus, even though intimal hyperplasia is an almost universal finding in restenosis lesions, intimal hyperplasia is not specific for restenosis because histologically identical hyperplasia may be found in nearly half of primary coronary artery stenoses. The finding of intimal hyperplasia in primary coronary stenoses, however, does not predict a different outcome from that seen in primary stenoses without intimal hyperplasia.

Brogan and associates,[158] from Washington, DC, evaluated the clinical and angiographic outcome of patients undergoing rotational coronary atherectomy after unsuccessful balloon PTCA using quantitative angiographic methods to provide insight into this procedure's mechanism of benefit. During the study period, 41 patients with 50 lesions were referred for rotational atherectomy after standard balloon PTCA was unsuccessful. After rotational atherectomy, percent diameter stenosis was reduced from 72% to 41%; adjunct balloon PTCA was performed in 44 lesions, resulting in a 25% final diameter stenosis. The acute gain in minimal lumen diameter was 1.2 mm. In lesions needing adjunct balloon dilatation, lesion stretch was 73% and elastic recoil was 22%, with no variation by etiology of the initial balloon failure. Overall angiographic success (<50% residual diameter stenosis) was obtained in 49 lesions (98%). Procedural success, defined as <50% residual diameter stenosis and the absence of major in-hospital complications (death, Q-wave AMI, or emergency CABG), was obtained in 37 of 41 procedures (90%); complications developed in 3 patients (7%), including 2 patients who needed emergency CABG after development of delayed abrupt closure. These authors concluded that rotational coronary atherectomy may be used in selected patients when standard balloon PTCA is unsuccessful. Its mechanism of benefit appears related, at least in part, to changes in plaque compliance resulting from partial atheroma ablation.

Medina and associates,[159] from Las Palmas and Córdoba, Spain, focused on the early and late angiographic evolution in 82 patients with CAD who were successfully treated by directional coronary atherectomy without adjunctive balloon angioplasty. Qualitative inspections and quantitative measurements were obtained from a selected angled-view projection in the following conditions: (1) before treatment, (2) immediately after treatment, (3) the day after atherectomy, (4) 1 month after, and (5) 6 months after. The appearance of the treated segment 24 hours after the procedure did not differ in 79 patients from that observed immediately after directional coronary atherectomy; silent total occlusion occurred in 2 patients, and 1 had an aneurysm at the site of resection (all 3 patients were excluded from the analysis). At the 1-month study, restenosis developed in 3 patients (3.6%); the remaining 76 patients had identical appearances, with no evidence of renarrowing of the lumen. However, from 1 to 6 months after the procedure, restenosis developed in 35 of the remaining 76 patients (46%), and 41 patients were free of restenosis and symptoms. These findings, which show that early elastic recoil does not occur after successful directional coronary atherectomy, are different from the changes observed after balloon angioplasty. At the

1-month observation, restenosis is an infrequent but possible phenomenon. From this point the healing of the arterial wall leads to no or mild renarrowing (late success); an exaggerated proliferative response produces restenosis.

In a study by Suneja and associates,[160] from Cleveland, Ohio, to assess the mechanisms of luminal improvement, 40 patients undergoing directional coronary atherectomy and a matched control group of 25 patients undergoing PTCA were evaluated with intracoronary ultrasound imaging before and after intervention. Despite similar sized vessels, a similar angiographic severity of diameter stenosis (75% ± 12% for the PTCA group v 69% ± 15% for the atherectomy group), and a similar plaque burden (percent plaque area) before intervention (84% ± 5% in the PTCA group v 85% ± 13% in the atherectomy group), the residual plaque area after intervention was significantly smaller in the atherectomy group (54% ± 14%) compared with the PTCA group (65% ± 13%). Despite excellent angiographic results, significant residual plaque was noted after either successful intervention. Based on the absolute changes in lumen area, plaque area, and vessel area, improvement in the lumen area in the atherectomy group occurred as a result of plaque compression (48%), plaque removal (37%), and vessel expansion (15%). In the PTCA group, plaque compression accounted for 94% of the improvement in lumen area, whereas vessel expansion contributed 6%. Thus, compression of plaque remains the major mechanism of luminal improvement during atherectomy.

Intravascular ultrasound provides a unique method for characterizing the results of interventions for CAD. Kovach and associates,[161] from Washington, DC, reported on 48 lesions in 46 patients treated with rotational atherectomy, followed by adjunct balloon angioplasty in 44. Before intervention, target lesion external elastic membrane area measured 17.3 mm^2. After atherectomy, lumen area increased, plaque plus media area decreased, and 26% of the target lesion had dissection planes. After adjunct balloon angioplasty, external elastic membrane area increased and 77% of the target lesions had dissection planes. Arterial expansion was seen in 80% of lesions. The pattern of dissection plane location, which was predominantly within calcified plaque after rotational atherectomy, became predominantly adjacent to calcified plaque after adjunct balloon angioplasty. These authors concluded that high speed rotational atherectomy causes lumen enlargement by selective ablation of hard, especially calcific, atherosclerotic plaque with little tissue disruption and rare arterial expansion. Adjunct balloon angioplasty further increases lumen area by a combination of arterial dissection and arterial expansion, especially of compliant noncalcified plaque elements.

Coronary Stenting

Although intracoronary stenting has been advocated as an adjunct to balloon PTCA to circumvent late restenosis, its effectiveness has not yet been verified. Therefore the aim of the study by de Jaegere and associates,[162] from Rotterdam, The Netherlands, was to determine the differences in the immediate and long-term changes in stenosis geometry between Wallstent implantation and balloon PTCA in native coronary artery lesions. To obtain two study populations with identical baseline stenosis characteristics, patients were matched for lesion site, vessel size, and minimal luminal diameter. Only patients undergoing elective and successful coronary intervention of a native coronary artery, in whom a control angiographic study had been performed, were included. A total of 186 patients (93 in each group) were selected. The coronary angiograms were analyzed with the computer-assisted cardiovascular angiographic analysis system. Matching was considered adequate, because there was an equal number of lesion sites in each study population and there were no differences in baseline reference diameter and minimal luminal diameter. Wallstent implantation resulted in a significantly greater increase in minimal luminal diameter (from 1.22 ± 0.34 mm to 2.49 ± 0.40 mm) compared with balloon PTCA (from 1.21 ± 0.29 mm to 1.92 ± 0.35 mm). Despite a greater decrease in minimal luminal diameter after Wallstent implantation (0.48 ± 0.74 mm) than after balloon PTCA (0.20 ± 0.46 mm), the minimal luminal diameter at follow-up was significantly greater after stent implantation (2.01 ± 0.75 mm v 1.72 ± 0.54). It was concluded that Wallstent implantation results in a superior immediate and long-term increase in minimal luminal diameter compared with balloon PTCA. The larger initial gain after stent implantation compensates for the late loss, and thus, an improved initial result and not lessened neointimal hyperplasia is responsible for a reduced incidence of restenosis. Studies based on matching of angiographic variables are a surrogate for randomized studies, forecasting their results and offering insight into the effects of different interventional techniques. Moreover, these studies yield statistical information that may be helpful for the proper design of a randomized study.

To determine whether patients with diabetes mellitus, when compared with nondiabetic patients, have a higher frequency of restenosis after coronary stenting and, if so, whether restenosis is attributable to lesion or procedural differences or to a greater biologic tendency for late loss of minimum diameter in diabetic patients, Carrozza and associates,[163] from Boston, Mass, studied 220 consecutive patients with CAD referred for placement of a Palmaz-Schatz stent in either a native coronary artery or a saphenous vein graft. Based on traditional dichotomous definition of restenosis (≥50% stenosis at follow-up), lesions in diabetic patients had a significantly greater restenosis rate (55%) than lesions in nondiabetic patients (20%). Vessel size, lesion length, preprocedure lesion severity, procedural outcome, and acute gain (the difference between minimum lumen diameter before and after the procedure) were similar in the diabetic and nondiabetic groups. However, at follow-up, stents in diabetic patients had a smaller lumen diameter (1.66 ± 1.18 mm), as well as a greater percent stenosis (49% v 32%). Thus, the increased restenosis rate in stents in diabetic patients (55% v 20%) is secondary to increased late loss of minimum lumen diameter (1.66 ± 1.28 mm v 1.23 ± 0.97 mm). After arterial injury produced by stent placement, diabetic patients have a significantly greater incidence of restenosis because of greater late loss at the treatment site. Because elastic recoil or vasospasm contributes little to stent restenosis, the increased late loss of minimum lumen diameter in diabetic patients suggests that they have a greater predisposition to intimal hyperplasia.

Abrupt vessel closure complicates 6% to 8% of coronary angioplasty procedures. This leads to death, myocardial infarction, or emergency CABG in more than half of these patients. Previous studies have suggested that stents may be helpful in preventing these complications. Lincoff and associates,[164] from Cleveland, Ohio, carried out a case-control analysis to compare the clinical outcome after intracoronary stenting with that after conventional therapy for abrupt vessel closure. Sixty-one of 92 consecutive patients treated at two clinical sites by intracoronary stenting for abrupt vessel closure were matched according to angiographic features of closure and estimated LV mass threatened by ischemia with patients treated conventionally during the 18 months before stent availability. In 33 pairs of matched patients, vessel closure was established; in 28, vessel closure was threatened. The baseline clinical and angiographic characteristics were similar in the two matched groups. Stents were successfully deployed in 60 of 61 patients at a median time of 52 minutes. When compared with conventional treatment, stenting resulted in less residual stenosis (26% v 49% diameter stenosis), a greater likelihood of restoration of TIMI grade 3 blood flow (97% v 72%), and a reduction in the need for emergency bypass surgery (4.9% v 18%). The incidence of Q-wave myocardial infarction, however, was nearly the same in the two groups (32% v 20%). At a mean time of 6.3 months after hospital discharge, survival, free from late cardiac death, myocardial infarction, bypass surgery, or coronary angioplasty, was 75% and 81% in the stent and control treatment groups, respectively (p = NS). These authors concluded that although early treatment of established vessel closure by intracoronary stenting was associated with a low incidence of both myocardial infarction and emergency bypass surgery, the likelihood or severity of an infarction was not reduced. Furthermore patients with threatened vessel closure could not be shown to benefit from stent treatment.

Foley and associates,[165] from London, Canada, reported the immediate safety, efficacy, and 6-month angiographic follow-up after elective implantation of the Palmaz-Schatz stent in the first 100 consecutive patients at a single center. Patients with suitable cardiac anatomy and no contraindications to anticoagulation were prospectively entered into the study. One hundred two stents were successfully implanted in 99 patients. The mean diameter stenosis was 70% ± 11% before implantation and was reduced to 20% ± 11% after stent implantation. There were no deaths, Q-wave AMIs, urgent CABGs, or strokes during the procedure or follow-up period. Stent thrombosis occurred in 2 patients; in both, vessel patency was successfully accomplished by balloon angioplasty. There were three gastrointestinal hemorrhages, two of which required transfusion. Angiographic follow-up was performed in 98% of patients at 6.3 ± 2.6 months after the procedure. Restenosis (≥50% stenosis within or immediately adjacent to the stent) occurred in 32% of patients. Stent restenosis was associated with male sex (36% v 7% for female patients) and stent implantation in a restenosis lesion (47% v 25% for de novo lesions). In conclusion, the Palmaz-Schatz stent can be electively implanted with high success and low complication rates; the restenosis rate appears to be similar to that of balloon angioplasty.

Kastrati and associates,[166] Heidelberg, Germany, determined the time course of luminal changes during the first year after emergency placement of coronary stents. From June 1989 to May 1991, 82 patients who received Palmaz-Schatz stents and did not have early vessel occlusion after stenting were enrolled into a serial angiographic follow-up study. Coronary normal reference diameter and minimal luminal diameter were measured with an automated edge detection technique. Patients who underwent repeat PTCA for restenosis were excluded from further analyses. The restudy rate at 3, 6, and 12 months was 96%, 81%, and 90% of the eligible patients, respectively. The incidence of restenosis, defined as a diameter stenosis ≥50%, was 22% at 3 months, 32% at 6 months, and 33% at 12 months. Minimal luminal diameter was increased from 0.66 + 0.32 mm before to 2.85 + 0.43 mm immediately after stenting. It was 0.46 + 0.31 mm smaller than the diameter of the maximally inflated balloon during the procedure. The reduction in minimal luminal diameter was 0.80 + 0.69 mm for the first 3 months, 0.29 + 0.52 mm between 3 and 6 months, and 0.13 + 0.32 mm for the last 6 months. The percentage of patients presenting with a significant change in minimal luminal diameter declined from 51% during the first 3 months and 19% between 3 and 6 months to 7% for the period between 6 and 12 months. Thus, after emergency coronary stenting, the incidence and time course of restenosis is similar to that reported for PTCA. Coronary lumen diameters demonstrated a peak change at 3 months and remained generally stable after the first 6 months.

Restenosis is a major limitation following balloon angioplasty. Kimura and associates,[167] from Kitakyushu, Japan, used the Palmaz-Schatz balloon expandable coronary stent as one therapeutic option to attenuate restenosis. Ninety-six patients who had 97 lesions treated with a stent were compared to a cohort of 179 patients with 192 lesions who received balloon angioplasty. Serial angiographic follow-up studies were performed the day after stent implantation and at 1, 3, and 6 months after the procedure. A significantly larger lumen diameter was obtained immediately after stent implantation (2.9 v 2.1 mm in the balloon group). At 3 to 6 months of follow-up a significantly larger lumen diameter was maintained in the stent group (2.2 v 1.5 mm). The late restenosis rate was significantly lower in the stent group (13% v 39%). The greatest tendency to restenosis was observed between 1 and 3 months after the procedure. These authors concluded that the Palmaz-Schatz stent was effective in reducing the restenosis rate in this highly selected group of patients. The final role of the stent in this subset of patients will depend on further prospective studies.

Maiello and associates,[168] from Milan, Italy, studied 32 patients (aged 58 ± 9 years) who had been treated with a Palmaz-Schatz stent after significant dissection complicating PTCA. The stents were placed in an attempt to cover the entire site of dissection with the prosthesis. The presence of dissection after PTCA was associated with Thrombolysis in Myocardial Infarction grade 0 to 1 flow in 19 patients and grade 2 flow in 13. The stented arteries were LAD in 19 patients, right coronary artery in 7 patients, and LC in 5 patients. A single stent was implanted in 11 patients and multiple stents in 21 patients. Angiographic success was achieved in 30 patients (94%). Two patients (6%) had urgent CABG, 2 patients (6%) had AMI, and 1 patient (3%) died. Subacute occlusion occurred in 1 patient (3%). Angiographic restenosis was found in 3 of 9 patients (33%) with a single stent and 11 of 17 patients (65%) with multiple stents. Clinical follow-up at 11 ± 3 months showed the necessity of CABG in 2 patients and repeat PTCA in 9 patients (31%). These authors concluded that coronary stenting is an effective treatment for significant coronary dissection after PTCA with an acceptable incidence of major cardiac events at follow-up.

Laskey and associates,[169] from Philadelphia, Pa, studied 12 patients undergoing elective coronary stent implantation for either recurrent restenosis or adverse lesion appearance. By use of a 4.8 French 20 MHz intravascular ultrasound catheter, the conventional angioplasty site was examined before and after coronary stent implantation. Quantitative angiographic analysis revealed the expected excellent final results with a group mean poststent diameter reduction of 14% ± 9% and a cross-sectional area reduction of 22% ± 13%. Angiographic analysis also indicated an increase in minimum stenosis diameter from 1.8 ± 0.6 mm after conventional balloon angioplasty to 2.8 ± 0.3 mm after coronary stent implantation. Quantitative analysis of the corresponding intravascular ultrasound images, however, revealed significant residual endoluminal obstruction. Fractional plaque area remained unchanged from 30% ± 12% after conventional balloon angioplasty to 32% ± 11% after stent implantation. The circumferential distribution of plaque increased significantly from 0.44 ± 0.17 to 0.55 ± 0.15 after stent implantation. Despite the lack of significant change in the ultrasound-determined minimum stenosis diameter after stent placement, there was a borderline significant increase in the plaque-free lumen area (before stent, 6.35 ± 1.55 mm^2; after stent, 7.25 ± 1.6 mm^2). Thus, in contrast to the substantial improvement in the angiographically assessed residual luminal obstruction after stent implantation compared with the prestent condition, considerably less improvement was found by intravascular ultrasound assessed examination. Morphometric analysis indicated a tendency toward circumferential remodeling of plaque. The inherently different approaches to vascular imaging represented by contrast angiography and intravascular ultrasound techniques appear to provide complementary information. Detailed endovascular anatomy, which was not apparent on contrast angiography, may provide additional useful information during interventional procedures in which plaque is neither removed nor ablated.

Abrupt or threatened vessel closure after PTCA is associated with increased risk of AMI, emergency CABG, and in-hospital death. Coronary stenting is a nonsurgical alternative to lesions that are unresponsive to additional prolonged balloon catheter inflation. George and associates,[170] from Columbus, Ohio, and West Lafayette, Ind, evaluated 518 patients who underwent attempted coronary stenting with a 20 mm long Gianturco-Roubin coronary stent. In 494 patients, one or more stents were deployed. Thirty-two percent of the patients received stents for acute closure and 69% for threatened closure. Successful deployment was achieved in 95% of patients, with improvement in the diameter stenosis from 63% before stenting to 15% after stenting. Emergency CABG was required in 4.3%. In-hospital AMI was 5.5%. At 6 months AMI was infrequent, occurring in 1.6% of patients. In-hospital death was 2.2%, and late death occurred in 7 patients (1.4%). Thirty-four patients required later bypass graft surgery. These authors concluded from this early multicenter experience that this stent is a useful adjunct to PTCA to prevent or minimize the complications associated with flow-limiting coronary artery dissections. Because this study was not randomized, a controlled study would be required to fully assess the value of this stent.

Despite excellent results as a bail-out procedure for the management of abrupt closure after balloon angioplasty and the potential beneficial effects on restenosis after angioplasty, intracoronary stenting is limited, especially by subacute stent thrombosis. In an investigation by Haude and associates,[171] from Essen and Mainz, Germany, carried out in 100 consecutive patients with intracoronary implantation of 118 Palmaz-Schatz stents, 10 patients (10%) developed subacute stent thrombosis during their hospital course three to nine days after implantation. Therapy included intravenous thrombolysis, mechanical recanalization by balloon angioplasty, and emergency CABG. Although successful recanalization was maintained in 8 of 9 nonsurgically treated patients <2 hours after the onset of symptoms, 7 patients developed AMI with 2 patients having Q-wave AMI and 5 patients having non-Q-wave AMI. By univariate analysis, several variables could be identified as risk factors for the development of subacute stent thrombosis: bail-out implantations, unstable angina, long and complex lesions with large plaque areas, symptomatic postangioplasty dissections, incomplete wrapping of the dissection after stenting, and vessel irregularities distal to the stented segment. These variables, except the variable large plaque area, were confirmed as independent predictors of subacute stent thrombosis by a stepwise multivariate logistic regression analysis. Optimal anticoagulation by intravenous heparin and overlapping warfarin and additional aspirin, according to the results of global coagulation tests (activated partial thromboplastin time and thrombin time >70 seconds, international normalized ratio >3), was not associated with a significantly reduced relative risk for subacute stent thrombosis. The results of this retrospective analysis indicate that subacute stent thrombosis is unpredictable and is associated with a high risk of AMI despite fast recanalization. The identified risk factors for subacute stent thrombosis should particularly be considered when stenting is performed. Because global anticoagulation tests are inadequate, improved and more sophisticated coagulation monitoring are required.

A study by Kiemeneij and associates,[172] from Amsterdam, The Netherlands, describes initial results of Palmaz-Schatz stent implantation to restore and maintain vessel patency in 52 patients with obstructive dissection, defined as an intraluminal filling defect with coronary flow impairment after PTCA. The majority of patients (62%) underwent PTCA for unstable angina (n = 28), defined as angina at rest with documented ST-segment changes resistant to nitrates, or AMI (n = 4). In 6 patients (11%), the stent could not be delivered. Seven of the remaining 46 patients (15%) had CABG performed because of increased risk for subacute stent occlusion, residual thrombosis, residual obstruction near the stent, coronary artery diameter <3.0 mm, or multiple and overlapping stents. One patient (3%) died in-hospital from intracranial bleeding. Nine patients (23%) had subacute stent occlusion, retrospectively unpredictable in 4 patients. Nine of 29 patients (29%) with an uncomplicated clinical course after stenting had angiographic restenosis at a mean follow-up of 6.0 ± 1.4 months (range, 12 days to 8.3 months). Two patients (7%) died 3 months after successful stenting: 1 patient because of stent thrombosis after stopping warfarin before an abdominal operation and 1 patient after acute vascular surgery for late traumatic groin bleeding. Of the 39 medically treated patients with a stent, 3 patients (8%) had major bleeding complications. These authors concluded that stent implantation is feasible in most patients with obstructive dissection after PTCA. After successful stent delivery, coronary flow is temporarily restored. However, during this early experience with emergency stenting, it was shown that nonsurgical treatment of these patients resulted in substantial subacute stent occlusion rates. Accordingly, stabilized patients should be considered as a high-risk population for sub-acute stent thrombosis, needing careful monitoring of anticoagulant treatment and ambulation. Semi-elective CABG after emergency stenting may be the treatment of choice. With a combination of an optimal angiographic result and an optimal clinical infrastructure and patient management, a more conservative treatment after emergency stent implantation may be advocated.

Implantation of coronary artery stents via the percutaneous femoral approach is associated with a high rate of vascular complications at the access site related to the size of the entry hole and the intense anticoagulation required to prevent stent thrombosis. Therefore, Resar and associates,[173] from Baltimore, Md, studied the feasibility of using the left brachial approach utilizing open arterial repair for implantation of coronary artery stents. Intracoronary stent implantation via the femoral approach in 24 patients (group A) was compared with implantation via the brachial approach in 16 patients (group B). Baseline lesion characteristics were similar in the two groups. All stents in group A (n = 27 stents) were successfully delivered to their target vessel. One stent in group B (n = 18 stents) could not be delivered because of an inability to engage the coronary artery from the brachial approach. There were no significant differences in the angiographic outcome between the two groups. Complications including hematomas, hemorrhage requiring blood transfusion, vascular injury requiring surgery, and pseudoaneurysm formation were significantly more common in group A than in group B (33% v 6%). In addition, the length of hospital stay was significantly longer for the femoral approach than the brachial approach (9.4 v 6.5 days). Thus, the left brachial approach for intracoronary stent implantation is technically feasible, safe, and associated with fewer local vascular complications and a shorter hospitalization than the femoral approach.

Hearn and associates,[174] in Atlanta, Ga, studied 116 patients who attempted stent placement for imminent or total acute closure after PTCA. In 103 patients (110 stents, 105 procedures), the stent was successfully deployed (89%). Angiographic success was achieved in 94 placements (85%). Seventy-one phase 2 procedures were angiographically successful without complications of death, Q-wave myocardial infarction, or CABG. Stent placement was associated with resolution of ST-segment deviation and angina in 84% of patients. Five deaths and five Q-wave myocardial infarctions occurred during hospitalization. Two deaths were related to pulmonary insufficiency from chronic lung disease, and one patient died after rescue stent placement for left main coronary artery occlusion during routine angiography. Another patient died after CABG. The final death occurred in an elderly patient who suffered a stroke while on intravenous heparin. During hospitalization, nine patients developed reocclusion after stent placement (95% of procedure) and six had a repeat PTCA. CABG was performed after 29 stent procedures (28%). The first nine patients underwent CABG as part of the phase 1 protocol, and in addition, nine patients had CABG after stenting with a good angiographic result but with a large amount of myocardium at risk. Clinical follow-up was obtained in all patients at a median of 14 months. There were 3 late deaths (3%), 2 Q-wave myocardial infarcts (2%), 16 repeat PTCAs (16%), and 15 CABG procedures (15%). Angiographic restenosis was found in 30 of 57 patients (53%) and a median of 4 months. A total of 41 procedures were successful and not accompanied

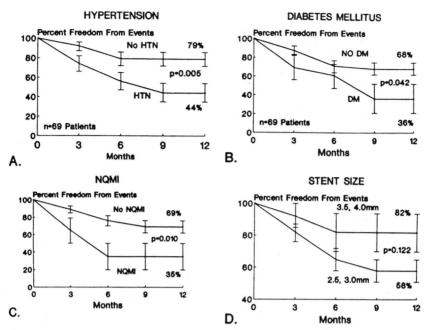

Figure 2-23. The effects of various clinical variables and stent size on cumulative freedom from events in patients with successful stent procedures (HTN = hypertension; DM = diabetes mellitus; NQMI = non-Q-wave myocardial infarction). Reproduced with permission from Hearn et al.[174]

by an important subsequent coronary event. Restenosis and/or clinical events were associated with non-Q-wave myocardial infarction, hypertension, diabetes, left circumflex coronary artery stenting, saphenous vein graft stenting, smaller caliber artery stenting, higher balloon to artery ratios, and shorter inflation times. Coronary artery stenting for acute closure after PTCA relieves myocardial ischemia and provides an alternative means of treatment. This early series includes a learning curve experience with stent placement, but even so, certain clinical and angiographic subsets of patients are at increased risk for restenosis and future cardiac events (Figure 2-23).

LASER ANGIOPLASTY

Recently, access to the coronary arteries became available to laser angioplasty because of a new technique utilizing a pulsed laser source and multifiber over-the-wire guided catheters. The aim of this study by Geschwind and associates,[175] from Creteil, France, was to evaluate the early and long-term results and the side effects of coronary angioplasty with an excimer or a holmium-yttrium aluminum garnet laser. Forty consecutive patients were treated with the holmium-yttrium aluminum garnet laser (group 1), and 46 consecutive patients were treated with the excimer laser (group 2). The primary laser angioplasty success rate was 55% and 72% for groups 1 and 2, respectively. This success rate was highest in saphenous vein grafts. It was similar in calcified and noncalcified lesions and in total occlusions and stenoses. It tended to be lower in long lesions than in short ones (40% v 60% and 44% v 78% for groups 1 and 2, respectively). Laser stand-alone therapy was performed in 5% of patients in group 1 versus 22% in group 2. Failures were due to the inability of the laser catheter tip to reach the lesion, to cross the obstruction, or to obtain a significant reduction in stenosis. They were more frequent in patients in group 1 than in those in group 2 (45% v 28%). There were no deaths, no AMIs, and no need for emergency CABG because most patients had total occlusions or a well-protected coronary artery. Complications included acute closure in 8% and 27% of patients in groups 1 and 2, respectively, and spasm in 10% and 13% of patients in groups 1 and 2, respectively. Dissection occurred more frequently in patients in group 2 than in those in group 1 (28% v 7%). The angiographic patency rate at 6-month follow-up was 33% and 29% for patients in groups 1 and 2, respectively. Multifiber, wire-guided catheters provide easy access to the coronary arteries. Excimer laser angioplasty is effective but induces a high rate of dissections. Technical improvements are required to ablate more tissue to possibly reduce the restenosis rate.

Eigler and the ELCA Investigators,[176] from Los Angeles, Calif, conducted a prospective multicenter trial of excimer laser coronary angioplasty of aorto-ostial stenosis involving coronary arteries and saphenous vein grafts between December 1989 and May 1992 in 206 aorto-ostial excimer laser coronary angioplasty procedures performed on 209 stenoses in 200 patients. Canadian Cardiovascular Society class III or IV angina was present in 76% of patients. The distribution of stenosis locations was left main coronary in 26 patients (12%), right coronary artery in 124 patients (59%), and vein grafts in 59 patients (28%). Adjunctive PTCA was performed in 72%. Procedure success defined as ≤50% diameter stenosis with major complication occurred in 90% of the treated patients, including 92% of those with left main stenoses, 89% of those with right coronary artery stenoses, and 90% of those with vein graft stenoses. Quantitative angiographic analysis documented an improvement in stenosis diameter from 76% ± 14% at baseline to 36% ± 15% at the completion of the procedure. Most of the acute gain was in diameter and resulted from the excimer laser coronary angioplasty. A major complication during hospitalization occurred in 4% of patients, including the development of Q-wave myocardial infarction in 0.5% and the need for CABG in 3%. The only predictor of procedure failure was female gender. Six-month angiographic follow-up, available in 51% of eligible patients, documented a mean diameter stenosis of 46% ± 26%. Restenosis occurred in 39% of patients, including 64% of those with left main disease. Restenosis was less likely when residual stenosis was <35%. Clinical events at follow-up were death, 3%; CABG, 7%; AMI, 2%; and the need for repeat PTCA, 16%. Seventy-eight percent of the remaining patients were asymptomatic. An adverse event during follow-up was more than twice as likely in the group with LM narrowing. These data suggest that excimer laser coronary angioplasty may be an effective and safe therapy in patients with aorto-ostial stenoses. However, 6-month restenosis, adverse event rates are higher and function status poorer in the group with LM stenosis. Excimer laser coronary angioplasty may be considered as an alternative to CABG in carefully selected patients, but with the understanding that the risk of restenosis and of adverse events is high.

CORONARY ARTERY BYPASS GRAFTING

In the United States v Canada

To compare overall rates of CABG in several jurisdictions in Canada and the United States and to compare use by age and income groups in the two countries, Anderson and associates,[177] from San Francisco and Santa Monica, Calif, and Winnipeg, Canada, surveyed all adult residents in five jurisdictions who underwent CABG in a hospital in their jurisdiction using computerized hospital discharge abstracts from all nonfederal hospitals in New York, California, Ontario, Manitoba, and British Columbia between 1983 and 1989. Between 1983 and 1989, the CABG rates were consistently highest in California and lowest in the Canadian jurisdictions. In 1989, the age-adjusted rate of CABG in California (112.5/100,000 adults) was 27% higher than in New York (88.4/100,000) and 80% higher than in the three Canadian provinces combined (62.4/100,000). The CABG rates increased for those aged 65 years and older and decreased for those aged 20 to 54 years in all five jurisdictions. In 1989, CABG rates were three times higher in California than in Canada for those aged 75 years and older, and the higher rates for those aged 65 years and older accounted for 75% of the overall difference in rates between California and Canada. In Canada, CABG rates for the nonelderly varied little by income of area of residence, but in New York and California, rates increased steadily with the income of area of residence. Control over the supply of resources in Canada is associated with markedly lower CABG rates for the elderly than found in the United States. Overall rates are lower in Canada, and the Canadian universal health insurance system reduces the influence of income on access to CABG found in the United States. However, even without universal health insurance, CABG rates for the nonelderly living in the poorest areas in California are similar to the rates for those living in the poorest parts of Canada.

APPROPRIATENESS IN NEW YORK

To determine the appropriateness of use of CABG in New York State, Leape and associates,[178] from several US medical centers, examined 1,338 patients undergoing isolated CABG in New York State in 1990 at 15 randomly selected hospitals in that state. The percentage of patients who had CABG for appropriate, inappropriate, or uncertain indications, and 30 day mortality and complications, were the main outcome measures. Nearly 91% of the CABG operations were rated appropriate; 7% were rated uncertain; and 2.4% were rated inappropriate. This low inappropriate rate differs substantially from the 14% rate found in a previous study of patients operated on in 1979, 1980, and 1982. The difference in rates was not due to more lenient criteria but to changes in practice, the most important being that the fraction of patients receiving CABGs for one- and two-vessel disease fell from 51% to 24%. Individual hospital rates of inappropriateness (0% to 5%) did not vary significantly. Rates of appropriateness also did not vary by hospital location, volume, or teaching status. Operative mortality was 1%; 17% of patients suffered a complication. Complication rates varied significantly among hospitals and were higher in downstate hospitals. The rates of inappropriate and uncertain use of CABG in New York State were very low. Rates of inappropriate use did not vary significantly among hospitals, or according to region, volume of bypass operations performed, or teaching status.

With Low Ejection Fractions

Lansman and associates,[179] from New York, NY, and Philadelphia, Pa, described 42 patients with an LVEF of 20% or less, and each underwent CABG using a method of myocardial protection termed "centigrade cardioplegia," combining single-dose, cold, crystalloid cardioplegia, systemic hypothermia, and local hypothermia. Thirty-day mortality was 4.8% (2/42 patients). Perioperative morbidity included AMI in 2 patients (5%) and stroke in 1 patient (2%). Postoperative LVEF rose from 0.16 to 0.23, NYHA classification decreased from 3.4 to 1.8, and Canadian class 3.3 to 0.61. Survival at 1 year was 88%, at 3 years, 68%, and at 6 years, 34%. Four clinical variables were associated with long-term survival: (1) chief complaint of pain only, (2) history of unstable angina, (3) Canadian class less than IV, and (4) NYHA class less than IV. These factors may help predict which patients with severe LV dysfunction will benefit from CABG.

Luciani and associates,[180] from Padova, Italy, reviewed data in 143 patients (137 men and 6 women) with CAD and a LVEF less than 0.30. Patients were divided into three groups according to therapy: medical only, 72 (group 1); CABG, 20 (group 2); and heart transplantation, 51 (group 3). Clinical status was poorer in group 3, with CHF as predominant symptom; angina was more frequent in group 2. No difference was noted in hemodynamic variables. Four early deaths (20%) occurred in group 2 and 7 early deaths (13.7%) in group 3. Follow-up ranged from 1 to 64 months (mean, 22 ± 19 months), with an actuarial survival of 28% ± 9%, 80% ± 8%, and 82% ± 5% at 5 years in groups 1, 2, and 3, respectively. Even though postoperative NYHA class was better in group 3 (1.0 v 2.3 in group 2), the difference in survival was not significant. Although in patients with CAD and low LVEF, heart transplantation offers the best clinical results, considering the donor shortage, CABG may still be performed with good mid-term results (Figure 2-24).

Milano and associates,[181] from Durham, NC, evaluated 118 consecutive patients with an EF ≤25% and performed CABG on each of them. Operative mortality was 11%. Ventricular arrhythmia requiring treatment was the most common postoperative complication (27%), followed by low cardiac output state (22%). Median length of postoperative hospitalization was nine days. Estimate of survival at 1 year and 5 years was 77% and 58%, respectively, and was better than estimated survival with medical therapy alone. Survivors experienced significant improvement in angina class, CHF class, and follow-up EF. Of 22 preoperative factors evaluated by univariate survival analysis, 5 were associated with significantly greater mortality: other vascular disease, female sex, hypertension, elevated LV end-diastolic pressure, and depressed cardiac index. Three factors showed significant adverse effect: time on cardiopulmonary bypass, acute presentation, and female sex. These data suggest that patients

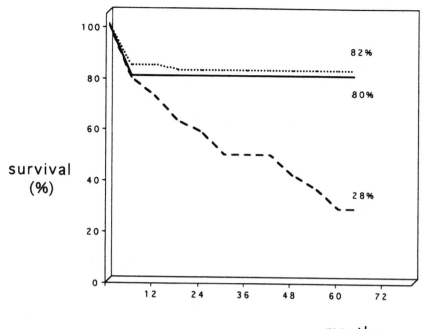

Figure 2-24. Actuarial survival of patients with severe ischemic left ventricular failure according to type of treatment. The dotted line depicts survival of patients undergoing heart transplantation (51); the solid line, survival of patients undergoing myocardial revascularization (20); and the broken line, survival of patients receiving medical therapy only (72). The percentage numbers at the end of each line represent actuarial survival for each group of patients at follow-up (64 months). Reproduced with permission from Luciani et al.[180]

with CAD and severely depressed LVEF benefit from CABG, and specific preoperative factors may help determine optimal survival.

In Familial Hypercholesterolemia

Takahashi and associates,[182] from Osaka and Nara, Japan, analyzed long-term results of CABG in 32 consecutive patients with familial hypercholesterolemia, 6 homozygotes and 26 heterozygotes studied between 1976 and 1990. Seventeen patients in the early series underwent CABG with vein grafts alone. Subsequently, 15 patients underwent CABG with internal mammary artery grafting to the LAD artery and received intensive lipid-lowering treatments early after CABG. All homozygotes and 1 heterozygote received intermittent LDL apheresis after CABG. There was only one late noncardiac death (3%), and the actuarial rates of freedom from cardiac events (AMI, cardiac death, and angina pectoris) were 60% at 5 and 10 years for homozygotes, and 87% and 73% for heterozygotes (Figure 2-25). The cardiac event-free curve for the heterozygous familial hypercholesterolemia group was comparable with that for the random age-matched subset of patients without familial hypercholesterolemia who underwent CABG during the same period. Two of 3 homozygotes and 4 of 14 heterozygotes in the early series had one or more cardiac

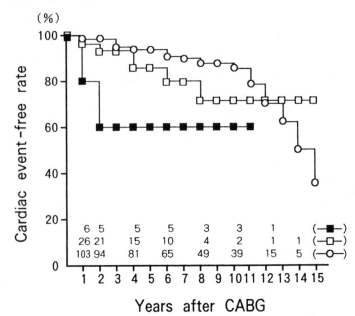

Figure 2-25. Actuarial rates of freedom from cardiac events for the homozygous familial hypercholesterolemia (FH) group (■: n = 6), heterozygous FH group (□: n = 26), and non-FH group (O: n = 103). There was no significant difference between the heterozygous FH group and non-FH group with respect to actuarial cardiac event-free curve. Reproduced with permission from Takahashi et al.[182]

events. The patency rate of internal mammary artery grafts to the LAD artery from 1 to 3 years after CABG was significantly higher than that of vein grafts to the LAD artery (92% v 45%). Abdominal aortic aneurysm developed postoperatively in 2 homozygotes and 2 heterozygotes without sufficient cholesterol reduction. The authors concluded that internal mammary artery grafting in combination with postoperative intensive lipid-lowering treatments, including LDL apheresis, may provide acceptably good long-term results of coronary revascularization in patients with familial hypercholesterolemia.

Brain Swelling Afterwards

Harris and associates,[183] from London, England, examined six patients undergoing routine CABG by magnetic resonance imaging of the brain before surgery, immediately afterwards, and 6 to 18 days later. Brain swelling was visible in all six patients on the immediate postoperative scan. In five patients who had later scans, the swelling had subsided. No major neurological deficits were seen, and the patients were extubated successfully within three hours of operation. The mechanism of the cerebral swelling is uncertain, but it may provide insight into the cause of neurophysiological deficits seen after CABG.

Bradyarrhythmias Afterwards

To evaluate clinical and electrocardiographic characteristics that may predict the occurrence of bradyarrhythmias after isolated CABG, 1,614 consecutive patients who had this procedure performed from January 1988 to December 1990 were reviewed by Emlein and associates,[184] from Worcester, Mass. Thirteen patients (0.8%) (7 males and 6 females) had prolonged (mean, 11 ± 6.5 days) postoperative bradyarrhythmias and required insertion of a permanent pacemaker. Complete heart block occurred in 8 patients and sinus node dysfunction in 5 patients. These 13 patients (group A) were compared with a group of 490 arbitrarily selected CABG patients (group B) without bradyarrhythmias whose preoperative electrocardiograms were reviewed. Patients in group A were older (mean age, 69 v 63 years) and had concomitant LV aneurysmectomy more frequently and internal mammary graft revascularization less frequently than group B patients. Review of preoperative electrocardiograms revealed a higher occurrence of complete left BBB (5 of 13 v 6 of 490) and a borderline, more leftward frontal plane QRS axis (-5.3 v 13 degrees) in group A patients. There were no differences between the groups with respect to gender, number of bypass grafts, location of prior myocardial infarction, and preoperative electrocardiographic intervals (PR, QRS, QTc). Multivariate analysis identified the presence of a preoperative left BBB, concomitant LV aneurysmectomy, and age >64 years as independent predictors of severe and prolonged postoperative bradyarrhythmias, mainly complete heart block. Follow-up (mean, 23 ± 12 months) of patients demonstrated no or only partial recovery of A-V conduction in patients with postoperative complete heart block (n = 8) and persistent sinus node dysfunction in 3 of 5 patients with postoperative severe sinus arrest. Eleven of 13 patients continued to benefit from pacing. It was concluded that preoperative left BBB, age ≥ 64 years, and concomitant LV aneurysmectomy are associated with a higher incidence of severe and prolonged postoperative bradyarrhythmias after isolated CABG and that the majority of patients continue to benefit from long-term pacing.

Angina Afterwards

In a prospective, angiographically-controlled study, Yli-Mayry and Huikuri,[185] in Oulu, Finland, examined 339 consecutive patients to evaluate the preoperative, perioperative, and postoperative risk factors for occurrence of AMI and recurrence of severe angina during 5 years after CABG. The incidence of AMI was 6% and the recurrence of severe angina was 13%. No preoperative or perioperative variable could predict the occurrence of AMI. Postoperative EF was significantly lower in patients with than without AMI (50% v 58%), and the Cox proportional-hazards method showed a low postoperative EF to be the only significant risk factor for the occurrence of AMI. Patients with a recurrence of severe angina had higher blood total cholesterol concentrations (7.7 v 7.0 mmol/L) and triglyceride levels (2.7 v 2.0 mmol/L) than did those without angina, and also more often had ≥1 occluded bypass graft 3 months after CABG. No other preoperative or postoperative variable could predict the recurrence of angina. Both total blood cholesterol concentration and triglyceride level were significant predictors of the risk of recurrent severe angina by the Cox proportional-hazards method. Thus, reduced EF is a risk factor for subsequent AMI, whereas blood lipid abnormalities predict the recurrence of severe angina during the 5 years after CABG. The dissimilarities in risk factors between these cardiac events may be explained by differences in their pathophysiologic trigger mechanisms.

Left Ventricular Perfusion and Function Afterwards

Cigarroa and associates,[186] from Dallas, Tex, determined whether dobutamine stress echocardiography might identify hibernating myocardium and predict improvement in regional systolic wall thickening after CABG. Dobutamine stress echocardiography was performed in 49 consecutive patients with multivessel CAD and depressed LVEF. Contractile reserve during dobutamine stress echocardiography was defined by the presence of two criteria: (1) improved systolic wall thickening in at least two adjacent abnormal segments and (2) >20% improvement in regional wall thickening score. Postoperative echocardiograms were evaluated for improvement in regional wall-thickening score. Postoperative echocardiograms were evaluated for improved regional wall thickening in 25 patients at least 4 weeks after successful CABG. All studies were read in blinded fashion. Contractile reserve during dobutamine stress echocardiography was present in 24 of 49 patients (49%). The presence or absence of contractile reserve on preoperative dobutamine stress echocardiography predicted recovery of ventricular function in 25 patients who underwent successful CABG. Therefore, 9 of 11 patients with contractile reserve had improved systolic wall thickening after CABG, whereas 12 of 14 patients without contractile reserve did not improve (Figure 2-26). Thus, dobutamine stress echocardiography provides a simple, cost-effective, and widely available method of identifying hibernating myocardium and predicting improvement in regional LV wall thickening after CABG. This technique may be clinically valuable in the selection of patients for CABG.

A study by Iskandrian and associates,[187] from Philadelphia, Pa, examined the LV perfusion and EF by using simultaneous single-photon emission computed tomography and first-pass radionuclide angiography with technetium-99m sestamibi in 95 patients after uncomplicated CABG.

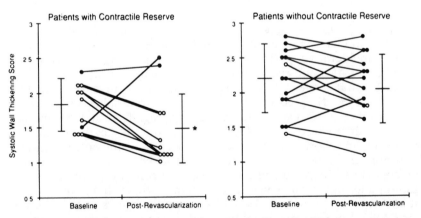

Figure 2-26. Plot of regional echocardiographic systolic wall-thickening scores at rest and after revascularization in patients with (left panel) and without (right panel) contractile reserve by dobutamine stress echocardiography. Open circles represent patients with improved regional left ventricular function after revascularization. Closed circles represent patients without improved regional left ventricular function after revascularization. Error bars show the mean ± SD. *P < .0001 compared with resting values. Reproduced with permission from Cigarroa et al.[186]

The patients were divided into those with normal EF and no previous myocardial infarction before surgery (group 1, n = 57), and those with abnormal EF or infarction (group 2, n = 38). The single-photon emission computed tomographic images were normal in 37 patients in group 1 and in 6 patients in group 2. The patients with normal single-photon emission computed tomographic images had a higher EF after surgery than those with abnormal images (65% ± 10% v 50% ± 14%) and was higher in group 1 than in group 2 (64% ± 8% v 46% ± 16%). There was a significant correlation between the EF and the extent of perfusion abnormality. The patients with normal single-photon emission computed tomographic images could not be separated from those with abnormal images based on peak creatine kinase, creatine kinase-MB, and the electrocardiographic changes. Of the 69 patients with postoperative EF ≥50%, the perfusion pattern was normal in 41 and abnormal in 28; of the 26 patients with EF <50%, 24 had abnormal single-photon emission computed tomography. There was no significant change in mean EF after surgery (55% ± 14% before v 56% ± 15% after). Thus, simultaneous assessment of LV perfusion and function after CABG showed that an abnormal perfusion pattern may exist despite a normal EF. These patients could not be predicted by enzymes or electrocardiographic changes.

Adverse Events Afterwards

To determine whether adverse events occurring after CABG in Medicare patients can be predicted from clinical variables representing illness severity at admission, Geraci and associates,[188] from Boston, Mass, retrospectively analyzed 2,213 Medicare patients 65 years of age or more who underwent CABG between January 1985 and June 1986. Thirty-three percent of patients had one or more postoperative adverse events or died within 30 days of admission. Mortality within 30 days of admission was 7%; each adverse event was associated with increased mortality (range, 8% to 67%). Admission predictors of the occurrence of an adverse event included a history of CABG, emergency surgery, a history of chronic obstructive pulmonary disease, the presence of an infiltrate on admission chest radiograph, a pulse of 110 beats/minute or more, age, blood urea nitrogen of 11 mmol/L (30 mg/dL) or more, AMI at admission, and a history of AMI; the presence of one- or two-vessel disease was negatively associated with the occurrence of an adverse event. The model c-statistic was 0.64. Severity of illness at admission has modest predictive power with respect to adverse-event occurrence in Medicare patients who undergo CABG.

Late Results

Rahimtoola and associates,[189] from Portland, Ore, evaluated the 15- to 20-year outcome of CABG in patients with angina. The patient population included 7,529 patients who were operated on from 1969 to 1988. The 5-, 10-, 15-, and 20-year survival rates were 88%, 73%, 53%, and 38%, respectively. The actuarial percentages of re-operation and myocardial infarction at 15 years were 33% and 26%, respectively, and did not differ significantly between men and women (Figure 2-27). Eighty-one percent of the men versus 74% of the women had no angina or mild

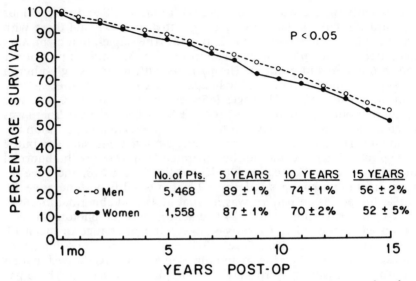

Figure 2-27. Late cohort. Actuarial survival by gender for patients operated on from 1974 to 1988. Reproduced with permission from Rahimtoola et al.[189]

angina at the most recent follow-up study. These authors concluded that these results of CABG after 20 years appear to be better than predictions based on the earlier studies of graft preclusion. Although women did experience a statistically significant higher operative mortality, reduced long-term survival probability, and less relief of angina than did men, the differences were small and not clinically significant.

Comparing With and Without Reoperation for Stenosis of Saphenous Vein Graft

Does coronary artery reoperation improve the survival of patients with stenoses in saphenous vein bypass grafts to coronary arteries? To examine this question, Lytle and associates,[190] from Cleveland, Ohio, retrospectively reviewed 1,117 patients who had CABG and then underwent a postoperative coronary angiogram that showed a stenosis (≥20%) of at least one vein graft. Reoperation within 1 month of the postoperative angiogram was performed for 394 patients (REOP group), whereas 723 patients (MED group) received initial medical therapy (no reoperation or PTCA within 1 year). Compared with the MED group, patients in the REOP group were older, more symptomatic, more likely to have LM stenosis, and had fewer patent bypass grafts. In-hospital mortality for the REOP group was 4.3%. Mean postangiogram follow-up of the entire group was 73 months. On the basis of the interval between the primary operation and the postoperative angiogram, patients were designated as having early (<5 years) or late (≥5 years) saphenous vein graft stenosis. Univariate and multivariate analyses were used to identify factors influencing the survival of these subgroups. Reoperation was not identified as a variable improving the survival of patients with early vein graft stenoses. For patients with late vein graft stenoses, moderate or severe impairment of LV function, advanced age, triple-vessel or LM stenosis, and stenosis in a vein graft to the LAD artery decreased survival, whereas reoperation improved survival. The improvement in survival with reoperation was particularly strong for patients with a stenotic vein graft to the LAD artery. For that subset, survival was 84% and 74% for the REOP group versus 76% and 53% for the MED group at 2 and 4 years after catheterization, respectively. For patients with stenotic vein grafts to the right coronary artery or circumflex coronary artery (or both), survival was 92% and 87% for the REOP group versus 89% and 78% for the MED group at 2 and 4 years after catheterization, respectively. Even for patients with class I and II symptoms, reoperation prolonged survival. Reoperation improves the survival of patients with late vein graft stenoses, those with stenotic grafts to the LAD coronary artery.

For a Third Time

Minimal data are available regarding the results of patients who have undergone CABG more than twice. Merrill and associates,[191] from Nashville, Tenn, reviewed the records of 13 consecutive patients who underwent CABG for the third time. All were operated on because of unstable angina. All patients were placed on cardiopulmonary bypass through a median sternotomy. The mean number of bypass grafts placed at the third operation was 1.9 (range, 1 to 3 grafts). A new internal mammary artery graft was placed in 6 patients (2 had prior internal mammary artery grafts). Hospital mortality was 7.7% (1/13). The single death was due to incomplete revascularization in a patient with poor distal vessels. Three patients required intra-aortic balloon pump support postoperatively, and 2 patients had prolonged ventilatory insufficiency. There were no late deaths. The 12 survivors have been followed up a mean of 44 months (range, 6 to 90 months). Four remain asymptomatic; 5 have mild angina easily controlled with medication. All except 1 are in improved condition compared with their preoperative status. The authors concluded that a third CABG can be performed with low mortality and morbidity and with the expectation of long-lasting symptomatic improvement.

Composition of Plaques in Men v Women in Saphenous Vein Conduits and Native Coronary Arteries

Plaque composition has been described in various manifestations of fatal CAD and after CABG, but no reports have investigated this composition according to gender. A total of 979 5-mm segments of native coronary arteries and 842 5-mm segments of saphenous vein grafts were examined by Mautner and associates,[192] from Bethesda, Md, by computerized planimetric techniques in 11 women and 11 men who were matched for survival time after CABG. The plaque components in women contained significantly more cellular fibrous tissue both in native coronary arteries and in saphenous vein grafts than in men. In contrast, the proportion of dense fibrous tissue was significantly less in the plaques of women than those in men both in native coronary arteries and in saphenous vein bypass grafts. The authors concluded that because cellular fibrous tissue is often found in the earlier stage of plaque development and dense fibrous tissue is a component in later stages, the plaques of the women appear younger than those of the men. This may be due to the later age at which atherosclerosis develops in women, or to other influences.

References

1. DeStefano F, Merritt RK, Anda RF, et al: Trends in nonfatal coronary artery disease in the USA, 1980 through 1989. Ann Intern Med 1993 (Nov 8);153:2489–2494.
2. Orencia A, Bailey K, Yawn BP, et al: Effect of gender on long-term outcome of angina pectoris and myocardial infarction/sudden unexpected death. JAMA 1993 (May 12);269:2392–2397.
3. Solymoss BC, Marcil M, Wesolowska E, et al: Relation of coronary artery disease in women <60 years of age to the combined elevation of serum lipoprotein(a) and total cholesterol to high-density cholesterol ratio. Am J Cardiol 1993 (Dec 1);72:1215–1219.
4. Kuhn FE, Rackley CE: Coronary artery disease in women. Arch Intern Med 1993 (Dec 13);153:2626–2636.
5. Mautner SL, Lin F, Mautner GC, et al: Comparison in women versus men of composition of atherosclerotic plaques in native coronary arteries and in saphenous veins used as aortocoronary conduits. J Am Coll Cardiol 1993 (May);21:1312–1318.
6. Johnson PA, Lee TH, Cook EF: Effect of race on the presentation and management of patients with acute chest pain. Ann Intern Med 1993 (April 15);118:593–601.
7. Stone PH, Gibson CM, Pasternak RC, for the Harvard Atherosclerosis Reversibility Project Study Group: Natural history of coronary atherosclerosis using quantitative angiography in men and implications for clinical trials of coronary regression. Am J Cardiol 1993 (Apr 1);71:766–772.
8. Waters D, Craven TE, Lesperance J: Prognostic significance of progression of coronary atherosclerosis. Circulation 1993 (April);87:1067–1075.
9. Jost S, Deckers JW, Nikutta P, and the INTACT investigators: Progression of coronary artery disease is dependent on anatomic location and diameter. J Am Coll Cardiol 1993 (May);21:1339–1346.
10. Guerra OR, Janowitz WR, Agatston AS, et al: Coronary artery diameter and coronary risk factors: A study with ultrafast computed tomography. Am Heart J 1993 (Sep);126:600–606.
11. Haskell WL, Sims C, Myll J, et al: Coronary artery size and dilating capacity in ultradistance runners. Circulation 1993 (April);87:1076–1082.
12. Hermiller JB, Tenaglia AN, Kisslo KB, et al: In vivo validation of compensatory enlargement of atherosclerotic coronary arteries. Am J Cardiol 1993 (Mar 15);71:665–668.
13. Stajduhar KC, Laird JR, Rogan KM, et al: Coronary arterial ectasia: Increased prevalence in patients with abdominal aortic aneurysm as compared to occlusive atherosclerotic peripheral vascular disease. Am Heart J 1993 (Jan);125:86–92.
14. Jiang W, Hayano J, Coleman ER, et al: Relation of cardiovascular responses to mental stress and cardiac vagal activity in coronary artery disease. Am J Cardiol 1993 (Sep 1);72:551–554.
15. Boltwood MD, Taylor CB, Burke MB, et al: Anger Report predicts coronary artery vasomotor response to mental stress in atherosclerotic segments. Am J Cardiol 1993 (Dec 15);72:1361–1365.
16. Carney RM, Freedland KE, Rich MW, et al: Ventricular tachycardia and psychiatric depression in coronary artery disease. Am J Med 1993 (July);95:23–28.

17. Michaelides A, Ryan JM, VanFossen D, et al: Exercise-induced QRS prolongation in patients with coronary artery disease: A marker of myocardial ischemia. Am Heart J 1993 (Dec);126:1320–1325.

18. Featherstone JF, Holly RG, Amsterdam EA: Physiologic Responses to Weight Lifting in Coronary Artery Disease. Am J Cardiol 1993 (Feb 1);71:287–292.

19. Collins P, Bulman J, Chung H-I, et al: Hemoglobin inhibitis endothelium-dependent relaxation to acetylcholine in human coronary arteries in vivo. Circulation 1993 (Jan);87:80–85.

20. Arbustini E, Grasso M, Diegoli M, et al: Morphologic changes induced by acetylcholine infusion in normal and atherosclerotic coronary arteries. Am J Cardiol 1993 (June 15);71:1382–1390.

21. Egashira K, Inou T, Hirooka Y, et al: Effects of age on endothelium dependent vasodilation of resistance coronary artery by acetylcholine in humans. Circulation 1993 (July);88:77–81.

22. Lefroy DC, Crake T, Uren NG, et al: Effect of inhibition of nitric oxide synthesis on epicardial coronary artery caliber and coronary blood flow in humans. Circulation 1993 (July);88:43–54.

23. Linnanmäki E, Leinonen M, Mattila K, et al: Chlamydia Pneumoniae—specific circulating immune complexes in patients with chronic coronary heart disease. Circulation 1993 (April);87:1130–1134.

24. Ernst SMPG, Tjonjoegin M, Schrader R, et al: Immediate sealing of arterial puncture sites after cardiac catheterization and coronary angioplasty using a biodegradable collagen plug: Results of an international registry. J Am Coll Cardiol 1993 (March 15);21:851–855.

25. Castro-Beiras A, Muniz J, Fernandez-Fuertes I, et al: Family history as an independent risk factor for ischaemic heart disease in a low incidence area (Galicia, Spain). Euro Heart J 1993 (Nov);14:1445–1450.

26. French JK, Elliott JM, Williams BF, et al: Association of angiographically detected coronary artery disease with low levels of high-density lipoprotein cholesterol and systemic hypertension. Am J Cardiol 1993 (March 1);71:505–510.

27. Fazio GP, Redberg RF, Winslow T, et al: Transesophageal echocardiographically detected atherosclerotic aortic plaque is a marker for coronary artery disease. J Am Coll Cardiol 1993 (Jan);21:144–150.

28. Ögren M, Hedblad B, Isacsson S-O, et al: Non-invasively detected carotid stenosis and coronary heart disease in mean with leg arteriosclerosis. Lancet 1993 (Nov 6);342:1138–1141.

29. Landesberg G, Luria MH, Cotev S, et al: Importance of long-duration postoperative ST-segment depression in cardiac morbidity after vascular surgery. Lancet 1993 (March 20);341:715–719.

30. Takase B, Younis LT, Byers SL, et al: Comparative prognostic value of clinical risk indexes, resting two-dimensional echocardiography, and dipyridamole stress thallium-201 myocardial imaging for perioperative cardiac events in major nonvascular surgery patients. Am Heart J 1993 (Nov);126:1099–1106.

31. Lebwohl M, Halperin J, Phelps, RG: Occult pseudoxanthoma elasticum in patients with premature cardiovascular disease. N Engl J Med 1993 (Oct 21);329:1237–1239.

32. Gorgels APM, Vos MA, Mulleneers R, et al: Value of the electrocardiogram in diagnosing the number of severely narrowed coronary arteries in rest angina pectoris. Am J Cardiol 1993 (Nov 1);72:999–1003.

33. Ribisl PM, Liu J, Mousa I, et al: Comparison of Computer ST criteria for diagnosis of severe coronary artery disease. Am J Cardiol 1993 (March 1);71:546–551.

34. Gallik DM, Mahmarian JJ, Verani MS: Therapeutic significance of exercise-induced ST-segment elevation in patients without previous myocardial infarction. Am J Cardiol 1993 (July 1);72:1–7.

35. Raby KE, Barry J, Treasure CB, et al: Usefulness of Holter monitoring for detecting myocardial ischemia in patients with nondiagnostic exercise treadmill test. Am J Cardiol 1993 (Oct 15);72:889–893.

36. Bernstein SJ, Hilborne LH, Leape LL, et al: The appropriateness of use of coronary angiography in New York State. JAMA 1993 (Feb 10); 269:766–769.

37. Poldermans D, Fioretti PM, Forster T, et al: Dobutamine stress echocardiography for assessment of perioperative cardiac risk in patients undergoing major vascular surgery. Circulation 1993 (May);87:1506–1512.

38. Bach DS, Hepner A, Marcovitz PA, et al: Dobutamine stress echocardiography: Prevalence of a nonischemic response in a low-risk population. Am Heart J 1993 (May);125:1257–1261.

39. Marwick T, D'hondt A, Baudhuin T, et al: Optimal use of dobutamine stress for the detection and evaluation of coronary artery disease: Combination with echocardiography or scintigraphy, or both? J Am Coll Cardiol 1993; (July);22:159–167.

40. Mertes H, Sawada SG, Ryan T, et al: Symptoms, adverse effects, and complications associated with dobutamine stress echocardiography. Experience in 1118 patients. Circulation 1993 (July);88:15–19.

41. Hoffmann R, Lethen H, Kleinhans E, et al: Comparative evaluation of bicycle and dobutamine stress echocardiography with perfusion scintigraphy and bicycle electrocardiogram for identification of coronary artery disease. Am J Cardiol 1993 (Sep 1);72:555–559.

42. Previtali M, Lanzarini L, Fetiveau R, et al: Comparison of dobutamine stress echocardiography, dipyridamole stress echocardiography and exercise stress testing for diagnosis of coronary artery disease. Am J Cardiol 1993 (Oct 15);72:865–870.

43. Hodgson JM, Reddy KG, Nair RN, et al: Intracoronary ultrasound imaging: Correlation of plaque morphology with angiography, clinical syndrome and procedural results in patients undergoing coronary angioplasty. J Am Coll Cardiol 1993 (Jan);21:35–44.

44. Hermiller JB, Buller CE, Tenaglia AN, et al: Unrecognized left main coronary artery disease in patients undergoing interventional procedures. Am J Cardiol 1993 (Jan 15);71:173–176.

45. Dupouy P, Geschwind HJ, Pelle G, et al: Assessment of coronary vasomotion by intracoronary ultrasound. Am Heart J 1993 (July);126:76–85.

46. Maublant JC, Lipiecki J, Citron B, et al: Reinjection as an alternative to rest imaging for detection of exercise-induced ischemia with thallium-201 emission tomography. Am Heart J 1993 (Feb);125:230–335.

47. Iskandrian AS, Heo J, Lemlek J, et al: Identification of high-risk patients with left main and three-vessel coronary artery disease by adenosine-single photon emission computed tomographic thallium imaging. Am Heart J 1993 (April);125:1130–1135.

48. O'Keefe JH, Bateman TM, Barnhart CS: Adenosine thallium-201 is superior to exercise thallium-201 for detecting coronary artery disease in patients with left bundle branch block. J Am Coll Cardiol 1993; (May)21:1332–1338.

49. Klein J, Rodrigues EA, Berman DS, et al: Prevalence and functional significance of transient ST-segment depression during daily life activity: Comparisons of ambulatory ECG with stress redistribution thallium 201 single-photon emission computed tomographic imaging. Am Heart J 1993 (May); 125:1247–1257.

50. Hays JT, Mahmarian JJ, Cochran AJ, et al: Dobutamine thallium-201 tomography for evaluating patients with suspected coronary artery disease unable to undergo exercise or vasodilator pharmacologic stress testing. J Am Coll Cardiol 1993 (June);21:1583–1590.

51. Matzer L, Kiat H, VanTrain K, et al: Quantitative severity of stress thallium-201 myocardial perfusion single-photon emission computed tomography

defects in one-vessel coronary artery disease. Am J Cardiol 1993 (Aug 1);72:273–279.

52. Dilsizian V, Perrone-Filardi P, Arrighi JA, et al: Concordance and discordance between stress-redistribution-reinjection and rest-redistribution thallium imaging for assessing viable myocardium. Comparison with metabolic activity by positron emission tomography. Circulation 1993 (Sep); 88:941–952.

53. Norris LP, Stewart RE, Jain AM, et al: Biplane transesophageal pacing echocardiography compared with dipyridamole thallium-201 single-photon emission computed tomography in detecting coronary artery disease. Am Heart J 1993 (Sep);126:676–685.

54. Manning WJ, Li W, Boyle NG, et al: Fat-suppressed breath-hold magnetic resonance coronary angiography. Circulation 1993 (Jan);87:94–104.

55. Manning WJ, Li W, Edelman RR: A preliminary report comparing magnetic resonance coronary angiography with conventional angiography. N Engl J Med 1993 (March 25);328:828–832.

56. Van Rugge FP, Van der Wall EE, De Roos A, et al: Dobutamine stress magnetic resonance imaging for detection of coronary artery disease. J Am Coll Cardiol 1993 (Aug);22:431–439.

57. Janowitz WR, Agatston AS, Kaplan G, et al: Differences in prevalence and extent of coronary artery calcium detected by ultrafast computed tomography in asymptomatic men and women. Am J Cardiol 1993 (Aug 1); 72:247–254.

58. Lawson W, BenEliyahu D, Meinken L, et al: Infrared thermography in the detection and management of coronary artery disease. Am J Cardiol 1993 (Oct 15);72:894–896.

59. Morrow K, Morris CK, Froelicher VF, et al: Prediction of cardiovascular death in men undergoing noninvasive evaluation for coronary artery disease. Ann Intern Med 1993 (May 1);118:689–695.

60. Morris CK, Morrow K, Froelicher VF, et al: Prediction of cardiovascular death by means of clinical and exercise test variables in patients selected for cardiac catheterization. Am Heart J 1993 (June);125:1717–1726.

61. Mazeika PK, Nadazdin A, Oakley CM: Prognostic value of dobutamine echocardiography in patients with high pretest likelihood of coronary artery disease. Am J Cardiol 1993 (Jan 1);71:33–39.

62. Krivokapich J, Child JS, Gerber RS, et al: Prognostic usefulness of positive or negative exercise stress echocardiography for predicting coronary events in ensuing twelve months. Am J Cardiol 1993 (March 15);71:646–651.

63. Travin MI, Boucher CA, Newell JB, et al: Variables associated with a poor prognosis in patients with an ischemic thallium-201 exercise test. Am Heart J 1993 (Feb);125:335–344.

64. Ahmed WH, Bittl JA, Braunwald E: Relation between clinical presentation and angiographic findings in unstable angina pectoris, and comparison with that in stable angina. Am J Cardiol 1993 (Sep 1);72:544–550.

65. Serneri GGN, Boddi M, Arata L, et al: Silent ischemia in unstable angina is related to an altered cardiac norepinephrine handling. Circulation 1993 (June);87:1928–1937.

66. Flugelman MY, Virmani R, Correa R, et al: Smooth muscle cell abundance and fibroblast growth factors in coronary lesions of patients with nonfatal unstable angina. A clue to the mechanism of transformation from the stable to the unstable clinical state. Circulation 1993 (Dec);88:2493–2500.

67. Mazzone A, De Servi S, Ricevuti G, et al: Increased expression of neutrophil and monocyte adhesion molecules in unstable coronary artery disease. Circulation 1993 (Aug);88:358–363.

68. Colles P, Juneau M, Gregoire J, et al: Effect of a standardized meal on the threshold of exercise-induced myocardial ischemia in patients with stable angina. J Am Coll Cardiol 1993 (April);21:1052–57.

69. Amanullah AM, Bevegård S, Lindvall K, et al: Assessment of left ventricular wall motion in angina pectoris by two-dimensional echocardiography and myocardial perfusion by technetium-99m sestamibi tomography during adenosine-induced coronary vasodilation and comparison with coronary angiography. Am J Cardiol 1993 (Nov 1);72:983–989.

70. Vanoverschelde J-L J, Wijns W, Depré C, et al: Mechanisms of chronic regional postischemic dysfunction in humans. New insights from the Study of Noninfarcted Collateral-Dependent Myocardium. Circulation 1993 (May); 87:1513–1523.

71. Tousoulis D, Davies G, McFadden E, et al: Coronary vasomotor effects of serotonin in patients with angina. Relation to coronary stenosis morphology. Circulation 1993 (Oct);88[part 1]:1518–1526.

72. Quyyumi AA, Panza JA, Callahan TS, et al: Prognostic implications of myocardial ischemia during daily life in low risk patients with coronary artery disease. J Am Coll Cardiol 1993 (March 1);21:700–708.

73. Andrews TC, Fenton T, Toyosaki N, et al, for the Angina and Silent Ischemia Study Group (ASIS): Subsets of ambulatory myocardial ischemia based on heart rate activity. Circadian distribution and response to anti-ischemic medication. Circulation 1993 (July);88:92–100.

74. Droste C, Ruf G, Greenlee MW, et al: Development of angina pectoris pain and cardiac events in asymptomatic patients with myocardial ischemia. Am J Cardiol 1993 (July 15);72:121–127.

75. Hikita H, Kurita A, Takase B, et al: Usefulness of plasma beta-endorphin level, pain threshold and automatic function in assessing silent myocardial ischemia in patients with and without diabetes mellitus. Am J Cardiol 1993 (July 15);72:140–143.

76. Thaulow E, Erikssen J, Sandvik L, et al: Initial clinical presentation of cardiac disease in asymptomatic men with silent myocardial ischemia and angiographically documented coronary artery disease (the Oslo Ischemia Study). Am J Cardiol 1993 (Sep 15);72:629–633.

77. Moss AJ, Goldstein RE, Hall WJ, et al: Detection and significance of myocardial ischemia in stable patients after recovery from an acute coronary event. JAMA 1993 (May 12);269:2379–2385.

78. Sugiishi M, Takatsu F: Cigarette smoking is a major risk factor for coronary spasm. Circulation 1993 (Jan);87:76–79.

79. Montorsi P, Agostoni PG, Annoni L, et al: Cardiopulmonary exercise testing in syndrome X. Am Heart J 1993 (March);125:711–717.

80. Romeo F, Rosano GMC, Martuscelli E, et al: Long-term follow-up of patients initially diagnosed with syndrome X. Am J Cardiol 1993 (March 15);71:669–673.

81. Chahine RA, Feldman RL, Giles TD, et al, and the Amlodipine Study 160 Group: Randomized placebo-controlled trial of amlodipine in vasopastic angina. J Am Coll Cardiol 1993 (May);21:1365–1370.

82. Egashira K, Inou T, Hirooka Y, et al: Evidence of impaired endothelium dependent coronary vasodilation in patients with angina pectoris and normal coronary angiograms. N Engl J Med 1993 (June 10);328:1659–1664.

83. Chauhan A, Mullins PA, Thuraisingham SI, et al: Clinical presentation and functional prognosis in syndrome X. Br Heart J 1993 (Oct);70:346–351.

84. Tousoulis D, Crake T, Lefroy DC, et al: Left ventricular hypercontractility and ST segment depression in patients with syndrome X. J Am Coll Cardiol 1993 (Nov 15);22:1607–1613.

85. Murray PM, Herrington DM, Pettus CW, et al: Should patients with heart disease exercise in the morning or afternoon? Arch Intern Med 1993 (April 12);833–836.

86. Lavie CJ, Milani RV: Factors predicting improvements in lipid values following cardiac rehabilitation and exercise training. Arch Intern Med 1993 (April 26);153:982–988.

87. Hambrecht R, Niebauer J, Marburger C, et al: Various intensities of leisure

time physical activity in patients with coronary artery disease: Effects on cardiorespiratory fitness and progression of coronary atherosclerotic lesions. J Am Coll Cardiol 1993 (Aug);22:468–477.

88. Théroux P, Waters D, Qiu S, et al: Aspirin versus heparin to prevent myocardial infarction during the acute phase of unstable angina. Circulation 1993 (Nov);88[part 1]:2045–2048.

89. Blankenhorn DH, Azen SP, Kramsch DM, et al: Coronary angiographic changes with lovastatin therapy (The Monitored Atherosclerosis Regression Study [MARS]). Ann Intern Med 1993 (Nov 15);119:969–976.

90. Chrysant SG, Glasser SP, Bittar N, et al: Efficacy and safety of extended-release isosorbide mononitrate for stable effort angina pectoris. Am J Cardiol 1993 (Dec 1);72:1249–1256.

91. Landau AJ, Frishman WH, Alturk N, et al: Improvement in exercise tolerance and immediate beta-adrenergic blockade with intranasal propranolol in patients with angina pectoris. Am J Cardiol 1993 (Nov 1);72:995–998.

92. Borzak S, Fenton T, Glasser SP, et al, for the Angina and Silent Ischemia Study Group (ASIS): Discordance between effects of anti-ischemic therapy on ambulatory ischemia, exercise performance and anginal symptoms in patients with stable angina pectoris. J Am Coll Cardiol 1993 (June); 21:1605–1611.

93. Raby KR, Vita JA, Pocci MB, et al: Changing vasomotor responses of coronary arteries to nifedipine. Am Heart J 1993 (Aug);126:333–338.

94. Pupita G, Mazzara D, Centanni M, et al: Ischemia in collateral-dependent myocardium: Effects of nifedipine and diltiazem in man. Am Heart J 1993 (July);126:86–94.

95. Quyyumi AA, Diodati JG, Lakatos E, et al: Angiogenic effects of low molecular weight heparin in patients with stable coronary artery disease: A pilot study. J Am Coll Cardiol 1993 (Sep);22:635–641.

96. Melandri G, Semprini F, Cervi V, et al: Benefit of adding low molecular weight heparin to the conventional treatment of stable angina pectoris. A double-blind, randomized, placebo-controlled trial. Circulation 1993 (Dec);88:2517–2523.

97. Zoldhelyi P, Webster MWI, Fuster V, et al: Recombinant hirudin in patients with chronic, stable coronary artery disease. Safety, half-life, and effect on coagulation parameters. Circulation 1993 (Nov);88[part 1]: 2015–2022.

98. van den Bos AA, Deckers JW, Heyndrickx GR, et al: Safety and efficacy of recombinant hirudin (CGP 39 393) versus heparin in patients with stable angina undergoing coronary angioplasty. Circulation 1993 (Nov);88[part 1]:2058–2066.

99. Cannon CP, Maraganore JM, Loscalzo J, et al: Anticoagulant effects of hirulog, a novel thrombin inhibitor in patients with coronary artery disease. Am J Cardiol 1993 (April 1);71:778–782.

100. Lidón RM, Théroux P, Juneau M, et al: Initial experience with a direct antithrombin, hirulog, in unstable angina. Circulation 1993 (Oct);88[part 1]:1495–1501.

101. Sharma GVRK, Lapsley D, Vita JA, et al: Usefulness and tolerability of hirulog, a direct thrombin-inhibitor, in unstable angina pectoris. Am J Cardiol 1993 (Dec 15);72:1357–1360.

102. Meyer BJ, Amann FW: Additional antianginal efficacy of amiodarone in patients with limiting angina pectoris. Am Heart J 1993 (April);125: 996–1001.

103. Langa KM, Sussman EJ: The effect of cost containment policies on rates of coronary revascularization in California. N Engl J Med 1993 (Dec 9);329:1784–1789.

104. Azanian JZ, Udvarhelyi IS, Gatsonis CA, et al: Racial differences in the use of revascularization procedures after coronary angiography. JAMA 1993 (May 26);269:2642–2646.

105. Whittle J, Conigliaro J, Good CB, et al: Racial differences in the use of invasive cardiovascular procedures in the department of veterans affairs medical system. N Engl J Med 1993 (Aug 26);329:621–627.

106. RITA Trial Participants: Coronary angioplasty versus coronary artery bypass grafting (the Randomised Intervention Treatment of Angina [RITA] trial). Lancet 1993 (March 6);341:573–580.

107. Weintraub WS, King SB III, Jones EL, et al: Coronary surgery and coronary angioplasty in patients with two-vessel coronary artery disease. Am J Cardiol 1993 (March 1);71:511–517.

108. O'Keefe JH Jr, Allan JJ, McCallister BD, et al: Angioplasty versus bypass surgery for multivessel coronary artery disease with left ventricular ejection fracion ≤40%. Am J Cardiol 1993 (April 15);71:897–901.

109. Rodriguez A, Boullon F, Perez-Balino N, et al, on behalf of the ERACI Group: Argentine randomized trial of percutaneous transluminal coronary angioplasty versus coronary artery bypass surgery in multivessel disease (ERACI): In-hospital results and 1 year follow-up. J Am Coll Cardiol 1993 (Oct);22:1060–1067.

110. Allen BS, Buckberg GD, Fontan FM, et al: Superiority of controlled surgical reperfusion versus percutaneous transluminal coronary angioplasty in acute coronary occlusion. J Thorac Cardiovas Surg 1993 (May);105: 864–884.

111. Lubitz JD, Gornick ME, Mentnech RM, et al: Rehospitalizations after coronary revascularization among Medicare beneficiaries. Am J Cardiol 1993 (July 1);72:26–30.

112. Hilborne LH, Leape LL, Bernstein SJ, et al: The appropriateness of use of percutaneous transluminal coronary angioplasty in New York State. JAMA 1993 (Feb 10);269:761–765.

113. Teirstein PS, Vogel RA, Dorros G, et al: Prophylactic versus standby cardiopulmonary support for high risk percutaneous transluminal coronary angioplasty. J Am Coll Cardiol 1993 (Mar 1);21:590–596.

114. Lamm C, Dohnal M, Serruys PW, et al: High-fidelity translesional pressure gradients during percutaneous transluminal coronary angioplasty: Correlation with quantitative coronary angiography. Am Heart J 1993 (July);126:66–75.

115. De Bruyne B, Sys SU, Heyndrickx GR: Percutaneous transluminal coronary angioplasty catheters versus fluid-filled pressure monitoring guidewires for coronary pressure measurements and correlation with quantitative coronary angiography. Am J Cardiol 1993 (Nov 15);72: 1101–1106.

116. Piek JJ, Koolen JJ, van Rijn ACM, et al: Spectral analysis of flow velocity in the contralateral artery during coronary angioplasty: A new method for assessing collateral flow. J Am Coll Cardiol 1993 (June);21:1574–1582.

117. Kelsey SF, James M, Holubkov AL, et al, and investigators from the National Heart, Lung, and Blood Institute Percutaneous Transluminal Coronary Angioplasty Registry: Results of percutaneous transluminal coronary angioplasty in women. 1985–1986 National Heart, Lung, and Blood Institute's Coronary Angioplasty Registry. Circulation 1993 (March);87: 720–727.

118. Bell MR, Holmes DR, Berger PB, et al: The changing in-hospital mortality of women undergoing percutaneous transluminal coronary angioplasty. JAMA 1993 (April 28);269:2091–2095.

119. Berger PB, Bell MR, Garratt KN, et al: Initial results and long-term outcome of coronary angioplasty in chronic mild angina pectoris. Am J Cardiol 1993 (June 15);71:1396–1401.

120. Holmes DR Jr, Detre KM, Williams DO, et al: Long-term outcome of patients with depressed left ventricular function undergoing percutaneous transluminal coronary angioplasty. The NHLBI PTCA Registry. Circulation 1993 (Jan);87:21–29.

121. Ofili EO, Kern MJ, Labovitz AJ, et al: Analysis of coronary blood flow velocity dynamics in angiographically normal and stenosed arteries before and after endolumen enlargement by angioplasty. J Am Coll Cardiol 1993 (Feb 21);2:308–316.

122. Tenaglia AN, Zidar JP, Jackman JD Jr, et al: Treatment of long coronary artery narrowing with long angioplasty balloon catheters. Am J Cardiol 1993 (June 1);71:1274–1277.

123. Nanto S, Nishida K, Hirayama A, et al: Supported angioplasty with synchronized retroperfusion in high-risk patients with left main trunk or near left main trunk obstruction. Am Heart J 1993 (Feb);125:301–309.

124. Topol EJ, Bonan R, Jewitt D, et al: Use of a direct antithrombin, hirulog, in place of heparin during coronary angioplasty. Circulation 1993 (May); 87:1622–1629.

125. Vemuri DN, Kochar GS, Maniet AR, et al: Angioplasty of the septal perforators: Acute outcome and long-term clinical efficacy. Am Heart J 1993 (March);125:682–686.

126. Buffet P, Danchin N, Marc MO, et al: Results of percutaneous transluminal coronary angioplasty of either the left anterior descending or left circumflex coronary artery in patients with chronic total occlusion of the right coronary artery. Am J Cardiol 1993 (Feb 15);71:382–385.

127. Liu MW, Douglas JS Jr, Lembo NJ, et al: Angiographic predictors of a rise in serum creatine kinase (distal embolization) after balloon angioplasty of saphenous vein coronary artery bypass grafts. Am J Cardiol 1993 (Sep 1);72:514–517.

128. Gasperetti CM, Gonias SL, Gimple LW, et al: Platelet activation during coronary angioplasty in humans. Circulation 1993 (Dec);88:2728–2734.

129. El-Tamimi H, Davies GJ, Crea F, et al: Response of human coronary arteries to acetylcholine after injury by coronary angioplasty. J Am Coll Cardiol 1993 (April);21:1152–1157.

130. McFadden EP, Bauters C, Lablanche J-M, et al: Response of human coronary arteries to serotonin after injury by coronary angioplasty. Circulation 1993 (Nov);88[part 1]:2076–2085.

131. Koning R, Cribier A, Korsatz L, et al: Progressive decrease in myocardial ischemia assessed by intracoronary electrocardiogram during successive and prolonged coronary occlusions in angioplasty. Am Heart J 1993 (Jan);125:56–61.

132. King SB, Schlumpf M: Ten-year completed follow-up of percutaneous transluminal coronary angioplasty: The early Zurich experience. J Am Coll Cardiol 1993 (Aug);22:353–360.

133. Le Feuvre C, Bonan R, Côté G, et al: Five- to ten-year outcome after multivessel percutaneous transluminal coronary angioplasty. Am J Cardiol 1993 (May 15);71:1153–1158.

134. Sharma SK, Israel DH, Kamean JI, et al: Clinical, angiographic, and procedural determinants of major and minor coronary dissection during angioplasty. Am Heart J 1993 (July);126:39–47.

135. Kern MJ, Aguirre F, Bach R, et al: Augmentation of coronary blood flow by intra-aortic balloon pumping in patients after coronary angioplasty. Circulation 1993 (Feb);87:500–511.

136. Fail PS, Maniet AR, Banka VS: Subcutaneous heparin in postangioplasty management: Comparative trial with intravenous heparin. Am Heart J 1993 (Nov);126:1059–1067.

137. Scott NA, Weintraub WS, Carlin SF, et al: Recent changes in the management and outcome of acute closure after percutaneous transluminal coronary angioplasty. Am J Cardiol 1993 (May 15);71:1159–1163.

138. Bell MR, Reeder GS, Garratt KN, et al: Predictors of major ischemic complications after coronary dissection following angioplasty. Am J Cardiol 1993 (Jun 15);71:1402–1407.

139. Tschoepe D, Schultheiss HP, Kolarov P, et al: Platelet membrane activation

markers are predictive for increased risk of acute ischemic events after PTCA. Circulation 1993 (July);88:37–42.

140. Hermans WRM, Foley DP, Rensing BJ, et al, on behalf of the CARPORT and MERCATOR Study Groups: Usefulness of quantitative and qualitative angiographic lesion morphology, and clinical characteristics in predicting major adverse cardiac events during and after native coronary balloon angioplasty. Am J Cardiol 1993 (July 1);72:14–20.

141. Van der Linden LP, Bakx ALM, Sedney MI, et al: Prolonged dilation with an autoperfusion balloon catheter for refractory acute occlusion related to percutaneous transluminal coronary angioplasty. J Am Coll Cardiol 1993;(Oct);22:1016–1023.

142. Hecht HS, DeBord L, Shaw R, et al: Usefulness of supine bicycle stress echocardiography for detection of restenosis after percutaneous transluminal coronary angioplasty. Am J Cardiol 1993 (Feb 1);71:293–296.

143. Weintraub WS, Ghazzal ZMB, Douglas JS Jr, et al: Long-term clinical follow-up in patients with angiographic restudy after successful angioplasty. Circulation 1993 (March);87:831–840.

144. Gapinski JP, VanRuiswyk JV, Heudebert GR, et al: Preventing restenosis following coronary angioplasty with fish oils. Arch Intern Med 1993 (July 12);153:1595–1601.

145. Bauters C, McFadden EP, Lablanche J-M, et al: Restenosis rate after multiple percutaneous transluminal coronary angioplasty procedures at the same site. A quantitative angiographic study in consecutive patients undergoing a third angioplasty procedure for a second restenosis. Circulation 1993 (Sep);88:969–974.

146. Rensing BJ, Hermans WRM, Vos J, et al, on behalf of the Coronary Artery Restenosis Prevention on Repeated Thromboxane Antagonism (CARPORT) Study Group: Luminal narrowing after percutaneous transluminal coronary angioplasty. A study of clinical, procedural, and lesional factors related to long-term angiographic outcome. Circulation 1993 (Sep); 88:975–985.

147. Serruys PW, Klein W, Tijssen JPG, et al: Evaluation of ketanserin in the prevention of restenosis after percutaneous transluminal coronary angioplasty. A multicenter randomized double-blind placebo-controlled trial. Circulation 1993 (Oct);88[part 1]:1588–1601.

148. Marie PY, Danchin N, Karcher G, et al: Usefulness of exercise SPECT-thallium to detect asymptomatic restenosis in patients who had angina before coronary angioplasty. Am Heart J 1993 (Sep);126:571–577.

149. Piessens JH, Stammen F, Desmet W, et al: Immediate and 6-month follow-up results of coronary angioplasty for restenosis: Analysis of factors predicting recurrent clinical restenosis. Am Heart J 1993 (Sep);126: 565–570.

150. Weintraub WS, Brown CL, Liberman HA, et al: Effect of restenosis at one previously dilated coronary site on the probability of restenosis at another previously dilated coronary site. Am J Cardiol 1993 (Nov 15);72: 1107–1113.

151. Heinle SK, Lieberman EB, Ancukiewicz M, et al: Usefulness of dobutamine echocardiography for detecting restenosis after percutaneous transluminal coronary angioplasty. Am J Cardiol 1993 (Dec 1);72: 1220–1225.

152. Kuntz RE, Gibson CM, Nobuyoshi M, et al: Generalized model of restenosis after conventional balloon angioplasty, stenting and directional atherectomy. J Am Coll Cardiol 1993 (Jan);21:15–25.

153. Stertzer SH, Rosenblum J, Shaw RE, et al: Coronary rotational ablation: Initial experience in 302 patients. J Am Coll Cardiol 1993 (Feb 21);2:287–295.

154. Suarez de Lezo J, Romero M, Medina A, et al: Intracoronary ultrasound

assessment of directional atherectomy: Immediate and follow-up findings. J Am Coll Cardiol 1993 (Feb 21);2:298–307.

155. Simons M, Leclerc G, Safian RD, et al: Relation between activated smooth-muscle cells in coronary-artery lesions and restenosis after atherectomy. N Engl J Med 1993 (March 4);328:608–613.

156. Popma JJ, De Cesare NB, Pinkerton CA, et al: Quantitative analysis of factors influencing late lumen loss and restenosis after directional coronary atherectomy. Am J Cardiol 1993 (March 1);71:552–557.

157. Miller MJ, Kuntz RE, Friedrich SP, et al: Frequency and consequences of intimal hyperplasia in specimens retrieved by directional atherectomy of native primary coronary artery stenoses and subsequent restenoses. Am J Cardiol 1993 (March 15);71:652–658.

158. Brogan WC III, Popma JJ, Pichard AD, et al: Rotational coronary atherectomy after unsuccessful coronary balloon angioplasty. Am J Cardiol 1993 (April 1);71:794–798.

159. Medina A, Suarez de Lezo J, Hernandez E, et al: Serial angiographic observations after successful directional coronary atherectomy. Am Heart J 1993 (May);125:1217–1220.

160. Suneja R, Nair RN, Reddy KG, et al: Mechanisms of angiographically successful directional coronary atherectomy: Evaluation by intracoronary ultrasound and comparison with transluminal coronary angioplasty. Am Heart J 1993 (Sep);126:507–514.

161. Kovach JA, Mintz GS, Pichard AD, et al: Sequential intravascular ultrasound characterization of the mechanisms of rotational atherectomy and adjunct balloon angioplasty. J Am Coll Cardiol 1993 (Oct);22:1024–1032.

162. de Jaegere PP, Hermans WR, Rensing BJ, et al: Matching based on quantitative coronary angiography as a surrogate for randomized studies: Comparison between stent implantation and balloon angioplasty of native coronary artery lesions. Am Heart J 1993 (Feb);125:310–319.

163. Carrozza JP, Kuntz RE, Fishman RF, et al: Restenosis after arterial injury caused by coronary stenting in patients with diabetes mellitus compared to those without. An Intern Med 1993 (March 1);118:344–349.

164. Lincoff AM, Topol EJ, Chapekis AT, et al: Intracoronary stenting compared with conventional therapy for abrupt vessel closure complicating coronary angioplasty: A matched case-control study. J Am Coll Cardiol 1993 (Mar 15);21:866–875.

165. Foley JB, Penn IM, Brown RIG, et al: Safety, success, and restenosis after elective coronary implantation of the Palmaz-Schatz stent in 100 patients at a single center. Am Heart J 1993 (March);125:686–694.

166. Kastrati A, Schomig A, Dietz R, et al: Time course of restenosis during the first year after emergency coronary stenting. Circulation 1993 (May);87:1498–1505.

167. Kimura T, Nosaka H, Yokoi H, et al: Serial angiographic follow-up after Palmaz-Schatz stent implantation: Comparison with conventional balloon angioplasty. J Am Coll Cardiol 1993 (June);21:1557–1563.

168. Maiello L, Colombo A, Gianrossi R, et al: Coronary stenting for treatment of acute or threatened closure following dissection after coronary balloon angioplasty. Am Heart J 1993 (June);125:1570–1575.

169. Laskey WX, Brady ST, Kussmaul WG, et al: Intravascular ultrasonographic assessment of the results of coronary artery stenting. Am Heart J 1993 (June);1576–1683.

170. George BS, Voorhees WD, Roubin GS, et al: Multicenter investigation of coronary stenting to treat acute or threatened closure after percutaneous transluminal coronary angioplasty: Clinical and angiographic outcomes. J Am Coll Cardiol 1993 (July);22:135–143.

171. Haude M, Erbel R, Issa H, et al: Subacute thrombotic complications after intracoronary implantation of Palmaz-Schatz stents. Am Heart J 1993 (July);126:15–22.

172. Kiemeneij F, Laarman GJ, van der Wieken P, et al: Emergency coronary stenting with the Palmaz-Schatz stent for failed transluminal coronary angioplasty: Results of a learning phase. Am Heart J 1993 (July);126:23–31.

173. Resar JR, Wolff MR, Blumenthal RS, et al: Brachial approach for intracoronary stent implantation: A feasibility study. Am Heart J 1993 (Aug);126:300–304.

174. Hearn JA, King SB III, Douglas JS Jr, et al: Clinical and angiographic outcomes after coronary artery stenting for acute or threatened closure after percutaneous transluminal coronary angioplasty. Initial results with a balloon expandable, stainless steel design. Circulation 1993 (Nov);88[part 1]:2086–2096.

175. Geschwind HJ, Nakamura F, Kvasicka J, et al: Excimer and holmium yttrium aluminum garnet laser coronary angioplasty. Am Heart J 1993 (Feb);125:510–522.

176. Eigler NL, Weinstock B, Douglas JS, et al, for the ELCA investigators: Excimer laser coronary angioplasty of aorto-ostial stenoses. Results of the Excimer Laser Coronary Angioplasty (ELCA) registry in the first 200 patients. Circulation 1993 (Nov);88[part 1]:2049–2057.

177. Anderson GM, Grumbach K, Luft HS, et al: Use of coronary artery bypass surgery in the United States and Canada. JAMA 1993 (April 7); 269:1661–1666.

178. Leape LL, Hilborne LH, Park RE, et al: The appropriateness of use of coronary artery bypass graft surgery in New York State. JAMA 1993 (Feb 10);269:753–760.

179. Lansman SL, Cohen M, Galla JD, et al: Effectiveness of cardiopulmonary bypass grafting with ejection fraction of 0.20 or less. Ann Thorac Surg 1993;56:480–486.

180. Luciani GB, Faggian G, Razzolini R, et al: Severe ischemic left ventricular failure—coronary bypass or heart transplantation? Ann Thorac Surg 1993;55:719–723.

181. Milano CA, White WD, Smith LR, et al: Usefulness of coronary artery bypass grafting in patients with severely depressed ventricular function. Ann Thorac Surg 1993;56:487–493.

182. Takahashi T, Nakano S, Shimazaki Y, et al: Long-term appraisal of coronary bypass operations in familial hypercholesterolemia. Ann Thorac Surg 1993;56:499–505.

183. Harris DNF, Bailey SM, Smith PLC, et al: Brain swelling in first hour after coronary artery bypass surgery. Lancet 1993 (Sep 4);342:586–587.

184. Emlein G, Huang SKS, Pires LA, et al: Prolonged bradyarrhythmias after isolated coronary artery bypass graft surgery. Am Heart J 1993 (Nov);126:1084–1090.

185. Yli-Mayry S, Huikuri HV: Clinical and angiographic prediction of myocardial and recurrence of severe angina during a five-year follow-up after coronary artery bypass grafting. Am J Cardiol 1993 (Dec 15);72: 1371–1375.

186. Cigarroa CG, deFilippi CR, Brickner E, et al: Dobutamine stress echocardiography identifies hibernating myocardium and predicts recovery of left ventricular function after coronary revascularization. Circulation 1993 (Aug);88:430–436.

187. Iskandrian AE, Kegel JG, Tecce MA, et al: Simultaneous assessment of left ventricular perfusion and function with technetium-99m sestamibi after coronary artery bypass grafting. Am Heart J 1993 (Nov);126:1199–1203.

188. Geraci JM, Rosen AK, Ash AS, et al: Predicting the occurrence of adverse events after coronary artery bypass surgery. Ann Intern Med 1993 (Jan 1);118:18–24.

189. Rahimtoola SH, Fessler CL, Grunkemeier GL, et al: Survival 15 to 20 years after coronary bypass surgery for angina. J Am Coll Cardiol 1993 (Jan);21: 151–157.

190. Lytle BW, Loop FD, Taylor PC, et al: The effect of coronary reoperation on the survival of patients with stenoses in saphenous vein bypass grafts to coronary arteries. J Thorac Cardiovasc Surg 1993 (April);105:605–614.

191. Merrill WH, Elkins CC, Stewart JR, et al: Third-time coronary artery bypass grafting. Ann Thorac Surg 1993;55:586–592.

192. Mautner SL, Lin F, Mautner GC, et al: Comparison in women versus men of composition of atherosclerotic plaques in native coronary arteries and saphenous veins used as aortocoronary conduits. J Am Coll Cardiol 1993 (May);21:1312–1318.

3

Acute Myocardial Infarction and Its Consequences

GENERAL TOPICS

Incidence Rates, Procedure Use, and Outcome by Gender and Age

Chiriboga and associates,[1] from Worcester, Mass, compared the overall use, as well as temporal trends, of various diagnostic and revascularization procedures for AMI in men and women. The study sample comprised a total of 2,924 men and 1,838 women with validated AMI admitted to any of the 16 teaching and community hospitals in the Worcester metropolitan area during 1975, 1978, 1981, 1984, 1986, and 1988. During the period under study, there was a significant increase in use of each of the examined procedures during hospitalization for AMI in both men and women. Increasing use of multiple procedures was also seen for each of the sexes. After controlling for a variety of demographic and clinical factors that might affect utilization rates, men were marginally more likely to undergo radionuclide ventriculography, and significantly more likely to undergo Holter monitoring, exercise treadmill testing, cardiac catheterization, and PTCA than women. However, there were no gender differences in the use of CABG. But, men were significantly less likely to undergo echocardiography. The results of this multi-hospital, population-based study suggest sex differences in the use of several diagnostic and revascularization procedures during hospitalization for AMI. These differences may be attributed to physicians' practice patterns, although gender bias in the delivery of medical care cannot be excluded.

Goldberg and associates,[2] from Amherst, Mass, carried out a prospective study in 16 teaching and community hospitals in Worcester in six time periods between 1975 and 1988. A total of 3,148 patients hospitalized with initial AMI comprised the study sample population. The age-adjusted incidence rates of initial AMI increased between 1975 and 1981 in the two sexes with a marked decrease thereafter. These rates declined by 26% in men and 22% in women between 1975 and 1988. Overall unadjusted in-hospital case-fatality rates after initial AMI were significantly higher in women (22%) than in men (13%) (Figure 3-1). Age- and multivariable-adjusted in-hospital case-fatality rates were not significantly different for men compared with women. There were no clear trends in in-hospital case-fatality rates between men and women. There were no significant sex differences in age-adjusted long-term survival rates of discharged survivors. The multivariate-adjusted risk of total mortality among discharged hospital survivors was significantly increased in men. The incidence rates of out-of-hospital deaths caused by coronary disease declined by 60% in men and 69% in women between 1975 and 1988. Therefore, in this multihospital, community-based study, there were declines in the incidence rates of AMI and out-of-hospital deaths caused by CAD in men and women. No significant sex differences in in-hospital survival were observed, whereas a poorer long-term survival experience after hospital discharge was observed for men compared with women (Figure 3-1).

To investigate changes between 1987 and 1990 in the care and outcomes associated with AMI in elderly patients, Pashos and associates,[3]

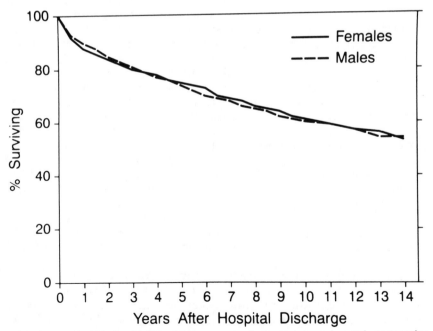

Figure 3-1. Graph of age-adjusted long-term survival rates among hospital survivors by sex (Worcester Heart Attack Study). Reproduced with permission from Goldberg et al.[2]

from Boston, performed a retrospective cohort study using a longitudinal database created from Medicare administrative files. A total of 856,847 AMI patients insured by Medicare between 1987 and 1990 were studied. Between 1987 and 1990, mortality rates decreased 10% overall from 26% to 23% at 30 days and from 40% to 36% at 1 year following AMI. Declines in mortality and adjusted risks of 1 year mortality were similar in men and women and in blacks and whites, but mortality declines were more evident in those aged less than 85 years. Meanwhile, the proportion of elderly AMI patients having angiography within the first 90 days after their index admission increased from 24% to 33%; proportions increased for both genders and all races. The proportion of patients undergoing revascularization procedures increased from 13% to 21%; rates of bypass surgery increased from 8% to 11%; and rates of angioplasty doubled from 5% to 10%. Between 1987 and 1990, survival of elderly patients following AMI improved significantly. Although changes in patients treatment may be responsible, the increased use of thrombolytic therapy appears to be only a partial explanation. Also, although the use of coronary angiography and revascularization procedures increased dramatically, the degree to which it caused the improvement in survival could not be determined.

External Triggers

To determine whether a circadian pattern in onset of symptoms existed and possible external triggers in the precipitation of AMI, Behar and associates,[4] of the SPRINT Study Group from Tel Hashomer, Israel, assessed 1,818 consecutive patients with AMI, hospitalized in 14 of the 21 existing coronary care units in Israel. The frequency of onset of symptoms by six-hour intervals showed a predominant morning peak (6 AM to noon) (32%) in comparison with the other 3 six-hour intervals of the day. The preponderance of the morning peak persisted for subgroup analysis by gender (males 32%, females 31%); age (≤65 years, 32%; >65 years, 33%); and diabetes mellitus (present or absent, 32%). However, patients with peripheral vascular disease and those with stroke in the past had a predominant evening peak. Possible external triggers of onset of AMI were present in 10% of patients. Exceptionally heavy physical work, violent quarrel at work or at home, and unusual mental stress were the three most frequent possible external triggers reported immediately before or within the 24 hours preceding pain onset. Patients with possible external triggers were more likely to be males (85%) and were somewhat but no significantly younger (63 years) in comparison with patients without external triggers (73% and 64 years, respectively). In a large group of consecutive patients with AMI, a predominant cyclic morning peak of pain onset was found in comparison with the other hours of the day. Possible external triggers precipitating AMI were involved in a minority of cases, suggesting that endogenous changes occurring in the morning hours are generally responsible for the increased rate of AMI occurring after awakening.

Although β-adrenergic blocking agents are known to reduce the risk of AMI, the mechanism of this protective effect is not well understood. The recent demonstration that β-blockers selectively blunt the increased morning risk of AMI suggests that these agents block the pathophysiologic consequences of stressors concentrated in the morning. Jimenez and associates,[5] from Boston, determined the effect of nadolol on the hemodynamic and hemostatic responses to mental stress and isometric exertion (handgrip), two potential triggers of AMI. The study was conducted in 15 subjects with mild systemic hypertension, using a placebo-controlled, double-blind, crossover design. Nadolol reduced systolic BP and heart rate after mental stress. Poststress systolic BP was 139 mm Hg during therapy with nadolol versus 161 mm Hg during placebo administration. Heart rate increased to 61 during nadolol therapy versus 89 beats/min during placebo therapy. The systolic BP increase was similar during therapy with nadolol and placebo; however, heart rate increase was less during nadolol therapy (4 v 12 beats/min). The responses to handgrip and their modification during nadolol therapy were similar to those observed after mental stress. Neither platelet aggregability nor fibrinolytic potential was altered by nadolol. Thus, nadolol modified hemodynamic indexes without altering the hemostatic indexes measured. This hemodynamic effect may contribute to the decrease in morning cardiovascular events by β-adrenergic blockers and their well-documented cardioprotective effect.

It is controversial whether the onset of AMI occurs randomly or is precipitated by identifiable stimuli. Previous studies have suggested a higher risk of cardiac events in association with exertion. Willich and associates,[6] for the Triggers and Mechanisms of Myocardial Infarction Study Group from Berlin and Augsburg, Germany, identified consecutive patients with AMI identified by recording all admissions to their hospital in Berlin and by monitoring a general population of 330,000 residents in Augsburg, Germany. Information on the circumstances of each AMI was obtained by means of standardized interviews. The data analysis included a comparison of patients with matched controls and a case-crossover comparison (one in which each patient serves as his or her own control) of the patient's usual frequency of exertion with the last episode of exertion before the onset of AMI. From January 1989 through December 1991, 1,194 patients (74% men; mean age, 61 ± 9 years) completed the interview 13 ± 6 days after AMI. These authors found that 7.1% of the case patients had engaged in physical exertion (≥6 metabolic equivalents) at the onset of AMI, as compared with 3.9% of the controls at the onset of the control event. For the patients as compared with the matched controls, the adjusted relative risk of having engaged in strenuous physical activity at the onset of AMI or the control event was 2.1. The case-crossover comparison yielded a similar relative risk of 2.1 for having engaged in strenuous physical activity within one hour before AMI. Patients whose frequency of regular exercise was <4 and 4 or more times per week had relative risks of 6.9 and 1.3, respectively. Thus, a period of strenuous physical activity is associated with a temporary increase in the risk of having an AMI, particularly among patients who exercise infrequently.

Despite anecdotal evidence suggesting that heavy physical exertion can trigger the onset of AMI, there have been no controlled studies of the risk of AMI during and after heavy exertion, the length of time between heavy exertion and the onset of symptoms (induction time), and whether the risk can be modified by regular physical exertion. To address these questions Mittleman and associates,[7] for the Determinants of Myocardial Infarction Onset Study Investigators from Boston and Worcester, Mass, collected data from patients with confirmed AMI on their activities one hour before the onset of AMI and during control periods. Interviews with 1,228 patients conducted an average of four days after AMI provided data on their usual annual frequency of physical activities and the time, type, and intensity of physical exertion in the 26 hours before the onset of AMI. These authors compared the observed frequency of heavy exertion (six or more metabolic equivalents) with the expected values using two types of self-matched analyses based on a new case-crossover study design. The low frequency of heavy exertion during the control periods was validated by data from a population-based control group of 218 subjects. Of the patients, 4.4% reported heavy exertion within one hour before the onset of AMI in the hour after heavy physical exertion, as compared with less strenuous physical exertion or none, was 5.9. Among people who usually exercised less than 1, 1 to 2, 3 to 4, or 5 or more times per week, the respective risks were 107, 19.4, 8.6, and 2.4 (Figures 3-2 and 3-3). Thus, increasing levels of habitual physical activity were associated with progressively lower

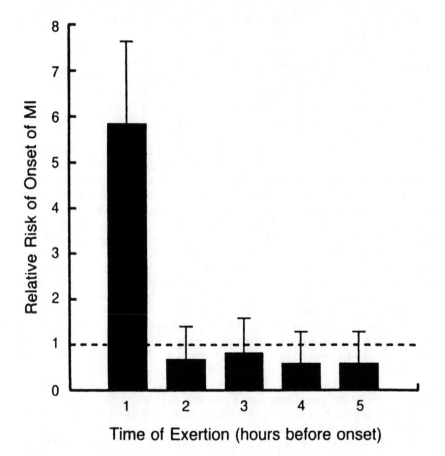

Figure 3-2. Time of onset of myocardial infarction (MI) after an episode of heavy physical exertion (induction time). Each of the five hours before the onset of myocardial infarction was assessed as an independent hazard period, and exertion during each hour was compared with that during the control period. Only exertion during the hour immediately before the onset of myocardial infarction was associated with an increase in the relative risk, suggesting that the induction time for myocardial infarction is less than one hour. The T bars indicate the 95% confidence limits. The dotted line indicates the base-line risk. Reproduced with permission from Mittleman et al.[7]

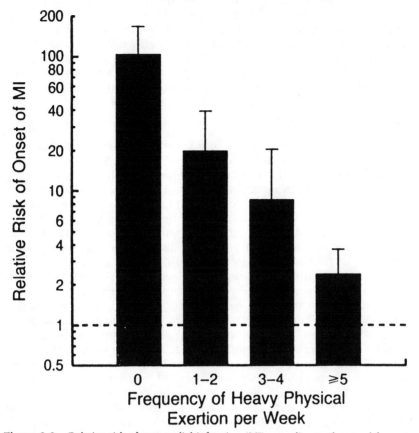

Figure 3-3. Relative risk of myocardial infarction (MI) according to the usual frequency of heavy exertion. Heavy exertion was defined as physical activity at a level of 6 MET or more. The relative risk is shown on a logarithmic scale. Habitually sedentary persons had an extreme relative risk (107), whereas those who reported heavy exertion five or more times per week had a risk only 2.4 times higher than the base-line risk (P < 0.001). The T bars indicate the 95% confidence limits. The dotted line indicates the base-line risk. Reproduced with permission from Mittleman et al.[7]

relative risks. The induction time from heavy exertion to the onset of AMI was <1 hour, and symptoms usually began during the activity. Thus, heavy physical exertion can trigger the onset of AMI, particularly in people who are habitually sedentary. Improved understanding of the mechanisms by which heavy physical exertion triggers the onset of AMI and the manner in which regular exertion protects against it would facilitate the design of new preventive approaches.

Secondary Peak in Onset 11 to 12 Hours After Awakening

Studies have shown that the symptoms of AMI have a primary peak one to two hours after awakening. Peters and associates,[8] from Baltimore, evaluated the time of onset of myocardial infarction in 3,549 patients in the CAST Trial. Of the patients, 3,309 had data on the onset of symptoms relative to the time of awakening. Eight hundred seventy patients (26.3%) were awakened by symptoms. Of the remaining 2,439 patients,

798 (32.7%) experienced the onset of symptoms in the first four hours after awakening with the highest number in the first hour. There was also a secondary peak in myocardial infarction 11 to 12 hours after awakening. These authors concluded that not only is there an early peak in myocardial infarction, but a secondary peak occurring 11 to 12 hours after awakening. This new observation may relate to an ingestion of the evening meal or other trigger factors concentrated in those hours.

ST Depression and Elevation

The mechanism and significance of precordial ST depression during inferior wall AMI is debated. Wong and associates,[9] from Sydney, Australia, assessed the location and extent of arterial perfusion distribution responsible for this electrocardiographic finding. Intracoronary thallium-201 was injected in 11 patients with one-vessel right CAD to delineate perfusion distribution that was quantitated by a new angiographic distribution score. The angiographic score correlated with posterior, posterolateral, and total extent of intracoronary thallium distribution. The angiographic distribution score was related to electrocardiographic changes in 16 patients showing an inferior ST-segment elevation during PTCA (7 with and 9 without precordial ST depression), of which 6 received intracoronary thallium injection. None had thallium distribution in the anterior or septal segment, but there was a trend toward a greater angiographic distribution score and posterior segment thallium score in patients with precordial ST depression. In another 77 patients with inferior wall AMI due to RC occlusion (24 with concomitant LAD narrowing), precordial ST depression was present in 16 with and 31 without LAD narrowing. The angiographic distribution score was higher in those with than those without precordial ST depression in both patients with and without LAD disease. The magnitude of both inferior ST elevation and precordial ST depression correlated with the angiographic distribution score, but only precordial ST depression was independently related in multivariate analysis. Precordial ST depression during inferior wall AMI indicates a larger extent of posterolateral and total perfusion of the infarct-related artery independent of the presence or absence of LAD narrowing, and identifies a subgroup who may derive greater benefit from reperfusion.

The purpose of this study by Fletcher and associates,[10] from Rochester, Minn, was to examine the relation between the presence or absence of ST-segment depression in inferior leads (II, III, and aV_F) and ST-segment elevation in lateral (I and aV_L) or left precordial (V_5 and V_6) leads with the amount and location of myocardium at risk for infarction in patients with AMI. Forty-three patients with anterior infarctions were injected with technetium 99m-sestamibi when they were first seen and underwent tomographic imaging to measure the amount and location of myocardium at risk. Patients with inferior ST depression (n = 10) compared with those without ST depression (n = 33) had perfusion defects that extended significantly further into the lateral wall (47° v 20°) and larger anterior injury vectors. There was no significant association with the percentage of myocardium at risk, disease of the right coronary artery, the presence of an inferior perfusion defect, or the size of the inferior injury vector. Among the patients with ST elevation in lateral leads (n = 16) compared with those without (n = 27), there was a significantly more lateral defect border (47° v 25°) and a larger anterior injury vector. There was no significant correlation with the percentage of myocardium at risk. A significant relation could not be demonstrated between the presence of ST elevation in the left precordial leads and any measure of the amount or location of myocardium at risk. These data support the theory that inferior ST depression in patients with transmural anterior ischemia is a reciprocal finding and does not represent inferior ischemia. The presence of inferior ST depression or lateral ST elevation is associated with a more lateral perfusion defect. Neither of these electrocardiographic findings is associated with the amount of myocardium at risk for infarction.

Patients with suspected AMI who present with ST depression have a high mortality that is not reduced by thrombolytic therapy. Despite this, there are few data on these patients. Lee and associates,[11] from Aberdeen, United Kingdom, studied the electrocardiographic and clinical characteristics of these patients, the diagnostic and prognostic value of the presenting electrocardiogram, and the reasons for the mortality and apparent lack of thrombolytic efficacy. These authors studied all patients with suspected AMI admitted during 1990 with ST depression. Of the 136 patients (84 men; mean age, 68 ±11 years), 74 (54%) had confirmed AMI and 73 (54%) had previous AMI. One-year mortality was 26% for all patients, 31% for those with confirmed AMIs, and 19% for those in whom AMI was subsequently excluded. Patients with AMI had more severe ST depression (mean, 2.5 mm) and more electrocardiogram leads with ST depression leads (mean, 4.7) compared with patients without AMI (1.4 mm). Sensitivity and specificity for the subsequent diagnosis of AMI with ST depression were 20% and 97%, respectively, for at least 4 mm; and 21% and 95%, respectively, for at least seven leads. One-year mortality was low in patients with 1 mm ST depression (14%) or no more than two leads (11%), but high in patients with at least 2 mm ST depression (39%) and at least three leads (30%). Patients with suspected AMI and ST depression had a high mean age, high incidence of previous AMI, and poor prognosis. The presenting electrocardiogram is helpful in predicting prognosis, and ST depression of at least 4 mm or involving at least seven leads is highly specific for diagnosis of AMI.

Infarct Artery Patency Assessment by 12-Lead ST-Segment Recovery Analysis

Early angiography may not adequately subgroup patients with AMI if cyclic changes in coronary flow occur frequently. From a pilot experience using a new 12-lead ST-segment monitor, Krucoff and associates,[12] in Durham, NC, developed a continuously updated, self-referenced ST-recovery analysis method to quantify both instantaneous recovery, as a noninvasive marker of patency, and cumulative ST recovery over time, as a marker of the speed, stability, and duration of reperfusion. In 22 patients with AMI in whom 44 observations of unique angiographic patency were noted within six hours of presentation, serial patency assessments simultaneous with all angiographic observations predicted coronary occlusion with 90% sensitivity and 92% specificity. Of the 22 patients, 11 had multiple ST-trend transitions suggesting cyclic changes in coronary flow before catheterization. Speed, stability, and duration of ST-segment recovery were defined by the time to first 50% ST recovery, total number of ST-trend transitions, and patent physiology index (percentage of monitoring period showing ST recovery), respectively. Sub-grouped angiographically, the median for cumulative ST parameters with patent versus occluded arteries were, respectively, time to 50% recovery, 1.6 versus 0.2 hours; number of reelevation/recovery events, 1.5 versus 3; and patent physiology index, 52 versus 50. Thus, continuous ST-segment recovery analysis appears to predict simultaneous angiographic patency over serial assessments, whereas cumulative parameters appear to contain independent information, probably because of patency changes before or after angiography.

Relation to Alcohol Intake and High-Density Lipoprotein Cholesterol

Previous studies have suggested that moderate alcohol intake exerts a protective effect against CAD. Alterations in plasma lipoprotein levels represent one plausible mechanism of this apparent protective effect. Gaziano and associates,[13] from Boston and West Roxbury, Mass, and New York, examined the interrelation among alcohol consumption, plasma lipoprotein levels, and the risk of AMI in 340 patients who had had AMI and an equal number of age- and sex-matched controls. The case patients were men or women less than 76 years of age with no history of CAD who were discharged from one of six hospitals in the Boston area with a diagnosis of a confirmed AMI. Alcohol consumption was estimated by means of a food-frequency questionnaire. These authors observed a significant inverse association between alcohol consumption and the risk of AMI. In multivariate analyses, the relative risk for the highest intake category (subjects who consumed ≥3 or more drinks per day) as compared with the lowest (those who had <1 drink a month) was 0.45 (Tables 3-1, 3-2, and 3-3). The levels of total LDL cholesterol and its HDL_2 and HDL_3 subfractions were strongly associated with alcohol consumption (P for trend, <0.001 for each). The addition of HDL or either of its subfractions to the multivariate model substantially reduced the inverse association between alcohol intake and AMI, whereas the addition of the other plasma lipid measurements did not materially alter the relation. These data confirm the inverse association of moderate alcohol intake with the risk of AMI and support the view that the effect is mediated, in large part, by increases in both HDL_2 and HDL_3.

Newer Biochemical Markers

In a substantial proportion of patients with suspected AMI, biochemical markers are needed for clinical decision making at the time of admission, because electrocardiographic recordings are inconclusive. Bakker and associates,[14] from Amsterdam, The Netherlands, assessed the usefulness for exclusion of AMI at admission of the newer markers creatine kinase MB (CK-MB) mass concentration, troponin T, and myoglobin in comparison with the routinely used markers creatine kinase (CK) and CK-MB activity. A total of 290 consecutive patients were enrolled. AMI was diagnosed on the basis of clinical history, ECG criteria, and time-dependent changes in CK and CK-MB activity. A total of 153 patients had definite AMI. Troponin T had the highest sensitivity for prediction of AMI; high concentrations (above the upper reference limits) were found in 98 (64%) of the patients with infarctions compared with 92 (60%) for CK-MB mass concentration, 76 (50%) for myoglobin, 61 (40%) for CK activity, and 53

Table 3-1. Coronary Risk Factors Among the Controls, According to Alcohol Consumption. Reproduced with permission from Gaziano et al.[13]

VARIABLE	No. of Drinks*			
	<1/MO (N = 85)	≥1/MO BUT <1/DAY (N = 98)	≥1/DAY BUT <3/DAY (N = 90)	≥3/DAY (N = 57)
Age (yr)	59.2±9.6	56.8±10.2	57.8±10.3	57.5±8.2
Male sex (%)	57.6	79.6	85.6	91.2
High blood pressure (%)	32.9	21.4	22.5	22.8
Body-mass index†	26.3±4.7	25.2±3.6	25.4±3.9	25.7±3.9
History of diabetes (%)	15.3	6.1	5.6	3.5
Family history of premature myocardial infarction (%)	23.5	15.3	11.1	10.5
Type A personality (%)	48.2	46.9	52.2	47.4
Physical-activity index ≥2500 kcal/wk (%)‡	48.2	57.1	55.6	57.9
Cigarette smoking (%)				
Never	37.6	41.2	25.6	19.3
Former	34.1	35.1	53.3	45.6
Current	28.2	23.7	21.1	35.1
Total calories/day	2165±763	2195±645	2372±646	2747±846
Calories as saturated fat (%)	12.0±3.0	12.7±3.0	12.0±2.7	11.5±3.0

*Plus–minus values are means ±SD. Ten subjects who had recently stopped drinking were excluded from the analysis. One drink was defined as 13.2 g of ethanol.

†The weight in kilograms divided by the square of the height in meters.

‡To convert kilocalories to kilojoules, multiply by 4.2.

Table 3-2. Plasma Lipid Levels, Adjusted for Age and Sex, According to Alcohol Consumption. Reproduced with permission from Gaziano et al.[13]

LIPID*	No. of Drinks†				P FOR TREND
	<1/MO	≥1/MO BUT <1/DAY	≥1/DAY BUT <3/DAY	≥3/DAY	
	milligrams/deciliter				
Total cholesterol	209.9±40.6	209.0±40.7	215.5±46.0	218.0±41.4	0.087
LDL	132.2±35.9	133.7±33.7	136.2±38.9	130.6±38.8	0.898
Triglycerides‡	150.6±83.7	149.4±94.6	144.0±95.8	185.7±176.7	0.099
VLDL	40.9±24.5	37.9±22.4	37.1±26.4	44.6±29.6	0.653
Total HDL	36.5±10.9	38.0±10.2	42.1±12.1	42.8±12.8	<0.001
HDL$_2$	13.4±9.2	14.2±8.3	17.2±8.8	16.3±9.1	<0.001
HDL$_3$	22.9±6.4	23.7±5.7	24.8±7.2	26.6±7.0	<0.001

*To convert cholesterol values to millimoles per liter, multiply by 0.02586; to convert triglyceride values to millimoles per liter, multiply by 0.01129.

†Values are means ±SD. One drink was defined as 13.2 g of ethanol.

‡Triglyceride values were used in logarithmic form for the multivariate analyses; for log(triglycerides), P = 0.651.

(35%) for CK-MB activity. However, troponin T also had the highest "false-positive" rate; of 137 patients without AMI, 36 (26%) had high troponin T concentrations. Sensitivity, specificity, and positive and negative predictive values were calculated in relation to time between onset of chest pain and hospital admission. Although CK-MB mass concentration

Table 3-3. Adjusted Relative Risk of Myocardial Infarction Among Subjects whose Lipid Levels were Measured, According to Alcohol Consumption.* Reproduced with permission from Gaziano et al.[13]

VARIABLES ADDED TO MODEL		No. OF DRINKS			P FOR TREND
	<1/MO†	≥1/MO BUT <1/DAY	≥1/DAY BUT <3/DAY	≥3/DAY	
		relative risk (95% confidence interval)			
No lipids	1.00	1.17 (0.71–1.90)	0.60 (0.36–1.02)	0.52 (0.28–0.99)	0.011
Total cholesterol	1.00	1.17 (0.71–1.91)	0.59 (0.35–1.00)	0.50 (0.27–0.96)	0.008
LDL	1.00	1.16 (0.71–1.90)	0.59 (0.34–0.99)	0.53 (0.28–1.00)	0.010
Triglycerides‡	1.00	1.11 (0.67–1.83)	0.63 (0.36–1.08)	0.43 (0.22–0.84)	0.005
Total VLDL	1.00	1.17 (0.72–1.92)	0.63 (0.37–1.06)	0.48 (0.25–0.92)	0.008
Total HDL	1.00	1.20 (0.72–2.00)	0.84 (0.48–1.48)	0.76 (0.38–1.51)	0.326
HDL$_2$	1.00	1.17 (0.71–1.95)	0.77 (0.44–1.34)	0.61 (0.31–1.20)	0.102
HDL$_3$	1.00	1.20 (0.73–1.98)	0.67 (0.39–1.15)	0.66 (0.34–1.29)	0.081
HDL$_2$ and HDL$_3$	1.00	1.21 (0.72–2.02)	0.86 (0.49–1.51)	0.77 (0.38–1.54)	0.361

*One drink was defined as 13.2 g of ethanol. The multivariate model was adjusted for sex, age (in 10-year groups), history of treatment for hypertension, history of diabetes mellitus, body-mass index, type A personality, family history of premature myocardial infarction, physical-activity level, smoking (never, former, or current [<1 pack per day, ≥1 but <2 packs per day, or ≥2 packs per day]), caloric intake, and percent of caloric intake as saturated fat.

†The reference category.   ‡Triglyceride values were used in logarithmic form.

was, by a small margin, the best marker in patients admitted within eight to ten hours of onset of chest pain, all the markers had negative predictive values too low to allow exclusion of AMI at admission in patients with symptoms suggestive of AMI of less than ten hours duration.

Plasma Endothelin-1

Endothelin-1 is a potent vasoconstricting substance that may aggravate circulatory dysfunction in AMI. In an investigation carried out by Tomoda,[15] from Kanagawa, Japan, in 59 patients with AMI, peripheral venous blood was sampled, and endothelin-1 was measured by radioimmunoassay. Hemodynamic measurements were performed with a flow-directed thermodilution catheter in 16 patients. Plasma endothelin-1 levels in Killip's classes were as follows: group I (no heart failure, n = 25) 1.97 ± 0.69 pg/mL; group II (heart failure, n = 16) 2.74 ± 1.02 pg/mL; group III (pulmonary edema, n = 13) 4.54 ± 1.17 pg/mL; group IV (cardiogenic shock, n = 5) 8.91 ± 3.16 pg/mL; normal control group (n = 12) 1.51 ± 0.39 pg/mL. There were significant correlations between the plasma endothelin-1 level and mean RA pressure, mean PA pressure, and cardiac index. There were closer correlations between plasma endothelin-1 level and mean PA wedge pressure and total pulmonary vascular resistance. These results indicate that endothelin-1 is elevated in accordance with cardiac and pulmonary circulatory distress in patients with AMI, which may further aggravate circulatory dysfunction.

Plasma Interleukin-6

Interleukin-6 plays a key role in the synthesis of human acute-phase protein and several acute-phase responses occur in patients with AMI.

Miyao and associates,[16] from Kumamoto, Japan, examined the plasma levels of interleukin-6 in 23 consecutive patients with AMI over the course of 4 weeks and in 30 control individuals. In patients with AMI, the plasma interleukin-6 levels (in picograms per milliliter) were increased at all sampling points from admission to discharge (range, 29 ± 6.6 to 47 ± 7.8) compared with levels in control individuals (12 ± 2.9). Cardiac catheterization did not influence plasma interleukin-6 levels. The plasma interleukin-6 level reached its peak approximately three days (47 ± 7.8) and approximately 1 week after admission in patients with AMI. There was a significant positive linear correlation between the peak level of plasma interleukin-6 minus the level on admission and the peak level of plasma C-reactive protein in patients with AMI. The peak interleukin-6 level did not correlate with the peak levels of creatine kinase, pulmonary capillary wedge pressure, or LVEF at 4 weeks. It was concluded that the plasma interleukin-6 level is increased over a time course of 4 weeks in patients with AMI.

Antioxidants in Adipose Tissue

Laboratory and epidemiologic studies suggest that the antioxidants, vitamin E and β-carotene, protect against CAD. In a European multicenter case-control study by Kardinaal and associates,[17] alpha-tocopherol and β-carotene concentrations were measured in adipose-tissue samples collected in 1991–1992 from 683 people with AMI and 727 controls. Mean adipose-tissue β-carotene concentrations were 0.35 µg/g and 0.42 µg/g for cases and controls, respectively, with age-adjusted and center-adjusted mean difference 0.07 µg/g. Mean alpha-tocopherol concentrations were 193 µg/g and 192 µg/g for cases and controls, respectively. The age-adjusted and center-adjusted odds ratio for risk of AMI in the lowest quintile of β-carotene, as compared with the highest, was 2.62. Additional control for body-mass index and smoking reduced the odds ratio to 1.78; other established risk factors did not substantially alter this ratio. The increased risk was mainly confined to current smokers: the multivariate odds ratio in the lowest β-carotene quintile in smokers was 2.39; it was 1.07 for people who had never smoked. A low alpha-tocopherol concentration was not associated with risk of AMI. Thus, the results support the hypothesis that high β-carotene concentrations within the normal range reduce the risk of a first AMI. The findings for alpha-tocopherol are compatible with previous observations of reduced risk among vitamin E supplement users only. The consumption of β-carotene-rich foods, such as carrots and green-leaf vegetables, may reduce the risk of AMI.

Ultrasound Wall-Motion Analysis to Predict Extent of Coronary Disease

Regional changes in LV size and function characterize LV remodeling and start very early after AMI. Shen and associates,[18] from Bronx, NY, studied the diagnostic value of LV dyssynergic patterns in predicting the presence of single- versus multi-vessel disease. Fifty-three consecutive patients with AMI were studied by electrocardiography, two-dimensional echocardiography, and angiography during the same hospitalization. Thirty-eight normal individuals served as the control group.

According to the angiographic findings, the patients were categorized as having: single-vessel disease (n = 17), two-vessel disease (n = 17), and three-vessel disease (n = 19). Two-dimensional echocardiography was performed and optimal frames from five cardiac cycles were digitized and quantitatively analyzed off-line with a microcomputer. Echocardiographic wall-motion analysis demonstrated a depressed regional segmental thickening in the infarcted area that was characteristic for each echocardiographic view. In the segments remote from the infarcted area, however, the three patient groups displayed differences in function that ranged from hyperkinetic in patients with single-vessel disease to hypokinetic in patients with multi-vessel disease. Patients with single-vessel disease constantly displayed a wider range of segmental thickening when compared with patients with multi-vessel disease and the control group. In conclusion, patients with single-vessel disease after myocardial infarction display compensatory hyperkinesis of remote segments, which is attenuated in patients with multi-vessel disease. The present study introduces new parameters of segmental myocardial function that might be helpful in predicting single-vessel disease and multi-vessel disease in patients after AMI.

Perioperative Infarction After Non-Cardiac Surgery

To determine the incidence of and risk factors for perioperative AMI with noncardiac surgery and to test the accuracy of a risk stratification system, Aston and associates,[19] from Houston, studied 1,487 men older than 40 years undergoing major, nonemergent, non-cardiac operations. Patients with CAD (high-risk stratum) had a 4.1% incidence of AMI (13 of 319); patients with peripheral vascular disease with no evidence of CAD (intermediate-risk stratum) had a 0.8% incidence (2 of 260); patients with high atherogenic risk factor profiles with no clinical atherosclerosis (low-risk stratum) had a 0% incidence (0 of 256). No cardiac deaths occurred in 652 men who had no atherosclerosis and low atherogenic risk factor profiles (the negligible-risk stratum). Factors independently associated with AMI included age more than 75 years (adjusted odds ratio, 4.77), signs of CHF on the preoperative examination (adjusted odds ratio, 3.31), CAD (10.39), and a planned vascular operation (3.72). CAD is the major risk factor for perioperative AMI. The stratification scheme identifies subsets of patients with different risks, and finer within-stratum distinctions can be made using additional variables.

Apolipoprotein E Phenotype

The apolipoprotein E polymorphism is a genetic determinant of LDL cholesterol. Its status as a risk factor for CAD, either through a causal relation with LDL cholesterol level or independently, is less clearly established. Eichner and associates,[20] from Pittsburgh, used data from the Multiple Risk Factor Intervention Trial to examine the influence of apolipoprotein E phenotype on risk of coronary events. Of the 12,866 randomized participants, 619 were studied in a nested case-control design. CAD deaths (93) and nonfatal AMI (113) were matched to 412 controls. The allele frequencies of apolipoprotein E in the white subset were very similar to other nonselected white American populations, and the relation of apolipoprotein E on total and LDL cholesterol was generally similar to that seen in other studies, with the ε2 allele being associated with lower and the ε4 allele with higher total and LDL cholesterol. Allele frequencies were not the same for patients and control subjects. The presence of ε4 was associated with an increased risk of CAD that was most evident for fatal cases. There was no relation between changes in LDL cholesterol over time during the trial and apolipoprotein E phenotypes.

Relation of Infarct-Artery Patency to Lipoprotein(a)

Moliterno and associates,[21] from Dallas and Houston, evaluated 105 survivors of myocardial infarction, including 75 men and 30 women, aged 30 to 80 years, not given thrombolytic therapy to relate the presence of coronary artery patency with lipoprotein(a) concentrations. Coronary angiography revealed a patent (group 1, n = 52) or occluded (group 2, n = 53) infarct-related artery. Plasma concentrations of plasminogen, fibrinogen, tissue plasminogen activator activity, plasminogen activator inhibitor activity, cholesterol, triglycerides, and lipoproteins, including lipoprotein(a), were measured in blood obtained 23 ± 13 months after infarction. Groups 1 and 2 were similar with respect to age, sex, race, cardioactive medications, infarct artery, extent of CAD, and LV function. The groups were similar except that lipoprotein(a) averaged 19 ± 22 mg/dL in group 1 and 49 ± 45 mg/dL in group 2. This difference was evident in both Caucasian and African Americans. Therefore, survivors of myocardial infarction who failed to recanalize the infarct-related artery have higher lipoprotein(a) concentrations than those with a patent infarct artery. Lipoprotein(a) may inhibit intrinsic fibrinolysis.

Angiographic Differences from Angina

Bogaty and colleagues,[22] from London, England, evaluated coronary angiographic findings in 102 patients presenting with either AMI as a first manifestation of CAD or stable angina for at least two years with no history, ECG, or left ventriculographic evidence of an acute event, with an angiogram performed at least 2 years after initial symptoms. These angiograms were evaluated blindly for severity, extent of disease, and anatomic pattern. In patients with unheralded MI, there were fewer vessels diseased, fewer stenoses, and occlusions, and a lower extent index than in those patients with uncomplicated stable angina (Figure 3-4). A discrete pattern was present in 55% of patients with unheralded MI and only 9% of those with uncomplicated angina. Thus, these different angiographic findings suggest that unheralded AMI and uncomplicated stable angina do not occur randomly on a common atherosclerotic background but that other factors, such as varying susceptibility to thrombosis, may predispose to one or the other of these two clinical syndromes.

Effects of Diabetes Mellitus on Mortality

Previous studies have shown that diabetic patients have a high mortality rate after AMI. Zuanetti and associates,[23] from Milan, Italy, evaluated this question further in patients after AMI who had been treated with fibrinolytic agents. In the GISSI II studies, the prevalence of diabetes was higher in women than in men for insulin dependent (8.75% v 1.85%)

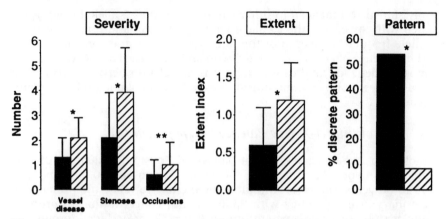

Figure 3-4. Severity, extent, and pattern of CAD compared in patients with unheralded acute MI and uncomplicated chronic stable angina. Solid bars demonstrate patients with unheralded acute MI. Hatched bars demonstrate patients with uncomplicated chronic stable angina. Reproduced with permission from Bogaty et al.[22]

and for noninsulin dependent (23.7% v 13.8%) diabetic patients. The type of fibrinolytic agent did not affect mortality rates. The increase in in-hospital mortality of diabetic patients was moderate and similar for men with insulin and noninsulin dependent diabetes (8.7% and 10.1%, respectively, v 5.8% in nondiabetic patients). In women, mortality was markedly higher for insulin-dependent and only slightly higher for non-insulin dependent diabetic patients (24% and 16%, respectively, v 14% for nondiabetic patients). The adjusted relative risks were 1.9 for insulin-dependent diabetic women and 1.4 for noninsulin-dependent men. The mortality rate after discharge showed a similar gender difference, and in insulin-dependent diabetic women the prognosis was ominous even in the absence of left ventricular damage before discharge. These authors concluded that a history of diabetes is associated with a worse prognosis after AMI, even in patients treated with thrombolytic agents. Gender and type of diabetes appear to be critical in affecting survival. In men, both insulin-dependent and noninsulin-dependent diabetes are associated with a moderately higher mortality rate. In women, insulin-dependent diabetes is in itself a strong risk factor for death after AMI.

On-Site Cardiac Catheterization Facilities and Their Use

During the past decade the use of coronary angiography after AMI has substantially increased. Among the possible contributing factors, the increasing availability of cardiac catheterization facilities was the focus of an investigation by Every and associates,[24] for the Myocardial Infarction Triage and Interventional Project Investigators. These authors investigated whether the availability of cardiac catheterization facilities at an admitting hospital was associated with the likelihood that a patient would undergo coronary angiography. After adjusting for age, sex, cardiac history, and cardiac complications during hospitalization, this association was evaluated in 5,867 consecutive patients with AMI admitted to 19 Seattle-area hospitals, as well as the association between the presence of on-site cardiac catheterization facilities and in-hospital mortality.

Table 3-4. Hospital Events and Procedures, According to the Availability of Cardiac Catheterization Facilities. Reproduced with permission from Every et al.[24]

Event	No Facilities (2122 Patients)	Facilities (3745 Patients)	P Value
Shock at time of admission (%)	1.8	2.2	0.24
Heart failure at time of admission (%)	21.3	21.4	0.96
Recurrent chest pain (%)	24.4	27.8	<0.01
Infarct extension (%)	4.0	4.3	0.68
Heart failure during hospitalization (%)	34.2	31.3	<0.05
Mean ejection fraction ±SD (%)	46.5±14.2	50.4±15.5	<0.001
Use of thrombolytic agents (%)	20.7	21.3	0.60
Use of coronary angiography (%)	36.3	65.7	<0.001
Use of bypass surgery (%)	8.5	12.3	<0.001
Use of coronary angioplasty (%)	9.1	28.2	<0.001

Patients admitted to hospitals with on-site cardiac catheterization facilities were far more likely to undergo coronary angiography (odds ratio, 3.21) than patients admitted to hospitals where transfer to another institution would be required to perform cardiac catheterization (Table 3-4). Admission to a hospital with on-site facilities was more strongly associated with the use of coronary angiography than any characteristic of the patient. Although our study had limited power to detect differences in mortality, the availability of coronary angiography had no discernible association with in-hospital mortality rates (odd ratio for mortality among patients admitted to hospitals with on-site facilities v patients admitted to hospitals without such facilities, 0.88). In this community-wide study, the availability of on-site cardiac catheterization facilities was associated with a higher likelihood that a patient would undergo coronary angiography. However, admission to hospitals with these facilities did not appear to be associated with lower short-term mortality.

Economics of Cardiac Rehabilitation

Although there are extensive clinical evaluations of cardiac rehabilitation after AMI, no full economic evaluation is available. Oldridge and associates,[25] from Ontario, Canada, randomized patients with AMI and mild to moderate anxiety or depression, or both, while still in hospital to either an 8-week rehabilitation intervention (99 patients) or usual care (102 patients). Comprehensive costs and health-related quality of life, measured with the time trade-off preference score, were obtained in a 12-month trial and, together with survival data derived from published meta-analyses, cost-utility, and cost-effectiveness of early cardiac rehabilitation, were estimated. The best estimate of the incremental net direct 12-month costs for patients randomized to rehabilitation was $480 (United States, 1991) per patient. During 1-year follow-up, rehabilitation patients had fewer "other rehabilitation visits" and gained 0.05 quality adjusted life-year more than did the group with usual care. The cost-utility ratio was $9,200/quality-adjusted life-year gained with cardiac rehabilitation during the year of follow-up. This economic evaluation of cardiac rehabilitation does not consider the important distinctions be-tween affordability and worth of alternative health-care services. The data provide evidence that brief cardiac rehabilitation initiated soon after AMI for patients with mild to moderate anxiety or depression, or both, is an efficient use of health-care resources and may be economically justi-fied.

Exercise and Quality of Life Afterwards

To determine whether a group program of light exercise could improve quality of life in patients after AMI to the same extent as a high intensity exercise training program, Worcester and associates,[26] from Melbourne, Australia, studied 224 men from a consecutive series of 339 men under 70 years of age admitted to a coronary care unit with Q-wave AMI. The main outcome measures were physical working capacity based on meta-bolic equivalents achieved from treadmill exercise tests at entry, after 11 weeks, and after 1 year. Quality of life based on self report scores of anxi-ety, depression, denial, and well-being and interview assessments of ac-tivities and psychosocial adjustment at entry, after 4 months, and after one year were other outcome measures. The two groups were well matched at entry. At 11 weeks the mean results of treadmill testing were 10.7 metabolic equivalents for exercise training and 9.7 for light exercise. Apart from this small temporary benefit in mean physical working capac-ity, there were no significant differences between groups. Improvement in occupational adjustment score from baseline to 4 months was greater after exercise training than after light exercise, but at 1 year, repeated measures analysis of variance showed no significant effects of treatment or interaction between treatment and time point. In conclusion, the ef-fects on quality of life of a low cost program of light exercise were similar to those obtained from a high intensity exercise training program.

Detection of Viable Myocardium After Healing

Reinjection imaging with thallium-201 may provide a convenient method of assessing myocardial viability. Lekakis and associates,[27] from Athens, Greece, examined 20 patients with a previous Q-wave healed AMI to evaluate the detection of viable tissue in infarcted segments. All patients underwent dipyridamole thallium-201 tomographic imaging with reinjection of 1 mCi of thallium-201 after redistribution. Radionu-clide ventriculography was performed before and after administration of 5 mg of dinitrate isosorbide sublingually for regional wall-motion analy-sis. Patients presented with 38 fixed defects, 12 of which demonstrated improved thallium-201 uptake on reinjection; 10 of 12 reinjection-re-versible segments were hypokinetic or normal after administration of ni-trates, and 22 of 26 nonreversible segments remained akinetic or dyskinetic. Of 20 patients, 9 had reinjection-reversible segments; coro-nary angiography revealed a patent infarct-related artery or collaterals, or both, in 7 of these patients. The infarct-related artery was patent or collaterals were present, or both, in 4 of 11 patients who did not improve with reinjection. These investigators concluded that reinjection of thal-lium-201 during dipyridamole thallium-201 scintigraphy may frequently detect viable tissue in infarcted segments in patients with a Q-wave in-farction. Segments with reinjection reversibility usually do not remain dyskinetic or akinetic after administration of nitrates and have some residual flow on coronary angiography.

Left Ventricular Filling After Healing

LV diastolic filling is impaired in hearts with healed AMI. Possible hemodynamic parameters related to impaired LV filling include LA pressure, time constant of isovolumic relaxation, chamber stiffness, and wall-motion asynchrony. Previous studies demonstrated univariate correlations between each of these parameters and LV filling. Aoyagi and associates,[28] from Boston, Mass, designed a study to compare relative importance of these parameters in patients with an AMI. Left ventriculograms with simultaneous LV pressure measurement were analyzed in 15 patients with an AMI and in 10 control subjects. Every frame of the left ventriculogram was divided into eight segments and the volume of each segment was obtained frame-by-frame by planimetry and area-length method. Asynchrony was quantitated as the sum of areas of discrepancy between each segmental and global volume-time curve. Patients with AMI had greater asynchrony, greater atrial filling fraction, and slower peak early filling rate than the control subjects. Multiple regression analyses with hemodynamic variables (asynchrony, LV pressure at mitral valve opening, time constant of LV isovolumic pressure decrease, and LV chamber stiffness constant) showed that asynchrony and LV pressure at mitral valve opening were significant determinants of LV filling in patients with AMI, whereas LV pressure at mitral valve opening was the only significant determinant in control subjects.

Management Patterns in the United States v Canada

There are major differences in the organization of the health care systems in the United States and Canada. Rouleau and associates,[29] from multiple North American medical centers and for the SAVE Investigators, hypothesized that these differences may be accompanied by differences in patient care. To test the hypothesis, these authors compared the treatment patterns for patients with AMI in 19 Canadian and 93 US hospitals participating in the Survival and Ventricular Enlargement (SAVE) study, which tested the effectiveness of captopril in this population of patients after AMI. In Canada, 51% of the patients admitted to a participating coronary care unit had AMIs, as compared with only 35% in the United States. Despite the similar clinical characteristics of the 1,573 US patients and the 658 Canadian patients participating in the study, coronary arteriography was more commonly performed in the United States than in Canada (68% v 35%), as were revascularized procedures before randomization (31% v 12%) (Table 3-5). During an average follow-up of 42 months, these procedures were also performed more commonly in the United States than in Canada. These differences were not associated with any apparent difference in mortality (22% in Canada and 23% in the United States) or rate of reinfarction (14% in Canada and 13% in the United States), but there was a higher incidence of activity-limiting angina in Canada than in the United States (33% v 27%). Drug usage was different (Table 3-6). The threshold for the admission of patients to a coronary care unit or for the use of invasive diagnostic and therapeutic interventions in the early and late periods after an AMI is higher in

Table 3-5. Coronary Arteriography and Revascularization Procedures after the Index Infarction.* Reproduced with permission from Rouleau et al.[29]

Procedure or Procedures	Before Randomization			During Follow-up after Randomization			Entire Period after Infarction		
	United States	Canada	Prevalence Ratio (95% CI)	United States	Canada	Prevalence Ratio (95% CI)	United States	Canada	Prevalence Ratio (95% CI)
	no. (%)			*no. (%)*			*no. (%)*		
Coronary arteriography	1069 (68)	232 (35)	1.93 (1.73–2.15) P<0.001	496 (32)	144 (22)	1.44 (1.23–1.69) P<0.001	1227 (78)	317 (48)	1.62 (1.49–1.76) P<0.001
PTCA	350 (22)	53 (8)	2.76 (2.10–3.63) P<0.001	112 (7)	32 (5)	1.46 (1.00–2.15) P = 0.033	417 (27)	75 (11)	2.33 (1.85–2.92) P = 0.001
CABG	159 (10)	32 (5)	2.08 (1.44–3.01) P<0.001	180 (11)	51 (8)	1.48 (1.10–1.99) P = 0.005	339 (22)	83 (13)	1.71 (1.37–2.13) P<0.001
Revascularization	482 (31)	80 (12)	2.52 (2.03–3.14) P<0.001	270 (17)	79 (12)	1.43 (1.13–1.81) P = 0.001	674 (43)	148 (22)	1.91 (1.63–2.22) P<0.001
PTCA per coronary arteriography	(33)	(23)	1.43 (1.11–1.84) P = 0.001	(23)	(22)	1.02 (0.72–1.44)	(34)	(24)	1.44 (1.16–1.78) P<0.001
CABG per coronary arteriography	(15)	(14)	1.08 (0.76–1.53)	(36)	(35)	1.02 (0.80–1.32)	(28)	(26)	1.06 (0.86–1.30)
Revascularization per coronary arteriography	(45)	(34)	1.31 (1.08–1.58) P = 0.002	(54)	(55)	0.99 (0.84–1.17)	(55)	(47)	1.18 (1.04–1.34) P = 0.009

*CI denotes confidence interval, PTCA percutaneous transluminal coronary angioplasty, and CABG coronary-artery bypass grafting.

Table 3-6. Drug Therapy 12 and 24 Months after Randomization. Reproduced with permission from Rouleau et al.[29]

Type of Drug	Drugs Used after 12 mo				Drugs Used after 24 mo			
	United States	Canada	Prevalence Ratio (95% CI)*	P Value	United States	Canada	Prevalence Ratio (95% CI)*	P Value
	% of patients				*% of patients*			
Nitrates	37	31	1.18 (1.03–1.36)	0.013	35	30	1.15 (0.99–1.33)	0.054
Beta-blockers	28	23	1.19 (1.01–1.41)	0.032	28	23	1.22 (1.02–1.46)	0.02
Calcium-channel blockers	32	27	1.20 (1.03–1.40)	0.015	31	25	1.21 (1.03–1.43)	0.017
Aspirin	58	63	0.92 (0.85–0.99)	0.026	59	62	0.95 (0.88–1.03)	0.221
Other antiplatelet agents	10	3	3.99 (2.36–6.73)	<0.001	8	2	3.19 (1.81–5.64)	<0.001
Anticoagulants	10	11	0.86 (0.65–1.14)	0.311	9	8	1.07 (0.78–1.49)	0.662
Digitalis	24	25	0.94 (0.80–1.12)	0.503	23	26	0.88 (0.75–1.05)	0.170
Diuretics	33	40	0.82 (0.72–0.92)	0.002	32	38	0.82 (0.72–0.94)	0.005
Antiarrhythmic agents	10	8	1.20 (0.88–1.63)	0.241	9	6	1.61 (1.10–2.36)	0.007
Cholesterol-lowering agents	12	13	0.93 (0.72–1.19)	0.565	18	18	1.01 (0.82–1.25)	0.903

*CI denotes confidence interval.

Canada than in the United States. This is not associated with any apparent difference in the rate of reinfarction or survival, but it is associated with a higher frequency of activity-limiting angina.

With Angiographically Normal Coronary Arteries

Brecker and associates,[30] from London, England, studied haematological variables associated with a prothrombotic tendency in patients with angiographically normal coronary arteries after an AMI and compared findings with those in patients whose AMI had been associated with obstructive CAD and in normal subjects. These authors studied 12 patients who had normal epicardial coronary arteries by angiogram after healing of AMI. The findings are summarized in Table 3-7. These authors found no specific coagulation defect, and standard haematological indices were normal.

The role of coronary vasospasm in the pathogenesis of AMI is unclarified. In this study by Fukai and associates,[31] from Fukuoka, Japan, among 212 patients with AMI in whom PTCA or coronary thrombolysis was not performed at the acute stage, 21 patients (10%) showed no significant coronary stenosis (the degree of stenosis was <50% of the luminal diameter) by coronary angiography 4 weeks after AMI. Among them, 11 (52%) had preinfarction angina at rest, including 2 with vari-

Table 3-7. Clinical Characteristics, Risk Factors, and Haematological Profiles of Patients with Myocardial Infarction and of Healthy Controls. Values are Means (SD) Unless Stated Otherwise. Reproduced with permission from Brecker et al.[31]

	Patients with:		
	Normal coronary arteries (n=12)	Stenosed or occluded artery (n=11)	Healthy controls (n=11)
Age (years)	40 (6)*	58 (9)**	37 (8)
No of men	9	10	8
Weight (kg)	73 (9)	74 (14)	
Site of infarction (No of subjects):			
Anterior	6	5	
Inferior	6	6	
No of current smokers	6	7	4
No taking contraceptive pill	2	0	
No with hypertension	1	0	0
No with family history of ischaemic heart disease	5	5	
No with previous angina or infarction	0*	7	0
Cholesterol (mmol/l)	5·2 (0·6)	5·6 (1·0)	
Triglyceride (mmol/l)	1·6 (0·4)	1·9 (1·0)	
Packed cell volume	0·43 (0·04)	0·43 (0·02)	0·42 (0·02)
Platelet count (× 10⁹/l)	276 (93)	267 (60)	268 (40)
International normalised ratio	1·1 (0·1)	1·0 (0·1)	1·0 (0·1)
Partial thromboplastin time (s)	34 (6)	32 (5)	31 (2)
Fibrinogen (g/l)	3·39 (1·86)	3·83 (1·11)	3·39 (1·30)
Antithrombin III (% activity)	104 (21)	109 (13)	118 (13)
Protein C (% activity)	90 (12)	92 (17)	94 (12)
Protein S (% activity)	95 (13)	89 (15)	94 (13)
Plasminogen (% activity)	119 (22)	125 (20)	123 (22)
α-2-Antiplasmin (% activity)	119 (16)	115 (16)	105 (30)
Whole blood viscosity (mPa.s)	9·1 (3·8)	7·4 (4·1)	8·5 (1·2)
Plasminogen activator inhibitor (U/ml)	5·5 (2·7)	8·6 (5·8)	6·6 (3·2)

*p < 0·05 compared with patients with a stenosed or occluded artery.
**p < 0·05 compared with healthy controls.

ant angina, and 9 (43%) had postinfarction angina at rest. Intracoronary ergonovine maleate induced coronary vasospasm in 12 (75%) of 16 patients examined. Coronary vasospasm occurred in the infarct-related coronary arteries in all patients, and importantly, multi-vessel coronary vasospasm occurred in 11 patients (69%). The infarct size was relatively small in these patients: (1) 7 patients (33%) had Q-wave AMI, and 14 patients (67%) had non-Q-wave AMI; (2) peak creatine phosphokinase was lower than 1000 IU/mL in all patients; and (3) thallium-201 scintigraphic study showed no perfusion defect in 8 of 18 patients. There was only 1 patient with CHF, and no patient died. These results suggest that coronary vasospasm may play an important role in the pathogenesis of AMI in patients without significant coronary stenosis. The relatively small infarct size suggests that coronary reperfusion occurred in the early stages of myocardial infarction.

PROGNOSTIC INDICES

Determinants of 6-Month Mortality

Volpi and associates,[32] from Milano, Italy, assessed risk prediction in 10,219 survivors of AMI, with follow-up data available, who had been enrolled in the GISSI-2 trial relying on a set of prespecified variables. The 3.5% 6-month all-cause mortality of these patients contrasted with a 4.6% mortality found in the GISSI-1 cohort, originally allocated to streptokinase therapy, indicating a 24% reduction in postdischarge 6-month mortality (Figure 3-5). With multivariate analysis, variables predictive of 6-month all-cause mortality were ineligibility for exercise test for both cardiac and noncardiac reasons, early LV CHF, echocardiographic evidence of recovery phase LV dysfunction, advanced age (i.e., more than 70 years of age), electrical instability, late LV CHF, previous AMI, and a history of treated hypertension. Early post-AMI angina, a positive exercise test, female sex, history of angina, history of insulin-dependent diabetes, and anterior site of myocardial infarction were not risk predictors. On multivariate analysis performed on 8,315 patients with the echocardiographic indicator of LV dysfunction, only previous AMI was not retained as an independent risk factor. Thus, a decline in 6-month mortality for AMI survivors seen within six hours of symptom onset has been observed in recent years. Ineligibility for exercise test, early LV CHF, and recovery-phase LV dysfunction are the most powerful predictors of 6-month mortality among patients recovering from AMI after thrombolysis. Qualitative variables reflecting residual myocardial ischemia do not appear to be risk predictors.

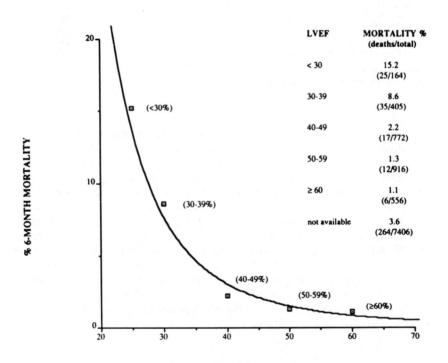

Figure 3-5. Plot of 6-month all-cause mortality in five categories of echocardiographically-determined LVEF. The LVEF mortality curve exhibits a hyperbolic trend with an upturn in mortality occurring at values of less than 40%. Reproduced with permission from Volpi et al.[32]

SINCE THROMBOLYSIS

To record prognosis and determinants of outcome in patients with AMI since thrombolysis was introduced, Stevenson and associates,[33] from London, England, studied 608 consecutive patients admitted to their coronary care unit with AMI between Jan 1, 1988 and Dec 21, 1991. Of the 608 patients, 89 (15%) died in hospital, and 596 patients were followed up after discharge from hospital. Mortality at 30 days, 1 year, and 3 years was 16% (13.4% to 19.2%), 21.7% (18.6% to 25.2%), and 29.4% (25.3% to 33.9%), respectively. Event free survival (survival without a nonfatal ischemic event) was 80.4% (77% to 83.4%) at 30 days, 66.8% (62.8% to 70.5%) at one year, and 56.1% (51.3% to 60.6%) at 3 years (Figure 3-6). Survival in patients treated with thrombolysis was considerably higher than in those not given thrombolysis (3-year survival, 76.7% v 54.3%), although the incidence of nonfatal ischemic events was the same in the two groups. Multivariate determinants of 6-month survival were LV failure, treatment with thrombolysis and aspirin, smoking history, bundle branch block, and age (Figure 3-7). For patients who survived 6 months, age was the only factor related to long-term survival. Although patients treated by thrombolysis had a relatively good prognosis, long-term mortality and the incidence of nonfatal recurrent ischemic events remained high. Effective strategies for the identification and treatment of high-risk patients need to be reassessed.

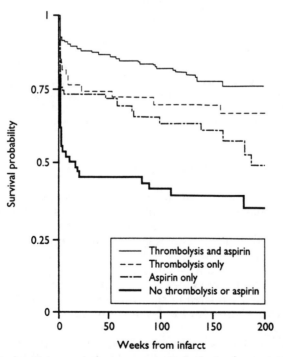

Figure 3-6. Kaplan-Meier survival curves comparing patients who received thrombolysis therapy and aspirin, thrombolysis only, aspirin only, and neither treatment. Reproduced with permission from Stevenson et al.[33]

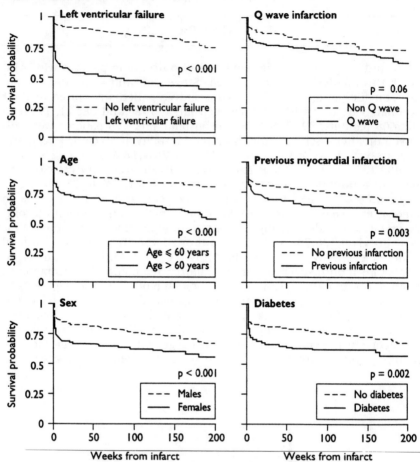

Figure 3-7. Kaplan-Meier survival curves illustrating the effects on prognosis after infarction of left ventricular failure, Q-wave infarction, age, sex, diabetes, and history of myocardial infarction. Reproduced with permission from Stevenson et al.[33]

Patency of the Infarct-Related Artery

One hundred seventy-two patients with one-vessel CAD documented at predischarge angiography who had been followed for 43 months after an initial Q-wave AMI were retrospectively evaluated by Galvani and associates,[34] from Forlí, Italy, to investigate the prognostic value of infarct-related artery patency and LV function. Multiple logistic regression analysis revealed that only infarct artery patency (thrombolysis in myocardial Infarction grades 2–3 v 0–1) and end-systolic volume index were independently related to survival. Sixteen cardiac deaths were observed; all 16 patients had LV dysfunction (defined as end-systolic volume index >40 mL/m²), and 15 had an occluded infarct-related artery. In the subgroup with LV dysfunction, the 10-year percent survival rate was 20% among patients with thrombolysis grade 0 to 1 versus 96% with grade 2–3. Patency of the infarct-related artery was also the only independent predictor of recurrent ischemia. In conclusion, both infarct-related artery patency and LV function are independent predictors of survival after Q-wave AMI. Patients with normal LV function have an excellent long-term prognosis, which is only partially counterbalanced by the tendency toward clinical instability observed in those with an open infarct-related vessel. However, when an occluded infarct-related artery is observed in the setting of LV dysfunction, the long-term outcome appears to be relatively poor.

There is emerging data that a patent infarct related artery is beneficial for short and long term survival. Vogt and associates,[35] from Kassel, Germany, analyzed four German multicenter studies to further assess this hypothesis. Nine hundred thirty-nine patients were treated less than six hours after the onset of AMI with thrombolytic therapy. Of these patients, 97% had an angiogram of the infarct related artery 90 minutes after the initiation of thrombolytic therapy. Complete reperfusion (TIMI grade 3) flow was found in 561 of 970 patients and partial reperfusion (TIMI grade 2) in 122 of 907. The in-hospital mortality rate was 4.6%. In patients with complete reperfusion of the infarct-related vessel, the mortality rate was only 2.7% versus 7.1% in patients with an occluded vessel at the 90 minute angiogram. In patients with partial perfusion of the infarct vessel, the mortality rate was 6.6%. These authors concluded that early perfusion status of the infarct-related artery is an independent predictor of short-term survival. However, only complete early reperfusion was associated with reduced in-hospital mortality rate, whereas patients with partial perfusion (TIMI grade 2) have a short-term prognosis similar to that of patients with a persistently occluded infarct vessel. Thus, complete reperfusion can potentially be used as a surrogate endpoint for mortality.

Occlusion of the infarct-related artery has recently been associated with an increased risk of sudden death, particularly in patients with poor LV function. Depressed heart rate variability also identifies postinfarction patients at an increased risk of sudden death. In an investigation by Odemuyiwa and associates,[36] from London, England, the correlation between infarct artery patency, LV function, and heart rate variability was examined in 186 survivors of a first myocardial infarction. Predischarge coronary angiography and Holter monitoring were carried out in 186 patients with a first AMI. Coronary angiography was performed because of abnormal predischarge exercise test findings. Mean age (56 ± 9 years) and the proportions of type and site of infarction did not differ between patients with occluded or patent arteries or between patients who did or did not undergo coronary angiography. The mean LVEF was 55 ± 15% in patients with patent and 49 ± 14% in those with occluded infarct arteries; and the LVEF was <40% in 17% and 28% of the respective groups. Heart rate variability was <20 U in 7 (18%) of the 39 patients with a LVEF <40% but in only 7 (5%) of the 147 patients with a LVEF >40%. Among patients with a LVEF <40%, there was no difference in the mean LVEF between patients with patent and those with occluded infarct arteries; but heart rate variability was <20 U in 6 (22%) of the 27 patients with an occluded artery but in only 1 (8%) of the 12 patients with a patent infarct artery. Moreover, mean heart rate variability was 25 ± 17 U and 37 ± 15 U, respectively. In patients with a LVEF ≥40%, heart rate variability <20 U was found in 6% of those with patent and in 4% of those with occluded infarct-related arteries. In conclusion, the status of the infarct-related artery appears to influence the severity of autonomic dysfunction in patients with LV dysfunction after a first AMI. This subgroup of patients may benefit from prophylactic revascularization or pharmacologic autonomic manipulation.

Signal-averaged high resolution electrocardiography is used to identify late potential in the terminal portion of the QRS complex of the ECG. These potentials when present are believed to increase the risk of serious arrhythmias and adverse outcome after AMI. Several studies have also suggested that the loss of vagal activity is associated with an increased incidence of arrhythmic death after AMI. Hermosillo and associates,[37] from Mexico City, evaluated short duration high resolution ECGs before hospital discharge in 175 patients with a first AMI. Of these patients, 73 received thrombolytic therapy, all underwent coronary angiography, and 88 (50%) had an occluded infarct-related artery. Sixty-two healthy subjects served as control subjects to determine the normal range of heart rate variability. The heart rate variability in patients with late potentials was lower than in those with a normal signal averaged ECG. Those patients with spontaneous or thrombolysis-induced reperfusion had less occurrence of late potentials and higher parasympathetic activity than patients with a closed artery. These authors concluded that patency of the infarct-related artery may cause both the absence of late potentials and preserve vagal tone and thus explain the reduction in mortality induced by thrombolytic therapy in AMI.

Persistent ST Depression or Elevation

In a study by Currie and Saltissi,[38] from Liverpool, United Kingdom, the significance of ST-segment elevation during ambulatory monitoring after AMI was examined in 203 patients. Ambulatory monitoring was performed both early (mean, 6.4 days [range 3 to 15]; n = 201) and late (38 days [range, 22 to 93]; n = 177), and 174 patients underwent exercise treadmill testing (38 days [range, 22 to 99]). Cardiac events (death, reinfarction, and coronary revascularization) were documented during a 1-year follow-up period. ST elevation (all silent) occurred in 25 of 201 patients (12%) on early monitoring but in only 4 of 177 (2%) on late monitoring. Compared with patients (n = 148) without any ST deviation, those with early ST elevation had more pericarditis (8/25 [32%] v 23/148 [16%]), but no more angina or exercise ischemia. The mortality rate tended to be higher in patients with early ST elevation (4/25 [l6%] v 10/148 [7%]), but ST elevation was too infrequent to be a valuable prognostic indicator. ST elevation is not uncommon during ambulatory monitoring early after AMI but is rare during later monitoring. Such ST elevation is almost always silent, does not usually reflect myocardial ischemia, and is not a useful prognostic indicator.

A number of markers have been used to stratify patients into high- and low-risk subgroups following AMI. Krone and associates,[39] from St. Louis, Mo, evaluated the long-term prognostic significance of ST-segment depression in the patient cohort of the MDPIT Trial. Admitting ECGs of 1,234 patients who survived the coronary care unit with Q-wave (n = 896) or non-Q-wave (n = 338) AMI were analyzed for the presence of ST-segment depression. Patients were followed for up to 4 years. Of these patients, 607 patients had ST depression and had a mortality rate of 10.3% compared with 5.6% for those without ST depression. This effect was present in both Q-wave and non-Q-wave AMI. Of the 437 patients with anterior ST-segment elevation, those with ST depression in other regions had a 13.6% one-year mortality rate compared with 6.9% for those with no ST-segment depression. Of the 514 patients with inferior ST-segment elevation, those with ST-segment depression in other leads had an 11.0% one-year mortality rate compared with a 1.8% rate for those with no ST-segment depression. These authors concluded that ST-segment depression on the admitting electrocardiogram in patients with AMI is a predictor of increased mortality in the year after infarction. Additional prospective studies of patients with ST depression to define coronary anatomy might be helpful to assess whether interventional strategies could be utilized to improve prognosis.

In a study by Gheorghiade and associates,[40] from Chicago, Ill, and Detroit, Mich, the prognostic significance of ST-segment depression in patients with their first AMI was investigated in 1,444 patients with an AMI, who were randomly assigned to the placebo arm of the Beta-Blocker Heart Attack Trial. Patients were divided retrospectively into three groups based on the presence or absence of 21 mm ST-segment depression in two contiguous leads of a 12-lead electrocardiogram obtained during the first few days after admission and at the time of randomization, which occurred at 9.7 ± 3.3 days after the index AMI. Group 1 included 392 patients with no ST-segment depression, group 2 comprised 713 patients with transient ST-segment depression in the first few days after admission or at the time of randomization, and group 3 included 339 patients with persistent ST-segment depression in the first few days after admission and at the time of randomization. At a median follow-up of 26 months, the mortality rate was 4.9% in group 1, 7.6% in group 2, and 14% in group 3. When Cox regression was used to adjust for baseline differences in other variables, the differences between the three groups continued to be highly significant. It was concluded that persistent and transient ST-segment depression in patients with their first myocardial infarction are strong predictors of increased long-term mortality when compared with patients without ST-segment depression. These findings should be taken into consideration when stratifying patients at risk in the postmyocardial infarction period.

Various Noninvasive Studies

Mickley and associates,[41] from Odense, Denmark, determined the relation between early out-of-hospital ambulatory ST-segment monitoring, clinical characteristics, predischarge maximal exercise testing, and cardiac events in 123 consecutive men with a first AMI. During 36 hours of ambulatory recording 11 days after AMI, 23 patients (19%) had 123 ischemic episodes (group 1), whereas 100 patients demonstrated no ischemia (group 2). Exercise-induced ST-segment depression was more prevalent in group 1 (83%) than in group 2 (47%). Group 1 patients also had more severe ischemia as judged from a shorter exercise duration before significant ST-segment depression and more pronounced ST-segment depression on exercise testing. Furthermore, exercise test results revealed an impaired hemodynamic response in group 1 compared with group 2: systolic BP at maximal work load (160 v 176 mm Hg) and systolic BP increase during exercise (41 v 56 mm Hg). Within 368 days of follow-up, the frequency of cardiac events (cardiac death, nonfatal reinfarction, and severe angina including the need of revascularization) was 52% in group

1 compared with 22% in group 2. Exercise-induced ischemia did not predict an adverse outcome: event rate.30% v 25% in patients without residual ischemia. None of the 5 patients who died had residual ischemia on either ambulatory monitoring or exercise testing. Patients having cardiac death had a significantly lower LVEF, 32%, than the 118 survivors, 49%. The study once again demonstrates the prognostic significance of LV function in the post-AMI patient.

Many of the studies of signal-averaged electrocardiography, radionuclide ventriculography and Holter ECG monitoring in risk stratification after AMI preceded the introduction of thrombolytic therapy. McClements and Adgey,[42] from Belfast, Ireland, evaluated a consecutive series of 301 survivors of AMI, 205 of whom received thrombolytic agents. Patients underwent signal-averaged electrocardiography, Holter ECG monitoring, and radionuclide left ventriculography. The median follow-up time was about 1 year. Of these patients, 4.3% had an arrhythmic event (sudden death in one, sustained VT in two). The signal-averaged ECG was 64% sensitive and 81% specific for these episodes. High-grade ventricular ectopic activity on the Holter ECG was only 38% sensitive and 74% specific. A left ventricular EF less than .40 was the best test for prediction of arrhythmia events (sensitivity 75% and specificity 81%). In a multivariate analysis in rank order, digoxin therapy at discharge, an abnormal signal-averaged ECG before discharge, absence of angina before infarction, and previous infarction were predictors of arrhythmic events. With digoxin therapy excluded, EF was an independent predictor. These authors concluded that the signal-averaged ECG and left ventricular EF are each independently predictive of arrhythmia events after myocardial infarction but the Holter ECG is not. A combination of clinical descriptors and selected tests, including the signal-averaged ECG, best identified the patients at highest risk.

Many patients with AMI undergo tests to identify myocardial ischemia, LV dysfunction, and arrhythmias. Myers and associates,[43] from Toronto, Canada, examined the usefulness of these tests in clinical practice by comparing the ability of a cardiologist to predict outcome at 1 year after AMI with and without knowledge of the results of an exercise test, radionuclide angiogram, and 24-hour Holter electrocardiographic recording. The study was limited to patients older than 65 years, who have a greater risk of cardiovascular sequelae and undergo fewer interventional procedures. The patients' own cardiologist predicted outcome on a standard rating scale, based on clinical findings and routine hospital tests and then made a second prediction after seeing the noninvasive test results. Two other cardiologists not involved in the care of the patient independently made similar predictions. Success in predicting outcome was assessed by comparison of differences between the first and second predictions in the area under receiver operating characteristic curves. During 1-year follow-up, there were 24 cardiovascular deaths and 3 recurrent AMIs among the 147 patients. There were no significant differences in mean curve areas between the first and second predictions for the patients' own cardiologist (0.62 v 0.60) or the other cardiologists (0.63 v 0.64 and 0.61 v 0.65). All predictions were significantly better than chance. Prediction of outcome in older patients after AMI is not improved by knowledge of the results of an exercise test, radionuclide angiogram, or 24-hour Holter ECG recording.

Early Exercise Testing

Early exercise testing after AMI is a well-established means of detecting patients at high risk for subsequent cardiac events. However, the value of this test is not well documented in elderly patients. Ciaroni and associates,[44] from Geneva, Switzerland, evaluated the clinical and prognostic significance of early exercise testing in 188 patients, aged 70 years or more, 14 ± 3 days after an uncomplicated AMI. The mean follow-up period was 3.6 years (range, 1 to 6 years) in 95% of the patients. The total mortality rate was 14% (24/178) and the cardiac-related mortality rate was 7.8% (14/178), with 65% of the deaths occurring in the first 3 years. There were no complications during early exercise testing. The following parameters measured during early exercise testing on a bicycle ergometer were predictive of subsequent cardiac death: an increase in systolic BP of <30 mm Hg, an increase in the double product of <12,500 mm Hg ■ beats/min, a maximal load <60 W, and a total duration of exercise <5 minutes. The combination of these four parameters increased the predictive value of the test. ST-segment depression and ventricular arrhythmias during exercise were not correlated with the incidence of subsequent cardiac death, but the degree of ST-segment depression was directly and significantly associated with the incidence of subsequent nonlethal cardiac events (CABG, PTCA, reinfarction, or unstable angina). Early exercise testing after AMI appears to be a safe and useful method for evaluating elderly patients (≥70 years) who remain asymptomatic. The discrimination of patients who are at high risk for subsequent cardiac-related mortality is possible with parameters reflecting cardiac performance during exercise (systolic BP, double product, duration of exercise, and maximal load), whereas detection of patients who are at high risk for subsequent nonlethal cardiac events is possible based on the degree of ST-segment depression.

Dipyridamole Echocardiography

To determine the prognostic capability of the dipyridamole echocardiography test (DET) early after an AMI, Picano and associates,[45] for the EPIC Study Group from 11 different echocardiographic laboratories, evaluated 925 patients after a mean of ten days from AMI onset and followed the patients up for a mean of 14 months. During the follow-up, there were 34 deaths and 37 nonfatal AMIs; 104 patients developed class III or IV angina, and 149 had CABG or PTCA. Considering all spontaneous events (angina, reinfarction, and death), the most important univariate predictor was the presence of an inducible wall-motion abnormality after dipyridamole administration. With a Cox analysis, echocardiographic positivity, age, and male gender were found to have an independent and additive value. Considering survival (and, therefore, death as the only event), age was the most meaningful parameter, followed by the wall-motion score index during dipyridamole administration. Among other parameters, the resting wall-motion score index was a significant predictor of death. In a multivariate analysis, the prognostic contributions of age (relative risk estimate = 1.08) and wall-motion score index during dipyridamole administration (relative risk estimate = 4.1) were independent and additive. In particular, considering death only, the event rate was 2% in patients with negative DET results, 4% in patients with positive high dose DET results, and 7% in patients with positive low dose DET results. Thus, DET is feasible and safe early after uncomplicated AMI and allows effective risk stratification on the basis of the presence, severity, extent, and timing of the induced dyssynergy.

Heart Rate Variability

Data suggests that diminished heart rate variability assessed 1 to 2 weeks after AMI is associated with an increased risk of cardiac death in the subsequent years. Bigger and associates,[46] from New York, NY, assessed the prognostic value of measurements of heart rate variability measured one year after AMI. They studied 331 patients who had been admitted to the cardiac arrhythmia pilot study (CAPS) who survived for one year. The 24-hour power spectral density was computed from ECG recordings using fast Fourier transforms. They analyzed ultra low frequency (<.0033 Hz), very low frequency (.0033 to <0.04 Hz), low frequency (0.04 to <0.15 Hz), and high frequency power (0.15 to <0.40 Hz), plus total power (1.157×10^{-5} to <0.40 Hz) and the ratio of low to high frequency power. Each of these measures of RR variability had a strong and significant univariate association with mortality. The relative risk for these variables ranged from 2.5 to 5.6. After adjustment for New York Heart Association functional class, rales in the coronary care unit, LVEF, and ventricular arrhythmias, some measures of heart rate variability still had a strong and significant independent association with all-cause mortality. These authors concluded that measurements of heart period variability one year after AMI still had prognostic significance for the subsequent time period.

Bigger and associates,[47] from New York, NY, studied 715 patients 2 weeks after myocardial infarction to test the hypothesis that short-term power spectral measurements of RR variability calculated from 2 to 15 minutes of normal RR interval data predict all-cause mortality or arrhythmic death. Power spectral analyses on the entire 24-hour RR interval time was obtained. For comparison, short segments of ECG recordings from two time periods available for analysis, including 8 AM to 4 PM and midnight to 5 AM, were also obtained. The former corresponds to the time interval during which short-term measures of RR variability would most likely be obtained. The latter, during sleep, represents a period of increased vagal tone, which may simulate the conditions existing when patients have a signal-averaged ECG recorded. Four frequency domain measures were calculated from the spectral analysis of heart period data over a 24-hour interval. Investigators computed the 24-hour power spectral density and calculated the power within three frequency bands. In addition, they calculated the ratio of low to high frequency power. Mean power spectral values from short periods during the day and night were similar to 24-hour values, and the correlations between short-segment values and 24-hour values were strong. Survival experience of patients with low values for RR variability in short segments of ECG recordings were compared with those with high values. Power spectral measurements of RR variability were excellent predictors of all-cause, cardiac, and arrhythmic mortality and sudden death. Patients with low values were two to four times as likely to die over an average follow-up of 31 months as were patients with high values. Power spectral measures of RR variability did not predict arrhythmic or sudden death substantially better than all-cause mortality. Thus, power spectral measures of RR variability calculated from short ECG recordings are remarkably similar to those calculated over 24 hours. Power spectral measures of RR variability are excellent predictors of all-cause mortality and sudden cardiac death.

Location of the Infarct

In a study by Behar and associates,[48] from Tel Hashomer, Israel, of 3,981 patients with a first Q-wave AMI, 1,929 (48%) had an anterior and 1,724 (43%) an inferior-wall AMI. These two groups were well matched with respect to age, gender, and relevant history. The registry dated back to the early 1980s, and accordingly, no patient was treated with thrombolytic agents, PTCA, or CABG during AMI. The in-hospital mortality rate was 18%; and the 1- and 5-year postdischarge mortality rates were 9% and 25%, respectively, in patients with anterior-wall AMI compared with the corresponding rates of 11%, 6%, and 19% in those with inferior-wall AMI. The frequency of recurrent nonfatal AMI in the year after the index AMI was 8% in the patients with anterior-wall AMI compared with 4% in those with inferior-wall AMI. By multiple logistic regression analysis of events, anterior-wall AMI was an independent predictor of in-hospital mortality only. The findings indicate that the anatomic location of a Q-wave AMI influences immediate and short-term survival of patients with a first Q-wave AMI.

With Large Infarcts

McCallister and associates,[49] from Rochester, Minn, studied patients with previous AMI to determine the influence of reperfusion on patients whose infarcts involve more than 40% of their LV. Technetium-99m Sestamibi tomography was used to measure infarct size at discharge in 166 patients with acute myocardial infarction. Patients with previous myocardial infarction or revascularizations were excluded from the trial. Sixteen patients were identified with final infarct sizes >40% of the LV despite acute reperfusion therapy. These 16 patients, including 13 men, had a mean age of 63 ± 10 years. Forty-four percent had a previous history of angina. Ten patients had emergent coronary angioplasty only with a mean time to PTCA of 6 ± 3 hours. Six patients had thrombolytic therapy with a mean time to tissue plasminogen activator of 4 ± 1.5 hours and 2 of these had rescue PTCA at 5 and 3 hours from onset of pain, respectively. Among 15 patients who had angiograms after therapy, 15 had open infarct-related arteries. The LAD was the infarct-related artery in 14 and there were 9 proximal and 5 distal lesions. Half the patients had only single-vessel disease. Infarct size measured 50% ± 7% of the LV with ranges of 42% to 68%. LVEF by radionuclide ventriculogram was 0.33 ± 0.09 and 0.38 ± 0.07 at discharge and at 6 weeks, respectively. Hospital complications included shock in 1 patient, pulmonary edema in 2 patients, angina in 3 patients, symptomatic nonsustained VT in 1 patient, transient complete heart block in 2 patients, and transient bifascicular block in 1 patient. At follow-up of 13 + 9 months, the patient with shock had died, but the remaining 15 patients were asymptomatic, although 1 had late PTCA for angina. Thus, in patients with large residual myocardial infarctions treated by PTCA or thrombolytic therapy, many survive without CHF.

Early Postinfarction Angina

In an investigation by Galjee and associates,[50] from Amsterdam, The Netherlands, to evaluate the prognostic value of early postinfarction angina and its relationship to clinical and angiographic variables, 231 consecutive patients who had had a first AMI were studied. All underwent cardiac catheterization within 10 weeks after admission to the hospital. There were no differences in basic characteristics or in EF, extent or severity of CAD, or collateral circulation between the patients with early postinfarction angina (n = 27) and those without early postinfarction angina (n = 204) except for the incidence of angina before myocardial infarction. Patients with early postinfarction angina had exercise-induced angina (42% v 21%) more frequently and shorter exercise duration (6.9 ± 2.5 min v 8.3 ± 2.5 min). Early postinfarction angina was associated with a significantly higher event rate (15% v 4%) and a significantly higher mortality rate (15% v 3%) in the first year after infarction but not during the subsequent 4-year follow-up. In patients with early postinfarction angina, stress test results had no predictive value for future cardiac events in contrast to patients without early postinfarction angina in whom ST-segment depression as observed on the stress test ECG and exercise duration had predictive value for future cardiac events. In patients with early postinfarction angina, there was no relationship between the incidence of events and the number of diseased vessels in contrast to patients without early postinfarction angina who had a high incidence of events when three-vessel disease was present (16% v 62%). Logistic regression analysis demonstrated that early postinfarction angina was the strongest predictor of cardiac death in the first year after a first AMI. Thus, it was concluded that early postinfarction angina has no relationship to the extent or severity of vessel disease and is an independent prognostic variable in patients who have had a first myocardial infarction.

Preexisting Cardiovascular Conditions

In an investigation performed by Cupples and associates,[51] from Boston, Mass, preexisting cardiovascular conditions (angina pectoris, intermittent claudication, stroke or transient ischemic attack, and CHF) were evaluated in relation to long-term prognosis after an initial AMI in 828 participants from the Framingham Heart Study. Preexisting angina pectoris and intermittent claudication in men were associated with increased risk of coronary mortality and recurrent AMI, whereas CHP increased coronary mortality. In women, prior angina pectoris increased the risk of recurrent AMI, and CHF increased the coronary mortality. Adjusting for the major cardiovascular risk factors measured before AMI, these results held for men but no significant adverse effects persisted in women. Among subjects who survived to return for subsequent examinations, only prior CHF in men increased the risk after adjusting for post-AMI risk factors. In women who returned, angina pectoris and intermittent claudication were associated with poor post-AMI prognosis. These results suggest that atherosclerosis is a diffuse disease of the circulatory system, and one in which post-AMI prognosis is influenced by the presence of other preexisting cardiovascular conditions. Hence, a patient who has an AMI after prior expression of cardiovascular disease requires more vigorous preventive management.

Educational Level

Tofler and associates,[52] from Boston, compared the clinical course of 363 patients with AMI who did not complete high school education with that of 453 who completed at least high school. Both the in-hospital and 4-year mortality rates were markedly greater for the less educated than for the more educated patients. Adverse baseline characteristics were partially responsible for the increased in-hospital and long-term mortality. The less educated patients were not as likely to quit smoking after AMI as were the more educated patients. Patients who continued smoking had a greater mortality than did those who quit (24% v 15% for less educated and 10% v 4% for better educated). Therefore, greater effort should be directed to smoking cessation among the high-risk group of less educated patients. However, the smoking continuation was responsible for only a small portion of the mortality difference, suggesting unidentified causes of mortality, such as lack of compliance with therapy and possible social isolation. Despite the high-risk status of the less educated patients, cardiac catheterization tended not to be performed as frequently as in the more educated patients after discharge from the hospital.

Ventricular Dilation and Late Potentials

Zaman and associates,[53] from Leeds, United Kingdom, performed a prospective study to assess the relation between ventricular dilatation and the development of late potentials after myocardial infarction. Echocardiograms and signal-averaged ECGs were recorded on days 1, 3, 7, and 42 in 52 patients with a first anterior myocardial infarction. Twenty-nine percent of patients with late potential-positive on their initial signal-averaged ECGs were identified on the day of admission. The incidence of late potentials rose during the next week to a peak of 42% at day 7, declining to 13% by day 42. Late potentials on the day of admission were associated with an increase in end-diastolic volume index of 16 ± 6 mL/m^2 compared with a decrease of 5 ± 3 mL/m^2 among late potential-negative patients. Similar results were evident for late potentials on days 3 and 7. There was no association between late potentials on day 42 and ventricular dilatation. Marked dynamic changes in late potentials were evident during the first week. Patients with persistent late potentials on all three recordings in the first week showed a marked increase in end-diastolic volume index of 21 ± 8 mL/m^2 in comparison with patients who were still negative. Thus, these data indicate that late potentials during the first week after myocardial infarction are associated with a subsequent development of ventricular dilatation.

Depression Afterwards

To determine if the diagnosis of major depression in patients hospitalized following AMI would have an independent impact on cardiac mortality over the first 6 months after discharge, Frasure-Smith and associates,[54]

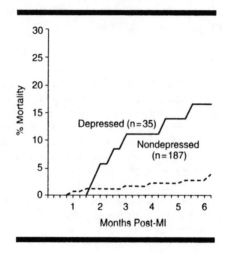

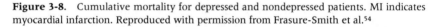

Figure 3-8. Cumulative mortality for depressed and nondepressed patients. MI indicates myocardial infarction. Reproduced with permission from Frasure-Smith et al.[54]

from Montreal, Canada, performed a prospective evaluation of the impact of depression assessed using a modified version of the National Institute of Mental Health Diagnostic Interview Schedule for major depressive episode. All 222 consenting patients met established criteria for AMI between August 1991 and July 1992 and survived to be discharged from the hospital. Patients were interviewed between 5 and 15 days following the AMI and were followed up for 6 months. There were no age limits (range, 24 to 88 years; mean, 60 years). The sample was 78% male. By 6 months, 12 patients had died. All deaths were due to cardiac causes. Depression was a significant predictor of mortality (hazard ratio, 5.74). The impact of depression remained after control for LV dysfunction (Killip class) and previous AMI, the multivariate significant predictors of mortality in the data set (adjusted hazard ratio, 4.29). Major depression in patients hospitalized following an AMI is an independent risk factor for mortality at 6 months (Figure 3-8). Its impact is at least equivalent to that of LV dysfunction (Killip class) and history of previous AMI. Additional study is needed to determine whether treatment of depression can influence post-AMI survival and to assess possible underlying mechanisms.

With Prior Coronary Bypass

Little is known concerning the influence of remote prior CABG on the outcome of patients with AMI. Dittrich and associates,[55] from San Diego, Calif, evaluated 2,494 patients with AMI of whom 219 (9%) had a history of CABG a mean of 7 years before the index AMI. Compared with all other patients, those with a history of CABG had an increased prevalence of a history of prior AMI, CHF, and angina pectoris. There was no difference in age, but patients with prior CABG were often men. During the hospitalization for AMI, patients with prior CABG had more recurrent ischemic pain and more frequently developed non-Q-wave AMI.

In-hospital mortality did not differ among patients with or without prior CABG. At hospital discharge, more patients with prior CABG had complex ventricular ectopic activity on 24-hour ambulatory electrocardiographic monitoring, and radionuclide EF <0.45. Among patients undergoing coronary angiography during the first two months, multivessel CAD was more prevalent among patients with prior CABG. Among patients with prior CABG, 25 of 133 (19%) had all grafts occluded, whereas 40 of 133 (30%) had only minor narrowing in any graft. The proportion with totally occluded grafts increased from 11% in patients who underwent operation <7 years before their AMI to 24% in patients with prior CABG 27 years before the index AMI. One-year cardiac mortality after hospital discharge was significantly higher in patients with prior CABG (16% v 8%). On multivariate analysis, prior CABG was of borderline independent importance to 1-year cardiac mortality. Thus, patients with prior CABG constitute a group at high risk for death after hospital discharge for AMI. This fact exists principally because of increased severity of underlying CAD and reduced LVEF.

COMPLICATIONS

Ventricular Arrhythmias

Hertzeanu and associates,[56] from Tel Hashomer, Israel, assessed the incidence of ventricular arrhythmias in rehabilitated post-AMI patients with LV dysfunction in a long-term rehabilitation program and compared the findings with those in similar patients who were not in such a program. Thirty-eight post-AMI patients (2 to 19 years after the acute event) with EF <40% were investigated by 48-hour Holter monitoring. They were divided into the following three groups: group I, 11 patients who underwent arm training for 60 months; group II, 11 patients who underwent calisthenics for 36 months; and group III, 16 patients who were not in any rehabilitation program; the average age of the patients was 61 years in all three groups. EF at rest was 31 for group I, 29 for group II, and 29 for group III. There were no significant differences concerning the location of AMI and antiarrhythmic treatment received by patients from all groups. At the conclusion of 48-hour Holter monitoring, two blood samples were obtained for assessment of norepinephrine (at rest and after postural change). Quality of life was determined by a detailed questionnaire, including questions concerning social activity, life satisfaction, and sexual function. After 36 and 60 months, an improvement in hemodynamic condition of patients in group I was noted. Quality of life was higher in the rehabilitated patients, with enhanced emotional stability, satisfaction with work and social life, and a high percentage of return to work (82% v 40%). The lowest levels of norepinephrine were found in group I and the highest in group III, whereas they were within normal limits in group II. Isolated PVCs were found in 1, 2, and 9 patients, and complex ventricular arrhythmias in 4, 3, and 12 patients in groups I, II, and III, respectively. Nonsustained VT was recorded in 2 patients from group I with 4 episodes, 2 patients from group II with 7 episodes, and 6 patients from group III with 24 episodes; 3 of the latter patients had complex ventricular arrhythmias also. Thus, it appeared that a long-term comprehensive rehabilitation program decreases neuroadrenergic activity, the arrhythmogenic effect of catecholamines and, consequently, the incidence of ventricular arrhythmias.

Pfisterer and associates,[57] from Basel, Switzerland, determined whether low-dose amiodarone improved 1-year survival in patients with asymptomatic complex ventricular arrhythmias continuing 2 weeks after MI. In this study, the investigators attempted to determine whether a beneficial effect of amiodarone persisted beyond discontinuation of amiodarone after 1 year by studying 98 amiodarone-treated patients and 114 control patients. Low dose amiodarone therapy included 200 mg per day after an initial loading dose of 1,000 mg for 5 days. After a mean follow-up of 72 months, information on 96% of patients was obtained regarding survival, death, and cause of death. Probability of death after 84 months was 30% for the amiodarone-treated 7 patients and 45% for control patients (Figure 3-9). For the total group, mortality remained significantly lower in the amiodarone group as compared to the control group for all deaths as well as cardiac deaths. The mortality reduction was due to the first-year amiodarone effect, because there was no significant mortality difference between groups when considering survival after discontinuation of amiodarone only. Therefore, these data demonstrate that the beneficial effect of amiodarone on survival in high-risk patients persists for several years, but not beyond the period of amiodarone usage. The results stress the importance of early treatment after MI for patients with asymptomatic but complex ventricular arrhythmias.

Maggioni and associates,[58] from Milan, Italy, used 24-hour Holter recordings obtained prior to discharge from the hospital in 8,676 post-AMI patients studied in the GISSI-2 evaluation to determine the presence of ventricular arrhythmias. Patients were followed for 6 months from the acute event. Total and sudden cardiovascular mortality rates were computed and relative risks in univariate and multivariate analyses calculated. The aim of the study was to establish the prevalence and

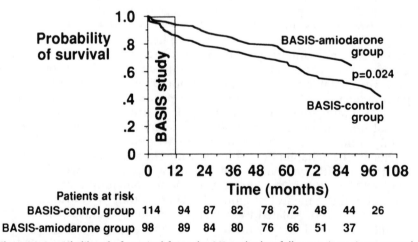

Patients at risk									
BASIS-control group	114	94	87	82	78	72	48	44	26
BASIS-amiodarone group	98	89	84	80	76	66	51	37	

Figure 3-9. Likelihood of survival from the MI to the last follow-up in patients treated with low-dose amiodarone for 1 year and in control patients. Reproduced with permission from Pfisterer et al.[57]

prognostic significance of ventricular arrhythmias in post AMI patients treated with fibrinolytic agents during the acute phase. Ventricular arrhythmias were identified in 64% of patients, including more than ten VPCs per hour in 20% of patients and nonsustained VT in 7% of patients. Ventricular arrhythmias were more frequent when there was clinical evidence of extensive LV damage. During follow-up, there was a total of 256 deaths (3%), 84 of which (33% of total deaths) were sudden deaths. Mortality rates were 2% in patients without ventricular arrhythmias, 3% in patients with one to ten VPCs per hour, 6% in those with more than ten VPCs per hour, and 5% in those with complex VPCs. The presence of frequent, i.e., more than ten VPCs per hour was a significant predictor of total and sudden mortality. The presence of nonsustained VT was not associated with the worsening of the prognosis (Figure 3-10). This study demonstrates that approximately 36% of patient recovering from AMI presented with less than one VPC per hour prior to discharge, but almost 20% of patients showed frequent ventricular arrhythmias. Frequent VPCs are an independent risk factor for total and sudden cardiac death in the first 6 months following AMI.

Hii and associates,[59] from Alberta, Canada, postulated that effective antiarrhythmic drug therapy selected during serial electrophysiologic studies in patients with VT after an AMI would be identified more frequently when the infarct-related artery is patent than when it is chronically occluded. In 64 consecutive patients with documented CAD and remote AMI presenting with spontaneous sustained VT or VF, 4 ± 2 electropharmacological studies identifying effective antiarrhythmic drug therapy in 16 patients (25%) occurred. Drug responders did not differ significantly from nonresponders in demographic, electrocardiographic, angiographic, or hemodynamic measurements. However, a patent infarct-related artery was associated with antiarrhythmic drug response significantly more frequently than an occluded infarct-related artery (45% v 9%) (Figure 3-11). Patency of the infarct-related artery was the

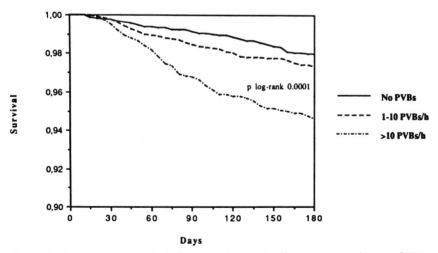

Figure 3-10. Six-month survival of patients characterized by presence or absence of VPCs per hour is shown. There was a significantly higher risk of death in the subgroup of patients with more than ten VPCs per hour. Reproduced with permission from Maggioni et al.[58]

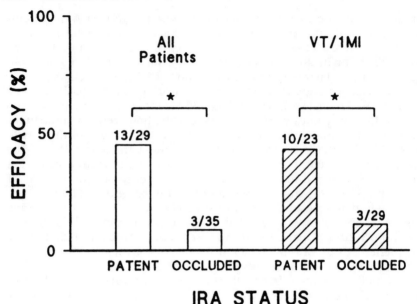

Figure 3-11. The effect of infarct-related artery patency on the results of drug testing in patients with inducible ventricular arrhythmias (VT and VF). Drug efficacy was enhanced with patients with patency infarct-related arteries in preventing VT and VF. Reproduced with permission from Hii et al.[59]

only independent predictor of response to antiarrhythmic drug therapy in this study population. The sensitivity and specificity of a patent infarct-related artery to predict successful drug testing were 81% and 67%, respectively. Therefore, the outcome of electropharmacological studies is predicted by the patency of an infarct-related artery after remote AMI.

Navarro-López and associates,[60] from Barcelona, Spain, conducted a randomized trial to assess the efficacy of amiodarone versus metoprolol or no antiarrhythmic treatment to suppress asymptomatic ectopic activity and improve survival in patients who have had AMI with LVEF of 20% to 45% and ≥3 VPCs per hour (pairs or runs). Patients (n = 368) were randomly assigned to receive amiodarone 200 mg/day (n = 115) 10 to 60 days after the acute episode and metoprolol 100 to 200 mg/day (n = 130), or no antiarrhythmic therapy (n = 123). After a median follow-up of 2.8 years, mortality in the amiodarone-treated patients (3.5%) did not differ significantly from that of untreated control subjects (7.7%), but was lower than that in the metoprolol group (15.4%) (Figure 3-12). Patients treated with metoprolol had twice the mortality seen in control subjects, even though the differences were not statistically significant. Holter studies performed at 1, 6, and 12 months showed that both amiodarone and metoprolol were equally effective in reducing heart rate, whereas only amiodarone significantly reduced ectopic activity. Thus, long-term treatment with amiodarone was clearly safe in patients with an EF of 20% to 45%, was effective in suppressing arrhythmias, and was associated with a lower mortality than metoprolol; corroboration is required in a larger trial.

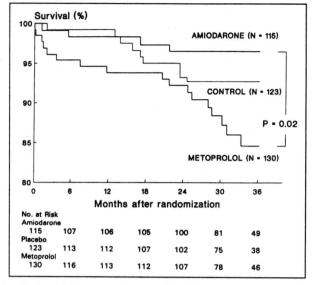

Figure 3-12. Kaplan-Meier survival curves of the three treatment groups. Survival in patients assigned to amiodarone (n = 115) differed significantly (p = 0.02, adjusted for multiple groups) from that of patients receiving metoprolol (n = 130), but was no different from that of untreated patients (n = 123). The number of patients at risk in each group at the end of each 6-month period are shown at the *bottom*. Reproduced with permission from Navarro-López et al.[60]

Shock

In this report by Champagnac and associates,[61] from Lyon, France, 15 patients (mean age, 49 ± 7 years) with AMI and cardiogenic shock underwent emergency cardiac transplantation after medical treatment failed to improve their hemodynamic status. The infarction was anterior in 12 cases, inferoposterior in 2 cases, and septal in 1 case. Shock occurred within three days after the onset of chest pain in 9 patients and during the first day in 6 patients. Mechanical circulatory assistance was used in 6 patients as a bridge to transplantation when their hemodynamic status could not be stabilized pharmacologically. Orthotopic cardiac transplantation was performed an average of 16 ± 14 days after onset of infarction. Three patients died during the early postoperative period. Another died 7 months after transplantation. During the mean follow-up period of 31 ± 20 months, there were three acute rejections, all successfully treated, and one chronic rejection. The survival rate for this series is 70%. Thus, emergency cardiac transplantation may be the best option for selected patients with AMI and cardiogenic shock refractory to conventional therapy.

Left and/or Right Ventricular Dilatation and Remodeling

Gaudron and associates,[62] from Würzburg, Germany, defined the relation between LV dilatation and global and regional cardiac dysfunction to identify early predictors of enlargement and chronic CHF in patients after AMI. LV volumes, regional area shrinkage fraction in 18 predefined sectors, global LVEF, and hemodynamics at rest and during exercise were assessed prospectively 4 days, 4 weeks, 6 months, and 2 and 3 years after first AMI. Seventy patients were assigned to groups with progressive, limited, or no dilatation of the LV. Patients without dilatation (n = 38) maintained normal volumes and hemodynamics for 3 years after AMI. With limited dilatation (n = 18), LV volumes increased up to 4 weeks after AMI and stabilized thereafter. Depressed stroke volume was restored at 4 weeks after AMI and remained stable at rest. However, pulmonary capillary wedge pressures during exercise progressively increased. In the patients with progressive LV dilatation (n = 14), depressed cardiac and stroke indexes were restored by 4 weeks but deteriorated thereafter. Area shrinkage fraction as an estimate of regional LV function in normokinetic sectors at 4 days gradually deteriorated during 3 years, but hypokinetic and dyskinetic sectors remained unchanged. Global LVEF fell after 2 years, whereas right atrial pressure, pulmonary capillary wedge pressure, and systemic vascular resistance increased. Using multivariate analysis, LVEF, and stroke index at 4 days, ventriculographic AMI size, AMI location, and Thrombolysis in Myocardial Infarction trial grade of infarct artery perfusion were predictors of progressive LV enlargement and chronic LV dysfunction. Therefore, almost 26% of patients may develop limited LV dilatation within 4 weeks after first AMI, which helps to restore cardiac index and stroke index at rest and preserve exercise performance. A small group, perhaps 20% of patients, developed progressive structural LV dilatation, which is compensatory first and then progresses to noncompensatory dilatation and finally results in severe global LV dysfunction. In these patients, depression of LVEF probably results from impairment of function of initially normally contracting myocardium. Multivariate analysis allows the early prediction of patients at high risk for progressive LV dilatation and chronic LV dysfunction within 4 weeks after AMI.

Activation of neurohumoral systems occurs in both acute and chronic heart failure. Rouleau and associates,[63] from Sherbrooke, Quebec, Canada, evaluated data from 519 patients enrolled in the Survival and Ventricular Enlargement (SAVE) Study. These patients had plasma neurohormones measured before randomization at a mean of 12 days after infarction. All patients had an LVEF less than 40% but no overt CHF. All neurohormones were increased compared with values from age-matched control subjects, except epinephrine. Plasma norepinephrine was 301 versus 222 pg/mL, renin activity was 3 versus 1.2 ng/mL per hour, arginine vasopressin was 1.9 versus 0.7 pg/mL, and atrial natriuretic peptide was 75 versus 21 pg/mL. Values ranged from normal to very high, indicating a wide spectrum of neurohumoral activation. The clinical and laboratory variables most closely associated with neurohumoral activation were Killip class, left ventricular EF, age, and use of diuretic drugs. These authors concluded that neurohumoral activation occurs in a significant proportion of patients at the time of hospital discharge after infarction. There is considerable variability, however, between individual patients.

LV remodeling after Q-wave anterior AMI was examined by Mallavarapu and associates,[64] from Philadelphia, Pa, with single-photon emission computed tomographic thallium imaging. Initial (after adenosine infusion) and 4-hour delayed reinjection images were obtained in

34 patients with a mean age of 65 years. Short-axis slices from the delayed images were quantitatively analyzed by measuring the outer and inner diameters, and wall thickness. The results were compared with those in a group of normal subjects. The outer diameter was greater in patients than in normal subjects at the apical, mid-, and basal levels; the average outer diameter was 17 mm in patients, and 12 mm in normal subjects. Similarly, the inner diameter was greater in patients than in normal subjects at the three levels; the average inner diameter was 7 mm in patients and 5 mm in normal subjects. Wall thickness was greater in patients than in normal subjects (5.2 v 3.8 mm). There were significant correlations between LV dilation and time elapsed (in weeks) since AMI, and the size of the perfusion abnormality. Thus, LV dilation occurs after Q-wave anterior AMI and is related to infarct size and duration. These changes can be studied by single-photon emission computed tomographic thallium imaging.

LV remodeling after LV AMI has been described previously. Little is known regarding concomitant adaptation, if any, in RV volumes after LV AMI. To examine this issue, Hirose and associates,[65] from Rochester, Minn, used cine-computed tomography to determine serial changes in absolute global LV and RV volumes in 27 patients without clinical CHF during the first year after an initial Q-wave AMI (14 anterior and 13 inferior). The patient group with anterior wall LV infarction showed progressive increases in LV and RV volumes from hospital discharge to 1 year (end-diastolic volumes ±25% and ±13%, respectively; end-systolic volumes ±35% and ±15%, respectively) (Figure 3-13) . In patients with inferior wall LV infarction, both LV end-diastolic and end-systolic vol-

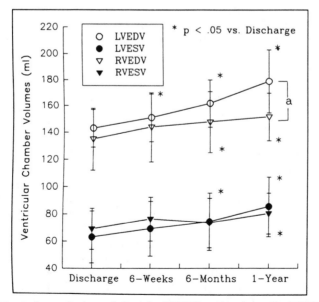

Figure 3-13. Left ventricular end-diastolic (LVEDV) and end-systolic (LVESV) chamber volumes, and right ventricular end-diastolic (RVEDV) and end-systolic (RVESV) chamber volumes during first year after anterior wall left ventricular myocardial infarction (n = 14). Data are presented as mean ± SD. *a*, p = 0.003 for left versus right ventricular end-diastolic volume. Reproduced with permission from Hirose et al.[65]

umes increased significantly during the study period (±13% and ±15%, respectively). Despite a trend for RV end-diastolic volume to be increased at 1 year, neither end-diastolic nor end-systolic volume increased significantly after hospital discharge following inferior wall LV infarction. Absolute RV end-diastolic volume was not significantly different between the infarct groups at any time after infarction. In conclusion, global changes occur in both LV and RV volumes during the first year after an initial infarction regardless of infarct location. The magnitude of these changes was greater after anterior than inferior wall LV infarction.

Left Ventricular Thrombus

The management of mural thrombus complicating anterior wall AMI remains controversial. Vaitkus and Barnathan,[66] from Burlington, Vt, performed a meta-analysis of published studies to evaluate the embolic risk of mural thrombi after AMI, the impact of systemic anticoagulation in reducing this risk, and the benefit of anticoagulation, thrombolytic therapy, and antiplatelet therapy in preventing mural thrombus formation. In 11 studies comprising 856 patients, the odds ratio for increased risk of emboli in the presence of echocardiographically demonstrated mural thrombus was 5.45. The odds ratio of anticoagulation versus no anticoagulation in preventing embolization (7 studies, 270 patients) was 0.14. The odds ratio of anticoagulation versus control in preventing mural thrombus formation was 0.32. The odds ratio for thrombolytic therapy in preventing mural thrombus was 0.48. For antiplatelet agents, the odds ratio was 1.43. They concluded that mural thrombus after AMI poses a significant increased risk of embolization. The risk of embolization is reduced by systemic anticoagulation. Anticoagulation can also prevent mural thrombus formation. Thrombolytic therapy may prevent mural thrombus formation, but antiplatelet therapy is of no benefit.

Right Ventricular Infarction

Inferior wall AMI frequently involves the RV wall. Zehender and associates,[67] from Freiburg, Germany, hypothesized that RV involvement, as diagnosed by ST-segment elevation of the right precordial lead V_{4R}, may affect the prognosis of patients with inferior AMI. In 200 consecutive patients admitted to the hospital with inferior wall AMI, these authors assessed the prevalence and diagnostic accuracy of ST-segment elevation in lead V_{4R} (as compared with four other diagnostic procedures) to identify RV involvement and its prognostic implications for in-hospital and long-term results (Table 3-8). The in-hospital mortality after AMI was 19%, and major complications occurred in 47% of the patients. The presence of ST-segment elevation in lead V_{4R} in 107 patients (54%) was highly predictive of RV AMI (sensitivity, 88%; specificity, 78%; diagnostic accuracy, 83%) as compared with the other diagnostic procedures. The patients with ST-segment elevation in lead V_{4R} had a higher in-hospital mortality rate (31% v 6%) and a higher incidence of major in-hospital complications (64% v 28%) than did those without ST elevation in V_{4R}. Multiple logistic-regression analysis showed ST elevation in V_{4R} to be independent of and superior to all other clinical variables available on admission for the prediction of in-hospital mortality (relative risk, 7.7)

Table 3-8. Clinical Characteristics, Mortality, and Complications During Hospitalization after an Acute Inferior Myocardial Infarction, According to the Presence or Absence of ST-Segment Elevation in Lead V_{4R}.* Reproduced with permission from Zehender et al.[67]

VARIABLE	ST-SEGMENT ELEVATION		P VALUE
	ABSENT (N = 93)	PRESENT (N = 107)	
Clinical characteristics			
Sex (M/F)	69/24	84/23	0.51
Age (yr)	62.3±5	60.8±6	0.66
Previous infarction — no. (%)	13 (14)	20 (19)	0.45
Thrombolytic therapy — no. (%)	30 (32)	41 (38)	0.38
Maximal CK >1000 U/liter — no. (%)	21 (23)	40 (37)	0.03
Shock at time of admission — no. (%)	7 (8)	15 (14)	0.18
LV ejection fraction (%)†	43±8	44±7	0.35
During hospitalization (no. of patients)‡			
Death	5	33	<0.001
Cardiogenic shock	4	27	<0.001
Ventricular fibrillation	9	22	0.05
Sustained ventricular tachycardia	7	17	0.08
Complete AV block	4	18	0.006
Severe bradycardia	3	10	0.09
Requirement for pacing	3	19	0.001
Myocardial rupture, tamponade	2	7	0.18

*CK denotes creatine kinase, LV left ventricular, and AV atrioventricular. Plus–minus values are means ±SD.

†Ten days after myocardial infarction, the mean left ventricular ejection fractions measured in 89 patients were 50±10 percent in the patients in whom ST-segment elevation was absent and 49±8 percent in those in whom it was present (P not significant).

‡Some patients had more than one major complication.

and major complications (relative risk, 4.7). The posthospital course (follow-up, at least 1 year; mean follow-up, 37 months) was similar in patients with and in those without electrocardiographic evidence of RV AMI. RV involvement during AMI can be accurately diagnosed by the presence of ST-segment elevation in lead V_{4R}, a finding that is a strong, independent predictor of major complications and in-hospital mortality. Electrocardiographic assessment of RV AMI should be routinely performed in all patients with AMI.

Pericardial Involvement

Correale and associates,[68] from Milan, Italy, reviewed data from the Gruppo Italiano per lo Studio della Sopravvivenza nell'Infarto Miocardico (GISSI) trial to describe the epidemiology of pericardial involvement in patients treated with or without thrombolysis and to establish its role as a marker of the extent of AMI and its prognostic value. In both GISSI-1 (n = 11,806) and GISSI-2 (n = 12,381), a specific item regarding presence/absence of clinically detected pericardial involvement was included in the study forms. In GISSI-1, patients with ST elevation and depression at the onset of AMI were admitted, whereas GISSI-2 included only those with ST elevation. Results of univariate analysis are presented as Mantel-Haenszel-Peto odds ratios with 95% confidence intervals. Cox proportional hazards models were used to assess the independent prognostic significance of pericardial involvement for in-hospital and long-term mortality. The main results indicate that (1) the incidence of pericardial involvement in patients treated with thrombolytic agents is approximately half of that in the control group (7% v 12%); (2) the earlier the treatment, the lower the incidence of pericardial involvement; (3) pericardial involvement is strongly associated with infarction size, evaluated by electrocardiograms, creatine kinase peak, and echo assessments; and (4) pericardial involvement is associated with a higher long-term mortality but is not an independent prognostic factor. Pericardial involvement is a reliable bedside, cost-free marker of AMI size and poorer outcome. Because it may elude detection owing to its transitory and often short duration, it should be given greater attention.

Oliva and associates,[69] from Denver, Colo, analyzed the clinical courses and serial ECGs of 200 consecutive patients with acute myocardial infarction. Among 43 patients with postinfarction pericarditis, the pattern of T-wave evolution consistently differed from the customary postinfarction pattern of T-wave evolution. This unusual evolutionary course was expressed as either persistently positive T-wave 48 hours or more after infarction (67%) or premature, gradual reversal of inverted T-waves to positive deflections (33%). The sensitivity and specificity of these T-wave alterations were 100% and 77%, respectively. Other processes identified that caused this type of postinfarction T-wave evolution were cardiopulmonary resuscitation, reinfarction, and very small infarcts (Figure 3-14). Ninety percent of patients with reperfusion had a maximum T-wave negativity of 3 mm or more within 48 hours after the onset of chest pain in the lead that initially demonstrated the greatest ST-segment elevation. Seventy-six percent of patients without reperfusion had a maximum negativity of 2 mm or less within 72 hours. Therefore, like the ST segment, accelerated evolution and deepening of the T-wave may be noninvasive markers of reperfusion. Thus, premature alterations of the ST and T-wave after acute myocardial infarction are a sensitive and easily recognizable ECG manifestation of postinfarction regional pericarditis. In addition, reperfusion is associated with accelerated evolution and deepening of the T-waves following myocardial infarction.

Cardiac Rupture

Rupture of the LV free wall is generally sudden and unanticipated. Oliva and associates,[70] from Denver, Colo, and Rochester, Minn, evaluated the clinical course of evolutionary electrocardiographic changes in 70 consecutive patients with rupture and 100 comparison patients with AMI but without rupture. Patients with rupture had a significantly greater incidence of pericarditis, repetitive emesis, and restlessness and agitation than did patients without rupture. More than 80% of patients with rupture had two or more symptoms compared with 3% of patients without rupture. A deviation from expected evolutionary T-wave pattern occurred in 94% of patients with rupture and 34% of control patients. An abrupt transient episode of hypotension and bradycardia probably secondary to the initial tearing of the epicardium with a resultant small hemopericardium was observed in 21% of patients with rupture. Rupture of the midlateral wall was most common and usually occurred in the setting of an inferoposterolateral infarction related to an acute left circum-

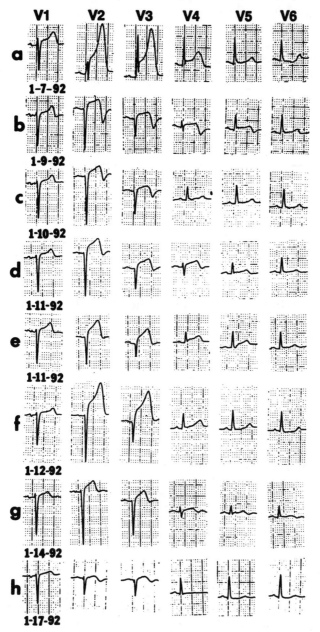

Figure 3-14. Serial ECGs of a patient with an acute anterior infarction followed by pericarditis between days 3 and 6. Panel a, ST-segment elevation and tall peak T-waves characteristic of the hyperacute phase of myocardial infarction are shown. Panel b, recorded 48 hours later, after reperfusion with thrombolytic therapy, discloses T-wave inversions with a maximum T-wave negativity existing in lead V_2. Subsequently, the patient developed pleural pericardial pain, which persisted for 3 days, accompanied by an intermittent friction rub. Panel c, d, e, and f show gradual reversal of the T-wave polarity and a gradual reelevation of the ST segment without reelevation of the creatine kinase-MB. Maximal reversal of the T-wave occurred on January 12, and the pain disappeared over the next 24 to 36 hours. The ECGs on January 14 and 17 showed gradual reduction of the accentuated T-waves with their becoming inverted again. Reproduced with permission from Oliva et al.[69]

flex coronary artery occlusion. In the two most recent patients, the event was recognized by the changes listed above and the defects successfully repaired. These authors concluded that cardiac rupture is often preceded by particular symptoms and signs and that the utilization of a bedside echocardiogram and echocardiographically-guided pericardiocentesis, if fluid is visualized, may identify patients early enough so that immediate surgery may be life-saving.

GENERAL TREATMENT

Mail-Out Intervention Program

Heller and associates,[71] from Newcastle, Australia, tested the hypothesis that 6 months after AMI, adoption of secondary prevention activities would be higher, quality of life better, and blood cholesterol lower in patients randomly allocated to a mail-out intervention program than in those receiving usual care. Patients were aged <70 years, admitted to hospitals in and around Newcastle, Australia with a suspected heart attack, and discharged alive from the hospital. Cluster randomization, based on the patient's family practitioner, was used to allocate consenting patients to an intervention or usual care group. A low-cost mail-out program was designed to help patients reduce dietary fat, to obtain regular exercise by walking, and (for smokers only) to quit smoking. Supplementary telephone contact was also used. In addition, a letter was sent to the family doctor regarding the benefit of aspirin and β-blockers for secondary prevention. Of eligible patients, 71% participated, and 79% of the 213 intervention subjects and 87% of the 237 usual care subjects returned a 6-month follow-up questionnaire. Self-reported fat intake was significantly lower, an "emotional" score obtained from a quality-of-life questionnaire was significantly higher in the intervention than in the usual care group, and "physical" and "social" scores for quality of life were slightly higher. Blood cholesterol level and other variables were not different between the groups at 6 months. Simple low-cost programs providing support and advice on lifestyle change may be beneficial, particularly in improving patients' perceived quality of life.

Smoking Cessation

Krumholz and associates,[72] from New Haven, Conn, and Boston, Mass, developed a model to examine the cost-effectiveness of a smoking cessation program after MI. The cost-effectiveness of the nurse-managed smoking cessation program was estimated to be $220/year of life saved. Over a wide range of estimates of costs and effectiveness, a nurse-managed smoking cessation program after AMI was extremely cost-effective intervention. By comparison the program was more cost effective than beta-adrenergic antagonist therapy after AMI.

Scopolamine

In 41 survivors of AMI, Pedretti and associates,[73] from Tradate, Italy, performed a prospective study in two sequential phases. In phase 1, the role of baroreflex sensitivity and heart rate variability as predictors of inducible and spontaneous sustained ventricular tachyarrhythmias was evaluated. In phase 2, the effects of transdermal scopolamine on baroreflex sensitivity and spectral and nonspectral measures of heart rate variability were investigated. At a mean follow-up of 10 months after AMI, 5 of 41 patients (12%) developed a late arrhythmic event. Of these, all had inducibility of sustained monomorphic VT at programmed stimulation compared with 3 of 36 patients (8%) without events. At multivariate analysis, baroreflex sensitivity had the strongest relation to both inducibility of sustained monomorphic VT and occurrence of arrhythmic events. Of 41 patients, 28 consented to undergo phase 2 of the investigation. Baroreflex sensitivity significantly increased after transdermal scopolamine as well as heart rate variability indexes. Of these, the mean of standard deviations of normal RR intervals for 5-minute segments and the total power had the most significant improvement after scopolamine. The present investigation confirms that assessment of autonomic function is an essential part of arrhythmic risk evaluation after AMI. Transdermal scopolamine, administered to survivors of a recent AMI, reverses the autonomic indexes that independently predict arrhythmic event occurrence. On the basis of these data, transdermal scopolamine could be a potentially useful tool in the prophylaxis of life-threatening ventricular arrhythmias after AMI.

Low heart rate variability is associated with increased mortality after AMI. Vybiral and associates,[74] from Houston, hypothesized that by enhancing parasympathetic activity, that low-dose transdermal scopolamine would increase heart rate variability after myocardial infarction. Conventional time domain heart rate variability was measured from 24-hour Holter recordings of 61 consecutive male patients six days after AMI. Patients were then randomly assigned to wear a patch of transdermal scopolamine or a matching placebo patch for 24 hours, during which their 24-hour heart rate variability was remeasured. Compared with placebo, transdermal scopolamine caused a significant increase in time domain measures of 24-hour heart rate variability by 26% to 35% above baseline. The medication was well tolerated. These authors conclude that low-dose transdermal scopolamine can safely increase cardiac parasympathetic activity and short-term heart rate variability after AMI. This sets the stage for a prospective trial of this approach to see if restoration of heart rate variability can reduce long-term morbidity and mortality.

Magnesium

To investigate the effect of long-term oral magnesium treatment on incidence of cardiac events among survivors of an AMI, Galløe and associates,[75] from Charlottenlund, Denmark, performed a double-blind, placebo-controlled parallel study in which patients were randomized to treatment or placebo. The patients received one tablet of 15 mmol magnesium hydroxide or placebo daily for 1 year. Among the 468 survivors of AMI (aged 31 to 92 years) there was no significant difference between treatment and placebo groups in the incidence of each of the three cardiac events, namely reinfarction, sudden death, and CABG within 1 year; but when the events were combined and dropouts were excluded from calculations, there was a significantly higher incidence of events in the treatment group (56/167 v 33/153; relative risk, 1.55). Long-term oral treatment with 15 mmol magnesium daily does not reduce the incidence of cardiac events in survivors of an AMI and, indeed, seems to increase the risk of developing a cardiac event. Consequently, this treatment cannot be recommended as secondary prophylaxis for such patients.

Encainide v Flecainide v Moricizine

To test the hypothesis that in survivors of AMI, the suppression VPCs improves survival free of cardiac arrest and arrhythmic death, Epstein and associates,[76] from CAST, studied a total of 3,549 patients with AMI and subsequently LV dysfunction. Overall survival and survival free of cardiac arrest or arrhythmic death were compared in patients randomized to long-term, active antiarrhythmic drug therapy versus corresponding placebo, using the stratified long-rank statistic. At 1 year from the time of randomization to blinded therapy, 95% of placebo-treated patients versus 90% of active drug-treated patients remained alive. Similarly, at 1 year, 96% of placebo-treated patients versus 93% of active drug-treated patients remained free of cardiac arrest or arrhythmic death. Thus, the suppression of asymptomatic or mildly symptomatic ventricular arrhythmias after AMI does not improve survival and can increase mortality. Treatment strategies designed solely to suppress these arrhythmias should no longer be followed.

Amiodarone

The prophylactic administration of amiodarone following AMI has been investigated in several small trials. Zarembski and associates,[77] from Tucson, Ariz, combined by meta-analysis these small trials to determine the effects of prophylactic low-dose amiodarone on mortality following AMI. Four prospective, randomized, placebo-controlled trials, which investigated the prophylactic administration of low-dose amiodarone (200 to 400 mg/dL) to patients after AMI, were selected from the current literature according to strict inclusion criteria. A total of 1,140 patients, 566 in the amiodarone-treated group and 574 in placebo-treated group, were included in the analysis. Sudden cardiac death, cardiac mortality, and total mortality were the endpoints of interest. In addition, the effect of impaired LV function (EF, <45%) on total mortality was assessed. Data were aggregated by using the Mantel-Haenszel method to obtain final summary statistics for these endpoints. Patients treated with low-dose amiodarone had a lower incidence of sudden death (3.1%) and total mortality (6.1%) compared with patients treated with placebo (6.9% and 11.2%, respectively). There was not significant difference between the amiodarone- and placebo-treated groups with respect to cardiac mortality (2.6% v 3.7%). For patients with a LVEF of <45%, total mortality was 5.5% in the amiodarone-treated group and 9.4% in the placebo-treated group. Thus, this meta-analysis suggests that the prophylactic administration of low-dose amiodarone to patients following AMI reduces the incidence of both sudden death and total mortality. The benefits of low-dose amiodarone may be limited to patients with preserved LV function.

Aspirin v Aspirin + Heparin v Aspirin + Warfarin

Antithrombotic therapy has been generally useful in patients with unstable angina and non-Q-wave myocardial infarction. Cohen and associates,[78] from Philadelphia, Pa, reported a multicenter trial of antithrombotic therapy in unstable angina or non-Q-wave AMI. Three hundred fifty-eight patients admitted with 48 hours of chest pain were randomized to antithrombotic therapy with either (1) aspirin alone or (2) aspirin plus heparin followed by aspirin plus warfarin, and were prospectively followed for 12 weeks. Admission cardiac enzyme analyses revealed unstable angina in 268 patients and non-Q-wave AMI in 62 patients. Patients in the two groups were similar with regard to age, gender, coronary risk factors, and prior antianginal medication. These authors found that patients with unstable angina or non-Q-wave AMI on antithrombotic therapy have a similar total number of ischemic events by 12 weeks. Despite maximal medical therapy with antianginal and antithrombotic medication, patients with non-Q-wave AMI have a significantly higher rate of reinfarction and death (16% v 7%).

Captopril

Motwani and associates,[79] from Dundee, Scotland, investigated whether favorable renal effects might contribute to the influence of captopril in offsetting ventricular dilation after AMI. Effective renal plasma flow and glomerular filtration rate were estimated by isotope injection methods in 20 patients on days 2, 7, 8, 42, and 180 after a first transmural anterior AMI. After measurements on day 7, patients were randomized to receive either captopril 25 mg three times daily or placebo for the remainder of the study. At baseline (day 7), there were no differences between the two treatment groups in radionuclide LVEF, effective renal plasma flow, glomerular filtration rate, or neurohormones. LVEF (40% at baseline) were higher in the captopril- than the placebo-treated patients on days 42 and 180 after AMI. Effective renal plasma flow became significantly higher at all time points after randomization in the captopril-treated group than in the placebo group. A similar but lesser trend was observed for glomerular filtration rate. Plasma atrial natriuretic factor and aldosterone were significantly higher in the placebo group. Renal hemodynamic indexes were directly correlated with and neurohumoral indexes inversely correlated with EFs. In a second group of 12 patients with higher baseline EF after an inferior AMI, none of these beneficial effects of captopril were demonstrable. It is proposed that in the setting of LV dysfunction after AMI, a prompt and sustained improvement in renal hemodynamics, by reducing inappropriate fluid retention and thus ventricular preload, may be one contributory mechanism by which captopril prevents progression of LV dilatation.

Søgaard and associates,[80] from Aarhus, Denmark, evaluated the effects of captopril in 64 patients with LV dysfunction after MI. Patients were randomized at day 7 to either placebo or captopril (50 mg daily) in a double-blind parallel study over a period of 6 months. The patients were followed up with ambulatory ECG monitoring, bicycle ergometer testing, and echocardiographic examinations. The duration of ST-segment depression detected during the ambulatory ECG monitoring was lower in patients treated with captopril (87 minutes) than in those

Table 3-9.   Twenty-Four–Hour Ambulatory ECG Monitoring after Myocardial Infarction: Duration of ST Segment Depression. Reproduced with permission from Sogaard et al.[80]

	Baseline	Day 30	Day 90	Day 180
Duration (minutes)				
Placebo	32 (0–84)	13 (0–66)‡	21 (0–74) ⎤	22 (0–69) ⎤
Captopril	35 (0–86)	13 (0–85)‡	6 (0–60) ⎦*	3 (0–26)§ ⎦†
No. of patients				
Placebo	21	18	21 ⎤	22 ⎤
Captopril	22	14	10‖ ⎦*	7‖ ⎦*

Mean duration of significant ST segment depressions are shown with ranges in parentheses.
*p<0.01, †p<0.001 between groups.
‡p<0.05 compared with baseline.
§p=0.02 compared with day 30.
‖p<0.01 compared with inclusion.

treated with placebo (638 minutes), and the number of patients in the captopril group with exercise-induced ST-segment depression was less at the completion of the study (Table 3-9). Work capacity increased during the study in the captopril-treated group and was higher than in the placebo group. Significant dilation of the LV end-diastolic and end-systolic volumes was observed in the placebo group but was prevented in the captopril group (Figure 3-15). These data confirm that captopril has a favorable effect on dysfunctioning myocardium after MI.

Captopril v Isosorbide Mononitrate

The administration of captopril beginning several days after AMI has been shown to attenuate the dilatation and remodelling process and to reduce mortality. Pipilis and associates,[81] from Oxford, England, evaluated the early treatment of patients with AMI using captopril and isosorbide mononitrate. In a double-blind study, 81 patients were randomized within 36 hours of the onset of symptoms of suspected AMI to 1 month of oral captopril (6.25 mg initial dose followed by 12.5 mg three times daily), isosorbide mononitrate (20 mg three times daily), or matching placebo. One hour after treatment, blood pressure was reduced by about 10% with both captopril and isosorbide mononitrate. Captopril was associated with an increase in stroke volume and cardiac output. Both captopril and isosorbide mononitrate reduced systemic vascular resistance within one hour, but only captopril's effect was sustained, perhaps because the three times daily nitrate regimen induced tolerance. These authors concluded that the hemodynamic effects of both captopril and isosorbide mononitrate are well tolerated in the acute phase of MI and that captopril favorably influences cardiac function. This trial has set the stage for the, as yet, unpublished ISIS 4 Trial.

Ramipril

Survival after AMI has been enhanced by treatment with thrombolytic agents, aspirin, and β-adrenoceptor blockade. There are, however, a substantial subgroup of patients who manifest clinical evidence of CHF despite the first two of these treatments, and for whom β-adrenoceptor antagonist are relatively or absolutely contraindicated. These patients have a greatly increased risk of fatal and nonfatal ischemic, arrhythmic,

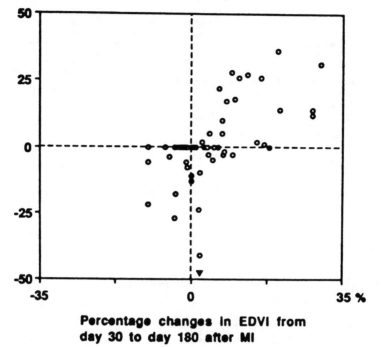

Figure 3-15. Scatterplot shows correlation between percentage changes in end-diastolic volume index (EDVI) and changes in ST-segment depression (minutes) from day 30 to day 180 after MI. The point marked with a triangle represents a value of +3%, -85 minutes, $p = 0.63$, $p < 0.001$, n = 58. Reproduced with permission from Søgaard et al.[80]

and hemodynamic events. In this selected high-risk subset of patients, the Acute Infarction Ramipril Efficacy (AIRE) Study Investigators[82] investigated the effect of therapy with the angiotensin converting enzyme inhibitor ramipril, postulating that it would lengthen survival. A total of 2,006 patients who showed clinical evidence of CHF at any time after an AMI were recruited from 144 centers in 14 countries. Patients were randomly allocated to double-blind treatment with either placebo (992 patients) or ramipril (1,014 patients) on day 3 to day 10 after AMI (day 1). Patients with severe CAD resistant to conventional therapy, in whom the attending physician considered the use of an angiotensin converting enzyme inhibitor to be mandatory, were excluded. Follow-up was continued for a minimum of 6 months and an average of 15 months. On intention-to-treat analysis, mortality from all causes was significantly lower for patients randomized to receive ramipril (170 deaths [17%]) than for those randomized to receive placebo (222 deaths [23%]) (Table 3-10). The observed risk reduction was 27%. Analysis of prespecified secondary outcomes revealed a risk reduction of 19% for the first validated outcome (ie, first event in an individual patient)—namely, death, severe/resistant CHF, AMI, or stroke. Oral administration of ramipril to patients with clinical evidence of either transient or ongoing CHF, initiated between the second and ninth day after AMI, resulted in a substantial reduction in premature death from all causes. This benefit was

Table 3-10. Summary of Primary Endpoints, Validated Secondary Events, and Secondary Endpoints. Reproduced with permission from the Acute Infarction Ramipril Efficacy Study Investigators.[82]

	Ramipril (n = 1004)	Placebo (n = 982)	Total (n = 1986)
Primary endpoint			
Death	170 (17%)	222 (23%)	392 (20%)
Secondary events validated by outcomes subcommittee			
Severe/resistant heart failure	143 (14%)	178 (18%)	321 (16%)
Reinfarction	81 (8%)	88 (9%)	169 (9%)
Stroke	25 (2%)	17 (2%)	42 (2%)
Secondary endpoint (ie, first validated event)			
Death	94 (9%)	118 (12%)	212 (11%)
Severe/resistant heart failure	103 (10%)	133 (14%)	236 (12%)
Reinfarction	68 (7%)	71 (7%)	139 (7%)
Stroke	21 (2%)	15 (2%)	36 (2%)
Any event	286 (28%)	337 (34%)	623 (31%)

apparent as early as 30 days and was consistent across a range of subgroups.

Class I Agents v Beta Blockers v Amiodarone v Calcium Antagonists

To investigate the effects of prophylactic therapy with antiarrhythmic agents on mortality in patients with AMI, Teo and associates,[83] from Bethesda, Md, Edmonton, Canada, and Winston-Salem, NC, obtained mortality data from 138 trials of 98,000 patients and combined them by the Yusuf-Peto adaptation of the Mantel-Haenszel method. There were 660 deaths among 11,712 patients allocated to receive class I agents and 571 deaths among 11,517 corresponding control patients (51 trials; odds ratio, 1.14). Of 26,973 patients allocated to receive β-blockers (class II agents), 1,464 died compared with 1,727 deaths among 26,295 control patients (55 trials; odds ratio, 0.81). Of 778 patients allocated to receive amiodarone (class III agent), 77 died compared with 101 deaths of 779 control patients (8 trials; odds ratio, 0.71). There were 982 deaths in 10,154 patients allocated to receive a class IV agent (calcium channel blockers) and 949 deaths in 10,188 control patients (24 trials; odds ratio, 1.04). The routine use of class I antiarrhythmic agents after AMI is associated with increased mortality. β-Blockers have been conclusively demonstrated to reduce mortality. The limited data on amiodarone appears promising. Data on calcium channel blockers remain unpromising.

THROMBOLYSIS

Review

Anderson and Willerson,[84] from Houston, Tex, provided an excellent review on thrombolysis in AMI. The thrombolytic agents currently available are summarized in Table 3–11. The risk factors for bleeding with

Table 3-11. Thrombolytic Agents Currently Available.* Reproduced with permission from Anderson HV and Willerson JT.[84]

CHARACTERISTIC	STREPTOKINASE	ANISTREPLASE	UROKINASE	t-PA
Molecular weight (daltons)	47,000	131,000	31,000–55,000	70,000
Plasma clearance time (min)	15–25	50–90	15–20	4–8
Fibrin specificity	Minimal	Minimal	Moderate	Moderate
Plasminogen binding	Indirect	Indirect	Direct	Direct
Potential allergic reaction	Yes	Yes	No	No
Typical dose	1.5 million units	30 units	2 million units	100 mg
Administration	1-hr IV infusion	5-min IV infusion	1-million-unit IV bolus, then 1 million units IV over 1 hr	10-mg IV bolus, with the remainder over 90 min
Approximate cost ($)	500	1,500	1,500	2,200

*Current recommendations are that a thrombolytic agent be administered with oral aspirin (160 to 325 mg per day) and intravenous heparin (at a dosage adjusted to keep the activated partial-thromboplastin time 1.5 to 2 times the control value). See the text for details. IV denotes intravenous.

thrombolytic regimens are summarized in Table 3-12. Criteria for thrombolysis in AMI are summarized in Table 3-13. The authors concluded that the use of thrombolytic therapy in patients with Q-wave AMI has resulted in better short-term and medium-term survival and better recovery of LV function. Many people are alive today, functioning at levels of physical activity that would not otherwise have been possible, because of this therapy.

Impact on Clinical Practices

The treatment of AMI changed when several trials reported that thrombolytic agents given within a few hours of AMI improved outcome. Gray and associates,[85] from Nottingham, United Kingdom, presented data from the Nottingham Heart Attack Register comparing 1982 to 1984, when thrombolysis was not available, and 1989 to 1990, when it was hospital policy to give thrombolysis to all patients who arrived within 6 hours of onset of symptoms, in the absence of a specific contraindication.

Table 3-12. Risk Factors for Bleeding with Thrombolytic Regimens.* Reproduced with permission from Anderson HV and Willerson JT.[84]

RISK CATEGORY	PERIPHERAL OR SYSTEMIC BLEEDING	INTRACRANIAL BLEEDING
Major (thrombolytic therapy contraindicated)	Major surgery or organ biopsy within 6 wk Major trauma within 6 wk Gastrointestinal or genitourinary bleeding within 6 mo History of a bleeding diathesis Known or suspected aortic dissection Known or suspected pericarditis	Known intracranial tumor Previous neurosurgery Stroke within 6 mo Head trauma within 1 mo
Important (a relative contraindication to thrombolysis)	Puncture of a noncompressible vessel Cardiopulmonary resuscitation for >10 min	Acute severe hypertension Remote thrombotic stroke Recent transient ischemic attacks
Minor (increased risk of bleeding, but no definite contraindication to thrombolysis)	Diabetic retinopathy Cardiopulmonary resuscitation for <10 min Older age Female sex Small body size	Older age History of hypertension Small body size Female sex

*The data have been adapted with modifications from Califf et al.[48] with the permission of the publisher.

Table 3-13. Criteria for Thrombolysis in Acute Myocardial Infarction. Reproduced with permission from Anderson HV and Willerson JT.[84]

Chest pain consistent with acute myocardial infarction
Electrocardiographic changes
    ST-segment elevation >0.1 mV in at least 2 contiguous
      leads
    New or presumably new left bundle-branch block
    ST-segment depression with prominent R wave in leads V_2
      and V_3, if this is thought to indicate a posterior infarction
      (benefit is doubtful if it is thought to indicate unstable
      angina)
Time from onset of symptoms
    <6 hours: most beneficial
    6–12 hours: lesser but still important benefits
    >12 hours: diminishing benefits but possibly still useful
      for continuing chest pain or "stuttering" pain course
Age
    Physiologic age more important than chronologic age
    <75 yr: clear-cut benefits
    ≥75 yr: fewer clear-cut benefits

The number of patients referred with symptoms suggestive of AMI increased by 75% from 1982 to 1990; a diagnosis of "possible infarction" was made in about half of all patients in 1982 to 1984 and 23% in 1989 to 1990. Our current thrombolytic policy has had little impact on patient and general practitioner behavior. The general practitioner was contacted by most patients. The median time between the onset of a patient's symptoms and admission to hospital, when the general practitioner was involved, was 229 minutes in 1982 to 1984 and 210 minutes in 1989 to 1990; when he was not involved in arranging the admission, median times to admission were 89 minutes and 75 minutes, respectively. By 6 hours from symptom onset, 60% of patients had been admitted; by 12 hours, about 70% were in hospital; and by 24 hours, 80% were in hospital. Of 7,855 patients admitted with suspected AMI in 1989 to 1990, 4,465 were admitted within 6 hours of symptom onset. Of these, 736 patients (16%) received a thrombolytic drug; 389 patients (9%) had a specific, documented contraindication to thrombolysis. Although these authors estimated that the policy has saved about eight lives per year, it is not surprising that there has been no improvement in overall case fatality after AMI.

Little is known about incorporation of new knowledge from randomized clinical trials into clinical practice. Thrombolytic therapy was shown to reduce the mortality of AMI in several large trials published during 1986 to 1988. To examine the effect of these data on clinical practice, Ketley and Woods,[86] from Leicester, United Kingdom, analyzed the supply of thrombolytic drugs in an English region of nearly 5 million persons in 1987 to 1992 (Figure 3-16). During the study period there were over 10,000 hospital admissions per year in the region for AMI. From a very low initial level, thrombolytic drug use rose slowly for several years after publication of the trial results and reached a plateau in 1991 to 1992. Rates of use per 1,000 patients admitted with AMI varied almost 6-fold between districts in 1989 to 1990 and over 2-fold in 1991 to 1992. Level of use attained by districts in the latter period was strongly associated with the extent of their previous participation in multicenter trials

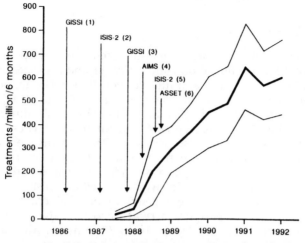

Figure 3-16. Supply of thrombolytic drugs in Trent region from district pharmacy services and trial organizations. Mean value for districts (bold line) and standard deviation are plotted by financial half-year. Dates of journal publication of the major trial results are also shown. Reproduced with permission from Ketley et al.[86]

of thrombolysis; the authors estimated that 35% to 50% of patients admitted with AMI were receiving thrombolytics. The full potential of thrombolytic treatment has still not been achieved in routine care and the limiting factors need to be defined.

In Different Countries

Many trials of thrombolytic agents have been conducted in a variety of different countries. It is unclear, however, that patient populations or morbidity and mortality are necessarily the same in different countries. Accordingly, Barbash and associates,[87] from Tel Hashomer, Israel, looked at the variation in mortality rates among countries participating in the International Tissue Plasminogen Activator/Streptokinase Mortality Trial. Risk factors were identified by a multivariate logistic model. Expected mortality rates based on these risk factors were then calculated and compared with actual mortality for each decile of the total study group and for each country.

The overall mortality rate among the 1,612 patients in risk deciles 9 and 10 was 26%, and for the 1,606 patients in deciles 1 and 2, 1.2%. The observed mortality in the different countries varied between 2.9% and 15%. The logistic model closely predicted and explained the different mortality rates for most countries except for the difference between the two lowest and highest mortality rates. They concluded that recognized risk factors in acute myocardial infarction can only account in part for mortality differences across populations of different countries. They postulated that genetic and environmental factors may interact with other patient characteristics in explaining these results. Several studies, for example, have demonstrated racial differences in endogenous fibrinolytic activity and have suggested that some populations may be more sensitive to thrombolytic therapy.

Prehospital Administration

To determine the effect of prehospital-initiated versus hospital-initiated treatment of AMI on clinical outcome, Weaver and associates,[88] for the Myocardial Infarction Triage and Intervention Project Group, performed a randomized, controlled clinical trial involving 360 patients with symptoms for six hours or less, no risk factors for serious bleeding, and ST-segment elevation. They represented 4% of patients with chest pain who were screened and 21% of those with AMI. The patients were allocated to have aspirin and alteplase treatment initiated before or after hospital arrival. Intravenous sodium heparin was administered to both groups in the hospital. The primary endpoint was a ranked composite score (combining death, stroke, serious bleeding, and myocardial infarct size). Initiating treatment before hospital arrival decreased the interval from symptom onset to treatment from 110 to 77 minutes. Although more patients whose therapy was initiated before hospital arrival had resolution of pain by admission (23% v 7%), there were no significant differences in the composite score, mortality (5.7% v 8.1%), EF (53% v 54%), or infarct size (6.1% v 6.5%) than later treatment. Identification of patients eligible for thrombolysis by paramedics reduced the hospital treatment time from 60 minutes (for patients not in the study) to 20 minutes (for study patients allocated to begin treatment in the hospital). There was no improvement in outcome associated with initiating treatment before hospital arrival; however, treatment within 70 minutes of symptom onset—whether in the hospital or in the field—minimized the infarct process and its complications.

The efficacy of thrombolytic therapy for AMI depends partly on how soon after the onset of symptoms it is administered. The European Myocardial Infarction Project Group[89] studied the efficacy and safety of thrombolytic therapy administered before hospital admission in patients with suspected AMI. In a multicenter, double-blind study, patients who were seen within six hours of the onset of symptoms and who had a qualifying 12-lead electrocardiogram were randomly assigned to receive either anistreplase before admission, followed by placebo in the hospital (prehospital group), or placebo before admission, followed by anistreplase in the hospital (hospital group). Prehospital therapy was administered by emergency medical personnel. A total of 2,750 patients were randomly assigned to the prehospital group and 2,719 to the hospital group. The patients in the prehospital group received thrombolytic therapy a median of 55 minutes earlier than those in the hospital group. There was an observation of a nonsignificant reduction in overall mortality at 30 days in the prehospital groups (9.7% v 11.1% in the hospital group; reduction in risk, 13%). Death from cardiac causes was significantly less frequent in the prehospital group than in the hospital group (8.3% v 9.8%; reduction in risk, 16%). Particular adverse events occurred more frequently in the prehospital group during the period before hospitalization; among these events were VF, shock, symptomatic hypotension, and symptomatic bradycardia. With the exception of symptomatic hypotension, however, the overall incidence of these events was similar for both groups. Prehospital thrombolytic therapy for patients with suspected AMI is both feasible and safe when administered by well-equipped, well-trained mobile emergency medical staff. Although such therapy appears to reduce mortality from cardiac causes, the data do not definitely establish that it reduces overall mortality.

The time window for salvage of myocardial tissue in AMI is narrow. Prehospital administration of thrombolytic agents can potentially reduce the time to treatment and thus be more efficacious. Linderer and associates,[90] from Berlin, Germany, reported on 170 patients who received 30 mg of anistreplase up to four hours from symptom onset by a mobile ICU physician. The decision to treat on scene was correct in 98% of patients. There were no bleeding complications or deaths outside of the hospital. In therapy initiated less than 1.5 hours (96 patients) versus greater than 1.5 hours (74 patients), there was reduced cardiac enzyme release (646 v 886 IU/L), improved EF (57% v 51%) and reduced 21 day mortality (1% v 7%). These authors concluded that the start of thrombolytic therapy at less than 1.5 hours in the prehospital setting limits infarct size, preserves LV function, and may reduce mortality compared with thrombolysis greater than 1.5 hours in the same setting.

Chest Pain Before and After

It is frequently difficult to determine noninvasively whether reperfusion has occurred in patients receiving thrombolytic therapy for AMI. Christian and associates,[91] from Rochester, Minn, evaluated the perception of chest pain severity to see if it was predictive of the amount of myocardium at risk and whether the response of pain during thrombolysis was associated with myocardial salvage during AMI. Sixty-two patients with AMI had evaluation of myocardium at risk with a technetium-99m sestamibi study before thrombolysis and again at hospital discharge. Chest pain severity was graded before thrombolysis as none, mild, moderate, or severe and during thrombolysis was graded as none, partial, or completely resolved. There was no association between chest pain severity and myocardium at risk. There was a significant association between chest pain, response to therapy, and myocardial salvage. By multivariate analysis, chest pain severity and response to chest pain during thrombolysis were significant independent predictors of myocardial salvage and infarct size. Thrombolysis was most effective in the 20 patients (32%) with moderate or severe chest pain and complete resolution of symptoms during thrombolysis. These authors concluded that the assessment of chest pain before and after thrombolytic therapy is a readily available and useful indicator of the efficacy of the therapy.

In Men v Women

White and associates,[92] from Auckland, New Zealand, analyzed data from 8,261 of the 8,387 randomized patients with AMI who received thrombolytic therapy in the International Tissue Plasminogen Activator/Streptokinase Mortality Study; patients were followed for 6 months. Women made up 23% (n = 1,944) of the study population. Baseline characteristics were worse in women. They were 6 years older; and they were more likely to have a history of prior infarction and antecedent angina, hypertension, and diabetes. They were also in a higher Killip class on admission, and they received thrombolytic therapy 18 minutes later than men after symptom onset with myocardial infarction. Fewer women were smokers and more women had a higher hospital mortality (12% v 7%) and 6 month mortality (17% v 10%). Women were also more likely to develop cardiogenic shock (9% v 6%), bleeding (7% v 5%), and hemorrhagic stroke (1% v 0.3%) or total stroke (2% v 1%) during hospitalization. Reinfarction rates and requirement for PTCA or surgery did not differ. After correction for worse baseline characteristics, women had similar morbidity and mortality apart from a significantly higher incidence of hemorrhagic stroke, which remained significant even when accounting for weight and treatment allocation (Table 3-14).

Several studies have suggested that there are gender differences in the management and prognosis of acute coronary artery syndromes. Lincoff and associates,[93] from Cleveland, Ohio, and Durham, NC, evaluated whether female gender portended an adverse prognosis independent of the severity of the underlying disease in patients with AMI treated with thrombolysis. A total of 348 women were compared with 1,271 men enrolled in the Thrombolysis and Angioplasty in AMI (TAMI) Trials. There were no differences in baseline hemodynamic variables among the group. Rates of in-hospital PTCA in men and women (52.6% v 54.1%) and bypass graft surgery (20.4% v 22.0%) were comparable. Women had higher unadjusted rates of mortality (9.2% v 5.4%), reinfarction (6.4% v 2.6%), and hemorrhagic stroke (2.0% v 0.55%) than did men during the hospital period. When adjusted for clinical and angiographic variables, differences in mortality and hemorrhagic stroke did not reach statistical significance and the risk of reinfarction was only marginally associated with gender. These authors concluded that the adjusted mortality rates and utilization of postlysis revascularization are similar in men and women. However women may be at increased risk for infarction.

On Right Ventricular Function

To determine the effect of thrombolytic therapy on the frequency of RV dysfunction, and whether RV dysfunction is a risk factor for morbidity and mortality after discharge from the hospital, 1,110 patients in the Thrombolysis in Myocardial Infarction (TIMI) II Trial with acute inferior

Table 3-14. Reproduced with permission from White et al.[92]

Group	rt-PA	Streptokinase	Odds Ratio*	95% Confidence Intervals	P
Men					
<80 kg	8/1890 (0.5%)	1/1860 (0.1%)	7.90	0.99-63.2	<.05
>80 kg	1/1261 (0.1%)	6/1306 (0.5%)	0.17	0.02-1.43	.14
Women					
<70 kg	9/692 (1.3%)	1/710 (0.1%)	9.34	1.71-51.05	<.05
>70 kg	1/287 (0.3%)	3/254 (1.2%)	0.29	0.03-2.83	.53

rt-PA indicates recombinant tissue plasminogen activator.

*Odds ratios >1 indicate a greater risk of hemorrhagic stroke for rt-PA compared with streptokinase. A test for interaction is significant ($P < .001$) indicating a relatively higher stroke rate for rt-PA than streptokinase in lighter patients and/or a relatively higher stroke rate for streptokinase than rt-PA in heavier patients.

wall LV AMI were studied by Berger and associates,[94] from Rochester, Minn. RV dysfunction was defined as an RV wall-motion abnormality on equilibrium radionuclide ventriculography performed a mean of nine days after admission to the hospital. Fifty-eight patients (5%) had RV dysfunction. Baseline clinical characteristics among patients with and without RV dysfunction were similar. However, patients with RV dysfunction had a lower mean LVEF (51% v 56%) and a greater frequency of in-hospital complications. Angiographic data from patients undergoing protocol catheterization 18 to 48 hours after hospital admission showed that the infarct-related artery was more likely to be occluded in those with RV dysfunction (48% v 14%). There was no difference in the frequency of multi-vessel disease between the two groups. In patients with RV dysfunction in whom radionuclide ventriculography was repeated 6 weeks after hospital discharge, RV wall-motion abnormalities persisted in only 18% (8 of 45). Mortality in the year after discharge was 3.5% among patients with RV dysfunction compared with 1.7% among those without RV dysfunction. Thus, RV dysfunction occurs infrequently after thrombolytic therapy, particularly in patients with patency of the infarct-related artery 18 to 24 hours after such therapy. Among surviving patients who undergo predischarge radionuclide ventriculography, RV dysfunction is not associated with a significantly increased mortality in the year after discharge from the hospital.

Administered Late (>6 Hours)

Early reperfusion (4 to 6 hours) after AMI reduces mortality and reduces the incidence of late potentials on a signal-averaged electrocardiogram. Recent reports suggest that reperfusion accomplished after >6 hours also may reduce mortality. The effect of such later reperfusion on the signal-averaged electrocardiogram is not known. Ragosta and associates,[95] from Charlottesville, Va, hypothesized that reperfusion by PTCA accomplished >24 hours after onset of AMI would reduce late potentials and improve the parameters on the signal-averaged electrocardiogram. Forty-one patients with a totally occluded infarct-related artery an average of 12 days after AMI underwent attempted PTCA. Signal-averaged electrocardiogram, echocardiography, and thallium-201 imaging were performed before and 1 month after attempted PTCA. PTCA resulted in successful reperfusion in 32 patients and was unsuccessful in 9 patients. No change in the incidence of late potentials occurred after successful reperfusion or after unsuccessful reperfusion. Among patients with successful reperfusion, no significant change occurred in the QRS duration or the terminal signal duration <40 µV. The terminal root-mean-square voltage in microvolts improved significantly at 1 month. Twenty-two of 32 patients with successful reperfusion had improved wall motion in the infarct zone at 1 month. Despite an improvement in function in these patients, no change in the incidence of late potentials occurred by 1 month. Among patients with successful reperfusion, those without late potentials at baseline had improved wall motion to a greater extent than those with late potentials. These authors concluded that late reperfusion after AMI has little effect on the signal-averaged electrocardiogram, and a normal signal-averaged electrocardiogram in patients with a totally occluded artery after AMI may signify the presence of viable myocardium.

In 1985, an overview of clinical trials confirmed that patients treated within six hours of the onset of symptoms of AMI benefited from thrombolytic therapy. Doubt remained about treatment later than this and this uncertainty prompted further randomized studies. In the South American Multicenter Trial (EMERAS),[96] a total of 4,534 patients entering hospital up to 24 hours after the onset of pain suspected of being due to AMI were randomized with intravenous streptokinase 1.5 mU and placebo, during the period January 1988 to January 1991. Once the results of ISIS-2 were known, only patients presenting more than six hours after symptom onset were randomized. There was not significant difference in mortality during the hospital stay (268/2,257 [11.9%] deaths among streptokinase patients v 282/2,277 [12.4] in controls). Among the 2,080 patients presenting 7 to 12 hours from symptom onset, there was a nonsignificant trend towards fewer deaths with streptokinase (11.7% streptokinase v 13.2% control; 14% [SD 12] reduction), whereas there was little difference among the 1,791 patients presenting after 12 to 24 hours (11.4% v 10.7%; 8% [16] increase). The EMERAS results, though not conclusive on their own, do contribute substantially to accumulating evidence on the question of whether fibrinolytic therapy really does produce any worthwhile improvement in survival among such patients.

Accessing Reperfusion

Ito and associates,[97] from Osaka, Japan, determined the risk area using myocardial contrast echocardiography and investigated the time course of functional recovery of postischemic myocardium within the risk area in patients with reperfused anterior MIs. The study population consisted of 21 patients with anterior MIs who demonstrated coronary reflow within six hours of onset following thrombolysis or PrCA. Myocardial contrast echocardiography was performed with the injection of hand-agitated Haemaccel (5 mL) into the right and left coronary arteries before coronary flow. The risk area was defined as the area of contrast perfusion defect in the apical long-axis view. The ratio of the endocardial length of abnormal contraction segment to that of contrast defect segment was determined at days 1, 2, 3, 7, 14, and 28 of reflow. Before reflow, the length of contrast defect correlated well with the segment length of dyskinesis/akinesis. The values for the same area progressively decreased in patient with successful perfusion until day 14. Greater improvement in segmental function was obtained in patients reperfused within 4 hours than in those reperfused at ≥4 hours. Thus, a significant amount of myocardium is salvaged in patients with a reperfused anterior MI. Major functional improvement seems to be achieved within 14 days of reperfusion.

Experimental data suggest that reperfusion injury involving free radicals contributes to the impairment of LV function after successful thrombolysis. Thus, Davies and associates,[98] from London, England, in 72 patients presenting with AMI, measured markers of free radical activity before streptokinase and two hours later. Thiobarbituric acid reactive material reflects lipid peroxidation by free radicals, and the concentration of plasma total thiols (34 patients) reflects oxidative stress. Coronary arteriography was performed at 18 to 72 hours after thrombolysis to determine coronary patency, and LV function was assessed by ventriculography and from QRS scoring of the electrocardiogram. The infarct-related artery was patent (Thrombolysis in Myocardial Infarction Trial grade 2 or better) in 60 patients (83%) and occluded in 12 patients. In the 60 patients with a patent artery, the concentration of thiobarbituric acid reactive material increased after streptokinase by 9.2 nmol/g albumin, whereas in the 12 patients with an occluded artery thiobarbituric acid reactive material decreased by 7 nmol/g albumin. In those with a patent artery, the rise in thiobarbituric acid reactive material associated with thrombolysis correlated with LVEF and with the QRS score. Plasma total thiol concentrations decreased by 13 µmol/L in those with a patent artery, and this decrease associated with thrombolysis correlated with LVEF but not with the QRS score. These findings suggest that reperfusion injury mediated by free radicals may be of clinical importance in humans.

Depressed baroreceptor sensitivity has been associated with an increased risk of ventricular arrhythmias and sudden cardiac death after AMI, but the influence of thrombolytic therapy on baroreceptor sensitivity has not been examined. In a study by Odemuyiwa and associates,[99] from London, England, to determine the effect of thrombolytic therapy on the evolution of baroreceptor sensitivity after AMI, baroreceptor sensitivity was assessed at 6 days, 6 weeks, and 3 months in 76 patients, 53 (70%) of whom had received thrombolytic therapy. The mean age (57 v 57 years), sites of infarction, and proportion of patients taking β-blockers (68% v 52%) did not differ between patients who did and patients who did not receive thrombolytic therapy. There was no difference in predischarge mean LVEF (42% v 46%) between the two groups of patients, but mean baseline baroreceptor sensitivity was 9.2 ms/mm Hg in patients who were treated with thrombolysis and 5.9 ms/mm Hg in those who were not. At 6 weeks, the corresponding values were 9.7 and 11.1 ms/mm Hg and at 3 months 9.1 and 6.5 ms/mm Hg. At baseline, 13% of patients who were treated with thrombolysis and 13% of those who were not had baroreceptor sensitivity <3.0 ms/mm Hg; but at 3 months, there were 9% of treated patients compared with 17% of untreated patients with baroreceptor sensitivity <3.0 ms/mm Hg. In conclusion, early after AMI, mean baroreceptor sensitivity was higher in patients treated with thrombolysis compared with nontreated patients. Similar trends were noted 3 months later, and the proportion of patients with lower baroreceptor sensitivity was smaller in those given thrombolytic therapy compared with those who were not. Thrombolytic therapy should reduce the incidence of early and late sudden cardiac death after AMI.

A number of studies have demonstrated that ventricular size is a good predictor of outcome after AMI. It is also clear that patients with a patent artery to the infarct zone have less dilatation and a better long-term outcome after AMI than those with a closed artery. It is uncertain, however, whether reestablishment of flow early during AMI is necessary to gain this benefit or whether one can open the artery after the infarction has been completed and still obtain the same long-term benefit. Nidorf and associates,[100] from Boston, Mass, used an echocardiographic mapping technique to evaluate this question over a 3 month period in 91 patients. Patients were classified as those who had no anterograde or collateral flow to the infarct bed; only collateral flow to the infarct bed; early restoration of anterograde flow within hours of chest pain; or late restoration of flow within a mean of five days after the AMI. Over 3 months, a progressive and significant increase in endocardial surface area was observed only in the patients without anterograde or collateral flow. A progressive reduction in wall motion was evident in the patients in whom anterograde flow to the infarct bed was restored within hours or days. Thus, the benefits seen in improvement in wall motion in the patients with anterograde flow was independent of the timing of reperfusion. This data supports the hypothesis that opening of the artery can be beneficial even if it is not done within the first several hours of the infarction. This retrospective analysis sets the stage for a prospective study to evaluate this question further.

Abe and associates,[101] from Kagoshima and Kyoto, Japan, measured creatine kinase isoforms by a new immunoinhibition method to evaluate their usefulness in detecting early coronary reperfusion. Blood samples were collected at 15-minute intervals from 50 patients with AMI. Creatine kinase isoforms were determined by a 10-minute immunoinhibition method with an autoanalyzer. Values for inhibited isoforms were divided by those of noninhibited isoforms to calculate the isoform ratio. In the reperfused group, the increase in the isoform ratio was 2.69 ± 1.80 at 30 minutes after reperfusion and 2.41 ± 2.01 at 60 minutes, which was significantly higher than the corresponding values in the nonreperfused group (0.17 ± 0.16 and 0.32 ± 0.26, respectively). When an increase of 0.70 or more in the isoform ratio was used as the criterion for reperfusion, the sensitivity and specificity were 92% and 100% at 30 minutes and 100% and 100% at 60 minutes after recanalization, respectively. It was concluded that the isoform ratio obtained by the new 10-minute assay of creatine kinase isoforms is useful for the noninvasive detection of reperfusion 30 and 60 minutes after recanalization in AMI.

In an investigation carried out by Luria and associates,[102] from Jerusalem, Israel, to assess early changes in heart rate variability, 81 patients with AMI during the initial 24 hours after thrombolytic therapy were studied. The standard deviation of the mean heart rate and the low- (0 to 0.5 Hz), mid- (0.05 to 0.20 Hz), and high- (0.20 to 0.35 Hz) frequency band power were evaluated with 24-hour Holter recordings. Found were diminished variance in the time domain and reduced power spectrum in the frequency domain, compared with a group of 41 normal individuals. Patients with anterior AMI had significantly higher heart rates and lower heart rate variability values than patients with inferior AMI. Reduction in heart rate variability occurred within the first eight hours in patients with anterior AMI; a significant fall was especially noted in the high-frequency band after a decline in ST-segment elevation. Heart rate variability alterations in patients with inferior AMI were most evident in the final eight-hour interval. These findings indicate sympathovagal imbalance and are related to clinical signs of intense autonomic nervous system activity that are observed early in the course of anterior and inferior AMI.

Harrison and associates[103] used contrast ventriculograms in 542 patients treated with intravenous thrombolytic agents for acute MIs to define changes in LVEF and regional wall motion that occur during the first week after reperfusion therapy and to elucidate clinical, acute angiographic, and treatment variables related to improvement in global and regional LVEF. Intravenous tissue-type plasminogen activator and/or urokinase were administered to 805 patients during AMI. Mean time from symptom onset to thrombolytic therapy was three hours. Acute and seven-day catheterizations were performed. Paired LVEF and analyses of regional wall motion were available in 542 patients. Stepwise, multivariate analysis of clinical, acute angiographic, and treatment variables were used to develop two models: one related to improvement in LVEF and the other related to improvement in infarct zone regional function. LVEF did not change acutely. Improvement in infarct zone regional function was modest at 1 week. Subgroup analysis demonstrated modest improvement in LVEF and greater improvement in infarct zone function in patients with sustained reperfusion at 1 week. Reductions in LVEF and infarct zone regional function during the acute study were associated with improvement in these variables at 1 week. Resolution of chest pain before catheterization, infarct-related artery flow at catheterization, and depressed regional wall motion in the noninfarct zone were associated with improvement in LVEF and regional infarct zone function at 1 week. In this study, the time from the onset of symptoms to initiation of thrombolytic therapy could not be demonstrated to be associated with subsequent improvement in LVEF. Important improvement in LV systolic function is not common after thrombolytic therapy for AMI. However, improvement in global and regional systolic function is most related to depressed LVEF and successful thrombolytic therapy. In patients with the most myocardium in jeopardy who have successful coronary reperfusion, one may expect improvement in global and regional ventricular function, but the magnitude of improvement is modest.

Zabel and associates,[104] from Bad Nauheim, Germany, studied 63 consecutive patients undergoing thrombolysis for their first MI and made serial determinations of creatine kinase, its CK-MB isoenzyme, myoglobin, and troponin T to determine their value for noninvasive prediction of coronary artery patency. Blood samples were drawn every 15 minutes during the first 90 minutes, every 30 minutes during the first 4 hours, every 4 hours during the first 24 hours, and every 8 hours during the first 72 hours. The perfusion status of the infarct-related artery was assessed angiographically 90 minutes after initiation of thrombolysis. For each marker, the time to its peak concentration and its earliest initial slope was determined. Areas under receiver operator characteristic curves were determined. The corresponding values for early slopes of disappearance were also measured. Sensitivity, specificity, and positive and negative predictive values regarding noninvasive prediction of coronary artery patency after 90 minutes were 80%, 82%, 95%, and 61% for time to CK maximums; 91%, 77%, 91%, and 77% for time to myoglobin maximums; 87%, 71%, 89%, and 67% for early CK slope; and 94%, 88%, 94%, and 82% for myoglobin slope, respectively. When myoglobin slope was assessed together with other clinical reperfusion markers, including the resolution of chest pain or ST-segment elevation or development of reperfusion arrhythmias by logistic regression analysis, only the myoglobin slope was an independent predictor of coronary artery patency. These data suggest that measurement of myoglobin appears to have advantages over the other markers evaluated because of its earlier rise.

Yamashita and associates,[105] from Kagoshima, Japan, evaluated how early and accurately infarct size can be estimated from serial plasma myoglobin measurements in patients with successful reperfusion. They measured plasma myoglobin and creatine kinase in 35 patients in whom reperfusion therapy was successfully performed. Blood samples were collected at 15-minute intervals for 2 hours after reperfusion, at 30-

minute intervals for the subsequent 2 hours, and at 3 to 6 hour intervals until 52 hours after reperfusion. Plasma myoglobin was measured by a newly developed latex agglutination assay. Total myoglobin and creatine kinase release were calculated with a one-compartment model. The mean chord motion in the most hypokinetic of the infarct-related artery territory was calculated from follow-up ventriculograms as an index of the severity of regional hypokinesis. There were significant correlations between total myoglobin and total creatine kinase and the severity of regional hypokinesis. The time required for cumulative myoglobin release to reach a plateau was 64 ± 28 minutes. An additional 53 minutes was required to calculate the disappearance rate constant of myoglobin and 15 minutes was necessary for the assay. Therefore, the total time required for calculating peak myoglobin was 132 ± 40 minutes, significantly shorter than the time required to calculate peak creatine kinase concentration. Infarct size could be estimated from the total myoglobin release in 34 of 35 patients within four hours of reperfusion. Thus, infarct size may be estimated four hours after reperfusion by calculating the peak myoglobin release in patients with successful reperfusion.

Scant data are available concerning the application and results of exercise thallium-201 scintigraphy after AMI treated with thrombolytic therapy. The goals in a study by Haber and associates,[106] from Charlottesville, Va, were to determine the ability of exercise thallium-201 scintigraphy to detect inducible ischemia and to identify multi-vessel CAD in 88 consecutive post-AMI patients who received thrombolytic therapy and underwent both predischarge noninvasive testing and coronary angiography. Exercise-induced thallium-201 redistribution on quantitative scintigraphy was significantly more prevalent than exercise ST-segment depression (48% v 14%). Sensitivity and specificity of exercise ST depression alone for identification of multi-vessel disease was 29% and 96%, respectively. Sensitivity of a remote thallium-201 defect for multi-vessel CAD detection was 35% and 87%, respectively—not significantly different from values for ST depression alone. When considered as a single variable, the presence of either ST depression or a remote thallium-201 defect was associated with a 58% sensitivity (compared with either ST depression or thallium redistribution alone) but a somewhat diminished specificity of 78%. There was no difference in extent or severity of angiographic CAD in patients with multi-vessel CAD with or without inducible ischemia. These authors concluded that exercise thallium-201 imaging is more sensitive than exercise ST depression for detection of residual ischemia during submaximal exercise in patients who received thrombolytic therapy for AMI. The combination of the presence of either thallium-201 redistribution or ischemic ST depression was better than either variable alone for identifying patients with multi-vessel CAD.

In an investigation by Crea and associates,[107] from London, England, to establish whether abnormal function of small coronary vessels might limit the advantages of thrombolytic treatment, coronary flow reserve in the infarct-related artery was measured in nine patients with AMI early after successful coronary thrombolysis by using a Doppler catheter and intracoronary adenosine infusion. In each patient, coronary flow reserve was calculated as the ratio between coronary blood flow velocity during the highest tolerated intracoronary dose of adenosine (0.6 mg/min in five patients and 1 mg/min in four patients) and baseline velocity. Coronary flow reserve ranged from 1 to 3 (mean, 2 ± 0.7). No correlation was found between coronary flow reserve and the interval between pain onset and administration of the thrombolytic treatment, which ranged between 2.2 and 6 hours (mean, 4.2 ± 1.4 hours). Thus, in patients with AMI, coronary flow reserve early after successful thrombolysis is strikingly variable and may be extremely low despite widely patent epicardial coronary arteries. This restriction of coronary blood flow, probably caused by abnormal function of small coronary vessels, might limit the potential benefit from successful coronary thrombolysis.

In an investigation by Picard and associates,[108] from Boston, to evaluate the influence of thrombolytic therapy on the natural history of LV size and regional function after AMI, 32 patients treated with acute thrombolytic therapy (treatment group) were studied by echocardiography on admission to the hospital and at 1 week, 3 months, and 1 year after AMI; they were compared with 40 patients who did not receive acute intervention (control group). The endocardial surface area index (cm^2/m^2) and the area of abnormal wall motion (cm^2) were calculated from LV dimensions and measurements of abnormal wall motion. Although no differences in the endocardial surface area index were noted over the year for the groups as a whole, a significant difference was noted in treated anterior infarctions with early functional infarct expansion compared with untreated infarct expansion: treatment group, 86 ± 2.0 cm^2/m^2 (entry) to 77 ± 2.7 cm^2/m^2 (1 week) to 70 ± 4.2 cm^2/m^2 (3 months) to 67 ± 6.4 cm^2/m^2 (1 year) versus control group, 84 ± 6.4 cm^2/m^2 (entry) to 84 ± 8.5 cm^2/m^2 (1 week) to 96 ± 8.6 cm^2/m^2 (3 months) to 82 ± 4.2 cm^2/m^2 (1 year). When early expansion was present, those receiving thrombolysis exhibited a consistent decrease in the initially enlarged endocardial surface area in contrast to control patients, who demonstrated continued increases in endocardial surface area during the first 3 months. In all groups, a decrease in the area of abnormal wall motion was observed during the year of follow-up. However, the magnitude and timing of the improvement was accelerated in the treatment group. Thus, acute thrombolytic therapy alters the natural history of LV size and function with a more rapid recovery of abnormal endocardial segments and reversal of functional infarct expansion.

To evaluate noninvasive markers for determining the reperfusion status without coronary angiography or serial blood sampling in patients with AMI, Abe and associates,[109] from Tokyo, Japan, examined two markers: serum myoglobin level and serum myoglobin/creatine kinase ratio. Before emergency coronary angiography, a blood sample was drawn from 72 AMI patients within six hours after the onset of AMI. Coronary angiography revealed Thrombolysis in Myocardial Infarction grades 0 to 1 in 56 patients and Thrombolysis in Myocardial Infarction grades 2 to 3 in 16 patients (spontaneous reperfusion). No patients had received thrombolytic therapy before admission. Thrombolysis in Myocardial Infarction grade 0 to 1 patients were characterized with lower myoglobin levels than Thrombolysis in Myocardial Infarction grade 2 to 3 patients at admission (346 ± 476 v 1558 ± 2005). Furthermore, the mean myoglobin/creatine kinase ratio in Thrombolysis in Myocardial Infarction grade 2 to 3 patients, who had already achieved the reperfusion at admission, was significantly higher than that in patients with Thrombolysis in Myocardial Infarction grade 0 to 1 patients (6.5 ± 3.9 v 2.1 ± 1.8). When myoglobin/creatine kinase ratio >5.0 was assumed to indicate sufficient reperfusion at admission, the sensitivity, specificity, and accuracy evaluating the reperfusion status were 75%, 96%, and 92%, respectively. It can be concluded that the reperfusion status can be predicted satisfactorily by a single blood sample obtained at the time of admission without coronary angiography.

Smart and associates[110] determined whether dobutamine-responsive wall motion accurately detects reversible postischemic dysfunction in patients with AMI. Dobutamine echocardiography was performed within seven days of thrombolytic therapy. Resting echocardiography was repeated ≥4 weeks after AMI and reversible dysfunction defined as improved wall motion. The accuracy of dobutamine-responsive wall motion was compared with that of early signs of reperfusion, non-Q-wave MI, and peak creatine kinase. Sixty-three patients underwent dobutamine echocardiography without complications. Follow-up echocardiograms were obtained in 51 patients (81%) and wall motion improved in 22 patients (41%). Dobutamine-responsive wall motion during all stages of dobutamine echocardiography was specific for reversible dysfunction (90% to 93%) but sensitive (86%) only when hemodynamics were not altered. Non-Q-wave AMI and a low peak CK were also specific (89% to 93%) but less sensitive. Signs of early reperfusion did not identify postischemic dysfunction. Low-dose dobutamine-responsive wall motion and non-Q-wave AMI independently identified reversible dysfunction, but only dobutamine-responsive wall motion was sensitive to all infarct locations. Non-Q-wave AMI was sensitive only in anterior infarcts. Therefore, multistage dobutamine echocardiography can be performed safely early after thrombolytic therapy. Low-dose dobutamine-responsive wall motion accurately detected reversible dysfunction in all infarct locations. Dobutamine-responsive wall motion and non-Q-wave AMI may be useful for accurately identifying reversible dysfunction after thrombolytic therapy for AMI.

Hirai and associates,[111] from Toyama, Japan, studied the effects of myocardial ischemic preconditioning and preexistent collateral circulation on the preservation of LV function in 30 patients who had successful intracoronary thrombolysis within six hours after the onset of a first anterior AMI. The existence of ischemic preconditioning was defined as the episode of recurrent ischemic chest pain within four hours before the onset of AMI. In 16 patients with ischemic preconditioning (group A), the LVEF during the convalescence of myocardial infarction was 57% ± 11%; regional wall motion in the infarct area was 13% ± 9%. In 14 patients without ischemic preconditioning (group B), the LVEF and regional wall motion in the infarct area were 46% ± 9% and 5% ± 9%, respectively. Moreover, among group A patients, 7 patients having a well-developed collateral circulation during the acute stage of myocardial infarction showed a more prominent improvement in regional wall motion in the infarct area compared with 9 patients having poor or no collateral circulation (18% ± 8% v 9% ± 7%). These data indicate that ischemic preconditioning is effective for the preservation of LV function in patients with successful intracoronary thrombolysis and that preexistent coronary collateral circulation potentiates this favorable effect of ischemic preconditioning.

Within four hours from the onset of symptoms in 61 patients with AMI and intravenous thrombolysis, ST-segment elevation and creatine phosphokinase were measured every 15 minutes in an investigation by

Dissmann and associates,[112] from Berlin, Germany. Because of a premature enzyme rise, 42 patients (69%) were reperfused early (group 1). Immediately following reperfusion, 8 of them (13%, group 1a) showed a marked increase of the ST elevation, in 6 of whom it was associated with clearly intensified chest pain. These patients exhibited a much steeper enzyme release and developed a larger enzymatic infarct size than patients (group 1b) without an additional transient ST elevation at reperfusion (creatine phosphokinase peak, 5.1 ± 1.6 v 9.8 ± 4.2 hours after the start of thrombolysis). At angiography 11 days later, LV function was significantly worse in group 1a than in group 1b (EF, 39 ± 14 v 58 ± 11). During intravenous thrombolysis in AMI, some patients showed a marked transient increase of the ST-segment elevation at reperfusion. Their enzyme rise was very rapid, suggesting a special reperfusion pattern. Most of these patients suffer large infarcts.

Stevenson and associates,[113] from London, England, carried out this investigation to evaluate the role of a treadmill stress test for identifying patients at risk of recurrent ischemic events after AMI treated by thrombolysis. The natural history of AMI has changed with the introduction of thrombolytic treatment; there is a lower mortality but a higher incidence of recurrent thrombotic events (reinfarction and unstable angina). The treadmill stress test continues to be recommended for risk stratification after AMI even though its value has never been formally reassessed in the thrombolytic era. A prospective observational study was performed in which 256 consecutive patients who presented with AMI treated by thrombolysis underwent an early treadmill stress test and were followed up for 10 months (range, 6 to 12). Recurrent ischemic events occurred in 41 patients (unstable angina, 15; reinfarction, 21; death, 5) and a further 21 patients required revascularization. Both ST depression at a low workload and low exercise tolerance (<7 metabolic equivalents of the tasks) were predictive of recurrent events. These variables, respectively, identified 50% and 70% of patients who subsequently sustained a recurrent ischemic event, but the corresponding values for positive predictive accuracy were only 26% and 21%. Thus, they are of limited value as a screening measure for identifying patients likely to benefit from invasive investigation and revascularization. None of the other variables (ST elevation, hemodynamic responses, ventricular extrasystoles, and angina) were significantly associated with recurrent ischemic events. These authors concluded that the treadmill stress test is of limited value for identifying patients at risk of recurrent ischemic events after AMI treated by thrombolysis.

Hirayama and associates,[114] from Osaka, Japan, studied 89 patients with an initial anterior AMI in whom reperfusion was successful in 69 patients to evaluate the impact of reperfusion on progressive dilatation of the LV. These 69 patients were divided into three groups according to the time required to achieve reperfusion at the onset of symptoms: early-reperfused (<3 hours from the onset of reperfusion, n = 22); intermediate-reperfused (3 to 6 hours from onset to reperfusion, n = 28); and late-reperfused (>6 hours from the onset to reperfusion, n = 19). The 20 patients whose infarct-related artery was occluded in the acute phase as well as 1 month later were classified as nonreperfused. Infarct size, evaluated as defect volume by thallium-201 single-photon emission computed tomography 1 month after the event, was 1,593 ± 652 units in the late-reperfused group, which was significantly larger than in the intermediate-reperfused (1,066 ± 546 U) or early-reperfused groups (372 ± 453 U) but not different from the nonreperfused group. The abnormalities in wall motion as well as in global LVEF evaluated by left ventriculography 1 month after the event showed that late perfusion did not preserve LV wall motion and LVEF. Earlier reperfusion decreased the size of the infarction and preserved LV function, whereas late reperfusion (>6 hours after onset) did not limit infarct size or preserve LVEF. The LV end-diastolic volumes did not differ significantly among the early-reperfused, intermediate-reperfused, and late-reperfused groups. All of these LV end-diastolic volumes were significantly smaller than in the nonreperfused group. LV hemodynamic data obtained in both acute and chronic phases in 39 patients showed that LV volumes increased significantly during the course of MI only in the nonreperfused group. Therefore, late reperfusion prevents ventricular dilatation following AMI independent of the limitation of infarct size.

Streptokinase

There are differences in the risk factor profile and coronary anatomy of young patients who develop CAD compared with those of older patients. There is an absence of data in published reports regarding the response to thrombolytic therapy and the outcome of AMI in young patients. Chouhan and associates,[115] from Doha, Qatar, compared 62 patients aged <35 years (group 1) with 58 patients aged >55 years (group 2) who presented with AMI and were treated with intravenous streptokinase. Group 1 had a significantly higher incidence of smoking and a lower incidence of diabetes mellitus than did group 2. Fifty-eight patients in group 1 and 40 in group 2 were studied by angiography at a similar time (five to six days) after admission. Patients in group 1 had a better LVEF (55% v 49%) but similar patency rates of the infarct vessel compared with those of group 2. Group 1 also had a higher incidence of insignificant disease and a lower incidence of three-vessel disease. This suggests that there are differences in the risk factor profiles and coronary anatomy of young patients compared with those of older ones. Despite similar benefits from thrombolytic therapy in the form of a patent infarct vessel, there may be differences in the long-term outcome among these patients.

Neutralization antibodies to streptokinase increase to high levels within several days of administration. It is not known how long these high levels persist. The time course of antibody levels needs to be further characterized owing to the increasing need to readminister thrombolytic therapy and to the possibility that these antibodies may compromise the safety and efficacy of a further dose of streptokinase or streptokinase-containing compounds. Elliott and associates,[116] from Auckland, New Zealand, measured paired streptokinase neutralization titers (in vitro functional assay) and specific antistreptokinase immunoglobulin G antibody levels in 145 patients who received streptokinase between 10 and 48 months previously. Serologic evidence of recent streptococcal infection was also sought. Neutralization titers sufficient to inactivate a conventional dose of 1,500,000 units of streptokinase were still present in 50% of patients at 24 months, 48% at 36 months, and 51% at 48 months after streptokinase administration. Levels of specific antistreptokinase immunoglobulin G antibodies also remained constant over the

1- to 4-year period. Neutralization titers were weakly correlated with specific immunoglobulin G levels. Antistreptolysin titers ≥250 and ≥333 IU/mL were present in 30% and 12% of these patients, respectively. Neutralization titers were not correlated with antistreptolysin titers. Neutralizing antibodies (assessed by an in vitro functional assay) remained high in 51% of patients 4 years after intravenous streptokinase administration. It is not known whether persisting high in vitro neutralization titers affect the efficacy and safety of repeat administration of streptokinase or streptokinase-containing compounds.

Herlitz and associates, [117] from Göteborg, Sweden, described and related to prognosis the occurrence of hypotension during infusion of streptokinase for strongly suspected AMI in one hospital during 1989 to 1990. In 54% of patients, the β-blocker metoprolol was simultaneously administered intravenously. The median systolic BP before infusion was 135 mm Hg, and the median value for the lowest systolic BP recorded during infusion was 100 mg Hg. A positive correlation between systolic BP before streptokinase and the lowest systolic BP during infusion was found. Among patients administered streptokinase and metoprolol, 23% had systolic BP <90 mm Hg, and 12% had <80 mm Hg at any time during infusion; corresponding values for patients administered streptokinase only were 47% and 30%, respectively. Patients with the lowest systolic BP <80 mm Hg during infusion had a mortality during the first 2 weeks of 22% v 11% for those with between 80 and 100 mm Hg, and 8% for those with >100 mm Hg. However, in a multivariate analysis, the systolic BP before infusion rather than the lowest systolic BP during infusion was independently associated with death. Therefore, the investigators concluded that although patients with low systolic BP during streptokinase infusion have a high mortality, the level of systolic BP before infusion is more strongly associated with the outcome. Simultaneous use of intravenous β-blockade does not increase the occurrence of hypotension during streptokinase infusion.

Although a number of studies have shown that the incidence of late potentials is lower after thrombolytic therapy, it is not known whether this is paralleled by fewer arrhythmic events during long-term follow-up. In patients with first AMI, Tobé and associates,[118] from Groningen, The Netherlands, found that filtered QRS duration was significantly shorter when treated with streptokinase (95 ms) than when treated with conventional therapy (99 ms). The low-amplitude signal was shorter after thrombolysis (28 v 33 ms). Terminal root-mean-square voltage did not differ significantly. Irrespective of treatment, late potentials were predictive in the complete group for arrhythmic events during follow-up, but treatment (streptokinase v conventional) did not significantly affect outcome when added to the model. These investigators concluded that thrombolysis prevents the development of late potentials. However, this study does not confirm the hypothesis that prevention of late potentials leads to a decrease in arrhythmic events.

Smokers have been reported to have an improved short-term prognosis after AMI when compared with nonsmokers. Gomez and associates,[119] from Salt Lake City, examined the effect of smoking status on infarct-related artery patency, a determinant of outcome, following thrombolytic therapy for AMI. To evaluate patency outcome by smoking status, the database of the Second Thrombolytic Trial of Eminase in Acute Myocardial Infarction was reviewed, and baseline characteristics were compared with infarct-related artery patency early (90 to 240 minutes) after thrombolysis in smokers versus nonsmokers. Smokers were younger, more likely to be men, normotensive, and more likely to have an inferior AMI and tended to have higher hematocrits and fibrinogen levels than nonsmokers. Smokers had a significantly greater chance of achieving complete perfusion (Thrombolysis in Myocardial Infarction trial grade 3) (66% v 51%) than nonsmokers, although the combination of grades 2 and 3 did not differ (Figure 3-17). After correcting for imbalances in baseline and angiographic variables, multivariate logistic regression identified smoking and infarct location as independent predictors of achieving grade 3 flow. The independent predictive component of smoking for achieving grade 3 patency after thrombolysis suggests the hypothesis that more active thrombogenic mechanisms may be operative in smokers, leading to a larger thrombus component that is more susceptible to lytic therapy.

Montrucchio and associates,[120] from Torino, Italy, evaluated whether streptokinase treatment enhances intravascular activation of platelets limiting the initial response to thrombolytic therapy. Specifically, they determined whether platelet activating factor, and ether lipid mediator with multiple potent biologic activities, is synthesized during therapy with streptokinase. These investigators extracted and quantified platelet activating factor in blood of patients with AMI treated or untreated with streptokinase, and they also determined whether cultured human endothelial cells synthesize platelet activating factor after stimulation with streptokinase or plasmin. Platelet activating factor was extracted from blood samples immediately after acidification to destroy the acid-labile platelet activating factor acetylhydrolase in 25 patients with AMI treated

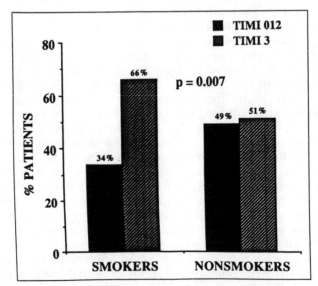

Figure 3-17. Comparison of early (90 to 240 minutes) "complete" Thrombolysis in Myocardial Infarction trial (TIMI) grade 3 infarct-related artery perfusion versus TIMI grade 0, 1, or 2 in smokers and nonsmokers. The proportion of smokers who achieved complete (TIMI grade 3) perfusion was significantly higher than that of nonsmokers (66% v 51%, p = 0.007). Reproduced with permission from Gomez et al.[119]

(n = 14) and untreated (n = 11) with intravenous infusion of streptokinase. Platelet activating factor was detected in 10 of 14 patients treated with streptokinase and in none of the patients untreated with streptokinase. Platelet activating factor was detectable within 60 to 90 minutes after streptokinase infusion and disappeared from the circulation within 120 to 180 minutes. Percent variation of platelet count over basal values correlated negatively with the amount of platelet activating factor present in the circulation at 90 minutes. Cultured human umbilical cord vein-derived endothelial cells synthesized platelet activating factor in a dose-dependent manner in response to streptokinase and plasmin with a synthesis that peaked at 15 minutes and persisted up to 30 minutes for streptokinase and 2 hours for plasmin. Thus, platelet activating factor was detectable in blood of patients treated with streptokinase but not in patients with a comparable infarct not treated with streptokinase, suggesting that streptokinase stimulates the synthesis of this mediator either directly or through plasmin generation. Studies done in cultured endothelial cells, both with streptokinase and plasmin, induce the production of platelet activating factor. Platelet activating factor's production following streptokinase treatment may promote platelet aggregation and vasoconstriction and limit the initial beneficial effect of thrombolytic therapy with this agent.

Recombinant Tissue Plasminogen Activator

Taylor and associates,[121] from Birmingham, Ala, compared clinical and laboratory data, responses to thrombolytic therapy, and clinical outcome in 2,885 patients participating in the Thrombolysis in Myocardial Infarction Phase II (TIMI II) Trial among three groups of patients, including 2,564 whites, 174 blacks, and 147 Hispanics. Differences were found in baseline characteristics among the three groups, including age, sex, and risk factor prevalence. The mean age for whites with myocardial infarction was older (57 years in whites v 55 years in blacks and 53 years in Hispanics), the percentage of women with infarcts was higher for blacks than whites or Hispanics (29% for blacks v 18% for whites v 14% for Hispanics), and the risk factors for frequency of smoking were higher for blacks and Hispanics (62% for blacks, 55% for Hispanics, and 49% for whites). In addition, the frequency of hypertension was higher in blacks (56% in blacks v 37% in whites and 40% in Hispanics) as was the history of diabetes mellitus (22% for blacks, 20% for Hispanics, and 12% for whites). Five hours after the infusion of recombinant tissue plasminogen activator, there was a profound fall in fibrinogen levels in black patients compared to that seen in Hispanics or whites without more frequent infarct-related artery patency or hemorrhagic complications. Mortality rates were similar in whites, blacks, and Hispanics through the first year after adjustment for baseline variables. Thus, the TIMI II database yields evidence suggesting (1) a high prevalence of classic cardiovascular risk factors among minority patients with AMI; (2) a greater decrease in fibrinogen level five hours after the start of tissue plasminogen activator among black as compared to white and Hispanic patients without more frequent infarct-related artery patency or hemorrhage; and (3) thrombolytic therapy with appropriate supplemental measures is associated with comparable 1 year mortality in white, black, and Hispanic patients.

Sometimes malignant arrhythmias have been reported to occur during the reperfusion phase after thrombolytic therapy. Berger and associates,[122] from Bethesda, Md, evaluated the incidence of VT and VF without hypotension or heart failure after rt-PA in patients in the TIMI II Trial. They analyzed 2,546 patients without CHF or hypotension during the first 24 hours after study entry. Of these patients, 1.9% developed sustained VT or VF within 24 hours of study entry and 98.1% did not. In the group 2 patients who did not have a serious arrhythmia, there was an 87% patency of the infarct-related artery 18 to 48 hours after thrombolysis. This was actually greater than in the group with arrhythmias (68%). For patients surviving to 21 days, there was no difference in mortality between the two groups of patients. These authors concluded that VT and VF are not markers for reperfusion after thrombolytic therapy.

To assess the effects of reperfusion therapy on acute RV AMI, Kalan and associates,[123] from Bethesda, Md, and Boston, Mass, studied at necropsy the hearts from 51 patients who died after receiving intravenous recombinant tissue plasminogen activator for acute LV AMI as part of the Thrombolysis in Myocardial Infarction (TIMI) study. RV infarction occurred in none of 29 patients with infarction of the anterior wall of the LV and in 8 of 22 patients (36%) with infarction of the posterior (inferior) wall of the LV. Of the 22 patients with posterior wall infarction, the 8 patients with RV infarction were compared with the 14 patients without RV infarction. The patients with RV infarction had a longer mean interval from tissue plasminogen activator infusion to peak creatine phosphokinase level (19 v 11 hours), a lower frequency of hemorrhagic necrosis (2 of 8 v 10 of 14), and higher frequency of liminal thrombus in the infarct-related coronary artery (6 of 8 v 3 of 14). Each of these findings is associated with the absence of coronary reperfusion. Thus, successful reperfusion following LV AMI appears to be associated with a decreased frequency of concomitant RV AMI.

Alteplase or Anistreplase

Anderson and associates,[124] from Salt Lake City, evaluated the functional significance of the Thrombolysis in Myocardial Infarction study group (TIMI) perfusion grades in 298 patients treated with anistreplase or alteplase within four hours of MI symptom onset. Using the grading scheme developed by the TIMI investigators, grade 0 is no obvious distal flow in the infarct-related artery; grade 1 perfusion is minimal flow in the distal part of the infarct-related artery; grade 2 is partial perfusion; and grade 3 is complete perfusion to the distal part of the infarct-related coronary artery. Investigators compared one-day coronary patency status with ventriculographic, enzymatic, and ECG indexes of AMI in patients treated within four hours of symptom onset and evaluated LVEF by radionuclide ventriculography at 1 week and at 1 month. Perfusion grades for the entire study population were distributed as grade 0/1 in 12% of patients, grade 2 in 13% of patients, and grade 3 in 74% of patients. Patency profile did not differ between the two thrombolytic regimens. Further coronary interventions were performed after the one-day patency determination in 43% of patients. The clinical outcome in patients with grade 2 perfusion did not differ from grade 0/1 perfusion as regards LVEFs, enzyme peaks, ECG markers, or other morbidity indicators. However, patients with grade 3 perfusion demonstrated a greater global LVEF at 1 week (54% v 49% for patients with 0 to 2 perfusion) and at 1 month (54% v 49%). They also demonstrated a greater infarct zone EF at 1 week and at 1 month, smaller enzyme peaks, and a trend toward lower morbidity index. Thus, the degree of coronary artery perfusion following thrombolytic therapy is a key variable as regards subsequent improvement in ventricular function.

The effect of late thrombolysis in AMI (ie, treatment beginning more than 6 hours after the onset of symptoms) remains controversial. The Late Assessment of Thrombolytic Efficacy (LATE) study[125] is a large randomized trial designed to resolve this question. A total of 5,711 patients with symptoms and electrocardiographic criteria consistent with AMI were randomized double-blind to intravenous alteplase (100 mg over 3 hours) or matching placebo, between 6 and 24 hours from symptom onset. Both groups received immediate oral aspirin and for later recruits, intravenous heparin for 48 hours was recommended. All patients were followed up for at least 6 months, and 73% were followed up for 1 year. Intention-to-treat analysis of survival revealed a nonsignificant reduction in the alteplase group (397/2,836 deaths) compared with placebo (444/2,857). Thirty-five day mortality was 8.86% and 10.31%, respectively, a relative reduction of 14.1%. Prespecified survival analysis according to treatment within 12 hours of symptom onset, however, showed a significant reduction in mortality in favor of alteplase: 35-day mortality was 8.9% v 11.9% for placebo, a relative reduction of 25.6%. Rates were 8.7% and 9.2%, respectively, for those treated at 12 to 24 hours, but subgroup analysis suggests that some patients may benefit even when treated after 12 hours. Although treatment with alteplase resulted in an excess of hemorrhagic strokes, by 6 months the number of disabled survivors was the same in both treatment groups and other clinical events were observed with similar frequency in the two groups. These authors concluded that the time window for thrombolysis with alteplase should be extended to at least 12 hours from symptom onset in patients with AMI.

Recombinant Staphylokinase

Collen and Van de Werf,[126] from Leuven, Belgium, determined the ability of staphylokinase, a protein with known profibrinolytic properties produced by staphylococcus aureus strains, to result in thrombolysis in humans with AMI. Ten milligrams of staphylokinase given intravenously over 30 minutes caused coronary artery thrombolysis within 40 minutes in four of five patients with AMI. Plasma fibrinogen and α_2-antiplasmin levels were not affected. Postinfusion disappearance of staphylokinase antigen followed a biphasic clearance. Neutralizing antibodies against staphylokinase were not demonstrated at baseline and for 6 days after infusion, but staphylokinase neutralizing antibodies cross-reacting with streptokinase were consistently demonstrable in plasma at 14 to 35 days. Therefore, staphylokinase may induce clot-selective coronary thrombolysis in patients with evolving AMI without concomitant induction of a systemic lytic state. Staphylokinase, a small protein that can be easily produced by recombinant DNA technology, may offer promise for thrombolytic therapy in patients with coronary thrombosis.

Streptokinase + Subcutaneous Heparin v Streptokinase + Intravenous Heparin v Tissue Plasminogen Activator + Intravenous Heparin v Streptokinase + Tissue Plasminogen Activator + Intravenous Heparin

The relative efficacy of streptokinase and tissue plasminogen activator (TPA) and the roles of intravenous as compared with subcutaneous heparin as adjunctive therapy in AMI are unresolved questions. The GUSTO (Global Utilization of Streptokinase and Tissue Plasminogen Activator for Occluded Coronary Arteries) Investigators[127] compared new, aggressive thrombolytic strategies with standard thrombolytic regimens in the treatment of AMI. The hypothesis of the GUSTO Investigators was that newer thrombolytic strategies would produce earlier and sustained reperfusion and therefore improve survival. In 15 countries and 1,081 hospitals, 41,021 patients with evolving AMI were randomly assigned to four different thrombolytic strategies, consisting of the use of streptokinase and subcutaneous heparin, streptokinase and intravenous heparin, accelerated tissue plasminogen activator (t-PA) and intravenous heparin, or a combination of streptokinase plus t-PA with intravenous heparin. ("Accelerated" refers to the administration of t-PA over a period of 90 minutes—with two thirds of the dose given in the first 30 minutes—rather than the conventional period of 3 hours.) The primary endpoint was 30-day mortality. The mortality rates in the four treatment groups were as follows: streptokinase and subcutaneous heparin, 7.2%; streptokinase and intravenous heparin, 7.4%; accelerated t-PA and intravenous heparin, 6.3%; and the combination of both thrombolytic agents with intravenous heparin, 7.0% (Table 3-15). This represented a 14% reduction in mortality for accelerated t-PA as compared with the two streptokinase-only strategies. The rates of hemorrhagic stroke were 0.49%, 0.54%, 0.72%, and 0.94% in the four groups, respectively, which represented a significant excess of hemorrhagic strokes for accelerated t-PA and for the combination strategy, as compared with streptokinase only (Figure 3-18). A combined endpoint of death or disabling stroke was significantly lower in the accelerated t-PA group than in the streptokinase only groups (6.9% v 7.8%). The findings of this large-scale trial indicate

Table 3-15. Major Clinical Outcomes. Reproduced with permission from the GUSTO Investigators.[127]

Outcome	Streptokinase and Subcutaneous Heparin (N = 9796)	Streptokinase and Intravenous Heparin (N = 10,377)	Accelerated t-PA and Intravenous Heparin (N = 10,344)	Both Thrombolytic Agents and Intravenous Heparin (N = 10,328)	P Value, Accelerated t-PA vs. Both Streptokinase Groups
	percent of patients				
24-hr mortality	2.8	2.9	2.3	2.8	0.005
30-day mortality	7.2	7.4	6.3	7.0	0.001
Or nonfatal stroke	7.9	8.2	7.2	7.9	0.006
Or nonfatal hemorrhagic stroke	7.4	7.6	6.6	7.4	0.004
Or nonfatal disabling stroke	7.7	7.9	6.9	7.6	0.006

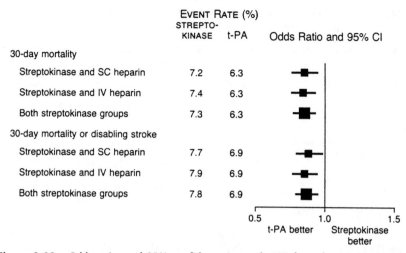

Figure 3-18. Odds ratios and 95% confidence intervals (CI) for reduction in mortality and net benefit, defined as reduction in mortality and disabling stroke, in the group assigned to accelerated t-PA as compared with the streptokinase groups. Reproduced with permission from The GUSTO Investigators.[127]

that accelerated t-PA given with intravenous heparin provides a survival benefit over previous standard thrombolytic regimes.

Although it is known that thrombolytic therapy improves survival after AMI, it has been debated whether the speed with which coronary-artery patency is restored after the initiation of therapy further affects outcome. To study this question, the GUSTO Angiographic Investigators,[128] chaired by Allen M. Ross, randomly assigned 2,431 patients to one of four treatment strategies for reperfusion: streptokinase with subcutaneous heparin; streptokinase with intravenous heparin; accelerated-dose tissue plasminogen activator (t-PA) with intravenous heparin; or a combination of both activators plus intravenous heparin. Patients were also randomly assigned to cardiac angiography at one of four times after the initiation of thrombolytic therapy: 90 minutes, 180 minutes, 24 hours, or 5 to 7 days. The group that underwent angiography at 90 minutes underwent it again after 5 to 7 days. The rate of patency of the infarct-related artery at 90 minutes was highest in the group given accelerated-dose t-PA and heparin (81%), as compared with the group given streptokinase and subcutaneous heparin (54%), the group given streptokinase and intravenous heparin (60%), and the group given combination therapy (73%) (Table 3-16). Flow through the infarct-related artery at 90 minutes was normal in 54% of the group given t-PA and heparin but in less than 40% of the three other groups. By 180 minutes, the patency rates were the same in the four treatment groups. Reocclusion was infrequent and was similar in all four groups (range, 4.9% to 6.4%). Measures of LV function paralleled the rate of patency at 90 minutes; ventricular function was best in the group given t-PA with heparin and in patients with normal flow through the infarct-related artery irrespective of treatment group (Table 3-17). Mortality at 30 days was lowest (4.4%) among patients with normal coronary flow at 90 minutes and highest (8.9%) among patients with no flow. This study supports the hy-

Table 3-16. Patency and Reocclusion of the Infarct-Related Artery, According to Treatment Group. Reproduced with permission from the GUSTO Angiographic Investigators.[128]

VARIABLE	STREPTO-KINASE + SC HEPARIN	STREPTO-KINASE + IV HEPARIN	ACCELERATED t-PA	t-PA + STREPTO-KINASE
	patients with feature/patients examined (%)			
Patency				
Open vessels, TIMI grades 2 and 3 combined				
At 90 min	159/293 (54)	170/283 (60)	236/292 (81)*†	218/299 (73)†
At 180 min	77/106 (73)	72/97 (74)	71/93 (76)	77/91 (85)
At 24 hr	64/83 (77)	74/92 (80)	89/104 (86)	87/93 (94)‡
At 5–7 days	67/93 (72)	81/96 (84)	70/83 (84)§	71/89 (80)
Complete reperfusion, TIMI grade 3				
At 90 min	85/293 (29)	91/283 (32)	157/292 (54)†¶	114/299 (38)
At 180 min	37/106 (35)	40/97 (41)	40/93 (43)	48/91 (53)
At 24 hr	42/83 (51)	38/92 (41)	47/104 (45)	56/93 (60)
At 5–7 days	47/93 (51)	56/96 (58)	48/83 (58)	49/89 (55)
Reocclusion				
From TIMI grade 2 at 90 min to grade 0 or 1 at follow-up	3/56 (5.4)	6/58 (10.3)	2/64 (3.1)	4/72 (5.6)
From TIMI grade 3 at 90 min to grade 0 or 1 at follow-up	4/54 (7.4)	1/69 (1.4)	9/121 (7.4)	4/92 (4.3)
Overall reocclusion	7/110 (6.4)	7/127 (5.5)	11/185 (5.9)	8/164 (4.9)

*P = 0.032 for the comparison of this group with the group given t-PA with streptokinase.

†P<0.001 for the comparison of this group with the groups given streptokinase with subcutaneous or intravenous heparin.

‡P<0.001 for the comparison of this group with the group given streptokinase with subcutaneous heparin.

§P = 0.032 for the comparison of this group with the group given streptokinase with subcutaneous heparin.

¶P<0.001 for the comparison of this group with the group given t-PA with streptokinase.

pothesis that more rapid and complete restoration of coronary flow through the infarct-related artery results in improved ventricular performance and lower mortality among patients with AMI. This would appear to be the mechanism by which accelerated t-PA therapy produced the most favorable outcome in the GUSTO trial.

Aspirin, Heparin, or Warfarin Afterwards

Meijer and associates,[129] from The Netherlands, studied the effects of three antithrombotic regimens on the angiographic and clinical courses after successful thrombolysis. Patients were treated with intravenous thrombolytic therapy followed by intravenous heparin when a patent infarct-related artery was demonstrated at angiography <48 hours later. Three hundred patients were randomized to either 325 mg aspirin daily or placebo with discontinuation of heparin or to Warfarin with continuation of heparin until oral anticoagulation was established. After 3 months, in which conservative treatment was intended, vessel patency and ventricular function were reassessed in 248 patients. Reocclusion rates were not significantly different, 25% with aspirin, 30% with Warfarin, and 32% with placebo. Reinfarction was seen in 3% of patients on aspirin, in 8% on Warfarin, and in 11% on placebo. Revascularization rates were 6% with aspirin, 13% with Warfarin, and 16% with placebo.

Table 3-17. Left Ventricular Function, According to Group. Reproduced with permission from the GUSTO Angiographic Investigators.[128]

Variable	Strepto-kinase + SC Heparin	Strepto-kinase + IV Heparin	Accelerated t-PA	t-PA + Strepto-kinase
At 90 min	**N = 242**	**N = 231**	**N = 246**	**N = 248**
Ejection fraction (%)	58±15	57±15	59±15	58±15
ESVI (ml/m²)	28±15	30±17	27±16†	29±16
Wall motion (SD/ chord)	−2.5±1.5	−2.7±1.4‡	−2.4±1.4‡	−2.4±1.5
Abnormal chords (no.)	23±17	25±18	21±19§¶	24±19
Preserved RWM (% of group)	18	19	29¶‖	21
At 5–7 days	**N = 186**	**N = 171**	**N = 197**	**N = 179**
Ejection fraction (%)	57±14	58±14	59±14	58±16
ESVI (ml/m²)	31±14	29±15	28±13	30±16
Wall motion (SD/ chord)	−2.4±1.4	−2.1±1.5**	−2.0±1.5††	−2.2±1.6
Abnormal chords (no.)	21±17	20±19	17±16‡‡	21±19
Preserved RWM (% of group)	21	34§§	31	30

*Plus–minus values are means ±SD. ESVI denotes end-systolic volume index, and RWM regional wall motion. Wall motion is expressed as the mean magnitude of depressed infarct-zone chords; wall motion was considered preserved if all infarct-zone chords were normal. Chords in the infarct zone were considered abnormal if they were more than 2 SD below the norm.

†P = 0.037 for the comparison of this group with the group given streptokinase with intravenous heparin.

‡P = 0.018 for the comparison of this group with the groups given streptokinase with subcutaneous or intravenous heparin.

§P = 0.027 for the comparison of this group with the groups given streptokinase with subcutaneous or intravenous heparin.

¶P = 0.035 for the comparison of this group with the group given t-PA with streptokinase.

‖P<0.001 for the comparison of this group with the groups given streptokinase with intravenous or subcutaneous heparin.

**P = 0.014 for the comparison of this group with the group given streptokinase with subcutaneous heparin.

††P = 0.05 for the comparison of this group with the group given streptokinase with subcutaneous heparin.

‡‡P = 0.05 for the comparison of this group with the group given streptokinase with intravenous or subcutaneous heparin.

§§P = 0.006 for the comparison of this group with the groups given streptokinase with subcutaneous heparin.

Mortality was 2% and did not differ between groups. An event-free clinical course was found in 93% of patients with aspirin, in 82% with Warfarin, and in 76% with placebo (Figure 3-19). An event-free course without reocclusion occurred in 73% of patients with aspirin, in 63% with Warfarin, and in 59% with placebo. An increase in LVEF was only found in the aspirin group. Therefore, at 3 months after successful thrombolysis, reocclusion occurs in about 30% of patients regardless of the use of antithrombotics. Compared with placebo, aspirin significantly reduces reinfarction rate and revascularization and reduces the risk of

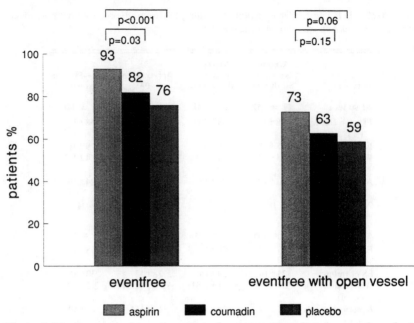

Figure 3-19. Bar graph shows proportion of patients with a clinical course free of reinfarction, revascularization, and death in the three treatment groups after 3 months of follow-up (left-hand side of the panel) and the proportion of patients with a clinical course both without events and without reocclusion who had follow-up coronary angiography (panel on the right). Reproduced with permission from Meijer et al.[129]

future events while better preserving LVEF. The efficacy of Coumadin appears less than that of aspirin but better than placebo.

Intracranial Hemorrhage

Thrombolytic therapy improves outcome in patients with AMI but is associated with an increased risk of intracranial hemorrhage. For some patients, this risk may outweigh the potential benefits of thrombolytic treatment. Using data from other studies, Simoons and associates,[130] from Rotterdam, The Netherlands, developed a model for the assessment of an individual's risk of intracranial hemorrhage during thrombolysis. Data were available from 150 patients with documented intracranial hemorrhage and 294 matched controls. Forty-nine patients with intracranial hemorrhage and 122 controls had been treated with streptokinase, whereas 88 cases and 148 controls had received alteplase. By multivariate analysis, four factors were identified as independent predictors of intracranial hemorrhage: age over 65 years (odds ratio, 2.2), body weight below 70 kg (2.1), hypertension on hospital admission (2.0), and administration of alteplase (1.6). If the overall incidence of intracranial hemorrhage is assumed to be 0.75%, patients without risk factors who receive streptokinase have a 0.26% probability of intracranial hemorrhage. The risk was 0.96%, 1.32%, and 2.17% in patients with one, two, or three risk factors, respectively. The authors present a model for individual risk assessment that can be used easily in clinical practice.

Effects of Angioplasty Afterwards

Predischarge supine bicycle ergometry was used by Chaitman and associates,[131] in Baltimore, to assess persistent myocardial ischemia in post-AMI patients who received thrombolytic therapy and were randomized to an invasive versus conservative strategy in the Thrombolysis in Myocardial Infarction (TIMI) II Trial. The frequency of ischemic responses in both strategies and the l-year prognostic importance of the different exercise test outcomes were examined. At 14 days, the percentage of patients with any adverse outcome (including death, presence of exercise-induced ST-segment depression, or inability to perform the exercise test) was 34% of 1,681 randomly assigned to the invasive strategy compared with 35% of 1,658 randomly assigned to the conservative strategy. The l-year mortality was greater in patients who did not perform the predischarge exercise test (8%) than in those who did (2%); the former were older, were a greater proportion of women, had a more frequent history of AMI, and had more extensive CAD. The l-year mortality in patients with exercise-induced ST-segment depression or chest pain was only 1% among those randomly assigned to the conservative strategy where coronary angiography and revascularization were recommended if the test result was abnormal. Among patients randomly assigned to the invasive strategy, exercise-induced ST-segment depression or chest pain was associated with a 1-year mortality of 3%. Thus, in post-AMI patients treated with thrombolytic therapy and a conservative strategy, the recommendation of performing cardiac catheterization and coronary revascularization when the predischarge exercise test is abnormal results in a low l-year mortality for those with exercise-induced angina or ST-segment depression, which is comparable with that for patients who do not have these findings.

In the previously published TIMI II Trial, patients were randomly assigned to an invasive (1,681 patients) or a conservative (1,658 patients) management strategy after receiving thrombolytic therapy for AMI. Terrin and associates,[132] from Baltimore, reported the survival and reinfarction rates for two- and three-year follow-up in the TIMI II clinical trial. Cumulative life-table death rates of death or reinfarction were 17.6% for the invasive strategy group and 17.9% for the conservative strategy group at the end of two years. At the end of three years, the rates of death or reinfarction were 21.0% for the invasive strategy group and 20.0% for the conservative strategy group. These authors concluded that invasive and conservative strategies resulted in similar favorable outcomes after 2 and 3 years. Mortality and reinfarction rates in the two strategies were comparable.

Thrombolysis v Angioplasty

The success of thrombolytic therapy for AMI is limited by bleeding complications, the impossibility of reperfusing all occluded coronary arteries, recurrent AMI, and the relatively small number of patients who are appropriate candidates for this therapy. Grines and associates,[133] for the Primary Angioplasty in Myocardial Infarction Study Group, hypothesized that these problems could be overcome by the use of immediate percutaneous transluminal coronary angioplasty (PTCA), without previous thrombolytic therapy. At 12 clinical centers, 395 patients who presented within 12 hours of the onset of AMI were treated with intravenous heparin and aspirin and then randomly assigned to undergo immediate PTCA (without previous thrombolytic therapy, 195 patients) or to receive intravenous tissue plasminogen activator (t-PA, 200 patients) followed by conservative care. Radionuclide ventriculography was performed to assess ventricular function within 24 hours and at 6 weeks. Among the patients randomly assigned to PTCA, 90% underwent the procedure; the success rate was 97%, and no patient required emergency CABG. The inhospital mortality rates in the t-PA and PTCA groups were 6.5% and 2.6%, respectively. In a post hoc analysis, the mortality rates in the subgroups classified as "not low risk" were 10.4% and 2.0%, respectively. Reinfarction or death in the hospital occurred in 12% of the patients treated with t-PA and in 5% of those treated with PTCA. Intracranial bleeding occurred more frequently among patients who received t-PA than among those who underwent PTCA (2% v 0%). The mean EF at rest (53% ± 13% v 53% ± 13%) and during exercise (56% ± 13% v 56% ± 14%) were similar in the t-PA and PTCA groups at 6 weeks. By 6 months, reinfarction or death had occurred in 32 patients who received t-PA (16.8%) and 16 treated with PTCA (8.5%). As compared with t-PA therapy for AMI, immediate PTCA reduced the combined occurrence of nonfatal reinfarction or death, was associated with a lower rate of intracranial hemorrhage, and resulted in similar LV systolic function.

Despite the widespread use of intravenous thrombolytic therapy and of immediate PTCA for the treatment of AMI, randomized comparison of the two approaches to reperfusion are lacking. Zijlstra and associates,[134] from Leiden, The Netherlands, reported the results of a prospective, randomized trial comparing immediate PTCA (without previous thrombolytic therapy) with intravenous streptokinase treatment. A total of 142 patients with AMI were randomly assigned to receive one of the two treatments. The LVEF was measured by radionuclide scanning before hospital discharge. Quantitative PTCA was performed to assess the degree of residual stenosis in the infarct-related arteries. A total of 72 patients were assigned to receive streptokinase and 70 patients to undergo immediate angioplasty. Angioplasty was technically successful in 64 of the 65 patients who underwent the procedure. Infarction recurred in 9 patients assigned to receive streptokinase but in none of those assigned to receive angioplasty. Fourteen patients in the streptokinase group had unstable angina after their AMI but only 4 in the angioplasty group. The mean LVEF as measured before discharge was 45% ± 12% in the streptokinase group and 51% ± 11% in the angioplasty group. The infarct-related artery was patent in 68% of the patients in the streptokinase group and 91% of those in the angioplasty group. Quantitative PTCA revealed stenosis of 36% ± 20% of the luminal diameter in the angioplasty group, as compared with 76% ± 19% in the streptokinase group. Immediate angioplasty after AMI was associated with a higher rate of patency of the infarct-related artery, a less severe residual stenotic lesion, better LV function, and less recurrent AMI and infarction than was intravenous streptokinase.

Maynard and associates,[135] from Seattle, Wash, conducted a study in 19 hospitals in the metropolitan Seattle area that included 6,270 unselected patients who had AMI between January 1988 and April 1991. Hospital mortality was determined and related to patient demographic and clinical characteristics, the use of reperfusion therapies, and compli-

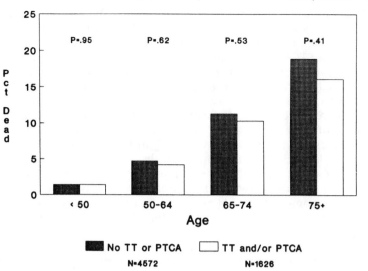

Figure 3-20. In-hospital mortality by age for patients treated with direct angioplasty or thrombolytic therapy (TT), or both, < 6 hours from onset of symptoms versus those not so treated. Pct = percent; PTCA = direct percutaneous transluminal coronary angioplasty. Reproduced with permission from Maynard et al.[135]

cations after AMI. Thrombolytic therapy or direct PTCA <6 hours from symptom onset was used to treat 1,185 patients (19%) and 524 patients (9%), respectively (Figure 3-20). There were 629 (10%) hospital deaths; most occurred during the first three days of hospitalization. Factors affecting mortality after admission included recurrent chest pain, recurrent AMI, development of CHF, and the occurrence of stroke. After adjustment for age, treatment with thrombolytic therapy or direct PTCA had no independent effect on reducing the overall mortality rate. Hospital mortality rates for AMI have improved considerably since 1970, although recurrent myocardial ischemic events continue to have an adverse effect on outcome. The current use of reperfusion treatments has had minimal causal impact on overall mortality rates, principally because less than one third of patients, who are relatively "low risk," are eligible and receive these treatments.

DIRECT ANGIOPLASTY

Patients with AMI and contraindication to thrombolysis have a high mortality and morbidity with conventional medical treatment. Himbert and associates,[136] from Paris, studied 226 consecutive patients hospitalized within six hours of the onset of Q-wave AMI, and 45 (20%) had contraindications to thrombolysis. All 45 were treated by emergent primary PTCA. Mean age of the 45 patients was 60 years and 8 patients (18%) were ≥70 years old. Seventeen patients (38%) had multi-vessel disease, and 5 patients (11%) presented with cardiogenic shock. Successful PTCA was achieved in 42 of the 45 patients (93%) 52 minutes after admission and 238 minutes after the onset of pain. Overall in-hospital mortality was 9% (4 of 45). Neither major bleeding nor stroke occurred. There was one case of early symptomatic reocclusion, treated with emergency repeat PTCA without reinfarction. Predischarge angiography in 33 patients showed only one silent reocclusion (3%). EF at discharge was 46%. Repeat catheterization at 6 months in 19 patients showed four restenoses (21%) and four reocclusions (21%) of the infarct-related artery. There were three late deaths (two noncardiac), which gave survival rates of 87% and 85% at 1 and 3 years, respectively, and event-free survival rates of 71% and 69% including in-hospital deaths. There were no cases of late reinfarction. Consequently, in this study, primary PTCA proved safe and highly effective in rapidly restoring sustained infarct-vessel patency during AMI and led to a greater improvement in early and late outcomes than that reported in the literature for medically treated subjects in this high-risk subset for which thrombolytic therapy is contraindicated.

In an investigation by Shirotani and associates,[137] from Kyoto, Japan, the factors responsible for early occlusion of the infarct vessel after emergency PTCA were retrospectively examined in 191 patients with AMI. During the 24-hour period after the initial balloon inflation, 47 patients (25%) had occlusion of the vessel (occlusion group), and 144 did not (nonocclusion group). The former patients immediately underwent repeat PTCA, which was successful in 37. Univariate correlates of early occlusion were a shorter time interval between the onset of symptoms and PTCA (3.5 ± 2.2 v 4.5 ± 2.9 hours), right coronary artery involvement (53% v 30%), prior thrombolytic therapy (49% v 32%), and undersized inflation (43% v 17%). With multivariate analysis, the three independent predictors were undersized inflation, right coronary artery involvement, and a shorter time interval until PTCA. Thus, patients undergoing early PTCA and having right coronary artery involvement appear to be at greater risk of having early occlusion. Thrombolytic agents and undersized inflation may also play an important role in its development.

Both thrombolytic therapy and PTCA have proven to be beneficial in patients with AMI. Ribeiro and associates,[138] from Sao Paulo, Brazil, directly compared these two techniques for achieving coronary revascularization in 100 patients with ST-segment elevation presenting to a single high volume interventional center within six hours of the onset of chest pain. Patients were randomized to receive either 1.2 million U streptokinase over one hour or immediate catheterization and direct coronary angioplasty. There was no difference in the baseline characteristics of the two treatment groups. Average patient age was 56 years, and 83% of patients were male. Ninety-seven percent were in Killip class I or II. Time to treatment was delayed in the angioplasty group (average 238 minutes v 179 minutes). Despite this time difference, there was no difference in 48 hour infarct related artery patency (74% v 80%) or left ventricular EF (59% v 57%) (angioplasty v streptokinase). There were no major bleeding events, and the mortality rate with angioplasty (6%) and streptokinase (2%) was not statistically different. These results suggest little difference between the techniques although the authors concluded that intravenous thrombolytic therapy might be preferred over angioplasty because of the shorter time to treatment with most patients.

Early reperfusion for AMI results in improved LV function and survival. There is a dearth of data on long-term survival (>5 years) after

PTCA performed either as a primary procedure or in conjunction with thrombolytic therapy. O'Murchu and associates,[139] from Rochester, Minn, studied 160 patients who underwent PTCA during AMI between 1981 and 1987 either with (101) or without (59) streptokinase therapy. Mean time to reperfusion was 4.6 hours, and patency was achieved in 134 patients (84%). Mean discharge EF was 46. CABG was performed before dismissal in 34 patients (21%), including 21 of 130 patients (16%) with one- or two-vessel disease and 13 of 30 patients (43%) with three-vessel disease. Eleven patients (7%) died in the hospital. The 149 hospital survivors were followed for a mean of 69 months. During follow-up, 22 patients (15%) died, 21 patients (14%) had reinfarction, 23 patients (15%) underwent CABG, and 21 patients (14%) underwent repeat PTCA of the infarct-related artery. On univariate analysis, age ≥62 years, multi-vessel disease, EF ≤40%, previous AMI, and being a non-smoker at the time of AMI were predictive of late mortality. On multivariate analysis, only EF <40% and prior AMI were predictive of late death. In patients treated with PTCA for AMI, late survival is excellent. Early surgical revascularization of high-risk patients may contribute to these encouraging results.

Important sex-related differences have been recognized in several CAD presentation and treatment subsets. Little data exist describing the relative findings and outcome in women versus men who received direct PTCA for AMI. Vacek and associates,[140] from Kansas City, Mo, studied 670 such patients of whom 464 (69%) were men and 206 were women. The women were significantly older (67 ± 11 years v 61 ± 11) but had undergone less prior CABG (6% v 12%), whereas prior AMI (17% women v 22% men) and CAD distribution were not significantly different. Forty-one percent of women and 43% of men had single-vessel disease. Both women and men had 1.5 lesions/patient dilated acutely, with similar success rates (95% women, 91% men). Mean EFs were similar (48% in both groups), and a similar percentage in each group had an EF <30% (10% women v 13% men). Over a mean follow-up period of 86 weeks, the need for repeat catheterization was frequent and was similar in both groups (44% women, 47% men), whereas documented restenosis was less common in women (20% v 28%). The need for CABG was similar (15% women, 17% men), as was the need for repeat PTCA in the infarct vessel (14% women, 18% men) and overall mortality (7% women, 9% men). It was concluded that other than older age, the clinical features of the women initially seen for direct PTCA for AMI are very similar to those of men. In spite of this age difference, PTCA success and outcomes are also very similar, other than a 29% lower incidence of documented restenosis in women.

Weaver and associates,[141] from Seattle, working in the Myocardial Infarction, Triage and Intervention (MITI) registry of patients with AMI, treated 441 (12%) of 3,750 patients with direct PTCA as initial treatment for their AMI. Approximately half (233) of these procedures were performed in hospital with no on-site surgery. Procedure success rates, use of emergent surgery, and factors influencing outcome were compared in both PTCA groups as well as with 653 patients treated with thrombolytic therapy in the same hospitals. There were no differences in baseline characteristics between patients treated by PTCA in the two types of hospitals. Patency was established in 88% of patients. Only 1% of patients underwent emergent CABG. Survival was 93% but was significantly worse after a failed procedure in all ECG and hemodynamic subsets as well as in those with prior CABG. In a multivariate analysis, age, initial heart rate, blood pressure, and prior CABG, but not type of hospital, were predictive of survival. Survival rates were similar, but there tended to be fewer strokes (0.6% v 2%), shorter hospital stays (7 v 8 days), and less recurrent ischemia (20% v 30%) in patients treated by PTCA compared with thrombolysis. Readmission and reinfarction rates were similar for both groups. Outcome in this registry study was dependent on initial hemodynamic findings and infarct location but not on the presence of on-site surgery. Compared with thrombolytic therapy, the incidence of complications was the same or lower in this study.

To determine the outcome of very elderly patients who had coronary revascularization during hospitalization for AMI, Krumholz and associates,[142] from Boston and West Roxbury, Mass, studied 1,215 consecutive patients aged 80 years and older who were hospitalized with an AMI between 1985 and 1990. The study sample included all 93 patients (8%) who had cardiac catheterization before discharge and had not been excluded from study because of the following: severe valvular disease, absence of significant CAD, or death before a decision about revascularization could be made. After catheterization, 41 patients had angioplasty, 18 patients had CABG, and 34 patients did not have revascularization procedure. Among the patients alive at discharge, those who had revascularization had a high likelihood of achieving a good or excellent quality of life (angioplasty, 86%; surgery, 89%; medical therapy, 44%). Mortality rates at 1 year were 24% for the angioplasty group, 6% for the surgery group, and 44% for the medical therapy group. In a Cox proportional hazards model that adjusted for clinical, demographic, hemodynamic, and anatomic differences between the groups, the performance of coronary revascularization was associated with increased survival (hazard ratio, 0.42). Thus, a small percentage of very elderly patients with complicated AMI, selected by their physicians for invasive cardiovascular procedures, can tolerate these procedures, avoid serious complications, return to independent living, and have excellent probability of survival. Although our results suggest that coronary revascularization may have benefited these patients, the study design did not permit definite conclusions, and future studies are needed to resolve this important question.

References

1. Chiriboga DE, Yarzebski J, Goldberg RJ, et al: A community-wide perspective of gender differences and temporal trends in the use of diagnostic and revascularization procedures for acute myocardial infarction. Am J Cardiol 1993 (Feb 1);71:268–273.
2. Goldberg RJ, Gorak EJ, Yarzebski J, et al: A communitywide perspective of sex differences and temporal trends in the incidence and survival rates after acute myocardial infarction and out-of-hospital deaths caused by coronary heart disease. Circulation 1993 (June);87:1947–1953.

3. Pashos CL, Newhouse JP, McNeil BJ: Temporal changes in the care and outcomes of elderly patients with AMI, 1987–1990. JAMA 1993 (Oct 20);270:1832–1836.

4. Behar S, Halabi M, Reicher-Reiss H, et al: Circadian variation and possible external triggers of onset of acute myocardial infarction. Am J Med 1993 (April);94:395–400.

5. Jimenez AH, Tofler GH, Chen X, et al: Effects of nadolol on hemodynamic and hemostatic responses to potential mental and physical triggers of myocardial infarction in subjects with mild systemic hypertension. Am J Cardiol 1993 (July 1);72:47–52.

6. Willich SN, Lewis M, Löwel H, et al: Physical exertion as a trigger of acute myocardial infarction. N Engl J Med 1993 (Dec 2);329:1684–1690.

7. Mittleman MA, Maclure M, Tofler GH, et al: Triggering of acute myocardial infarction by heavy physical exertion. N Engl J Med 1993 (Dec 1);329:1677–1683.

8. Peters RW, Zoble RG, Liebson PR, et al: Identification of a secondary peak in myocardial infarction onset 11 to 12 hours after awakening: The cardiac arrhythmia suppression trial (CAST) experience. J Am Coll Cardiol 1993 (Oct);22:998–1003.

9. Wong CK, Freedman SB, Bautovich G, et al: Mechanism and significance of precordial ST-segment depression during inferior wall acute myocardial infarction associated with severe narrowing of the dominant right coronary artery. Am J Cardiol 1993 (May 1);71:1025–1030.

10. Fletcher WO, Gibbons RJ, Clements IP: The relationship of inferior ST depression, lateral ST elevation, and left precordial ST elevation to myocardium at risk in acute anterior myocardial infarction. Am Heart J 1993 (Sep);126:526–535.

11. Lee HS, Cross SJ, Rawles JM, et al: Patients with suspected acute myocardial infarction who present with ST depression. Lancet 1993 (Nov 13);342:1204–1207.

12. Krucoff MW, Croll MA, Pope JE, et al: Continuously updated 12-lead ST-segment recovery analysis for myocardial infarct artery patency assessment and its correlation with multiple simultaneous early angiographic observations. Am J Cardiol 1993 (Jan 15);71:145–151.

13. Gaziano JM, Buring JE, Breslow JL, et al: Moderate alcohol intake, increased levels of high-density lipoprotein and its subfractions, and decreased risk of acute myocardial infarction. N Engl J Med 1993 (Dec 16);329:1829–1834.

14. Bakker AJ, Koelemay MJW, Gorgels JPMC, et al: Failure of new biochemical marker to exclude acute myocardial infarction at admission. Lancet 1993 (Nov 13);342:1220–1222.

15. Tomoda H: Plasma endothelin-1 in acute myocardial infarction with heart failure. Am Heart J 1993 (March);125:667–675.

16. Miyao Y, Yasue H, Ogawa H, et al: Elevated plasma interleukin-6 levels in patients with acute myocardial infarction. Am Heart J 1993 (Dec);126:1299–1304.

17. Kardinaal AFM, Kok FJ, Fingstad J, et al: Antioxidants in adipose tissue and risk of acute myocardial infarction (the EURAMIC study). Lancet 1993 (Dec 4);342:1379–1384.

18. Shen Z, Palma A, Rajachandran M, et al: Prediction of single and multivessel coronary disease in patients after myocardial infarction according to quantitative ultrasound wall-motion analysis. Am Heart J 1993 (April);125:949–957.

19. Aston CM, Petersen JJ, Wray NP, et al: The incidence of perioperative myocardial infarction in men undergoing noncardiac surgery. Ann Intern Med 1993 (April 1);118:504–510.

20. Eichner JE, Kuller LH, Orchard TJ, et al: Relation of apolipoprotein E phenotype to myocardial infarction and mortality from coronary artery disease. Am J Cardiol 1993 (Jan 15);71:160–165.

21. Moliterno DJ, Lange RA, Meidell RS, et al: Relation of plasma lipoprotein(a) to infarct artery patency in survivors of myocardial infarction. Circulation 1993 (Sep);88:935–940.

22. Bogaty P, Brecker SJ, White SE, et al: Comparison of coronary angiographic findings in acute and chronic first presentation of ischemic heart disease. Circulation 1993 (June);87:1938–1946.

23. Zuanetti G, Latini R, Maggioni AP, et al, on behalf of GISSI-2 Investigators: Influence of diabetes on mortality in acute myocardial infarction: data from the GISSI-2 Study. J Am Coll Cardiol 1993;(Dec);22:1788–1794.

24. Every NR, Larson EB, Litwin PE, et al: The association between on-site cardiac catheterization facilities and the use of coronary angiography after acute myocardial infarction. N Engl J Med 1993 (Aug 19);329:546–551.

25. Oldridge N, Furlong W, Feeny D, et al: Economic evaluation of cardiac rehabilitation soon after acute myocardial infarction. Am J Cardiol 1993 (July 15);72:154–161.

26. Worcester MC, Hare DL, Oliver RG, et al: Early programs of high and low intensity exercise and quality of life after acute myocardial infarction. Br Med J 1993 (Nov 13);307:1244–1247.

27. Lekakis J, Vassilopoulos N, Germanidis J, et al: detection of viable tissue in healed infarcted myocardium by dipyridamole thallium-201 reinjection and regional wall motion studies. Am J Cardiol 1993 (Feb 15);71:401–404.

28. Aoyagi T, Pouleur H, Van Eyll C, et al: Wall motion asynchrony is a major determinant of impaired left ventricular filling in patients with healed myocardial infarction. Am J Cardiol 1993 (Aug 1);72:268–272.

29. Rouleau JL, Moyé LA, Pfeffer MA, et al: A comparison of management patterns after acute myocardial infarction in Canada and the United States. N Engl J Med 1993 (March 18);328:779–784.

30. Brecker SJD, Stevenson RN, Roberts R, et al: Acute myocardial infarction in patients with angiographically normal coronary arteries. N Engl J Med 1993 (Nov 13);307:1255–1256.

31. Fukai T, Koyanagi S, Takeshita A: Role of coronary vasospasm in the pathogenesis of myocardial infarction: Study in patients with no significant coronary stenosis. Am Heart J 1993 (Dec);126:1305–1311.

32. Volpi A, De Vita C, Franzosi MG, et al, the Ad hoc Working Group of the Gruppo Italiano per lo Studio della Sopravvivenza nell'Infarto Miocardico (GISSI)-2 Data Base: Determinants of 6 month mortality in survivors of myocardial infarction after thrombolysis. Results of the GISSI-2 Data Base. Circulation 1993 (Aug);88:416–429.

33. Stevenson R, Ranjadayalan K, Wilkinson P, et al: Short and long term prognosis of acute myocardial infarction since introduction of thrombolysis. Br Med J 1993 (Aug 7);307:349–353.

34. Galvani M, Ottani F, Ferrini D, et al: Patency of the infarct-related artery and left ventricular function as the major determinants of survival after Q-Wave acute myocardial infarction. Am J Cardiol 1993 (Jan 1);71:1–7.

35. Vogt A, von Essen R, Tebbe U, et al: Impact of early perfusion status of the infarct-related artery on short-term mortality after thrombolysis for acute myocardial infarction: Retrospective analysis of four German multicenter studies. J Am Coll Cardiol 1993 (May);21:1391–1395.

36. Odemuyiwa O, Jordaan P, Malik M, et al: Autonomic correlates of late infarct artery patency after first myocardial infarction. Am Heart J 1993 (June);125:1597–1600.

37. Hermosillo AG, Dorado M, Casanova JM, et al: Influence of infarct-related artery patency on the indexes of parasympathetic activity and prevalence of late potentials in survivors of acute myocardial infarction. J Am Coll Cardiol 1993 (Sep);22:695–706.

38. Currie P, Saltissi S: Significance of ST-segment elevation during ambulatory monitoring after acute myocardial infarction. Am Heart J 1993 (Jan);125: 41–47.

39. Krone RJ, Greenberg H, Dwyer EM, et al, and the Multicenter Diltiazem Postinfarction Trial Research Group: Long-term prognostic significance of ST segment depression during acute myocardial infarction. J Am Coll Cardiol 1993 (Aug);22:361–367.

40. Gheorghiade M, Shivkumar K, Schultz L, et al: Prognostic significance of electrocardiographic persistent ST depression in patients with their first myocardial infarction in the placebo arm of the Beta-Blocker Heart Attack Trial. Am Heart J 1993 (Aug);126:271–278.

41. Mickley H, Pless P, Nielsen JR, et al: Transient myocardial ischemia after a first acute myocardial infarction and its relation to clinical characteristics, predischarge exercise testing and cardiac events at one-year follow-up. Am J Cardiol 1993 (Jan 15);71:139–144.

42. McClements BM, Adgey AJ: Value of signal-averaged electrocardiography, radionuclide ventriculography, Holter monitoring and clinical variables for prediction of arrhythmic events in survivors of acute myocardial infarction in the thrombolytic era. J Am Coll Cardiol 1993 (May);21:1419–1427.

43. Myers MG, Baigrie RS, Charlat ML, et al: Usefulness of routine non-invasive tests in predicting outcome after acute myocardial infarction in elderly people. Lancet 1993 (Oct 30);342:1069–1072.

44. Ciaroni S, Delonca J, Righetti A: Early exercise testing after acute myocardial infarction in the elderly: Clinical evaluation and prognostic significance. Am Heart J 1993 (Aug);304–311.

45. Picano E, Landi P, Bolognese L, et al: Prognostic value of dipyridamole echocardiography early after uncomplicated acute myocardial infarction. Am J Med 1993 (Dec 1993);95:608–618.

46. Bigger JT, Fleiss JL, Rolnitzky LM, et al: Frequency domain measures of heart period variability to assess risk late after myocardial infarction. J Am Coll Cardiol 1993 (Mar 1);21:729–736.

47. Bigger JT, Fleiss JL, Rolnitzky LM, et al: The ability of several short-term measures of RR variability to predict mortality after myocardial infarction. Circulation 1993 (Sep);88:927–934.

48. Behar S, Rabinowitz B, Zion M, et al, for the Secondary Prevention Reinfarction Israeli Nifedipine Trial (SPRINT) Study Group: Immediate and long-term prognostic significance of a first anterior versus first inferior wall Q-wave acute myocardial infarction. Am J Cardiol 1993 (Dec 15);72: 1366–1370.

49. McCallister BD, Chrstian TF, Gersh BJ, et al: Prognosis of myocardial infarctions involving more than 40% of the left ventricle after acute reperfusion therapy. Circulation 1993 (Oct);88[part 1]:1470–1475.

50. Galjee MA, Visser FC, De Cock CC, et al: The prognostic value, clinical, and angiographic characteristics of patients with early postinfarction angina after a first myocardial infarction. Am Heart J 1993 (Jan);l25:48–55.

51. Cupples LA, Gagnon DR, Wong ND, et al: Preexisting cardiovascular conditions and long-term prognosis after initial myocardial infarction: The Framingham Study. Am Heart J 1993 (March);125:863–872.

52. Tofler GH, Muller JE, Stone PH, et al, and the Multicenter Investigation of the Limitation of Infarct Size (MILIS): Comparison of long-term outcome after acute myocardial infarction in patients never graduated from high school with that in more educated patients. Am J Cardiol l993 (May 1);71: 1031–1035.

53. Zaman AG, Morris JL, Smyllie JH, et al: Late potentials and ventricular enlargement after myocardial infarction. A new role for high-resolution electrocardiology? Circulation 1993 (Sep);88:905–914.

54. Frasure-Smith N, Lespérance F, Talajic M: Depression following myocardial infarction. JAMA 1993 (Oct 20);270:1819–1825.

55. Dittrich HC, Gilpin E, Nicod P, et al: Outcome after acute myocardial infarction in patients with prior coronary artery bypass surgery. Am J Cardiol 1993 (Sep 1);72:507–513.

56. Hertzeanu HL, Shemesh J, Aron LA, et al: Ventricular arrhythmias in rehabilitated and nonrehabilitated post-myocardial infarction patients with left ventricular dysfunction. Am J Cardiol 1993 (Jan 1);71:24–27.

57. Pfisterer ME, Kiowski W, Brunner H, et al: Long-term benefit of 1 year amiodarone treatment for persistent complex ventricular arrhythmias after myocardial infarction. Circulation 1993 (Feb);87:309–311.

58. Maggioni AP, Zuanetti G, Franzosi MG, et al, on behalf of GISSI-2 Investigators: Prevalence and prognostic significance of ventricular arrhythmias after acute myocardial infarction in the fibrinolytic era. GISSI-2 results. Circulation 1993 (Feb);87:312–322.

59. Hii JTY, Traboulsi M, Mitchell B, et al: Infarct artery patency predicts outcome of serial electropharmacological studies in patients with malignant ventricular tachyarrhythmias. Circulation 1993 (March);87:764–772.

60. Navarro-López F, Cosin J, Marrugat J, et al, for the SSSD Investigators: Comparison of the effects of amiodarone versus metoprolol on the frequency of ventricular arrhythmias and on mortality after acute myocardial infarction. Am J Cardiol 1993 (Dec 1);72:1243–1248.

61. Champagnac D, Claudel J Ph, Desseigne P, et al: Primary cardiogenic shock during acute myocardial infarction: Results of emergency cardiac transplantation. Euro Heart J 1993 (July);14:925–929.

62. Gaudron P, Eilles C, Kugler I: Progressive left ventricular dysfunction and remodeling after myocardial infarction. Potential mechanisms and early predictors. Circulation 1993 (March);87:755–763.

63. Rouleau JL, Champlain J, Klein M, et al: Activation of neurohumoral systems in postinfarction left ventricular dysfunction. J Am Coll Cardiol 1993 (Aug);22:390–398.

64. Mallavarapu C, Pancholy S, Cave V, et al: Study of myocardial infarct remodeling by single-photon emission computed tomographic imaging. Am J Cardiol 1993 (Oct 1);72:747–752.

65. Hirose K, Shu NH, Reed JE, et al: Right ventricular dilatation and remodeling the first year after an initial transmural wall left ventricular myocardial infarction. Am J Cardiol 1993 (Nov 15);72:1126–1130.

66. Vaitkus PT, Barnathan ES: Embolic potential, prevention and management of mural thrombus complicating anterior myocardial infarction: A meta-analysis. J Am Coll Cardiol 1993 (Oct);22:1004–1009.

67. Zehender M, Kasper W, Kauder E, et al: Right ventricular infarction as an independent predictor of prognosis after inferior wall acute myocardial infarction. N Engl J Med 1993 (April 8);328:981–988.

68. Correale E, Maggioni AP, Romano S, et al, on behalf of the Gruppo Italiano per lo Studio della Sopraw ivenza nell'Infarto Miocardico (GISSI): Comparison of frequency, diagnostic and prognostic significance of pericardial involvement in acute myocardial infarction treated with and without thrombolytics. Am J Cardiol 1993 (June 15);71:1377–1381.

69. Oliva PB, Hammill SC, Edwards WD: Electrocardiographic diagnosis of postinfarction regional pericarditis. Ancillary observations regarding the effect of reperfusion on the rapidity and amplitude of T wave inversion after acute myocardial infarction. Circulation 1993 (Sep);88:896–904.

70. Oliva PB, Hammill SC, Edwards WD: Cardiac rupture, a clinically predictable complication of acute myocardial infarction: Report of 70 cases with clinicopathologic correlations. J Am Coll Cardiol 1993 (Sep);22:720–726.

71. Heller RF, Knapp JC, Valenti LA, et al: Secondary prevention after acute myocardial infarction. Am J Cardiol 1993 (Oct 1);72:759–762.

72. Krumholz HM, Cohen BJ, Tsevat J, et al: Cost-effectiveness of a smoking cessation program after myocardial infarction. J Am Coll Cardiol 1993 (Nov 15);22:1697–1702.

73. Pedretti R, Colombo E, Braga SS, et al: Influence of transdermal scopolamine on cardiac sympathovagal interaction after acute myocardial infarction. Am J Cardiol 1993 (Aug 15);72:384–392.

74. Vybiral T, Glaeser DH, Morris G, et al: Effects of low dose transdermal scopolamine on heart rate variability in acute myocardial infarction. J Am Coll Cardiol 1993 (Nov 1);22:1320–1326.

75. Galløe, Rasmussen HS, Jørgensen LN, et al: Influence of oral magnesium supplementation on cardiac events among survivors of an acute myocardial infarction. Br Med J 1993 (Sep 4);307:585–587.

76. Epstein AE, Hallstrom AP, Rogers WJ, et al: Mortality following ventricular arrhythmia suppression by encainide, flecainide, and moricizine after acute myocardial infarction (The Original Design Concept of the Cardiac Arrhythmia Suppression Trial [CAST]). JAMA 1993 (Nov 24);270:2451–2455.

77. Zarembski DG, Nolan PE Jr, Slack MK, et al: Empiric long-term amiodarone prophylaxis following acute myocardial infarction. Arch Intern Med 1993 (Dec 13);153:2661–2667.

78. Cohen M, Xiong J, Parry G, et al, and the Antithrombotic Therapy in Acute Coronary Syndromes Research Group: Prospective comparison of unstable angina versus non-Q wave myocardial infarction during antithrombotic therapy. J Am Coll Cardiol 1993 (Nov 1);22:1338–1343.

79. Motwani JG, Fenwick MK, McAlpine HM, et al: Effectiveness of captopril in reversing renal vasoconstriction after Q-wave acute myocardial infarction. Am J Cardiol 1993 (Feb 1);71:281–286.

80. Søgaard P, Gøtzsche C-O, Ravkilde J, et al: Effects of captopril on ischemia and dysfunction of the left ventricle after myocardial infarction. Circulation 1993 (April);87:1093–1099.

81. Pipilis A, Flather M, Collins R, et al: Hemodynamic effects of captopril and isosorbide mononitrate started early in acute myocardial infarction: A randomized placebo-controlled study. J Am Coll Cardiol 1993 (July);22:73–79.

82. The Acute Infarction Ramipril Efficacy (AIRE) Study Investigators: Effect of ramipril on mortality and morbidity of survivors of acute myocardial infarction with clinical evidence of congestive heart failure. Lancet 1993 (Oct 2);342:821–828.

83. Teo KK, Yusuf S, Furberg CD: Effects of prophylactic antiarrhythmic drug therapy in acute myocardial infarction. JAMA 1993. (Oct 6);270: 1589–1595.

84. Anderson HV, Willerson JT: Thrombolysis in acute myocardial infarction. N Engl J Med 1993 (Sep 2);329:703–709.

85. Gray D, Keating NA, Murdock J, et al: Impact of hospital thrombolysis policy on out-of-hospital response to suspected acute myocardial infarction. Lancet 1993 (March 13);341:654–657.

86. Ketley D, Woods KL: Impact of clinical trials on clinical practice as exemplified by thrombolysis for acute myocardial infarction. Lancet 1993 (Oct 9);342:891–894.

87. Barbash GI, Modan M, Goldbourt U, et al: Comparative case fatality analysis of the international tissue plasminogen activator/streptokinase mortality trial: Variation by country beyond predictive profile. J Am Coll Cardiol 1993 (Feb);21(2):281–286.

88. Weaver WD, Cerqueira M, Hallstrom AP, et al: Prehospital-initiated vs hospital-initiated thrombolytic therapy. The myocardial infarction triage and intervention trial. JAMA 1993 (Sep);270:1211–1216.

89. The European Myocardial Infarction Project Group: Prehospital thrombolytic therapy in patients with suspected acute myocardial infarction. N Engl J Med 1993 (Aug 5);329:383–389.

90. Linderer T, Schroder R, Arntz R, et al: Prehospital thrombolysis: Beneficial effects of very early treatment on infarct size and left ventricular function. J Am Coll Cardiol 1993 (Nov 1);22:1304–1310.

91. Christian TF, Gibbons RJ, Hopfenspirger MR: Severity and response of chest pain during thrombolytic therapy for acute myocardial infarction: A useful

indicator of myocardial salvage and infarct size. J Am Coll Cardiol 1993 (Nov 1);22:1311–1316.

92. White HD, Barbash GI, Modan M, et al, for the Investigators of the International Tissue Plasminogen Activator/Streptokinase Mortality Study. Circulation 1993 (Nov);88[part 1]:2097–2103.

93. Lincoff AM, Califf RM, Ellis SG, et al, for the Thrombolysis and Angioplasty in Myocardial Infarction Study Group: Thrombolytic therapy for women with myocardial infarction: Is there a gender gap? J Am Coll Cardiol 1993 (Dec);22:1780–1787.

94. Berger PB, Ruocco NA Jr, Ryan TJ, et al, and the TIMI Research Group: Frequency and significance of right ventricular dysfunction during inferior wall left ventricular myocardial infarction treated with thrombolytic therapy. Results from the Thrombolysis in Myocardial Infarction (TIMI) II Trial. Am J Cardiol 1993 (May 15);71:1148–1152.

95. Ragosta M, Sabia PJ, Kaul S, et al: Effects of late (1 to 30 days) reperfusion after acute myocardial infarction on the signal-averaged electrocardiogram. Am J Cardiol 1993 (Jan 1);71:19–23.

96. EMERAS Collaborative Group: Effectiveness of late thrombolysis in patients with suspected acute myocardial infarction. Lancet 1993 (Sep 25);342:767–772.

97. Ito H, Tomooka T, Sakai N, et al: Time course of functional improvement in stunned myocardium in risk area in patients with reperfused anterior infarction. Circulation 1993 (Feb);87:355–362.

98. Davies SW, Hanjadayalan K, Wickens DG, et al: Free radical activity and left ventricular function after thrombolysis for acute infarction. Br Heart J 1993 (Feb);69:114–120.

99. Odemuyiwa O, Farrell T, Staunton A, et al: Influence of thrombolytic therapy on the evolution of baroreflex sensitivity after myocardial infarction. Am Heart J 1993 (Feb);125:285–291.

100. Nidorf SM, Siu SC, Galambos G, et al: Benefit of late coronary perfusion on ventricular morphology and function after myocardial infarction. J Am Coll Cardiol 1993 (Mar 1);21:683–691.

101. Abe S, Nomoto K, Arima S, et al: Detection of reperfusion 30 and 60 minutes after coronary recanalization by a rapid new assay of creatine kinase isoforms in acute myocardial infarction. Am Heart J 1993 (March);125:649–656.

102. Luria MH, Sapoznikov D, Gilon D, et al: Early heart rate variability alterations after acute myocardial infarction. Am Heart J 1993 (March);125:676–681.

103. Harrison JK, Califf RM, Woodlief LH, et al, and the TAMI Study Group: Systolic left ventricular function after reperfusion therapy for acute myocardial infarction. An analysis of determinants of improvement. Circulation 1993 (May);87:1531–1541.

104. Zabel M, Hohnloser SH, Koster W, et al: Analysis of creatine kinase, CK-MB, myoglobin, and troponin T time-activity curves for early assessment of coronary artery reperfusion after intravenous thrombolysis. Circulation 1993 (May);87:1542–1550.

105. Yamashita T, Abe S, Arima S, et al: Myocardial infarct size can be estimated from serial plasma myoglobin measurements within 4 hours of reperfusion. Circulation 1993 (June);87:1840–1849.

106. Haber HL, Beller GA, Watson DD, et al: Exercise thallium-201 scintigraphy after thrombolytic therapy with or without angioplasty for acute myocardial infarction. Am J Cardiol 1993 (Jun 1);71:1257–1261.

107. Crea F, Davies G, Crake T, et al: Variability of coronary blood flow reserve assessed by Doppler catheter after successful thrombolysis in patients with acute myocardial infarction. Am Heart J 1993 (June);125:1547–1552.

108. Picard MX, Wilkins GT, Ray P, et al: Long-term effects of acute thrombolytic therapy on ventricular size and function. Am Heart J 1993 (July); 126:1–10.

109. Abe J, Yamaguchi T, Isshiki T, et al: Myocardial reperfusion can be predicted by myoglobin/creatine kinase ratio of a single blood sample obtained at the time of admission. Am Heart J 1993 (Aug);126:279–285.

110. Smart SC, Sawada S, Ryan T, et al: Low-dose dobutamine echocardiography detects reversible dysfunction after thrombolytic therapy of acute myocardial infarction. Circulation 1993 (Aug);88:405–415.

111. Hirai T, Fujita M, Yoshida N, et al: Importance of ischemic preconditioning and collateral circulation for left ventricular functional recovery in patients with successful intracoronary thrombolysis for acute myocardial infarction. Am Heart J 1993 (Oct);126:827–831.

112. Dissmann R, Linderer T, Goerke M, et al: Sudden increase of the ST segment elevation at time of reperfusion predicts extensive infarcts in patients with intravenous thrombolysis. Am Heart J 1993 (Oct);126: 832–839.

113. Stevenson R, Umachandran V, Ranjadayalan K, et al: Reassessment of treadmill stress testing for risk stratification in patients with acute myocardial infarction treated by thrombolysis. Br Heart J 1993 (Nov);70:415–420.

114. Hirayama A, Adachi T; Asada S, et al: Late reperfusion for acute myocardial infarction limits the dilatation of left ventricle without the reduction of infarct size. Circulation 1993 (Dec);2565–2574.

115. Chouhan L, Hajar HA, Pomposiello JC: Comparison of thrombolytic therapy for acute myocardial infarction in patients aged <35 and >55 years. Am J Cardiol 1993 (Jan 15);71:157–159.

116. Elliott JM, Cross DB, Cederholm-Williams SA, et al: Neutralizing antibodies to streptokinase four years after intravenous thrombolytic therapy. Am J Cardiol 1993 (March 15);71:640–645.

117. Herlitz J, Hartford M, Aune S, et al: Occurrence of hypotension during streptokinase infusion in suspected acute myocardial infarction, and its relation to prognosis and metoprolol therapy. Am J Cardiol 1993 (May 1);71:1021–1024.

118. Tobé TJM, de Langen CDJ, Crijns HJGM, et al: Effects of streptokinase during acute myocardial infarction on the signal-averaged electrocardiogram and on the frequency of late arrhythmias. Am J Cardiol 1993 (Sep 15);72:647–651.

119. Gomez MA, Karagounis LA, Allen A, et al, for the TEAM-2 Investigators: Effect of cigarette smoking on coronary patency after thrombolytic therapy for myocardial infarction. Am J Cardiol 1993 (Aug 15);72:373–378.

120. Montrucchio G, Bergerone S, Bussolino F, et al: Streptokinase induces intravascular release of platelet-activating factor in patients with acute myocardial infarction and stimulates its synthesis by cultured human endothelial cells. Circulation 1993 (Oct);88[part 1]:1476–1483.

121. Taylor HA, Chaitman BR, Rogers WJ, et al, and the TIMI Investigators: Race and prognosis after myocardial infarction. Results of the Thrombolysis in Myocardial Infarction (TIMI) phase II trial. Circulation 1993 (Oct);88[part 1]:1484–1494.

122. Berger PB, Ruocco NA, Ryan TJ, et al, and the TIMI Investigators: Incidence and significance of ventricular tachycardia and fibrillation in the absence of hypotension or heart failure in acute myocardial infarction treated with recombinant tissue-type plasminogen activator. Results from the thrombolysis in myocardial infarction (TIMI) phase II trial. J Am Coll Cardiol 1993 (Dec);22:1773–1779.

123. Kalan JM, Gertz SD, Kragel AH, et al: Effects of tissue plasminogen activator therapy on the frequency of acute right ventricular myocardial infarction associated with acute left ventricular infarction. Internatl J Cardiol 1993;38:151–158.

124. Anderson JL, Karagounis LA, Becker LC, et al, for the TEAM-3 Investigators: TIMI perfusion grade 3 but not grade 2 results in improved outcome after thrombolysis for myocardial infarction. Ventriculographic, enzymatic, and electrocardiographic evidence from the TEAM-3 study. Circulation 1993 (June);87:1829–1839.

125. LATE Study Group: Late assessment of thrombolytic efficacy (LATE) study with alteplase 6–24 hours after onset of AMI. Lancet 1993 (Sep 25);342:759–766.

126. Collen D, Van de Werf F: Coronary thrombolysis with recombinant staphylokinase in patients with evolving myocardial infarction. Circulation 1993 (June);87:1850–1853.

127. The GUSTO Investigators: An international randomized trial comparing four thrombolytic strategies for acute myocardial infarction. N Engl J Med 1993 (Sep 2);329:673–682.

128. The GUSTO Angiographic Investigators: Effects of tissue plasminogen activator, streptokinase, or both on coronary-artery patency, ventricular function, and survival after acute myocardial infarction. N Engl J Med 1993 (Nov 25);329:1615–1622.

129. Meijer A, Verheugt FWA, Werter CJPJ, et al: Aspirin versus coumadin in the prevention of reocclusion and recurrent ischemia after successful thrombolysis: A prospective placebo-controlled angiographic study. Results of the APRICOT study. Circulation 1993 (May);87:1524–1530.

130. Simoons ML, Maggioni AP, Knatterud G, et al: Individual risk assessment for intracranial hemorrhage during thrombolytic therapy. Lancet 1993 (Dec 18/25);342:1523–1528.

131. Chaitman BR, McMahon RP, Terrin M, et al, for the TIMI Investigators: Impact of treatment strategy on predischarge exercise test in the thrombolysis in myocardial infarction (TIMI) II trial. Am J Cardiol 1993 (Jan 15);71:131–138.

132. Terrin ML, Williams DO, Kleinman NS, et al, for the TIMI II Investigators: Two- and three-year results of the thrombolysis in myocardial infarction (TIMI) phase II clinical trial. J Am Coll Cardiol 1993 (Dec);22:1763–1772.

133. Grines CL, Browne KF, Marco J, et al: A comparison of immediate angioplasty with thrombolytic therapy for acute myocardial infarction. N Engl J Med 1993 (March 11);328:673–679.

134. Zijlstra F, Boer MJ, Hoorntje JCA, et al: A comparison of immediate coronary angioplasty with intravenous streptokinase in acute myocardial infarction. N Engl J Med 1993 (March 11);328:680–684.

135. Maynard C, Weaver WD, Litwin PE, et al, for the MITI Project Investigators: Hospital mortality in acute myocardial infarction in the era of reperfusion therapy. The Myocardial Infarction Triage and Intervention Project. Am J Cardiol 1993 (Oct 15);72:877–882.

136. Himbert D, Juliard JM, Steg PG, et al: Primary coronary angioplasty for acute myocardial infarction with contraindication to thrombolysis. Am J Cardiol 1993 (Feb 15);71:377–381.

137. Shirotani M, Yui Y, Hattori R, et al: Emergency coronary angioplasty for acute myocardial infarction: Predictors of early occlusion of the infarct-related artery after balloon inflation. Am Heart J 1993 (April);125:931–938.

138. Ribeiro EE, Silva LA, Carneiro R, et al: Randomized trial of direct coronary angioplasty versus intravenous streptokinase in acute myocardial infarction. J Am Coll Cardiol 1993 (Aug);22:376–380.

139. O'Murchu B, Gersh BJ, Reeder GS, et al: Late outcome after percutaneous transluminal coronary angioplasty during acute myocardial infarction. Am J Cardiol 1993 (Sep 15);72:634–639.

140. Vacek JL, Rosamond TL, Kramer PH, et al: Sex-related differences in patients undergoing direct angioplasty for acute myocardial infarction. Am Heart J 1993 (Sep);126:521–525.

141. Weaver WD, Litwin PE, Martin JS, for the Myocardial Infarction, Triage, and Intervention Project Investigators: Use of direct angioplasty for treatment of patients with acute myocardial infarction in hospitals with and without on-site cardiac surgery. Circulation 1993 (Nov);88[part 1]: 2067–2075.

142. Krumholz HM, Forman DE, Kuntz RE, et al: Outcomes and long-term follow-up of coronary revascularization after acute myocardial infarction in patients ≥80 years of age. Ann Intern Med 1993 (Dec 1);119:1084–1090.

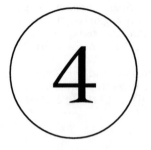

Arrhythmias, Conduction Disturbances, and Cardiac Arrest

Left Atrial Contrast Echoes

In an investigation by de Belder and associates,[1] from London, United Kingdom, a consecutive series of 80 patients with AF were studied with both precordial and transesophageal echocardiography. LA spontaneous contrast echoes were observed in 1 patient with precordial echocardiography and in 26 patients (33%) with transesophageal echocardiography. They were found most commonly in patients with rheumatic mitral valve disease (67%) but were observed in 28% of patients with lone AF. Their presence was unrelated to the age, gender, and therapy of the patient. Although they were more common in patients with a large left atrium, they were sometimes observed in a normal sized atrial chamber. They were more common in chronic (40%) than in paroxysmal AF (5% to 6%). No patient had severe MR, but contrast echoes were observed in some patients with mild or moderate MR. Of the 26 patients with spontaneous contrast echoes, 6 patients (23%) had echoes consistent with LA thrombus compared with 1 of the 54 patients without these echoes (1% to 9%); 17 patients (65%) had suffered a previous thromboembolic event compared with 17 of the 54 patients (32%) without these echoes. These data support the concept that spontaneous contrast echoes in the left atrium are associated with sluggish blood flow and a thrombogenic environment. Transesophageal echocardiography may thus be useful in assessing which patients with AF might most benefit from anticoagulation.

Prediction by P-Wave Signal Averaged Electrocardiogram

Steinberg and associates,[2] from New York, NY, evaluated consecutive patients undergoing cardiac surgery to determine whether the P-wave signal averaged ECG noninvasively detects atrial conduction delay. The P-wave signal averaged ECG was recorded before surgery from three orthogonal leads using a sinus P-wave template and a cross-correlation function. The averaged P wave was filtered with a least-squares-fit filter and combined into a vector magnitude. Total P-wave duration was measured. Patients were observed after cardiac surgery for the development of atrial fibrillation. One hundred thirty patients were enrolled, and 33 (25%) developed atrial fibrillation on average three days after surgery. Patients with atrial fibrillation more often had LV hypertrophy on ECG and lower LVEFs. The P-wave duration on the signal averaged ECG was significantly longer in those patients with atrial fibrillation than in those without. A signal averaged ECG P-wave duration >140 ms predicted atrial fibrillation with a sensitivity of 77%, specificity of 55%, positive predictive accuracy of 37%, and negative predictive accuracy of 87% (Figure 4-1). Therefore, the likelihood of experiencing atrial fibrillation was increased 4-fold if the signal averaged ECG P-wave duration was prolonged. P-wave signal averaged ECG results were independent of other clinical variables by multivariate analysis.

Hemodynamics

Ueshima and associates,[3] from Palo Alto, Long Beach, and Stanford, Calif, and Wakayama, Japan, evaluated the response of patients with chronic AF to exercise. Seventy-nine male patients (mean age, 64 ± 1 years) with AF underwent resting two-dimensional and M-mode echocardiography and symptom-limited treadmill testing with ventilatory gas exchange analysis. Patients were classified by underlying disease into five subgroups: no underlying disease and thereby lone AF (n = 17), hypertension (n = 11), ischemic heart disease (n = 13), cardiomyopathy or history of CHF (n = 26), and valvular disease (n = 12). A higher maximal heart rate than expected for age was observed (175 v 157 beats/min), which was most notable in the lone AF and hypertension subgroups. Maximal oxygen uptake was lower than expected for age in all groups. Patients with CHF had a lower resting EF than all other patients, a lower maximal oxygen uptake, and a lower maximal heart rate than lone AF and hypertension patients. Stepwise regression analysis demonstrated that echocardiographic measurements at rest were poor predictors of maximal oxygen uptake and oxygen uptake at the ventilatory threshold. Among clinical, morphologic, and exercise variables, maximal systolic BP accounted for the greatest variance in exercise capacity, but it explained only 35%. In patients with AF, the higher than predicted maximal heart rates may be a compensatory mechanism for maintaining exercise capacity after the loss of normal atrial function.

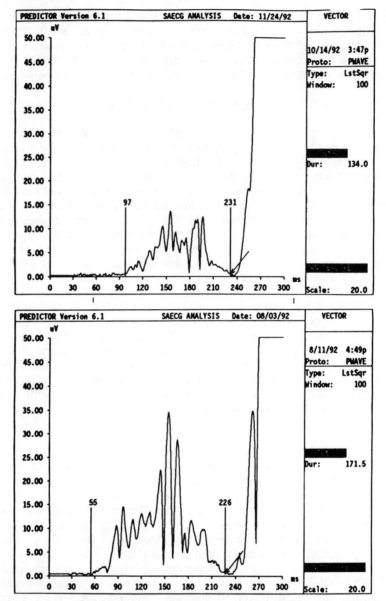

Figure 4-1. Examples of signal-averaged (SA) P waves. A, SAECG from a patient who did not develop atrial fibrillation (AF) with a measured P-wave duration of 134 milliseconds. B, SAECG from a patient who had AF on day 3 after coronary bypass graft surgery with a measured P-wave duration of 172 milliseconds. Reproduced with permission from Steinberg et al.[2]

However, even in the absence of underlying disease, it does not appear to compensate fully for a compromised exercise capacity. Although the exercise response was not strongly influenced by cardiac function at rest, the response of patients with AF without morphologic heart disease differed markedly from those with AF and underlying CHF. Although AF is associated with a reduced exercise capacity, the response to exercise in patients with AF is related more to the underlying heart disease than to AF itself.

Van Gelder and associates,[4] from Utrecht, The Netherlands, prospectively assessed the time course, magnitude, and mechanism of the hemodynamic changes after restoration of sinus rhythm in patients with chronic AF unassociated with valvular disease. Severe cardiac dysfunction may occur after chronic SVT in patients with and without underlying cardiac disease. Improvement may follow abolishment of the arrhythmia or adequate slowing of the ventricular rate. Eight patients were studied with a mean previous duration of AF of 10 months. EF, exercise capacity, and the atrial contribution to the LV filling (only during sinus rhythm) were studied before cardioversion and after cardioversion, and 1 week, 1 month, and 6 months thereafter. A significant improvement in EF from 36% to 53% occurred at 1 month after cardioversion. Concomitantly, peak oxygen consumption had increased at 1 month, from 20 to 25 mL/min/kg. Thereafter, no further improvement in hemodynamic parameters occurred. The atrial systole improved already at 1 week and remained unchanged thereafter. Thus, restoration of sinus rhythm was associated with a delayed improvement in EF and maximal exercise capacity, preceded by an early restoration of atrial contractility and an acute slowing of the heart rate. The discrepancy in time course of restoration of atrial and ventricular function parameters suggests that an intrinsic LV cardiomyopathy is present in patients with AF.

Transesophageal Echocardiogram Before and During Conversion

Because atrial thrombi are poorly detected by conventional noninvasive techniques such as transthoracic echocardiography, patients with prolonged AF usually receive several weeks of oral anticoagulation therapy before cardioversion is attempted. Manning and associates,[5] from Boston, Mass, investigated whether transesophageal echocardiography, an accurate method of detecting atrial thrombi, would allow early cardioversion to be performed safely if no thrombi were identified. A total of 669 consecutive patients admitted with the diagnosis of AF were screened. Patients were excluded if they were receiving long-term anticoagulation, if the duration of AF was two days or less, if they were not candidates for cardioversion, or if transesophageal echocardiography was contraindicated. Of 119 qualifying patients, 94 agreed to participate; the average duration of AF was 4.5 weeks. Participating patients underwent transthoracic echocardiography and transesophageal echocardiography followed by cardioversion if no thrombi were seen. Short-term anticoagulation with heparin was used in 80 patients before cardioversion, and 60 patients received warfarin for one month after cardioversion. Fourteen atrial thrombi were identified in 12 patients (13%), and 12 of the 14 thrombi were visualized only on transesophageal echocardiography. Cardioversion was deferred in all 12 patients. Two of these 12 patients died suddenly; 4 of the 10 surviving patients underwent uneventful cardioversion after prolonged oral anticoagulation. Seventy-eight of the 82 patients without thrombi underwent successful cardioversion to sinus rhythm (47 by means of antiarrhythmic drugs and 31 by electrical cardioversion), all without long-term oral anticoagulation. No patient had an embolic event. In patients with AF of unknown or prolonged duration who are not receiving long-term anticoagulation, atrial thrombi are detected by transesophageal echocardiography in only a small minority (13% in this study). The data suggest that if transesophageal echocardiography excludes the presence of thrombi, early cardioversion can be performed safely without the need for prolonged oral anticoagulation before the procedure.

A study by Black and associates,[6] from Sydney, Australia, prospectively evaluated the role of transesophageal echocardiography in screening for atrial thrombi before electrical cardioversion in 40 non-anticoagulated patients with nonvalvular AF (n = 33) or atrial flutter (n = 7). Transthoracic echocardiography did not detect atrial thrombus in any patient. Transesophageal echocardiography detected LA appendage thrombi in 5 patients (12%), significantly associated with LV systolic dysfunction and LA spontaneous echo contrast. Cardioversion was canceled in the 5 patients with thrombi and in 2 patients with spontaneous reversion before planned cardioversion. Cardioversion was successful in 25 (76%) of the 33 remaining patients. Cerebral embolism occurred 24 hours after successful cardioversion in 1 patient with AF and LV dysfunction, who had LA spontaneous echo contrast, but no thrombus was detected by transesophageal echocardiography before cardioversion. Repeat transesophageal echocardiography after embolism showed a fresh LA appendage thrombus and increased LA spontaneous echo contrast. These results indicate that transesophageal echocardiography improves the detection of LA appendage thrombi in candidates for cardioversion in whom the procedure may be deferred. The exclusion by transesophageal echocardiography of preexisting LA thrombi before cardioversion does not eliminate the risk of embolism after cardioversion because of persistent atrial stasis and de novo thrombosis.

Postoperatively

Between Jan 1, 1986, and Dec 31, 1991, 4,507 adult patients underwent cardiac surgical procedures requiring cardiopulmonary bypass at Barnes Hospital in St. Louis, Mo. Of these patients, 3,983 who did not undergo operation for SVT and who were normal sinus rhythm preoperatively were separated out and analyzed by Creswell and associates.[7] Postoperatively, all patients were monitored continuously for the development of arrhythmias until the time of hospital discharge. The incidence of atrial arrhythmias requiring treatment for the most commonly performed operative procedures were as follows: CABG, 31.9%; CABG and MVR, 63.6%; CABG and AVR, 48.8%; and heart transplantation, 11.1%. For all patients considered collectively, the risk factors associated with an increased incidence of postoperative atrial arrhythmias included increasing patient age, preoperative use of digoxin, history of rheumatic heart disease, chronic obstructive pulmonary disease, and increasing aortic cross-clamp time. Postoperative AF was associated with an increased incidence of postoperative stroke (3.3% v 1.4%), increased length of hospitalization in the intensive care unit (5.7 v 3.4 days) and postoperative nursing ward (10.9 v 7.5 days), increased incidence of postoperative VT or VF (9.2% v 4.0%), and an increased need for placement of a permanent pacemaker (3.7% v 1.6%). These data provide a basis for targeting specific patient subgroups for prospective, randomized trials of therapeutic modalities designed to decrease the incidence of postoperative atrial arrhythmias.

Atrial Function After Conversion

It is often suggested but never proven that atrial function is not affected during atrial flutter, nor after its conversion to normal sinus rhythm. To evaluate this hypothesis, Jordaens and associates,[8] from Ghent, Belgium, performed a prospective study in 22 patients (age range, 20 to 88 years) with atrial flutter. Diastolic transmitral flow was analyzed with echo-Doppler before and after conversion. After randomization, conversion was attempted with overdrive pacing or up to two 50 J shocks. If the initial method was unsuccessful, a 200 J shock was administered. All patients were converted to sinus rhythm with this protocol. Shortly after conversion (at 1 and 6 hours), atrial contribution to ventricular filling was absent in 4 of 22 patients. In the remaining 18 patients, atrial contribution to ventricular filling was small. Atrial contribution to transmitral flow improved from 20% to 27% within 24 hours and increased further to 38% at 6 weeks. Peak velocity of late diastolic filling increased from 0.28 m/s after 1 hour to 0.39 m/s after 24 hours and improved even further during later follow-up. In 1 patient, an effective atrial systole was not observed until the 14th day. Cardiac output did not change significantly during the study period. No differences were observed between the conversion modalities. In conclusion, atrial dysfunction is present immediately after conversion of atrial flutter to normal sinus rhythm. This dysfunction occurs also after overdrive pacing and can last >1 week. The findings suggested that stasis in the atria can remain temporarily present after successful conversion of atrial flutter to sinus rhythm.

Prevention After Cerebral Event

Several studies have established the value of anticoagulation for primary prevention of thromboembolic events in patients with nonrheumatic AF. In patients with a recent transient ischemic attack or minor ischemic stroke, the preventive benefit of anticoagulation or aspirin remains unclear. The European Atrial Fibrillation Trial study group[9] included physicians in 108 centers from 13 countries who collaborated in a study of 1,007 patients who had nonrheumatic AF with a recent transient ischemic attack or minor ischemic stroke randomized to open anticoagulation or double-blind treatment with either 300 mg aspirin per day or placebo (group 1, 669 patients); patients with contraindications to anticoagulation were randomized to receive aspirin or placebo (group 2, 338 patients). The measure of outcome was death from vascular disease, any stroke, AMI, or systemic embolism. During mean follow-up of 2.3 years, the annual rate of outcome events was 8% in patients assigned to anticoagulants versus 17% in placebo-treated patients in group 1 (Figure 4-2). The risk of stroke alone was reduced from 12% to 4% per year. Among all patients assigned to aspirin (groups 1 and 2), the annual incidence of outcome events was 15%, against 19% in those on placebo. Anticoagulation was significantly more effective than aspirin. The incidence of major bleeding events was low, both on anticoagulation (2.8% per year) and on aspirin (0.9% per year). No intracranial bleeds were identified in patients assigned to anticoagulation. These authors con-

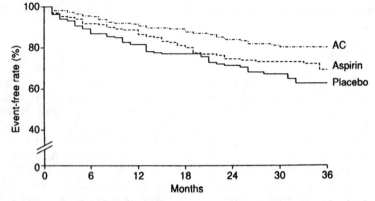

Figure 4-2. Survival analysis for primary outcome event: group 1. (Vascular death, non-fatal stroke, non-fatal myocardial infarction or non-fatal systemic embolism, whichever came first); anticoagulation (AC), aspirin, and placebo. Reproduced with permission from European Atrial Fibrillation Trial Study Group.[9]

cluded that anticoagulation is effective in reducing the risk of recurrent vascular events in nonrheumatic AF patients with recent transient ischemic attack or minor ischemic stroke. In absolute terms: 90 vascular events (mainly strokes) are prevented if 1,000 patients are treated with anticoagulation for one year. Aspirin is a safe, though less effective, alternative when anticoagulation is contraindicated; it prevents 40 vascular events each year for every 1,000 treated patients.

Propafenone v Sotalol

Because conventional antiarrhythmic therapy is often ineffective in maintaining sinus rhythm or is associated with adverse side effects in patients with AF, there is a clinical need to test newer agents. Reimold and associates,[10] from Boston, Mass, randomized 100 patients with AF who had unsuccessful therapy with two type IA antiarrhythmic agents to receive either propafenone or sotalol. Patients were stratified into four groups based on AF pattern (chronic v paroxysmal) and LA size (large [≥4.5 cm] v small [<4.5 cm]). The proportion of patients remaining in sinus rhythm on each agent was calculated for each group by the Kaplan-Meier method. For patients randomized to propafenone, 46%, 41%, and 30% remained in sinus rhythm at 3, 6, and 12 months, respectively, after cardioversion. A similar proportion of patients treated with sotalol remained in sinus rhythm at follow-up (49%, 46%, and 37% at 3, 6, and 12 months, respectively). The proportion of patients remaining in sinus rhythm on propafenone and sotalol was not dependent on arrhythmia pattern or LA dimension. Except for constipation that occurred more frequently in patients treated with propafenone, adverse side effects were equally distributed between the two therapies. Two patients receiving sotalol died during follow-up. Propafenone and sotalol, two new antiarrhythmic agents, were found to be equally effective in maintaining sinus rhythm in 100 patients with recurrent AF. Response rates were not affected by arrhythmia pattern, LA size, or unsuccessful prior drug therapy. These agents may be useful in the management of patients with recurrent symptomatic AF who have unsuccessful conventional therapy.

SUPRAVENTRICULAR TACHYCARDIA WITH AND WITHOUT SHORT P-R INTERVAL SYNDROME

Differential of Narrow QRS Complex Tachycardia

The 12-lead electrocardiogram is the basic diagnostic information available to evaluate different mechanisms producing paroxysmal narrow QRS complex tachycardias. Kalbfleisch and associates,[11] from Ann Arbor, Mich, analyzed 242 ECGs demonstrating paroxysmal narrow QRS complex tachycardia with a rate greater than 120 beats/min. The ECGs were examined in a blinded fashion and the mechanism of the tachycardia subsequently determined by standard electrophysiologic techniques. Three general types of paroxysmal supraventricular tachycardia exist including (1) atrial ventricular reciprocating tachycardia utilizing an accessory AV connection, (2) AV nodal reentrant tachycardia, and (3) atrial tachycardia. Of the 242 tachycardias, there were 137 atrial ventricular reciprocating tachycardias, 93 AV nodal reentrant tachycardias, and 12 atrial tachycardias. The criteria predictive of AV reciprocating tachycardia were the presence of a P wave distinct from the QRS complex and an RP/PR interval ratio <1, QRS alternans, and preexcitation during sinus rhythm. The criteria predictive of AV node reentrant tachycardia were the presence of a pseudo r' deflection in lead V, or pseudo S wave in the inferior leads. The criteria predictive of an atrial tachycardia were the presence of a P wave with an RP/PR interval ratio ≥1. These electrocardiographic criteria were able to accurately identify approximately 80% of AV node reentrant and AV reciprocating tachycardias, incorrectly characterized approximately 20% of paroxysmal supraventricular tachycardias, and were unable to differentiate atrial tachycardias from the other two types. Heart rate was not helpful in distinguishing the different mechanisms. The presence of a P wave separate from the QRS complex during tachycardia was found to be predictive of either AV reciprocating tachycardia or atrial tachycardia. The presence of a pseudo r' deflection in lead V_1 or a pseudo S wave in leads 2, 3, and AVF was highly predictive of AV node reentrant tachycardia.

Radiofrequency Catheter Ablation

In a report by Chen and associates,[12] from Taipei, Taiwan, 100 patients received selective radiofrequency ablation of retrograde fast pathway (32 patients, group I) or slow pathway (68 patients, group II) to treat drug-refractory AV nodal reentrant tachycardia. In group I, a mean of 6 ± 3 radiofrequency pulses eliminated the retrograde fast pathway. Thirty patients were free of symptoms and were not receiving antiarrhythmic drugs; 2 patients had accidental AV block. One patient had recurrent tachycardia and received a repeat ablation (slow pathway ablation). In group II, a mean of 9 ± 4 radiofrequency pulses eliminated the slow pathway in 68 patients. All patients were free of symptoms and were not receiving antiarrhythmic drugs. One patient had recurrent tachycardia and received a repeat ablation. Serial follow-up electrophysiologic studies (immediate [20 to 30 min], early [5 to 7 days], and late [3 to 6 months]) showed that selective ablation of retrograde fast pathway was associated with nonspecific injury on the antegrade fast pathway (increase of AH interval) without effects on the slow pathway. Selective ablation of slow pathway was associated with nonspecific injury on the retrograde fast pathway in 15 patients (22%), but the antegrade fast pathway conduction parameters did not change significantly. Thus, retrograde and antegrade fast pathway may be anatomically similar or have different sensitivities to radiofrequency energy, and slow pathway may be anatomically distinct from fast pathway. It was concluded (1) that selective radiofrequency ablation of retrograde fast or slow pathway could cure AV nodal reentrant tachycardia with a high success rate (98%) and a low recurrence rate (2%) during a follow-up period of 6 to 18 months, but fast pathway ablation was associated with accidental AV block (5%); and (2) that serial follow-up electrophysiologic studies elucidated the possible mechanisms of cure in AV nodal reentrant tachycardia.

Atrial ventricular node reentrant tachycardia is the most common form of paroxysmal SVT. The mechanism has been assumed to be reentry over two separate A-V node pathways with fast and slow conduction properties, although the anatomic location of these pathways has been less certain. Both direct current and radiofrequency energy have been used to treat these pathways by selectively ablating the fast pathway. Radiofrequency ablation has appeared to emerge as the preferred form of therapy. Mitrani and associates,[13] from Indianapolis, Ind, evaluated the effects of selected fast versus selected slow pathway radiofrequency ablation in 42 patients with drug resistant A-V node reentrant tachycardia who underwent 52 ablation attempts to prevent the tachycardia while preserving A-V conduction. Fast pathway ablation was attempted by delivering radiofrequency energy anteriorly across the tricuspid valve annulus, and slow pathway ablation was attempted by delivering radiofrequency energy posteriorly across the tricuspid valve annulus. Selective fast pathway ablation eliminated A-V node reentrant tachycardia without A-V block in 6 of 13 patients after one attempt and then an additional 3 patients (69% of total) after repeat attempts. Slow pathway ablation eliminated A-V reentrant tachycardia without A-V block in 26 (90%) of 29 patients after one ablation and in an additional 2 patients (97% of the total) after repeat ablation attempts. These authors concluded that slow pathway ablation produced more successful outcomes with a decreased prevalence of recurrent A-V node reentrant tachycardia or A-V block. Fast pathway radiofrequency ablation caused retrograde block in 7 of 11 patients, whereas no patients undergoing slow pathway ablation developed retrograde block. It should be pointed out, however, that this was not a randomized trial of ablation, and there may have been some learning curve in this series. It is also clear that recurrence of A-V node reentrant tachycardia may happen, and not all patients underwent follow-up study. Several reports have suggested that there may be multiple slow pathways in 31% to 37% of patients with A-V node reentrant tachycardia. Thus, even after successful ablation of one pathway, there may be other pathways that will lead to arrhythmias. Overall this data provides additional useful information about this effective treatment for this common arrhythmia.

In an investigation by Chen and associates,[14] from Taiwan, Republic of China, radiofrequency catheter ablation was performed in 142 patients with 166 accessory pathways. One hundred thirty-six patients with 160 accessory pathways underwent successful ablation in the first ablation session. Serial follow-up electrophysiologic studies were performed immediately (30 min), early (5 to 7 days), and late (3 to 6 months) after successful ablation to determine the recurrent accessory pathway conduction and possible new arrhythmias. After a minimum follow-up period of 6 months (mean, 14 ± 3 months), accessory pathway conduction recurred in 13 patients (9.6%), with recurrent tachycardia in 3 patients (2.2%). Five of the recurrent accessory pathways had decremental conduction properties. Incidence of recurrent accessory pathway conduction was similar in different accessory pathway locations (6.4% to 9.0%). Patients with concealed accessory pathways (12% v 2.9%) and patients without accessory pathway potentials in the ablation site (16% v 2.2%) had a higher recurrence rate. Patients without tachycardia in the late electrophysiologic study did not have recurrent tachycardia during follow-up. New arrhythmias including atrial and ventricular arrhythmias, which were detected by 24-hour Holter monitoring, were apparent only on the first day after ablation. The findings indicate that the overall incidence of recurrent accessory pathway conduction was low and that possible new arrhythmias were rare in the late follow-up period.

In an investigation by Chiang and associates,[15] from Taiwan, Republic of China, to evaluate arrhythmogenicity in patients who receive a modified direct-current shock ablation (distal pair of electrodes connected in common as the cathode) or radiofrequency ablation of SVT, a prospective study was performed with signal-averaged electrocardiography, 24-hour Holter monitoring, electrophysiologic study for VT, and treadmill exercise test. Sixty-nine consecutive patients with documented paroxysmal SVT were included. Twenty-eight patients proved to have AV nodal reentrant tachycardia, and 41 patients had AV reciprocating tachycardia that involved accessory AV pathways. The first 34 patients received direct-current shock ablation, and the other 35 patients received radiofrequency ablation. Signal-averaged electrocardiography, Holter monitoring, and electrophysiologic study for VT were performed before ablation and immediately after ablation, and then 1 week, 2 weeks (Holter monitoring), 1 month (except electrophysiologic study), and 3 months after ablation. Treadmill exercise testing was performed before ablation, and at 1 week and 3 months after ablation. The root mean square, low-amplitude signal, and QRS duration of signal-averaged electrocardiogram disclosed no significant change after either direct-current or radiofrequency ablation up to 3 months. Late potential developed in only 1 patient in the direct-current shock group, and it was considered to be innocuous because neither VT nor VF was noted or induced. Increases in the number of VPCs and in short-run VT were detected by Holter monitoring in the first week after either mode of ablation, which were greater and lasted longer in the direct-current shock group than in the radiofrequency group. Direct-current shock also caused an increased number of atrial premature contractions in the first week after ablation. No sustained VT, nonsustained VT, or sudden death was noted in either group during the follow-up period (3 months to 1 year). Sustained VT or VF was not induced by electrophysiologic study in either group up to 3 months after ablation. No exercise-induced VT was observed in either group in the study. In conclusion, these ablation methods were found to be relatively safe in treating patients with SVT, because only transient atrial and ventricular irritability were observed. Longer observation is required to evaluate long-term study.

Klein and associates,[16] from Indianapolis, Ind, determined the feasibility of radiofrequency catheter ablation of Mahaim fibers at the tricuspid annulus. Four patients who fulfilled criteria for having Mahaim fibers and preexcitation reciprocating tachycardia had radiofrequency catheter ablation. Three patients had atriofascicular connections, and one patient had an atrioventricular connection. The mean age of the patients was 27 years with a range of 11 to 48 years. All patients had highly symptomatic tachycardias resulting in syncope in one patient and presyncope in the remaining three individuals. Symptoms were present for a mean of 13 years. All pathways conducted only anterogradely, and preexcitation resulted in a left BBB block QRS morphology. Adenosine caused block in the accessory pathway in three patients in whom it was tested. The stimulus to delta interval increased by 75 ms during rapid atrial pacing. The atrial insertion of the Mahaim fiber was in the right lateral atrium in one patient, right posterolateral atrium in two patients, and right posterior atrium in one patient. The ventricular insertion was in the distal right bundle branch in three patients and in the posterolateral right ventricle near the tricuspid annulus in the patient with the AV connection. The stimulus to delta wave mapping was used to help localize the atrial insertion of the atriofascicular connection. A mean of 15 radiofrequency pulses delivered to the tricuspid annulus in the posterior to lateral regions eliminated accessory pathway conduction in all patients. No complications occurred. Tachycardia did not recur during a mean follow-up of 8 months. Thus, radiofrequency current applied to the tricuspid annulus may safely eliminate tachycardia in selected patients with Mahaim fibers.

In an investigation by Chen and associates,[17] from Taipei, Taiwan, complete electrophysiologic study and radiofrequency ablation were performed in 145 consecutive patients with WPW syndrome. Presence of multiple accessory A-V pathways was documented in 20 patients (14%); 17 patients had two, 2 patients had three, and 1 patient had four accessory pathways. Location of accessory pathways was posteroseptal in 18 patients, left free wall in 15 patients, right free wall in 9 patients, and right midseptal in 2 patients. Of the 44 pathways, 36 were found during baseline electrophysiologic study, and 8 were found after successful ablation of the initially attempted pathways. After delivering 20 ± 23 pulses (per patient) of radiofrequency energy (37 ± 6 W, 70 ± 30 sec), 43 accessory pathways were ablated successfully without complications. Duration of the procedure (4.5 ± 1.7 v 3.7 ± 1.6 hours) and radiation exposure time (53 ± 30 v 38 ± 18 min) were longer in patients with multiple pathways, whereas the success rate (95% v 95%) and incidence of recurrent conduction (11% v 11%) were similar in patients with single or multiple accessory pathways. These findings confirm that multiple accessory pathways are common in patients with WPW syndrome, and these pathways can be ablated successfully by radiofrequency energy with a success rate comparable to that of a single accessory pathway.

Radiofrequency ablation of accessory A-V connections has an efficacy of about 95% and a favorable cost-benefit ratio even though patients have been traditionally kept in the hospital for two to five days. Kalbfleisch and associates,[18] from Ann Arbor, Mich, prospectively evaluated 137 consecutive patients. Exclusionary criteria included an age less than 13 or greater than 70 years, anteroseptal location of the accessory A-V connection, obesity, or a clinical indication for hospitalization. Patients with venous punctures had a recovery period of three hours and those with arterial punctures had a recovery period of six hours. Thirty-seven of the 137 patients were excluded for the above reasons, which left 100 consecutive patients who underwent this procedure. The pathway was left-sided in 67 patients and right-sided or posteroseptal in 33 patients. The procedure was successful in 97 of 100 cases. In 70 cases, the patient was discharged the same day; in 30 cases, the patient required an overnight stay because the procedure was completed too late in the day for recovery in the outpatient facility. At follow-up, 2 patients had a clinically significant complication (femoral artery pseudoaneurysm). The mean cost of the procedure was slightly over $10,000. These authors concluded that this important technique can be performed in selected patients on an outpatient basis and thus, would be very cost-effective in the current health-care environment.

Primary atrial tachycardias are relatively uncommon arrhythmias that may be especially difficult to control with standard antiarrhythmic medications. Some preliminary data has suggested that radiofrequency ablation may be effective in their control. Kay and associates,[19] from Birmingham, Ala, further evaluated radiofrequency ablation in 15 consecutive patients with primary atrial arrhythmias that were refractory to medical treatment. Eleven patients had ectopic atrial tachycardia, and 4 patients had sinus node reentry. The origin of the tachycardia was the right atrium in 14 patients and the left atrium in 1 patient. Radiofrequency energy successfully terminated the primary atrial tachycardia in each of the patients, and all were discharged from the laboratory in sinus rhythm without inducible atrial tachycardia. A mean of 11 radiofrequency applications were delivered using 30 watts of power for 30 seconds. No complications were observed, although 1 patient with incessant ectopic atrial tachycardia had sinus pauses after ablation. During a mean follow-up time of 277 days, the arrhythmias recurred in 3 patients, including 2 patients with ectopic atrial tachycardia and 1 patient with sinus node reentry. One of these patients was successfully treated in a second ablation session. These authors concluded that radiofrequency catheter ablation is a safe and effective technique for the treatment of primary atrial arrhythmias that are refractory to anti-arrhythmic medication.

In a study by Chen and associates,[20] from Taipei, Taiwan, a total of 408 patients received radiofrequency catheter ablation for paroxysmal SVT; and 326 patients underwent serial follow-up electrophysiologic studies (early and late) after initially successful radiofrequency catheter ablation of accessory pathways (group 1, 186 patients with WPW) and slow A-V nodal pathways (group 2, 140 patients with A-V nodal reentrant tachycardia). Among the patients in group 1, early (4 ± 1 days) and late (129 ± 14 days) studies found recurrent conduction through the accessory pathways in 12 and 16 patients, respectively. During a follow-up period of 21 ± 7 months, recurrence of accessory pathway-mediated tachyarrhythmias was noted in 6 patients. Of these 6 patients, all had tachycardia inducible in the late study but not in the early study. Among the patients in group 2, four had recurrence of A-V nodal reentrant tachycardia during a follow-up of 16 ± 6 months. Of the 4 patients, 1 had tachycardia inducible in the early (4 ± 1 days) study and 3 in the late (130 ± 12 days) study. The results demonstrated that the early study was not as sensitive as the late follow-up electrophysiologic study in predicting late outcome of radiofrequency ablation, but both the early and late studies had a high total predictive accuracy (>90%) in groups 1 and 2. Furthermore, only 4 of the 326 patients had initial evidence of recurrent tachycardia activated by programmed electrical stimuli during follow-up studies, suggesting that follow-up electrophysiologic studies in asymptomatic patients are not warranted.

Surgical Treatment

Ectopic atrial tachycardia is an uncommon arrhythmia that is frequently unresponsive to medical therapy. Prager and associates,[21] from St. Louis, Mo, evaluated the effects of medical and then surgical therapy in 15 consecutive patients with ectopic atrial tachycardia. All 15 patients were initially treated with antiarrhythmic drugs (mean, 5.7). An effective drug regimen was identified in only 5 of the 15 patients. The remaining 10 patients were treated surgically. The procedure was guided by computer-assisted intraoperative mapping. Focal ablation was performed in 4 patients and atrial isolation procedures in 6. The patients were followed for a mean of 4 years. A permanent pacemaker was implanted in 2 patients, one of whom required re-operation for constrictive pericarditis. There were no operative deaths. Ectopic atrial tachycardia recurred in 3 of the 5 patients discharged on antiarrhythmic therapy. Map guided surgery abolished symptoms in 9 of 10 patients with ectopic atrial tachycardia. These authors concluded that surgery is an effective alternative for patients with ectopic atrial tachycardias that were not easily treated with antiarrhythmic drugs.

Verapamil

Lai and associates,[22] from Kaohsiung, Taiwan, studied the electrophysiologic effects of intravenous verapamil (0.15 mg/kg) and oral sustained-release verapamil (verapamil-SR) (240 mg once daily for 7 days) in 17 patients with paroxysmal SVT. Ten patients had AV nodal reentrant tachycardia, and 7 had AV reciprocating tachycardia involving an accessory AV pathway. Both preparations significantly prolonged anterograde effective refractory period of the AV node and depressed the retrograde AV nodal conduction system. The sinus cycle length and atrial and ventricular effective refractory periods were prolonged after oral verapamil-SR. Furthermore, oral verapamil-SR depressed retrograde accessory pathway conduction, which was not interfered with by intravenous verapamil. Intravenous verapamil and oral verapamil-SR prevented induction of sustained SVT in 12 of 17 and 10 of 17 patients, respectively. Follow-up study with oral verapamil-SR 240 mg once daily in 15 patients for 19 months revealed that among the 8 patients without induction of sustained SVT, 7 have been free of symptomatic arrhythmia; only one patient had occasional supraventricular tachycardia attacks. For the 7 patients with induction of sustained SVT, 3 patients failed to respond to oral verapamil-SR, 1 patient became symptom free, and the remaining 3 patients had less frequent supraventricular attacks. Thus, immediate intravenous verapamil testing predicts the electrophysiologic results of oral verapamil-SR therapy, and oral verapamil-SR once daily may be used for long-term prophylaxis of SVT with better patient compliance.

VENTRICULAR ARRHYTHMIAS

Self-Terminating

VF is generally regarded as being lethal unless promptly halted. There have been reports of self-terminating VF, but similar events are described by some cardiologists as polymorphic VT or even torsade de pointes. To examine how experienced cardiologists would diagnose such tachyarrhythmias, electrocardiograms of self-terminating ventricular tachyarrhythmias compatible with accepted definitions of VF (rate >300/min) were sent to 22 cardiologists by Clayton and associates.[23] During the study period of 19 months, 2,462 patients treated in a ten-bed coronary-care unit were monitored by use of a single bipolar chest lead. Forty-five (2%) had episodes of VF that were terminated by direct current shock. Twelve self-terminating tachyarrhythmias (duration 5.2 to 49.5) were recorded from 8 patients, 3 of whom also had sustained VF terminated by direct current shock. The cardiologists offered 264 diagnoses for the self-terminating events: 42 (15.9%) VF, 99 (37.5%) polymorphic VT, 98 (37.1%) torsade de pointes, and 25 (9.5%) "other." The cardiologists differed in their response patterns. The findings show that rapid self-terminating ventricular tachyarrhythmias are not uncommon in coronary-care unit patients and that the diagnostic categorization of these important events is highly subjective and inconsistent.

Right Ventricular Dysplasia

Metzger and associates,[24] from Maastricht, The Netherlands, studied the 12-lead electrocardiogram during sinus rhythm in 20 patients with arrhythmogenic RV dysplasia with symptomatic VT. Findings were analyzed, together with echocardiographic evaluation of site, extent, and progression of RV wall abnormalities. Electrocardiographic abnormalities were found in 90% of patients. No correlation was found between abnormalities on the initial 12-lead electrocardiogram and the echocardiographic extent and location of RV involvement. Over time, echocardiographic progression of the disease was observed; RV size increased in 6 of 7 patients from 34 to 39 mm, and there was progression in the extent of RV wall-motion abnormalities in 4 of 7 patients. Analysis of serial electrocardiographic recordings did not reveal changes indicative of progression of the disease during follow-up of 71 months. The investigators concluded that electrocardiographic abnormalities suggesting arrhythmogenic RV dysplasia are present in 90% of symptomatic patients on the first electrocardiogram recorded during sinus rhythm. Serial electrocardiographic recordings in these patients do not provide information regarding anatomic progression of the disease.

Electrophysiologic Study v Electrocardiographic Monitoring for Predicting Drug Efficacy

The ESVEM Investigators,[25] from Salt Lake City, Utah, determined the accuracy of predictors of antiarrhythmic drug efficacy using electrophysiological studies and compared them with Holter monitoring and exercise testing in 486 randomized patients. Patients with ventricular tachyarrhythmias were randomly assigned to undergo serial testing of up to six antiarrhythmic drugs by either electrophysiologic study or Holter monitoring and exercise testing. Efficacy predictions were achieved in 108 of 242 patients in the electrophysiologic limb and in 188 of 244 patients in the Holter monitoring limb (77%) after electrophysiologic limb (45%). LVEFs less than 0.25 and presence of CAD were negative correlates of drug efficacy predictions in the electrophysiologic limb. In the Holter monitoring limb, LVEF was the lone univariate correlate of efficacy, although it was only marginally significant. A multivariate model selected assessment by Holter monitoring and higher LVEF as independent predictors of drug efficacy. In this study, the drug evaluation process required a median time of 25 days in the electrophysiology limb and 10 days in the Holter monitoring limb. Thus, drug efficacy predictions were achieved more frequently by Holter monitoring and exercise testing than by electrophysiology study (Figure 4-3). Assessment by Holter monitoring and the severity of LV dysfunction are independent correlates of drug efficacy prediction. In this study, drug testing was considerably shorter for the Holter monitoring method.

Invasive electrophysiologic study and noninvasive Holter monitoring (in conjunction with exercise testing) have both been used to evaluate the efficacy of antiarrhythmic drugs in patients with sustained VT and in survivors of cardiac arrest. Mason,[26] for the Electrophysiologic Study

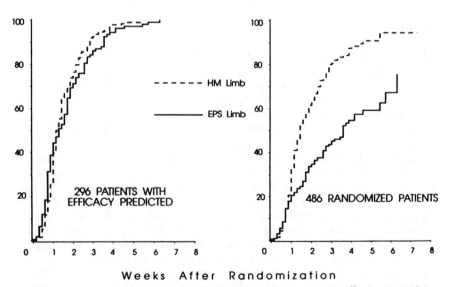

Weeks After Randomization

Figure 4-3. This figure demonstrates that Holter monitoring is more effective in predicting drug efficacy effect than electrophysiologic studies. Reproduced with permission from The ESVEM Investigators.[25]

Table 4-1. Categorization of Recurrences of Arrhythmia among Patients Receiving Drugs Predicted to be Effective. Reproduced with permission from Mason.[26]

CATEGORY*	ALL PATIENTS (N = 296)	HOLTER MONITORING (N = 188)	ELECTRO-PHYSIO-LOGIC STUDY (N = 108)
	no. (%) of patients		
Death from arrhythmia	34 (11)	18 (10)	16 (15)
Cardiac arrest	16 (5)	11 (6)	5 (5)
Sustained VT			
Terminated by DC shock	41 (14)	27 (14)	14 (13)
Terminated by intravenous drug	10 (3)	6 (3)	4 (4)
Terminated spontaneously	27 (9)	19 (10)	8 (7)
Unmonitored syncope	8 (3)	6 (3)	2 (2)
Unsustained VT	11 (4)	6 (3)	5 (5)
Torsade de pointes VT	3 (1)	1 (1)	2 (2)
All recurrences	150 (51)	94 (50)	56 (52)

*VT denotes ventricular tachycardia, and DC direct current.

versus Electrocardiographic Monitoring Investigators, directly compared these two approaches with the prediction of drug efficacy. A total of 486 patients who had documented VT that were inducible during electrophysiologic study and ten or more premature ventricular complexes per hour during Holter monitoring were randomly assigned to undergo serial testing of antiarrhythmic-drug efficacy by electrophysiologic study or Holter monitoring. The patients received up to six drugs in random order until one was predicted to be effective either in suppressing inducible arrhythmia (in the electrophysiologic-study group) or in suppressing premature ventricular complexes (in the Holter-monitoring group). The patients were then followed for recurrences of arrhythmia or death. In the electrophysiologic-study group, 108 of 242 patients (45%) received a prediction of efficacy, as compared with 188 of 244 patients (77%) in the Holter-monitoring group. Over a six-year follow-up period, there were 150 recurrences of arrhythmia and 46 deaths among the 296 patients receiving drugs predicted to be effective (Table 4-1). Thirty-four of the deaths were from arrhythmic causes, and 8 were from cardiac causes. There were no significant differences between the two study groups in the actuarial probabilities of these events. The risk of a recurrence of arrhythmia was significantly lower in patients who received sotalol than in those who received other antiarrhythmic drugs, and the risk was lower in those who had not previously failed to respond to antiarrhythmic drugs than in those who had. Although Holter monitoring led to predictions of antiarrhythmic-drug efficacy more often than did electrophysiologic study in patients with sustained ventricular tachyarrhythmias, there was no significant difference in the success of drug therapy as selected by the two methods.

Inducibility Without Structural Heart Disease

In a report by Brodsky and associates,[27] from Orange, Calif, 37 patients with symptomatic ventricular tachyarrhythmia and no apparent structural heart disease were evaluated with multiple cardiovascular tests to establish the relationship between the results of programmed electric stimulation and other clinical and arrhythmia variables. Of 37 patients, 12 (32%) had inducible sustained VT. Factors associated with the results of programmed electric stimulation included a history of VT ≥30 seconds requiring intervention for termination and global right heart abnormality documented by echocardiography. During treatment for a mean follow-up of 50 months, 29 patients did well, 6 patients had recurrences of major arrhythmia symptoms, 1 was lost to follow-up, and 1 had a noncardiac death. Those patients with an adverse outcome were more likely to have inducible VT. Thus, certain clinical and echocardiographic data are associated with the results of programmed electric stimulation, which in turn have important prognostic value in this group of patients. Sustained VT is unlikely to be induced in patients with no evidence of structural heart disease and clinical nonsustained VT.

Effects of Adenosine and Acetylcholine

Lerman,[28] from New York, NY, evaluated the response of nonreentrant catecholamine-mediated VT to endogenous adenosine and acetylcholine. Reentrant VT is known to be insensitive to adenosine. However, nonreentrant, catecholamine-mediated VT may be initiated with rapid pacing and is sensitive to exogenous adenosine as well as the Valsalva maneuver. The mechanism of this tachycardia is thought to be due to a catecholamine-induced, cyclic AMP-mediated increase in intracellular calcium, resulting in delayed after-depolarizations and triggered activity. Eight patients were studied who received dipyridamole, a transport blocker that potentiates the effects of adenosine; and it abolished sustained nonreentrant, nonautomatic, catecholamine-mediated VT in the five patients in whom it was evaluated. VT recurred with the addition of aminophylline, a competitive adenosine receptor antagonist. Edrophonium, a cholinesterase inhibitor that potentiates the effects of acetylcholine at the muscarinic cholinergic receptor, terminated VT in four of four patients, an effect that was reversed by atropine. In six patients with reentrant VT, dipyridamole and edrophonium had no effect on the VT. In four patients, adenosine and vagal maneuvers had no effect on catecholamine-mediated VT caused by automaticity. In one patient, adenosine transiently suppressed VT after which it spontaneously resumed. This study demonstrates the mechanism of a newly recognized form of VT. It can be identified by termination of the tachycardia in response to the activation of adenosine A_1 or muscarinic cholinergic receptors, which results in inhibition of adenylate cyclase. These receptor-mediated effects appear to be specific for identifying nonreentrant, nonautomatic, catecholamine-induced VT.

Inducibility After Amiodarone Therapy

The outcome of patients who receive intravenous amiodarone for suppression of incessant ventricular tachyarrhythmia has not been studied conclusively. Thus, Kowey and associates,[29] from Wynnewood and Philadelphia, Pa, conducted a prospective study in which all patients who responded acutely to intravenous amiodarone and went on to receive a subsequent oral loading dose were subjected to electrophysiologic testing before hospital discharge to determine whether additional or alternative therapy would be required. Among 18 patients (17 with ischemic heart disease) who entered the protocol, 16 had a clinical response to intravenous amiodarone alone (12 patients) or in combination with another antiarrhythmic drug (4 patients) and survived to study. Of these patients, 10 had monomorphic VT when first seen, 5 had polymorphous VT or VF, and 3 had both. In 7 patients, sustained monomorphic VT was inducible (group 1), and in 9 patients, it was not (group 2). The only clinical factor that distinguished group 1 from group 2 was age (group 1 > group 2). Five patients in group 1 and 1 in group 2 received an implantable cardioverterdefibrillator; 1 patient in group 1 had a successful endocardial resection. During a mean follow-up period of 11 months, 4 patients in group 1 have had appropriate implantable cardioverter-defibrillator discharges, whereas only 1 patient in group 2 has had a clinical event (sudden death). These investigators concluded that intravenous amiodarone is a highly effective drug used alone or in combination to suppress spontaneous incessant VT/VF. Predischarge electrophysiologic testing, even in patients who have polymorphous VT, has predictive value over and above the observed clinical response. These results favor predischarge testing and aggressive device treatment in this cohort.

Comparison of Seven Antiarrhythmic Drugs

The relative efficacies of various antiarrhythmic drugs in the treatment of ventricular tachyarrhythmias are not well known. Mason,[30] for the Electrophysiologic Study versus Electrocardiographic Monitoring Investigators, examined the effectiveness of imipramine, mexiletine, pirmenol, procainamide, propafenone, quinidine, and sotalol in patients with ventricular tachyarrhythmias who were enrolled in the Electrophysiologic Study versus Electrocardiographic Monitoring trial. Patients were randomly assigned to undergo serial testing of the efficacy of the seven antiarrhythmic drugs by one of two strategies: electrophysiologic study or Holter monitoring together with exercise testing. The seven drugs were then tested for efficacy in random order in patients who were eligible to receive them. The frequencies of predictions of drug efficacy and of adverse drug effects during the initial drug titration were tabulated for all 486 randomized subjects. Patients received long-term treatment with the first antiarrhythmic drug that was predicted to be effective on the basis of drug testing. Recurrences of arrhythmia, deaths, and adverse drug effects during long-term follow-up were recorded for the 296 patients in whom an antiarrhythmic drug was predicted to be effective. In the electrophysiologic-study group, the percentage of patients who had predictions of drug efficacy was higher with sotalol (35%) than with the other drugs (16%). There was not significant difference among the drugs in the Holter-monitoring group. The percentage of patients with adverse drug effects was lowest among those receiving sotalol. The actuarial probability of a recurrence of arrhythmia after a prediction of drug efficacy by either strategy was significantly lower for patients treated with sotalol than for patients treated with the other drugs (risk ratio, 0.43). With sotalol, as compared with the other drugs combined, there were lower risks of death from any cause (risk ratio, 0.50), death from cardiac causes (0.50), and death from arrhythmia (0.50). The cumulative percentage of patients in whom a drug was predicted to be effective and in whom it remained effective and tolerated was higher for sotalol than for the other drugs. Sotalol was more effective than the other 6 antiarrhythmic drugs in preventing death and recurrences of arrhythmia. In patients similar to those in this study, if antiarrhythmic-drug therapy is to be used to prevent recurrences of ventricular tachyarrhythmias, treatment with sotalol and assessment of its potential efficacy of Holter monitoring are a reasonable initial strategy.

Verapamil

A study by Gill and associates,[31] from London, United Kingdom, examines the efficacy of verapamil for the suppression of idiopathic VT of left BBB-like morphology. Forty-two patients (mean age, 36 ± 12 years; 20 men and 22 women) with VT and without any underlying cardiac abnormality on clinical examination and noninvasive investigation were studied. The inducibility of clinical VT was examined by treadmill exercise testing and programmed ventricular stimulation. VT was inducible in 19 patients by exercise testing and in 24 by programmed ventricular stimulation; and in 23 there was evidence of VT on Holter monitoring. After baseline testing, patients were treated with verapamil 120 mg three times daily for at least 5 half-lives, for the drug to load before evaluation. With Holter monitoring, 74% of patients with evidence of VT at baseline testing demonstrated a change of status from nonsustained VT to no VT or from sustained VT to nonsustained VT. Four patients had nonsustained VT during verapamil treatment but no VT at baseline. There was a significant reduction in the number of ventricular ectopic beats over 24 hours (baseline: 15,541 ± 17,599 v verapamil treatment: 8,892 ± 15,582). Exercise-induced VT was suppressed in 56% of patients with VT during baseline testing, but no effect of verapamil on the tachycardia was observed in 26%. The remaining patients demonstrated a partial response to verapamil; the rate of VT was unchanged, although the duration of the runs was reduced. Sustained monomorphic VT was inducible in only 5 patients, of whom 4 were rendered noninducible; 1 patient remained inducible. However, of the 13 patients with nonsustained VT inducible at baseline, 4 became sustained, of which 2 were hemodynamically unstable. There was no obvious difference in the age or sex distribution of the patients, axis of VT, presence of abnormal cardiac histology, or late potentials among patients responding to verapamil during Holter monitoring or exercise testing. VT of an inferior axis was more likely to respond to verapamil, whereas VT of a superior axis did not respond to verapamil during Holter monitoring. It was concluded that idiopathic VT of left BBB-like morphology can be suppressed in approximately two-thirds of patients by verapamil. In patients with a partial response, the rate of VT was unaffected. Some patients exhibit exacerbation of the arrhythmia, and verapamil should be avoided in these cases.

Sotalol ± Quinidine or Procainamide

In patients with VT, individual antiarrhythmic drugs are often ineffective in preventing the induction and recurrence of sustained VT. Dorian and associates,[32] from Toronto, Canada, reasoned that combination therapy with sotalol, which has β-blocking properties and prolongs ventricular refractoriness, and quinidine or procainamide, which slow conduction and prolong refractory period, would be effective therapy in such patients. They evaluated low dose sotalol (205 ± 84 mg/day) plus quinidine sulfate (1,278 ± 479 mg/day) or procainamide (2,393 ± 1,423 mg/day) in 50 patients with spontaneous sustained VT or fibrillation and inducible VT. In 46% of the patients, VT was rendered noninducible. In 37% of the patients, inducible VT was modified according to prospectively identified criteria for a combined 83% response rate. Ventricular refractory periods were increased. The cycle length of induced VT was slowed. Forty-two of the 50 patients were discharged on treatment with a drug combination. After an average of 25 months of follow-up, the recurrence rate of VT was 6%, 6%, and 11% at 1, 2, and 3 years, respectively. In patients in whom the drug combination was unsuccessful at electrophysiologic study and in those who received alternate therapy after combination therapy was discontinued because of side-effects, actuarial recurrence rates were 9%, 14%, and 32% at 1, 2, and 3 years, respectively. These authors concluded that the combination of sotalol plus quinidine or procainamide is an effective form of combined therapy for the treatment of sustained VT.

Amiodarone

In an investigation by Weinberg and associates,[33] from Indianapolis, Ind, between 1977 and 1986, 589 patients (aged 57 ± 13 years; 464 men and 125 women) received amiodarone for VF (147 patients), sustained VT (242 patients), or nonsustained VT (80 patients), or SVT (120 patients). Mean LVEF was 36% ± 17%, with 23% in New York Heart Association functional class I, 49% in class II, 25% in class III, and 3% in class IV. Sixty-two percent had ischemic heart disease. Follow-up was 32 ± 27 months. Life-table analysis revealed that patients with VF, sustained VT, and nonsustained VT had a cumulative incidence of sudden death of 9% at 1 year, increasing by about 3% per year. By years 2 and 5, the cumulative incidence of sudden death, VF or sustained VT recurrence, was 26% and 38% and the percent of patients still taking amiodarone was 54% and 32%. For patients with SVT at years 2 and 5, the cumulative incidence of sudden death was 1% and 3%; and of sudden death or SVT recurrence, the cumulative incidence was 20% and 29%. The percent of patients still taking amiodarone was 67% and 43%. Of 14 clinical variables assessed, New York Heart Association functional class was the best predictor of sudden death and arrhythmic failure, and no other variable added independent predictive power. Older age and lower LVEF were independent predictors of drug failure (sudden death or arrhythmic failure or need to discontinue amiodarone because of side effects). It was concluded that despite its side-effect profile, amiodarone is an effective and reasonably well-tolerated antiarrhythmic drug.

Olson and associates,[34] from Chapel Hill, NC, analyzed 122 patients treated chronically with amiodarone for sustained VT or VF after failing conventional antiarrhythmic therapy to determine which factors were predictive of sudden cardiac death during follow-up. The mean LVEF in the study group was 0.32, and 87% of the patients had CAD with a prior AMI. During a median follow-up of 19.5 months, 30 patients died suddenly. The only variable that was predictive of sudden death was LVEF.

Twenty-nine of the 84 patients with EF <0.40 died suddenly, compared with 1 of 35 patients with EF 20.40. The actuarial probability of sudden death at 5 years was 49% when the EF was <0.40 and 5% when the EF was 20.40. These results indicate that patients treated with amiodarone for sustained VT or VF whose EF are 20.40 are at low risk for sudden death. Patients with EF <0.40 remain at high risk for sudden death and should be considered for additional or alternative therapy.

Modifying Antiarrhythmic Therapy for Drug Intolerance or Efficacy

The incidence of recurrent VT and drug intolerance after therapy guided by electrophysiology study leading to a change in antiarrhythmic therapy is unknown. To explore this issue, Ujhelyi and associates,[35] from Hartford, Farmington, and Stors, Conn, studied 138 patients undergoing electrophysiology study with a serial drug testing protocol. Patients were followed for 24 ± 21 months (range, 1 to 91 months) for recurrent VT, drug intolerance, or both. At baseline electrophysiology study, sustained VT (76%), nonsustained VT (20%), and VF (4%) were induced. On discharge antiarrhythmic therapy, 70 patients (51%) were noninducible (<16 beats), and 68 patients (49%) remained inducible. Of the 138 patients, 56 (41%) required modification of antiarrhythmic therapy (change in drug or dose) for recurrent VT (n = 20) or drug intolerance (n = 36). These events occurred early during follow-up (8 ± 12 months). Patients who were rendered noninducible had a greater likelihood of remaining free of antiarrhythmic modification than patients who remained inducible at 1 year (68% and 60%, respectively) and 2-year (63% and 52%, respectively) follow-up examinations. Likewise, the noninducible patients had a greater likelihood of remaining free of recurrent VT than inducible patients at 1-year (95% and 80%, respectively) and 2-year (92% and 80%, respectively) follow-up testing. In contrast, the likelihood of remaining free of drug intolerance was similar between inducible and noninducible patients at 1-year (72% and 75%, respectively) and 2-year (69% and 65%, respectively) follow-up. It was concluded that antiarrhythmic therapy guided by electrophysiology study requires early modification in >40% of patients during follow-up. In addition, inducible patients require a change in antiarrhythmic therapy more frequently than noninducible patients because of higher incidence of recurrent VT.

Torsades de Pointes in Women

To test the hypothesis that female prevalence is greater than expected among reported cases of torsades de pointes associated with cardiovascular drugs that prolong cardiac repolarization, Makkar and associates,[36] from Detroit, Mich, did a MEDLINE search of the English-language literature for the period of 1980 to 1992, using the terms *torsade de pointes, polymorphic VT, atypical VT, proarrhythmia, and drug-induced VT*, supplemented by pertinent references (dating back to 1964). Ninety-three articles were identified describing at least one case of polymorphic VT (with gender specified) associated with quinidine, procainamide hydrochloride, disopyramide, amiodarone, sotalol hydrochloride, bepridil hydrochloride, or prenylamine. A total of 332 patients were included in the analysis following application of prospectively defined criteria (eg, corrected QT interval of 0.45 seconds or greater while receiving drug). Clinical and electrocardiographic descriptors were extracted for analysis. Expected female prevalence for torsades de pointes associated with quinidine, procainamide, disopyramide, and amiodarone was conservatively estimated from gender-specific data reported for antiarrhythmic drug prescriptions in 1986, as derived from the National Disease and Therapeutic Index, a large pharmaceutical database; expected female prevalence for torsades de pointes associated with sotalol, bepridil, and prenylamine was assumed to be 50% or less because these agents are prescribed for male-predominant cardiovascular conditions. Women made up 70% of the 332 reported cases of cardiovascular-drug-related torsades de pointes, and a female prevalence exceeding 50% was observed in 20 (83%) of 24 studies having at least four included cases. When analyzed according to various descriptors, women still constituted the majority (range, 51% to 94% of torsades de pointes cases), irrespective of the presence or absence of underlying coronary artery or rheumatic heart disease, LV dysfunction, type of underlying arrhythmia, hypokalemia, hypomagnesemia, bradycardia, concomitant digoxin treatment, or level of QT_c at baseline or while receiving drug. When cases or torsades de pointes were analyzed by individual drug, observed female prevalence was always greater than expected, representing a statistically significant difference for all agents except procainamide. These findings strongly suggest that women are more prone than men to develop torsades de pointes during administration of cardiovascular drugs that prolong cardiac repolarization.

Radiofrequency Catheter Ablation

Morady and associates,[37] from Ann Arbor, Mich, determined the feasibility of using radiofrequency ablation of VT in patients with CAD. Fifteen consecutive patients with CAD and a history of MI underwent an attempt at radiofrequency ablation of 16 hemodynamically stable monomorphic VTs documented clinically on a 12-lead ECG that had not been successfully managed by pharmacological or device therapy. One VT was incessant, 5 occurred more than 25 times, and the remainder occurred 2 to 20 times. An additional 4 VTs that had not been documented clinically also were targeted for ablation. The mean age of the patients was 68 ± 7 years. Their mean LVEFs were 0.27. The mean cycle length of 20 VTs targeted for ablation was 438 ± 82 ms. Ablation sites were identified based on endocardial activation mapping, pace mapping, identification of an isolated middiastolic potential, or concealed entrainment. Sixteen of the 20 VTs (80%) were ablated in 11 of 15 patients (73%), using a mean of 4 ± 3 applications of radiofrequency energy, and no recurrences of ablated VTs occurred during 9 ± 3 months of follow-up. The mean duration of the ablation procedure was 128 ± 30 minutes. There were no complications. This study demonstrates that radiofrequency ablation of hemodynamically stable VTs is feasible in selected patients with CAD.

Catheter ablation of VT with radiofrequency current is known to be safer than conventional ablation with direct current shocks. In an investigation by Aizawa and associates,[38] from Niigata, Japan, seven patients who had eight morphologically distinct symptomatic monomorphic VTs originating from the right ventricle underwent catheter ablation with radiofrequency current. The mean age was 52 ± 16 years, and the mean cycle length of the clinical VT was 298 ± 36 ms. Sustained VT was induced by programmed stimulation with or without isoproterenol in four patients and developed during the infusion of isoproterenol alone in two patients. Of these, four VTs were entrained with rapid pacing. The ablation was attempted at the site of earliest activation through the distal electrode and the external patch electrode on the back during VT in seven episodes in six patients. In the other patient, it was applied during sinus rhythm. Energy was 40 to 50 W in the first case and 30 to 40 W in the others, and was given for 30 seconds. All VTs were terminated within 6 seconds, 3.6 ± 0.8 seconds after the application of the radiofrequency current. Additional current was given to one to four predetermined sites by mapping. The mean number of applications was 4.0 ± 1.3 sites. Except in the first patient, VT was eliminated successfully and VT was not induced by programmed stimulation, by the administration of isoproterenol, or by treadmill exercise testing. VT did not recur during the follow-up period of 6.8 ± 1.1 months.

Nakagawa and associates,[39] from Oklahoma City, Okla, determined how frequently potentials generated by the Purkinje fiber network can be recorded preceding ventricular activation "P potential," and the role of the P potential in guiding radiofrequency catheter ablation. Eight patients with a mean age of 26 years and LV tachycardia cycle length of 346 ± 59 ms were evaluated. RV and LV endocardial mapping during tachycardia identified earliest ventricular activation at the posteroapical LV septum. In all patients, earliest ventricular activation during tachycardia was preceded by distinct potential. This potential also preceded ventricular activation during sinus rhythm consistent with activation of a segment of LV posterior fascicle. The earliest recorded P potential preceded the QRS during tachycardia of 15 to 42 ms. The application of radiofrequency current at one to four sites eliminated idiopathic left ventricular tachycardia in all patients. In the seven patients with P potentials recorded at multiple sites within the posteroapical septum, ablation was successful at the site of the earliest P potential and unrelated to the timing of ventricular activation. In the remaining patients, ablation was successful at a site recording a late P potential fusing with the earliest ventricular activation. During follow-up, idiopathic left ventricular tachycardia recurred only in the latter patient. Pace mapping during tachycardia at the successful ablation site in four patients produced a similar QRS with stimulus-QRS interval equal to P-QRS interval during tachycardia. These findings support the hypothesis that idiopathic LV tachycardia originates from the Purkinje network of the LV posterior fascicle. A P potential can be recorded at the posteroapical LV septum during idiopathic left ventricular tachycardia, and ablation is successful at the site recording the earliest P potential.

Coronary Bypass

The role of myocardial revascularization in the treatment of malignant ventricular arrhythmias is not well defined. Berntsen and associates,[40] from Tromsø, Norway, hypothesized that in patients with VT or VF exposed by exercise-induced ischemia, the acute transient ischemia plays a principal causal role, and that in these patients, surgical myocardial revascularization alone might be an effective treatment. Among 1,100 consecutive patients undergoing isolated CABG, 30 patients (2.7%) characterized by VT or VF at symptom-limited exercise test prior to revascularization were studied prospectively. All patients had exercise-induced angina pectoris or ischemic ST-segment depression preceding ≥1 of the arrhythmic events. In addition, 8 of these 30 patients had experienced syncope during out-of-hospital exertional activities. After surgical revascularization, the 28 patients surviving to hospital discharge were followed for 1.6 to 86 months (mean, 29 ± 29 months) as outpatients and underwent between 1 to 8 exercise tests (mean, 2.6 ± 1.9). One of these patients died suddenly of unknown cause at 14 months and another from cancer at 53 months. Twenty-six patients experienced a total of 34 episodes of VT before revascularization. Two patients, both having residual ischemia, had arrhythmia recurrences during follow-up. Exercise-induced VF occurred in 8 patients preoperatively. None of these had recurrence during follow-up, and none of the 8 who experienced a total of 15 episodes of syncope on exertion out-of-hospital preoperatively had any recurrences during the follow-up period. These results indicate that severe ventricular arrhythmias, including sustained monomorphic VT, exposed by exercise-induced ischemia, may effectively be abolished by surgical myocardial revascularization alone. The subjective maximal exercise test appears to be an effective means of identifying this subset of patients in which no additional antiarrhythmic treatment seems to be required.

CARDIAC ARREST

Review

To integrate information from the various disciplines that contribute to the understanding of the cause and prevention of sudden cardiac death, Myerburg and associates,[41] from Miami, Fla, reviewed a broad range of research reports and interpretations of data from English-language journal articles and reviews, published primarily between 1970 and 1993. These authors concluded that progress in the prevention of sudden death will require development of new approaches including epidemiologic techniques to address risk characteristics specific to the problem; characterization of triggering events and identification of specific persons at risk for responding adversely to these events; and methods of evaluating outcomes appropriate to the nature of sudden cardiac death.

Survival Rates

Survival rates from out-of-hospital cardiac arrest due to VF or pulseless VT vary greatly. The majority of published reports indicate a survival rate from 11% to 33%, depending on the area of observation. Two recent series from major metropolitan centers describe markedly less favorable outcomes and have led to speculation that dense urbanization may contribute to worse outcomes. Solomon,[42] from New Haven, Conn, reviewed a consecutive series of out-of-hospital cardiac arrests in New Haven, Conn, a city of 127,000 people and 55 km² with a two-tiered emergency response system. All cases of nontraumatic cardiac arrest due to VF or pulseless VT occurring outside of a hospital between January 1988 and June 1989 were considered. That city's emergency medical system employs emergency medical technicians and paramedics. Standard resuscitation techniques were employed; high-dose epinephrine and interposed abdominal counterpulsations were not routine interventions. The main outcome measure was survival to hospital discharge. Three (4%) of 75 patients survived cardiac arrest and were discharged alive from the hospital. Two (5.3%) of 38 witnessed arrests resulted in hospital discharges. Patient demographics were typical of those reported from other cities that have published outcomes data. Few patients (16%) received bystander-initiated cardiopulmonary resuscitation. There is increasing evidence that previously recognized standards for resuscitation success may not be present in certain types of municipalities, including this northeastern city.

Predicting Outcome After Resuscitation

Prediction of individual outcome after cardiopulmonary resuscitation is of major medical, ethical, and socioeconomic interest, but uncertain. Madl and associates,[43] from Vienna, Austria, studied the early predictive potency of evoked potential recording after cardiac arrest in 66 resuscitated patients who returned to spontaneous circulation but were unconscious and mechanically ventilated. Detailed long-latency and short-latency sensory evoked potentials were recorded, and neurological evaluations were done 4 to 48 hours after admission to intensive care. In all 17 patients with favorable outcome (cerebral performance categories 1 and 2), the cortical evoked potential N70 peak, a reliable measure of cortical function, was detected between 74 and 116 ms. In 49 patients with bad outcome (categories 4 and 5), the N70 peak was absent in 35 or found with a delay between 121 and 171 ms in 14. Thus, the predictive ability was 100% with cutoff of 118 ms. To confirm reproducibility and validity, repeated tracings and linked-earlobe referenced techniques were done and gave similar results. Early recordings of long-latency evoked potentials after cardiopulmonary resuscitation is highly predictive of outcome.

Tresch and associates,[44] from Milwaukee, Wis, analyzed a total of 196 patients who received cardiopulmonary resuscitation (CPR) at a nursing home in Milwaukee: 37 patients (19%) were successfully resuscitated and hospitalized, and 10 patients (5%) survived to be discharged. Of the patients who survived their cardiac arrest, which was witnessed and had demonstrated VF at the time of the arrest, 27% survived. In contrast, only 2% of all other nursing home patients who received CPR survived. Age, mental or functional status, hematocrit, renal dysfunction, pulmonary disease, cancer, and cardiovascular disease were not significant predictors of survival. At the time of hospital discharge, the functional status of most of the survivors (80%) was comparable to their pre-arrest status, and 40% of the survivors lived for greater than 12 months. These authors suggest that CPR should be initiated only in nursing home patients whose cardiac arrest was witnessed and should be continued in patients whose initial documented cardiac rhythm is VF or VT.

Racial Differences

Differences between blacks and whites have been reported in the incidence of several forms of cardiovascular disease, including hypertension and stroke. Becker and associates,[45] from Chicago, Ill, and Oklahoma City, Okla, examined racial differences in the incidence of cardiac arrest in a large urban population and in subsequent survival. They collected data on all nontraumatic, out-of-hospital cardiac arrests in Chicago from Jan 1, 1987, through Dec 31, 1988, and compared the incidence and survival rates for blacks and whites. These authors examined the association between survival and race and seven other known risk factors by logistic-regression analysis. They computed incidence rates by coupling our data with U.S. Census population data. The study population comprised 6,451 patients: 3,207 whites, 2,910 blacks, and 334 persons of other races. The incidence of cardiac arrest was significantly higher for blacks than for whites in every age group (Figure 4-4). The survival rate after cardiac arrest was 2.6% in whites, as compared with 0.8% in blacks. Blacks were significantly less likely to have a witnessed cardiac arrest, bystander-initiated cardiopulmonary resuscitation, or a "favorable" initial rhythm, or to be admitted to the hospital. When admitted, blacks were half as likely to survive. The association between race and survival persisted even when other recognized risk factors were taken into account. These authors did not find important differences between blacks and whites in the response time of the emergency medical services. The black community in the study was at higher risk for cardiac arrest and subsequent death than the white community, even after they controlled for other variables.

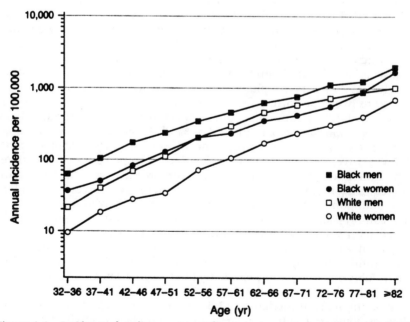

Figure 4-4. Incidence of cardiac arrest according to race, sex, and age. Reproduced with permission from Becker et al.[45]

Without Structural Heart Disease

Structural heart disease is absent in up to 5% of survivors of out-of-hospital cardiac arrest. Furthermore, 10% to 17% of forensic examinations fail to reveal the cause of sudden death in victims younger than 45 years of age. The prognosis among survivors of ventricular fibrillation with minimal or no structural cardiac abnormalities remains unclear. Meissner and associates,[46] from Detroit, Mich, evaluated the outcome of survivors of ventricular fibrillation with no or minimal structural heart disease who received an implantable cardioverter-defibrillator (ICD). Ventricular tachyarrhythmias were induced during baseline programmed stimulation in 39% of patients. During a median follow-up of 31 months after ICD implantation, there were no cardiac deaths and two noncardiac deaths. Sixteen patients experienced 36 shock episodes (total, 88 shocks). The majority of shocks were classified as indeterminant; one patient received 47 spurious shocks during one shock episode and each of four patients received 1 appropriate shock. Ventricular arrhythmias were not inducible in any of these latter four patients. These authors concluded that survivors of ventricular fibrillation with minimal or no structural cardiac abnormalities receiving an ICD have an excellent 3 year survival rate. The infrequent shocks during this 3-year time period suggest the potential benefit of an implantable cardioverter-defibrillator.

Methods of Resuscitation and Evaluation

Recent studies have demonstrated improved cardiopulmonary circulation during cardiac arrest with the use of a hand-held suction device (Ambu CardioPump) to perform active compression-decompression cardiopulmonary resuscitation. Cohen and associates,[47] from Manhasset, NY, enrolled all patients over 18 years of age who had a witnessed cardiac arrest while hospitalized at their medical center; they were randomly assigned according to their medical record numbers to receive either active compression-decompression or standard cardiopulmonary resuscitation. The study endpoints were the rates of initial resuscitation, survival at 24 hours, hospital discharge, and neurologic outcome. Compressions were performed according to the recommendations of the American Heart Association (80 to 100 compressions per minute; depth of compression, 3.8 to 5.1 cm; and 50% of the cycle spend in compression). Sixty-two patients (45 men and 17 women) with a mean age of 68 ± 2 years were entered into the trial. Sixty-two percent of the patients who underwent active compression-decompression were initially resuscitated, as compared with 30% of the patients who received standard cardiopulmonary resuscitation; 45% of the patients who underwent active compression-decompression survived for at least 24 hours, as compared with 9% of patients who underwent standard cardiopulmonary resuscitation. Two of the 62 patients survived to hospital discharge; both were randomly assigned to receive active compression-decompression. Neurologic outcome, as measured by the Glasgow coma score, was better with active compression-decompression (8.0 ± 1.3) than with standard cardiopulmonary resuscitation (3.5 ± 0.3). Thus, the authors concluded that, as compared with standard cardiopulmonary resuscitation, active compression-decompression cardiopulmonary resuscitation improved the rate of initial resuscitation, survival at 24 hours, and neurologic outcome after in-hospital cardiac arrest.

Tucker and associates,[48] from San Francisco, Calif, evaluated a new active compression-decompression device for cardiopulmonary resuscitation. This device was applied midsternum in five consecutive patients, and results compared sequentially with standard manual cardiopulmonary resuscitation both at a rate of 80 compressions per minute. Transesophageal echo data was obtained in each patient to evaluate transmitral flow and left ventricular volume. No difference was observed in end-compression volume between the two techniques. The new device increased end-decompression volume (81 v 69 mL), stroke volume (33 v 18 mL) and velocity time integral of transmitral flow (16 v 8 mL). These authors concluded that the use of active compression-decompression improved transmitral flow, end-decompression left ventricular volume, and stroke volume compared with standard CPR. This suggested a biphasic cardiothoracic cycle of flow with this new device. Further evaluation is warranted to evaluate this device as a better method than standard cardiopulmonary resuscitation, because it also has the advantage of improving air flow in these patients.

Criteria For Termination of Resuscitation

To identify distinct criteria for appropriate on-scene termination of resuscitation efforts for out-of-hospital cardiac arrest when on-scene interventions fail to restore spontaneous circulation, Bonnin and associates,[49] from Houston, Tex, evaluated for 18 months all out-of-hospital cardiac arrests prospectively for survival to hospital discharge and for all established survival predictors including age, gender, presenting cardiac rhythm, whether it was a witnessed event, performance of basic cardiopulmonary resuscitation by bystanders, and interval to paramedic arrival and return of spontaneous circulation. The number and circumstances of patients achieving survival to hospital discharge following failure to achieve on-scene return of spontaneous circulation were the main outcome measures. Of 1,461 consecutive primary arrest, 139 were monitored (paramedic witnessed), including 59 that occurred en route to the hospital. Of the 1,322 unmonitored patients, 370 achieved return of spontaneous circulation at the scene. Only 6 (0.6%) of the 952 who did not achieve return of spontaneous circulation at the scene survived, and all 6 were readily identifiable as having persistent VF. Excluding those patients with persistent VF, all survivors achieved return of spontaneous circulation within 25 minutes after paramedic arrival. Excluding patients with persistent VF, resuscitative efforts can be terminated at the scene when normothermic adults with unmonitored, out-of-hospital, primary cardiac arrest do not regain spontaneous circulation within 25 minutes following standard advanced cardiac life support (Table 4-2). These criteria should now be validated in several large centers with high survival rates.

Rehospitalization in Survivors

Surviving patients of out-of-hospital VF often need rehospitalization after initial hospital discharge, but little is known regarding the frequency of or reasons for rehospitalization. Maynard and associates,[50]

Table 4-2. Criteria for Termination of Resuscitation Efforts at the Scene Following Un-monitored, Out-of-Hospital, Adult, Primary Cardiac Arrest. Reproduced with permission from Bonnin et al.[49]

1. Adult cardiopulmonary arrest (not associated with trauma, body temperature aberration, respiratory etiology, or drug overdose)
2. Standard advanced cardiac life support[5] for 25 min
3. No restoration of spontaneous circulation (spontaneous pulse rate of >60 beats per min for at least one 5-min period)
4. Absence of persistently recurring or refractory ventricular fibrillation/tachycardia or any continued neurological activity (eg, spontaneous respiration, eye opening, or motor response)

from Seattle, Wash, examined 224 patients enrolled in the Cardiac Arrest in Seattle: Conventional Amiodarone Drug Evaluation (CASCADE) study, a randomized clinical trial comparing amiodarone with other antiarrhythmic drug therapies in survivors of out-of-hospital VF. The annual rate of rehospitalization was 79/100 patients/year; 168 of 224 patients (75%) were hospitalized at least once before censoring or cardiac mortality. Baseline LVEF was significantly lower in patients who were rehospitalized. Rehospitalization rates were lower in patients randomized to amiodarone therapy and in those with the automatic implantable cardioverter-defibrillator, although neither difference was statistically significant. However, length of stay for the first rehospitalization was shorter for patients with automatic implantable cardioverter-defibrillators. More than 50% of patients were rehospitalized in the first year after enrollment; 65% with EFs <0.3 were rehospitalized in the first year. Rehospitalization was a frequent occurrence for surviving patients of out-of-hospital VF, particularly in those with low EFs.

Neuropsychological Sequelae

Prospective and community-based studies on the cognitive outcome of out-of-hospital cardiac arrest have not been published. Roine and associates,[51] from Helsinki, Finland, studied prospectively the neuropsychological sequelae of cardiac arrest and evaluated the effects of nimodipine on them. They studied a total of 155 successfully resuscitated consecutive patients out of 677 resuscitation attempts during a 2.5 year period. Sixty-eight survivors were examined by a neuropsychologist and a neurologist. The neuropsychological outcome measures were at 3 months and at 12 months after cardiac arrest. Three months after cardiac arrest, 41 (60%) of 68 patients were found to have moderate to severe cognitive deficits. At 12 months, 26 (48%) of 54 survivors still had moderate to severe deficits, and the Symptom Check List 90-Revised score indicated the presence of depression in 22 patients (45%) and severe depression in 12 patients (24%). Moderate to severe neuropsychological sequelae of out-of-hospital cardiac arrest are still present in approximately one half of the survivors at 1 year and may be permanent. There seems to be no excess increased disability in the subgroup of patients with delayed advanced life support. Nimodipine failed to show any effect on the cognitive function tested.

Antiarrhythmic Drug Therapy

The Cardiac Arrest in Seattle: Conventional Versus Amiodarone Drug Evaluation (CASCADE) study[52] evaluated antiarrhythmic drug treatment of survivors of out-of-hospital VF not associated with a Q-wave AMI who were at especially high risk of recurrence of VF. Therapy was randomized to empiric treatment with amiodarone versus treatment with other antiarrhythmic drugs guided by electrophysiologic testing, Holter recording, or both (conventional therapy). The primary endpoints of the study were cardiac mortality, resuscitated cardiac arrest due to documented VF, or complete syncope followed by a shock from an implanted automatic defibrillator. Two hundred twenty-eight patients were enrolled in the study, and baseline characteristics were similar in the patients treated with amiodarone and with conventional therapy. Of these patients, 202 (89%) were men with an average age of 62 years. CAD was the most common underlying condition (82%); and in coronary patients, 81% had experienced a prior AMI before the index VF event. Mean LVEF was 0.35, and 45% of patients had a prior history of CHF. Survival free of cardiac death, resuscitated VF, or syncopal defibrillator shock for the entire population was 75% at 2 years (amiodarone, 82%; conventional, 69%), 59% at 4 years (amiodarone, 66%; conventional, 52%), and 46% at 6 years (amiodarone, 53%; conventional, 40%). The survival free of cardiac death and sustained ventricular arrhythmias was 65% at 2 years (amiodarone, 78%; conventional, 52%), 43% at 4 years (amiodarone, 52%; conventional, 36%), and 30% at 6 years (amiodarone, 41%; conventional, 20%).

Do-Not-Resuscitate Orders

The appropriate role of cardiopulmonary resuscitation in the hospital continues to be a topic of interest of physicians and patients alike. The use of do-not-resuscitate (DNR) orders reflects a growing expression of autonomy by patients to refuse medical treatment and also a growing recognition of its futility in many circumstances by physicians. Although it has been suggested that wider use of advance directives will lead to a reduction in health care costs near the end of life, little empiric data exist to support this prediction. Maksoud and associates,[53] from Cleveland, Ohio, retrospectively reviewed the hospital records of 852 of 953 hospital deaths that occurred at the Cleveland Clinic Foundation. Data were collected on resuscitation status, timing of DNR orders, participants in decision making, and physician and hospital charges. Of the 852 records reviewed, 625 (73%) had a DNR order at the time of death. The use of DNR orders for patients who died ranged from 97% of those on an oncology service to 43% of deaths on cardiology services. One hundred seven patients (17%) had the DNR order before admission. Of 512 patients who had a new DNR order in the hospital, approval was obtained from the patient in only 19%. Patients who died with a DNR order had longer hospital stays (median, 11 days) compared with those who died without a DNR order (6 days). The time from DNR order to death was 2 days overall with 2 days for medical patients and 1 day for surgical patients. Average charges for each patient who died were $61,215 with $10,631 for those admitted with a DNR order and $73,055 for those who had a DNR order made in the hospital. This study demonstrates high variability in the use of DNR orders between various medical and surgical services. These range from a high of 98% on an oncology service to a low of 43% on cardiology. Most patients have a DNR order at the time of death, but these typically occur late in the course of the hospital stay. Death in the hospital is costly and total hospital and professional charges are significantly lower when a patient is admitted with an established nonresuscitation order compared with those for whom a DNR is established while in the hospital. This study provides a basis against which to measure the impact of efforts such as the Patient Self-Determination Act of 1990 to increase the use of advance directives, as well as monitor their effect on health care expenditures.

To describe the characteristics of patients with do-not-resuscitate (DNR) orders and the frequency and timing of these orders in a representative sample of intensive care units (ICUs) and to compare practices from 1980 to 1990, Jayes and associates,[54] from Washington, DC, performed a perspective inception cohort study of 42 ICUs in 40 US hospitals with 200 or more beds; 26 randomly selected hospitals and 14 large, tertiary care hospitals that volunteered to be studied were used. A consecutive sample of 17,440 ICU admissions from 1988 to 1990 were studied. Physicians wrote DNR orders for 1,577 ICU admissions (9%). Patients with ICU DNR orders were older, were more functionally impaired, had more comorbid illness, had a higher severity of illness, and required the use of more ICU resources compared with patients without DNR orders. Compared with data from a similar survey from 1979 to 1982, ICU DNR orders were more frequent in 1988 to 1990 (9% v 5.4%) and preceded 60% of all in-unit deaths compared with only 39% in 1979 to 1982. Do-not-resuscitate orders were written sooner (for 3.6% v 2.0% of patients on day 1 in the ICU), and patients with DNR orders remained in the ICU longer in 1988 to 1990 (2.8 v 1.4 days) than in 1979 to 1982, and had lower ICU and hospital mortality rates (64% v 74%). Over the last decade, physicians and families of patients set limits earlier and more frequently in cases likely to have poor outcomes. These authors attribute this change to a greater dialogue about setting limits to care and a greater knowledge of treatment outcomes among physicians and families. These changes in practice preceded implementation of the Patient Self-Determination Act, designed to ensure patient autonomy for decisions about life-sustaining therapy.

Sudden Infant Death Syndrome

In several studies, the sudden infant death syndrome (SIDS) has been significantly associated with sleeping in the prone position. It is not known how the prone position increases the risk of SIDS. Ponsonby and associates,[55] from Tasmania, Australia, analyzed data from a case-control study (58 infants with SIDS and 120 control infants) and a prospective cohort study (22 infants with SIDS and 213 control infants) in Tasmania, Australia. Interactions were examined in matched analyses with a multiplicative model of interaction. In the case-control study, SIDS was significantly associated with sleeping in the prone position, as compared with other positions (unadjusted odds ratio, 4.5). The strength of this association was increased among infants who slept on natural-fiber mattresses, infants who were swaddled, infants who slept in heated rooms, and infants who had a recent illness. These variables had no significant effect on infants who did not sleep in the prone position. A history of recent illness was significantly associated with SIDS among infants who slept prone (odds ratio, 5.7) but not among infants who slept in other positions (0.83). In the cohort study, the risk of SIDS was greater among infants who slept prone on natural-fiber mattresses (6.6) than among infants who slept prone on other types of mattresses (1.8). When infants sleep prone, the elevated risk of SIDS is increased by each of four factors: the use of natural-fiber mattresses, swaddling, recent illness, and the use of heating in bedrooms.

SYNCOPE

A cardiac cause of syncope has been associated with increased sudden death risk, whereas unexplained syncope has a benign prognosis. However, in patients who have depressed LV function, the accuracy of diagnostic tests and the efficacy of therapy, such as antiarrhythmic drugs, are reduced. Previous studies of patients with syncope have not evaluated the contribution of LV performance in risk stratification for sudden death. The purpose of this investigation by Middlekauff and associates,[56] from Los Angeles, Calif, was to study a large population of patients with syncope to determine the impact of LV dysfunction on sudden death risk if syncope is caused by a cardiac cause or remains unexplained after electrophysiologic testing. The investigators retrospectively evaluated the relationship of LVEF to sudden death prognosis in 88 consecutive patients referred for electrophysiologic testing to determine a cause of syncope. The mean age was 57 ± 18 years, LVEF was 0.41 ± 0.20, and 66 patients (75%) had structural heart disease. In 49 patients (56%), a cardiac cause of syncope was diagnosed, and in 39 patients (44%), the cause of syncope remained unexplained after evaluation. Cardiac syncope was attributed to VT in 27 patients, bradyarrhythmia in 11 patients, and SVT in 11 patients. By logistic regression only structural heart disease was independently associated with cardiac cause of syncope. After a mean follow-up of 790 ± 688 days, 9 patients had died suddenly, 8 (89%) of whom had LVEF <0.30. In 51 patients who had LVEF >0.30, 3-year actuarial sudden death risk was similarly low for patients who had cardiac compared with unexplained causes of syncope. In 47 patients who had LVEF <0.30, sudden death risk was substantial for both patients who had cardiac syncope (58%) and for those who had unexplained syncope (50%). In the Cox multivariate analysis, reduced LVEF was the only independent predictor of sudden death. It was concluded that prognosis is excellent for patients with syncope who have preserved LV function, even if the cause of syncope is cardiac. In contrast, when LV function is markedly depressed, sudden death risk is high in patients who have cardiac or unexplained causes of syncope. More sensitive diagnostic tests and perhaps greater use of nonpharmacologic therapies may be needed in this high risk group.

There are few data regarding the immediate reproducibility of the tilt-table test. Therefore, de Buitleir and associates,[57] from Madison, Wis, examined the immediate reproducibility of the tilt-table test in 19 patients with syncope or presyncope. The mean number of episodes that patients had experienced was 14. After baseline supine observation for

10 minutes, patients were placed in 80° of head-up tilt until a positive response occurred or for a maximum of 10 minutes. Patients were then returned to the supine position for 5 minutes, followed by retilt for another 10 minutes. If the baseline tilt was negative, the study was repeated with intravenous isoproterenol, and immediate reproducibility was examined in the same manner. The 19 patients underwent a total of 31 tilt-table tests, and the tilt-table test was immediately reproducible in 24 of 31 tests performed (77%). Eight tests were reproducibly positive and 16 negative. The results of 7 tilt-table tests were not reproducible. In 6 of these studies, the positive result occurred first and the negative result second. The reproducibility of an initially negative tilt-table test result was much higher than that of an initially positive one. The immediate reproducibility of the tilt-table test in adult patients with unexplained syncope is approximately 75%. In studies that are not reproducible, most results are positive first and negative second. Therefore, in most patients it is not necessary to check immediate reproducibility. If a baseline tilt-table test is negative, it may be reasonable to repeat the test during the same session in some patients, because in 1 of 9 cases a positive result will be found on the second test. The performance of acute drug testing is limited by the relatively poor immediate reproducibility of positive tilt-table tests.

Müller and associates,[58] from Chicago, Ill, compared the efficacy of intravenous metoprolol in preventing symptoms during a repeat tilt test with the outcome of chronic oral treatment in 21 patients, aged 8 to 20 years, with unexplained syncope and a positive response to tilt testing. A positive response was defined as the development of either syncope or presyncope. During the initial tilt test, a positive response occurred during baseline or isoproterenol infusion with a cardioinhibitory, vasodepressor or mixed pattern. Metoprolol (0.1 to 0.2 mg/kg) was administered intravenously. During the repeat tilt test, response was negative in 18 patients, including 11 of 14 patients with a positive response in the baseline and 7 of 7 patients with a positive response during isoproterenol infusion. Metoprolol (0.8 to 2.8 mg/kg/day) was administered orally to 15 patients for an average of 10 months. Symptoms were absent in 7 patients and improved in 2 patients; metoprolol was discontinued because of adverse effects in 3 patients and recurrence of symptoms in 3 patients. In 7 of 12 patients with a negative response and 2 of 3 patients with a positive response after intravenous metoprolol, oral administration of metoprolol prevented or improved symptoms without adverse effects. Many young patients (60%) with recurrent syncope obtained symptomatic improvement from chronic oral metoprolol treatment without adverse effects; repeat tilt testing after intravenous metoprolol did not appear to offer any additional information than would have been obtained from a trial of chronic oral treatment.

The efficacy of permanent cardiac pacing in patients with neurocardiogenic (or vasovagal) syncope associated with bradycardia or asystole is not clear. Sra and associates,[59] from Milwaukee, Wis, compared the efficacy of cardiac pacing with that of oral drug therapy in the prevention of hypotension and syncopy during head-up tilt testing. Among 70 patients with a history of syncope in whom hypotension and syncope could be provoked during head-up tilt testing, 22 had bradycardia (a heart rate <60 beats/minute, with a decline in the rate by at least 20 beats/minute) or asystole along with hypotension during testing. There were 9 men and 13 women, with a mean age of 41 ± 17 years. Head-up tilt testing was repeated during A-V sequential pacing (in 20 patients with sinus rhythm) or ventricular pacing (in 2 patients with AF). Regardless of the results obtained during artificial pacing, all the patients subsequently had upright-tilt testing repeated during therapy with oral metoprolol, theophylline, or disopyramide. During the initial tilt test, 6 patients had asystole and 16 had bradycardia along with hypotension. Despite artificial pacing, the mean arterial pressure during head-up tilt testing still fell significantly, from 97 ± 19 to 57 ± 19 mm Hg; 5 patients had syncope, and 15 had presyncope. By contrast, 19 patients who later received only medical therapy (metoprolol in 10, theophylline in 3, and disopyramide in 6), 2 patients who received both metoprolol and A-V sequential pacing, and 1 patient who received only atrioventricular sequential pacing had negative head-up tilt tests. After a median follow-up of 16 months, 18 of the 19 patients who were treated with drugs alone (94%) remained free of recurrent syncope or presyncope, whereas the patient treated only with a permanent dual-chamber pacemaker had recurrent syncope.

To evaluate the day-to-day reproducibility of upright tilt-table testing, Brooks and associates,[60] from Boston, Mass, studied 109 patients with unexplained syncope prospectively who underwent testing on two consecutive days using a uniform protocol. Results of testing on two separate days were concordant in 69 of 109 patients (63%) and discordant in 40 of 109 patients (37%). Thirty-six of 109 patients (33%) had vasodepressor syncope on one or both days of testing. Nineteen of 30 patients (63%) with vasodepressor responses on the first day did not reproduce this response during the second day of testing. An additional 6 patients with an initial negative tilt test had a vasodepressor response on the second day. Only 11 of 36 patients (31%) had reproducible vasodepressor responses on both days of testing. Patients with reproducible vasodepressor responses had a significantly higher mean number of preceding clinical syncopal events than patients with two normal tests or nonreproducible results. In addition, these patients had a significantly longer duration of clinical symptoms relative to patients with two tests that yielded negative results and nonreproducible results. The elapsed time between the most recent clinical event and the performance of tilt-table testing was not significantly different among the three groups and did not appear to influence the outcome of testing. These data show that vasodepressor responses elicited by upright tilt-table testing show day-to-day variability in many patients, a finding that may limit the interpretation of initial and follow-up test results.

Carotid sinus syndrome (CSS) is frequently overlooked as a cause of syncope in the elderly. It is diagnosed when carotid sinus massage produces asystole exceeding 3 seconds (cardioinhibitory CSS), a reduction in systolic BP exceeding >50 mm Hg independent of heart rate slowing (vasodepressor CSS), or a combination of the two (mixed CSS). Most published data pertain to the cardioinhibitory subtype. The recent availability of noninvasive phasic BP monitoring has allowed accurate routine assessment of the vasodepressor response to carotid sinus massage. The aim of this study by McIntosh and associates,[61] from Newcastle, United Kingdom, was to assess the clinical characteristics of vasodepressor, cardioinhibitory, and mixed CSS. Carotid sinus massage was carried out on 132 consecutive patients over 65 years referred for investigation of dizziness, falls, or syncope. Massage was performed both supine and upright with continuous electrocardiographic and phasic BP monitoring. Patients exhibiting greater than 1.5 second asystole were give 600 μg of intravenous atropine to abolish heart rate slowing and allow assessment of the pure vasodepressor response. Carotid sinus hypersensitivity was documented in 64 patients (mean age, 81 ± 7 years; 31 male). The response was vasodepressor in 37%, cardioinhibitory in 29%, and mixed in 34%. Thirty-six patients had recurrent syncope, 17 presented with unexplained falls, and the remainder had dizziness alone. Symptoms had been present for a median of 24 months, and the median number of syncopal episodes was four. Twenty-five percent had sustained a fracture, and of these, 93% had not experienced a prodrome. Head movement precipitated symptoms in 47% and vagal stimuli in 73%. Episodes were unwitnessed in two thirds of patients. Twelve patients who presented with falls denied syncope but had witnessed loss of consciousness during carotid sinus massage. Mean cardioinhibition was 5 ± 2 seconds and mean vasodepression was 61 ± 9 mm Hg. The BP nadir occurred rapidly at 18 ± 3 seconds after massage, and baseline values were regained at 30 ± 6 seconds. The clinical characteristics of patients with vasodepressor, cardioinhibitory, and mixed responses were similar. CSS is an underdiagnosed cause of dizziness, falls, and syncope in the elderly. The vasodepressor form occurs more frequently than previously reported and has clinical characteristics similar to those of the cardioinhibitory and mixed subtypes. Elderly patients with this condition may deny syncope and present with recurrent unexplained falls. Carotid sinus massage, ideally with noninvasive phasic BP monitoring, should be routinely performed in elderly patients with unexplained bradycardic or hypotensive symptoms.

Neurally mediated syncope is a frequent cause of syncope and may be induced by head-up tilting. Some recent uncontrolled trials suggested that disopyramide might be an effective therapy in patients with neurally-mediated syncope. Morillo and associates,[62] from London, Ontario, Canada, evaluated 22 consecutive patients with recurrent neurally mediated syncope and two or more successive positive head-up tilt responses. The patients were randomly allocated to receive either intravenous disopyramide or placebo. Head-up tilt testing at 60 degrees was performed after 15 minutes. Head-up tilt test results were positive for syncope in 75% of patients receiving placebo and 60% of patients receiving disopyramide. After crossover, head-up tilt results were positive in 87% receiving placebo and 80% receiving disopyramide. A mean follow-up time of 29 months was obtained in 21 of the 22 patients. Syncope recurred in 27% of the patients receiving disopyramide and 30% of the patients not treated pharmacologically. These authors concluded that intravenous disopyramide was ineffective for the prevention of neurally mediated syncope provoked by head-up tilt testing. Furthermore, no significant effect was observed after oral therapy with disopyramide. There was a striking decrease in the incidence of positive tilt-tests over time regardless of the intervention. Thus, recurrence of syncope after the investigative protocol was infrequent in both groups.

Table 4-3. Causes of Pacemaker Malfunction. Reproduced with permission from Hayes et al.[63]

Malfunction	True Malfunction	Pseudomalfunction
Failure to output	Component failure (rare) Total battery depletion Lead fracture Lead disconnection Oversensing	Cross talk
Failure to capture	Lead dislodgment Lead insulation break Exit block Metabolic abnormalities Battery depletion	Inappropriately low energy output settings Pacemaker artifact in the myocardial refractory period (functional noncapture)
Undersensing	Lead dislodgment Poor lead position Lead insulation defect Low-amplitude intracardiac signal	Magnet application Environmental electrical noise Pacemaker refractory period (functional undersensing) Monitor artifact
Inappropriate pacemaker rate	Runaway pacemaker	Tracking atrial arrhythmias Pacemaker re-entrant tachycardia Resetting from electromagnetic interference Battery end-of-life indicator

PACEMAKERS

Hayes and Vlietstra,[63] from Rochester, Minn, and Lakeland, Fla, provided a review of pacemaker malfunction. They grouped the electrocardiographic signs of pacemaker malfunction into four categories: failure to output, failure to capture, undersensing, and inappropriate pacemaker rate (Table 4-3). For each of these four categories, there may be true malfunctions and pseudomalfunctions. In addition, environmental sources of electromagnetic interference, both within and outside the hospital environment, can result in pacemaker malfunction. These authors suggested that approaching pacemaker malfunction with these four categories in mind should help minimize confusion.

CARDIOVERTERS/DEFIBRILLATORS

Silka and associates,[64] from Portland, Ore, Minneapolis, Minn, and Ann Arbor, Mich, reported on 177 patients <20 years of age at the time of initial implantation of an implantable cardioverter-defibrillator. Detailed records were subsequently obtained from physicians involved in the care of 125 (75%) of these patients. The patients ranged in age from 2 to 20 years with a mean of 14.5 years and weighed 10 to 117 kg with a mean of 45 kg. Of the 125 patients, 76% were survivors of sudden cardiac death, 10% had drug refractory VT, and 10% had syncope with heart disease and inducible sustained VT. The most common types of associated disease were hypertrophic and dilated cardiomyopathies (54%), primary electrical diseases (26%), and congenital heart defects (18%). Ventricular function was abnormal in 46% of these patients. During a mean follow-up of 31 months, at least one defibrillator discharge occurred in 68% of the patients. One appropriate discharge occurred in 59%, and 20% had one or more spurious or indeterminate discharges. Duration of follow was >24 months, and inducibility of a sustained ventricular arrhythmia was correlated with appropriate defibrillator discharges. There were nine deaths during the study period: five sudden, two due to recurrent VT, and two related to CHF. Abnormal ventricular function and prior defibrillator discharge were univariate correlates of patient mortality by multivariate logistic regression. Abnormal ventricular function was the only significant correlate of death. The estimated overall post implant survival rates at 1, 2, and 5 years were 95%, 93%, and 85%, respectively. Implantable cardioverter-defibrillators can be effective in pediatric patients, as in adults with appropriate utilization as highlighted by these investigators.

Bardy and associates,[65] from Seattle, Wash, examined the safety, efficacy, and limitations associated with the use of a transvenously implanted cardioverter-defibrillator with antitachycardia pacing in a consecutive population of 84 patients with VF and sustained VT who had survived the arrhythmia. The arrhythmia promoting transvenous cardioverter-defibrillator implantation was VF in 41 patients, VT in 27, and both VF and VT in 16. Transvenous defibrillation through a coronary sinus, a right ventricular, a superior vena caval, and/or a subcutaneous chest patch lead system was attempted. The pulsing method used included two electrode single-pathway pulsing or three-electrode dual-pathway simultaneous or sequential pulsing. A transvenous cardioverter-defibrillator was inserted if the defibrillator threshold was <20 J. Successful implantation of a transvenous cardioverter-defibrillator was possible in 80 of 84 (95%) patients. The mean implant defibrillation threshold was 10.9 ± 4.8 J. After cardioverter-defibrillator implantation, all patients were extubated in the operating room and sent to a standard telemetry ward for monitoring. No patient suffered a postoperative pulmonary complication or perioperative flurry of cardiac arrhythmias. Postoperative complications included lead dislodgements in eight, transient long thoracic nerve injury in one, asymptomatic left subclavian vein occlusion in two, asymptomatic small pericardial effusion in one, subcutaneous patch pocket hematomas in four, pulse generator pocket infection in one, and lead fracture in one. It was routine to discharge patients three days after surgery, as experience was gained with the procedure. The mean hospital stay was 6 ± 2.4 days. At discharge, all patients returned to their prehospital activities including those with complications, except for the patient with the pocket infection who required intravenous antibody therapy. Patient survival using an intention-to-treat analysis was 98% over an 11 ± 7 month follow-up period. During this time period, 31 of 80 patients (39%) with transvenous lead systems were treated by their device for sustained VT or VF successfully. Antitachycardia pacing was used in 424 episodes of monomorphic VT and was successful in 88%. All episodes of VF were aborted by the device. Antiarrhythmic drugs were used after device implantation in only 10% of patients. Thus, transvenous cardioverter-defibrillator implantation is practical in most patients.

Survivors of sudden cardiac death in whom ventricular arrhythmias cannot be induced with programmed electrical stimulation remain at risk for recurrence of serious arrhythmias. Optimal protection to prevent sudden death in these patients is uncertain. Crandall and associates,[66] from Portland, Ore, Seattle, Wash, and Palo Alto, Calif, compared survival in this subset of survivors of sudden death with or without an implantable cardioverter-defibrillator. This retrospective study was performed on 194 consecutive survivors of primary sudden death who had less than six beats of ventricular tachycardia induced with programmed electrical stimulation with at least three extra stimuli. Ninety-nine patients received an implantable cardiac defibrillator (ICD), and 95 did not. Patients treated with an ICD were younger (55 v 59 years) and had a lesser incidence of CAD (48% v 63%) and a lower EF (.43 v .48). There were no significant differences between the groups in the use of revascularization procedures or antiarrhythmic agents after sudden cardiac death. Patients treated with an ICD had an improvement in sudden cardiac death-free survival, but the overall survival rate did not differ from that of the patients not so treated. These authors concluded that survivors of sudden cardiac death in whom no arrhythmias could be induced with programmed electrical stimulation remain at risk for arrhythmia recurrence. Although the proportion of deaths attributed to arrhythmia was lower in the patients treated with an ICD, this therapy did not significantly improve overall survival. It is possible that the selection of sicker patients to receive the ICD may have led to this result. Careful prospective trials will be needed to define the subgroups among these patients who will most benefit from the use of an intracardiac defibrillator.

Previous studies have suggested a remarkably low incidence of recurrent sudden death in patients with implantable cardioverter-defibrillators. Bocker and associates,[67] from Munster, Germany, further evaluated this question by evaluating the follow-up of 107 patients who had implantation of a third generation implantable cardioverter-defibrillator. Surgical mortality was 2.7% in all 107 patients and 1% in the 99 patients who qualified for endocardial leads. During a follow-up period of one year, actuarial survival rate free of events at 6, 12, and 18 months was 100% for sudden death, 97% for total arrhythmia related deaths, and 95% for total cardiac death. In contrast, after 6, 12, and 18 months the rate of survival free of fast ventricular tachycardia was only 83%, 74%, and 69%, respectively; and the rate of survival free of any ventricular tachyrhythmia was only 59%, 49%, and 40%, respectively. These authors concluded that the outcome of patients treated with an implantable cardioverter-defibrillator and endocardial defibrillation leads is excellent. Although not a controlled trial, it provides further evidence for the benefit of cardioverter-defibrillation, using transvenous endocardial leads.

Grimm and associates,[68] from Philadelphia, Pa, determined the incidence of clinical characteristics on shock occurrence and survival in 241 patients with implantable cardioverter-defibrillator therapy. Two hundred forty-one consecutive patients underwent implantable cardioverter-defibrillator implantation between November 1982 and November 1991 and were subsequently followed for 26 months. Actuarial incidence of appropriate shocks was 13%, 42%, and 63%, and the incidence of any spontaneous shocks was 15%, 51%, and 76% at 1, 3, and 5 years of follow-up, respectively. Poor LVEF with LVEFs ≤30% was associated with an earlier occurrence of both appropriate and any spontaneous defibrillator shocks. Appropriate and any spontaneous shocks occurred significantly later in patients who presented with cardiac arrest and in patients in whom only VF without VT was induced during preoperative programmed stimulation. Amiodarone treatment at implantation of the defibrillator was associated with later occurrence of any spontaneous shocks. Cumulative survival from all-cause mortality, including perioperative mortality was 84%, 62%, and 57%, and survival from arrhythmic death was 97%, 89%, and 83% at 1, 3, and 5 years, respectively. LVEF

≤30% was the best predictor of both total arrhythmic death and total mortality. Antiarrhythmic therapy with class 1 agents at implantation was also associated with a higher total mortality during follow-up but not with total arrhythmic death. Survival curves were similar for patients with and without spontaneous shocks. Thus, the majority of patients receiving shocks from an implantable defibrillator may not have these shocks associated with increased arrhythmic or total mortality, suggesting the effective prevention of sudden death with the implantable cardioverter-defibrillator. Although low LVEF is the strongest predictor of both shock occurrence and mortality, no easy algorithm can be derived from the analyzed clinical characteristics to predict which patients will benefit most from the implantable cardioverter-defibrillator implantation.

Powell and associates,[69] from Boston, Mass, studied 331 survivors of out-of-hospital cardiac arrest (mean age, 56 ± 14 years) who underwent electrophysiologically guided therapy. Implantable defibrillators were placed in 150 patients (45%) and 181 patients (55%) received pharmacological and/or surgical therapy alone. LVEF was 35% ± 17% in the defibrillator recipients and 45% ± 18% in the nondefibrillator patients. Median patient follow-up was 24 months in the defibrillator group and 46 months in the nondefibrillator group. The independent predictors of total cardiac mortality were LVEF of <0.40, absence of an implantable defibrillator, and persistence of inducible sustained VT. The 1- and 5-year probabilities of survival free of cardiac mortality in patients with LVEF of less than 40% were 94% and 70% with a defibrillator and 82% and 45% without a defibrillator, respectively. For patients with LVEF of 40% or more, the 1- and 5-year probabilities of survival free of cardiac mortality were 98% and 95% with a defibrillator and 95% and 87% without a defibrillator, respectively (Figure 4-5). Thus, in survivors of out-of-hospital cardiac arrest, the implantable defibrillator is associated with a reduction in cardiac mortality especially in patients with impaired LVEFs.

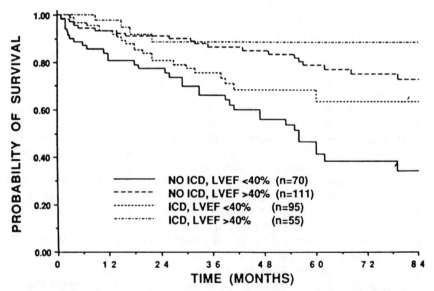

Figure 4-5. Total mortality in patients with and without an implantable defibrillator (ICD) stratified by LVEF is shown. Reproduced with permission from Powell et al.[69]

To determine the driving behavior of patients following the placement of automatic implantable cardioverter-defibrillators (AICDs), Finch and associates,[70] from Charleston, SC, sent questionnaires to 40 patients with AICDs (33 men and 7 women; mean age, 63 years) designed to ascertain driving behavior after hospital discharge. Despite medical advice never to drive again, 28 patients (70%) resumed driving, with the majority doing so by 8 months after AICD implantation. Of these, 11 (40%) identified themselves as the primary driver in their household. Fourteen (50%) drove daily. Two (7%) were driving and continued to drive during discharge of their AICDs. Twenty-five (91%) reported that they felt comfortable and safe while driving. A majority of patients with AICDs continue to drive after a proscription of this activity by health care workers.

New transvenous lead systems have made it more practical to place cardioverter-defibrillators in patients without the need of median sternotomy and general anesthesia. Brooks and associates,[71] from Boston, Mass, evaluated the determinants of successful cardioverter-defibrillator implantation in a total of 101 consecutive patients. Seventy-one percent of patients could have a nonthoracotomy system implanted. Twenty-nine patients required thoracotomy. Univariate predictors of successful nonthoracotomy implantation included smaller heart size, smaller cardiothoracic ratio, QRS duration <120 ms, female gender, VF as the presenting arrhythmia, and smaller echocardiographic LV size. Multivariate predictors included smaller cardiac size and female gender. Total survival over a mean of 12 months was 91% and was not different between the two groups. These authors concluded that a nonthoracotomy cardioverter-defibrillator system can be implanted in the majority of patients. Smaller heart size and female gender are associated with a high probability of successful implantation.

To determine the influence of LV function on survival and mode of death in patients with an implantable cardioverter-defibrillator, Kim and associates,[72] from the Bronx, NY, evaluated sudden death, surgical mortality, total arrhythmia-related death, total cardiac death, and total death in 377 consecutive patients. The outcomes were also compared between patients with an LVEF ≥30% (214 patients, group 1) and <30% (148 patients, group 2). Surgical mortality was 4% (2% in group 1, 7% in group 2). During the follow-up of 25 months, actuarial survival rates of all patients at 3 years were 96% for sudden deaths, 81% for total cardiac deaths, and 74% for total mortality. When the two groups were compared, survival rates of groups 1 and 2 at 3 years, respectively, were 99% and 90% for sudden death, 97% and 84% for sudden death and surgical mortality, 94% and 80% for total arrhythmia-related death, 88% and 68% for total cardiac death, and 81% and 62% for total mortality. In group 2, 73% of total cardiac deaths within 1 year were causally related to the arrhythmia. Thus, in patients with an implantable cardioverter-defibrillator, sudden death rates were very low. However, total cardiac death and total death rates were relatively higher. The outcomes of patients with an implantable cardioverter-defibrillator were strongly influenced by the degree of LV dysfunction. In group 2 patients, although the sudden death rate was relatively low (10% at 3 years), surgical mortality rate, total cardiac death rate, and total mortality rate were substantial. A significant majority of total cardiac deaths were causally related to the arrhythmia.

MISCELLANEOUS

Long Q-T Syndrome in Children

Garson and associates,[73] from Durham, NC, and the Pediatric Electrophysiology Society, studied patients <21 years old with long Q-T syndrome to define low-risk and high-risk subpopulations and to determine optimal treatment. Patients were included if QT_c was >0.44; they had unexplained syncope, seizures, or cardiac arrest preceded by emotion or exercise; or they had a family history of long Q-T syndrome. There were 287 patients from 26 centers identified with mean ± SD age at presentation of 6.8 ± 5.6 years. Cardiac arrest was the presentation in 9%, syncope in 26%, and seizures in 10%. Of those with symptoms, 67% were related to exercise. Family history was positive for long Q-T interval in 39% and for sudden death in 31%. Hearing loss was present in 5%. A normal QT_c was present in 6% and QT_c of >.6 was present in 13%. Heart block occurred in 5%; 13 of 15 had second degree block, and only 2 of 15 had complete block. Ventricular arrhythmias were found in 16% with 5% multiform PVCs, 1% monomorphic VT, and 6% torsade de pointes. Overall treatment was effective for symptoms in 76% and for ventricular arrhythmias in 60%. There was no difference between propranolol and other β-blockers in effective treatment. Left stellectomy was performed in 9 patients, and defibrillators were implanted in 4; no sudden death occurred in these 13 patients. In follow-up for an average duration for 5 years, 5% had cardiac arrest, 4% had syncope, and 1% had seizures. The two multivariate predictors of symptoms at follow-up were symptoms at presentation and propranolol failure. Sudden death occurred in 8%; multivariate predictors of sudden death were length of QT_c at presentation of more than .6 and medication noncompliance. The appearance of 2:1 AV block, multiple premature VPCs, and torsade de pointes are relatively more common in children with long Q-T syndrome than other children and should raise the suspicion for long Q-T syndrome. Because 9% of patients presented with cardiac arrest and no symptoms, prophylactic treatment in asymptomatic children may be indicated. Asymptomatic patients with normal QT_c and positive family history may be a low-risk group. Patients with QT_c of more than .6 are at particularly high risk for sudden death; and if treatment is not effective, consideration should be given to cardiac sympathetic denervation, pacemaker implantation, and/or defibrillator implantation. This study presents an excellent review of a fairly large number of patients with this problem. Determining optimal management for patients with a borderline long QT_c and vague symptoms continues to be difficult.

Global T-Wave Inversion

Symmetric global T-wave inversion is a striking finding in certain patients. Walder and Spodick[74] from Worcester, Mass, reported an 8-year prospective investigation of global T-wave inversion in a total of 118 patients who were followed for periods up to 11 years. The initial in-hospital death rate was approximately 8%. Long-term survival was shortened by digoxin, faster heart rates, atrial fibrillation, and especially malignancy. Seventy-eight percent of 23 patients with malignant condition died during the follow-up period with a mean survival time of only 12 months. Kaplan-Meier curves showed a poor prognosis for those taking digoxin (64% of 36 patients died). Eleven of the 12 patients with atrial fibrillation were taking digoxin, and 58% of these died demonstrating a worse prognosis than that of patients with sinus rhythm, 35% of whom died. Global T-wave inversion has an unexplained female preponderance. The long-term prognosis depends on the underlying or associated diseases, and the striking diffuse ECG changes do not in themselves imply a poor prognosis.

Electrophysiologic Study in Octogenarians

To assess the indications, diagnostic yield, and incidence of complications of electrophysiologic testing in the elderly, Wagshal and associates,[75] from Worcester, Mass, reviewed their experience with 60 procedures in 45 patients aged ≥80 years (range, 80 to 92 years; mean age, 83) undergoing full electrophysiologic evaluation over the past 7 years. The yield of inducible VT (31%), SVT (4%), and previously unsuspected conduction abnormalities significant enough to warrant permanent pacemaker implantation (9%), together with the low incidence of complications (1 patient had a deep venous thrombosis and femoral artery pseudoaneurysm, representing an incidence of 2.2% of patients undergoing studies or 3.3% incidence of complications per procedure), suggests that invasive electrophysiologic procedures in the elderly can provide useful information at a complication rate comparable with that of younger patients.

Myocardial Perfusion Scintigraphy in Left Bundle Branch Block

Among selected study populations, myocardial perfusion scintigraphy in patients with left BBB has been reported to show a low specificity for the diagnosis of CAD. However, the stress electrocardiogram is nondiagnostic in this setting. To place this method in its appropriate clinical context, Krishnan and associates,[76] from San Francisco, Calif, evaluated myocardial perfusion scintigraphy in all 69 consecutive patients with left BBB studied with scintigraphy for clinical reasons during a 4-year period. Among 32 patients who underwent coronary angiography for clinical indications, per patient sensitivity, 96%; per vessel sensitivity, 84%, 50%, and 100% for LAD, LC, and right coronary artery involvement, respectively; and per vessel specificity, 95% and 68% for LC and right coronary artery disease, respectively, were not significantly different from those previously published for the method in patients without left BBB. Although per patient specificity 38% and specificity 39% for LAD disease were low, the predictive value of a positive test remained relatively high (83%) owing to the small number of patients selected for angiography, in part based on scintigraphic findings, with normal coronary anatomy. In addition to a possible specific pathophysiologic cause related to left BBB, apparent perfusion abnormalities in the LAD distribution may relate to generic conditions that can make scintigraphic interpretation ambiguous, often in the anterior distribution, regardless of the clinical setting. Additionally, the apparent lack of scintigraphic specificity in the LAD distribution could relate in part to a selection of bias toward catheterization of patients with induced scintigraphic abnormalities, especially in the LAD distribution. The low incidence of coronary-related events among patients with limited defects or normal scintigrams is additional evidence of the true scintigraphic specificity and the clinical value of the method in patients with left BBB. The selective occurrence of false positive scintigrams in the LAD territory among patients undergoing dynamic exercise compared with the more specific findings in the subgroup undergoing pharmacologic stress scintigraphy suggest that the latter method may be preferred in this patient population regardless of the cause of this finding. The results demonstrate the full spectrum of scintigraphy in patients with left BBB and support an important clinical role for the method in this difficult diagnostic subgroup.

References

1. de Belder MA, Lovat LB, Tourikis L, et al: Left atrial spontaneous contrast echoes—markers of thromboembolic risk in patients with atrial fibrillation. Euro Heart J 1993 (March);14:326–335.

2. Steinberg JS, Zelenkofske S, Wong S-C, et al: Value of the P-wave signal-averaged ECG for predicting atrial fibrillation after cardiac surgery. Circulation 1993 (Dec);88:2618–2622.

3. Ueshima K, Myers J, Ribisl PM, et al: Hemodynamic determinants of exercise capacity in chronic atrial fibrillation. Am Heart J 1993 (May);125:1301–1305.

4. Van Gelder IC, Crijns HJGM, Blanksma PK, et al: Time course of hemodynamic changes and improvement of exercise tolerance after cardioversion of chronic atrial fibrillation unassociated with cardiac valve disease. Am J Cardiol 1993 (Sep 1);72:560–566.

5. Manning WJ, Silverman DI, Gordon SPF, et al: Cardioversion from atrial fibrillation without prolonged anticoagulation with use of transesophageal echocardiography to exclude the presence of atrial thrombi. N Engl J Med 1993 (March 18);328:750–755.

6. Black IW, Hopkins AP, Lee LCL, et al: Evaluation of transesophageal echocardiography before cardioversion of atrial fibrillation and flutter in nonanticoagulated patients. Am Heart J 1993 (Aug);126:375–381.

7. Creswell LL, Schuessler RB, Rosenbloom M, et al: Hazards of postoperative atrial arrhythmias. Ann Thorac Surg 1993;56:539–549.

8. Jordaens L, Missault L, Germonpré E, et al: Delayed restoration of atrial function after conversion of atrial flutter by pacing or electrical cardioversion. Am J Cardiol 1993 (Jan 1);71:63–67.

9. EAFT (European Atrial Fibrillation Trial) Study Group: Secondary prevention in non-rheumatic atrial fibrillation after transient ischemic attack or minor stroke. Lancet 1993 (Nov 20);342:1255–1262.

10. Reimold SC, Cantillon CO, Friedman PL, et al: Propafenone versus sotalol for suppression of recurrent symptomatic atrial fibrillation. Am J Cardiol 1993 (March 1);71:558–563.

11. Kalbfleisch SJ, El-Atassi R, Calkins H, et al: Differentiation of paroxysmal narrow QRS complex tachycardias using the 12-lead electrocardiogram. J Am Coll Cardiol 1993 (Jan);21:85–89.

12. Chen S-A, Chiang C-E, Tsang W-P, et al: Selective radiofrequency catheter ablation of fast and slow pathways in 100 patients with atrioventricular nodal reentrant tachycardia. Am Heart J 1993 (Jan);125:1–10.

13. Mitrani RD, Klein LS, Hackett K, et al: Radiofrequency ablation for atrioventricular node reentrant tachycardia: Comparison between fast (ante-

rior) and slow (posterior) pathway ablation. J Am Coll Cardiol 1993 (Feb);21(2):432–441.

14. Chen S-A, Chiang C-E, Tsang W-P, et al: Recurrent conduction in accessory pathway and possible new arrhythmias after radiofrequency catheter ablation. Am Heart J 1993 (Feb);125:381–387.

15. Chiang C-E, C'hen S-A, Wang D-C, et al: Arrhythmogenicity of catheter ablation in supraventricular tachycardia. Am Heart J 1993 (Feb);125:388–395.

16. Klein LS, Hackett FK, Zipes DP, et al: Radiofrequency catheter ablation of Mahaim fibers at the tricuspid annulus. Circulation 1993 (March);87: 738–747.

17. Chen S-A, Hsia C-P, Chiang C-E, et al: Reappraisal of radiofrequency ablation of multiple accessory pathways. Am Heart J 1993 (March);125: 760–771.

18. Kalbfleisch SJ, El-Atassi R, Calkins H, et al: Safety, feasibility and cost of outpatient radiofrequency catheter ablation of accessory atrioventricular connections. J Am Coll Cardiol 1993 (March 1);21:567–570.

19. Kay GN, Chong F, Epstein AE, et al: Radiofrequency ablation for treatment of primary atrial tachycardias. J Am Coll Cardiol 1993 (March 15);21: 901–909.

20. Chen S-A, Chiang C-E, Yang C-J, et al: Usefulness of serial follow-up electrophysiologic studies in predicting late outcome of radiofrequency ablation for accessory pathways and atrioventricular nodal reentrant tachycardia. Am Heart J 1993 (Sep);126:619–625.

21. Prager NA, Cox JL, Lindsay BD, et al: Long-term effectiveness of surgical treatment of ectopic atrial tachycardia. J Am Coll Cardiol 1993 (July);22: 85–92.

22. Lai WT, Voon WC, Yen HW, et al: Comparison of the electrophysiologic effects of oral sustained release and intravenous verapamil in patients with paroxysmal supraventricular tachycardia. Am J Cardiol 1993 (Feb 15);71:405–408.

23. Clayton RH, Murray A, Higham PD, et al: Self-terminating ventricular tachyarrhythmias. Lancet 1993 (Jan 9);341:93–95.

24. Metzger JT, de Chillou C, Cheriex E, et al: Value of the 12-lead electrocardiogram in arrhythmogenic right ventricular dysplasia, and absence of correlation with echocardiographic findings. Am J Cardiol 1993 (Oct 15);72:964–967.

25. The ESVEM Investigators: Determinants of predicted efficacy of antiarrhythmic drugs in the electrophysiologic study versus electrocardiographic monitoring trial. Circulation 1993 (Feb);87:323–329.

26. Mason JW: Comparison of electrophysiologic testing with Holter monitoring to predict antiarrhythmic-drug efficacy for ventricular tachyarrhythmias. N Engl J Med 1993 (Aug 12);329:445–451.

27. Brodsky MA, Orlov MV, Winters RJ, et al: Determinants of inducible ventricular tachycardia in patients with clinical ventricular tachyarrhythmia and no apparent structural heart disease. Am Heart J 1993 (Nov);126: 1113–1120.

28. Lerman BB: Response of nonreentrant catecholamine-mediated ventricular tachycardia to endogenous adenosine and acetylcholine: Evidence for myocardial receptor-mediated effects. Circulation 1993 (Feb);87:382–390.

29. Kowey PR, Marinchak RA, Pials SJ, et al: Electrophysiologic testing in patients who respond acutely to intravenous amiodarone for incessant ventricular tachyarrhythmias. Am Heart J 1993 (June);125:1628–1632.

30. Mason JW: A comparison of seven antiarrhythmic drugs in patients with ventricular tachyarrhythmias. N Engl J Med 1993 (Aug 12);329:452–458.

31. Gill JS, Blaszyk K, Ward DE, et al: Verapamil for the suppression of idiopathic ventricular tachycardia of left bundle branch block-like morphology. Am Heart J 1993 (Nov);126:1126–1133.

32. Dorian P, Newman D, Berman N, et al: Sotalol and type IA drugs in combination prevent recurrence of sustained ventricular tachycardia. J Am Coll Cardiol 1993 (July);22:106–113.

33. Weinberg BA, Miles WM, Klein IS, et al: Five-year follow-up of 589 patients treated with amiodarone. Am Heart J 1993 (Jan);125:109–120.

34. Olson PJ, Woelfel A, Simpson RJ, et al: Stratification of sudden death risk in patients receiving long-term amiodarone treatment for sustained ventricular tachycardia or ventricular fibrillation. Am J Cardiol 1993 (April 1);71:823–826.

35. Ujhelyi MR, Fisher JR, Chow MSS, et al: Evaluation of the need to modify antiarrhythmic therapy because of drug intolerance or inefficacy in patients evaluated by electrophysiology study. Am Heart J 1993 (Aug);126:352–359.

36. Makkar RR, Fromm BS, Steinman RT, et al: Female gender as a risk factor for torsades de pointes associated with cardiovascular drugs. JAMA 1993 (Dec 1);270:2590–2597.

37. Morady F, Harvey M, Kalbfleisch SJ, et al: Radiofrequency catheter ablation of ventricular tachycardia in patients with coronary artery disease. Circulation 1993 (Feb);87:363–372.

38. Aizawa Y, Chinushi M, Naitoh N, et al: Catheter ablation with radiofrequency current of ventricular tachycardia originating from the right ventricle. Am Heart J 1993 (May);125:1269–1275.

39. Nakagawa H, Beckman KJ, McClelland JH, et al: Radiofrequency catheter ablation of idiopathic left ventricular tachycardia guided by a Purkinje potential. Circulation 1993 (Dec);88:2607–2617.

40. Berntsen RF, Gunnes P, Lie M, et al: Surgical revascularization in the treatment of ventricular tachycardia and fibrillation exposed by exercise-induced ischaemia. Euro Heart J 1993 (Oct);14:1297–1393.

41. Myerburg RJ, Kessler KM, Castellanos A: Sudden cardiac death: Epidemiology, transient risk, and intervention assessment. Ann Intern Med 1993 (Dec 15);1187–1197.

42. Solomon NA. What are representative survival rates for out-of-hospital cardiac arrest as viewed from the New Haven, Connecticut experience. Arch Intern Med 1993 (May 24);153:1218–1221.

43. Madl C, Grimm G, Kramer L, et al: Early prediction of individual outcome after cardiopulmonary resuscitation. Lancet 1993 (April 3);341:855–858.

44. Tresch DD, Neahring JM, Duthie EH, et al: Outcomes of cardiopulmonary resuscitation in nursing homes. Am J Med 1993 (Aug);95:123–130.

45. Becker LB, Han BH, Meyer PM, et al, and the CPR Chicago Project: Racial differences in the incidence of cardiac arrest and subsequent survival. N Engl J Med 1993 (Aug 26);329:600–606.

46. Meissner MD, Lehmann MH, Steinman RT, et al: Ventricular fibrillation in patients without significant structural heart disease: A multicenter experience with implantable cardioverter-defibrillator therapy. J Am Coll Cardiol 1993 (May);21:1406–1412.

47. Cohen TJ, Goldner BG, Maccaro PC, et al: Comparison of active compression-decompression cardiopulmonary resuscitation with standard cardiopulmonary resuscitation for cardiac arrests occurring in the hospital. N Engl J Med 1993 (Dec 23);329:1918–1921.

48. Tucker KJ, Redberg RF, Schiller NB, et al, for the Cardiopulmonary Resuscitation Working Group, University of California, San Francisco: Active compression decompression resuscitation: Analysis of transmitral flow and left ventricular volume by transesophageal echocardiography in humans. J Am Coll Cardiol 1993 (Nov 1);22:1485–1493.

49. Bonnin MJ, Pepe PE, Kimball KT, et al: Distinct criteria for termination of resuscitation in the out-of-hospital setting. JAMA 1993 (Sep 22/29);270:1457–1462.

50. Maynard C, for the CASCADE Investigators: Rehospitalization in surviving patients of out-of-hospital ventricular fibrillation (the CASCADE Study). Am J Cardiol 1993 (Dec 1);72:1295–1300.

51. Roine RO, Kajaste S, Kaste M: Neuropsychological sequelae of cardiac arrest. JAMA 1993 (Jan 13);269:237–242.

52. The CASCADE Investigators: Randomized antiarrhythmic drug therapy in survivors of cardiac arrest (the CASCADE Study). Am J Cardiol 1993 (Aug 1);72:280–287.

53. Maksoud A, Jahnigen DW, Skibinski CI: Do not resuscitate orders and the cost of death. Arch Intern Med 1993 (May 24);153:1249–1253.

54. Jayes RL, Zimmerman JE, Wagner DP, et al: Do-not-resuscitate orders in intensive care units. JAMA 1993 (Nov 10);270:2213–2217.

55. Ponsonby A-L, Dwyer T, Gibbons LE, et al: Factors potentiating the risk of sudden infant death syndrome associated with the prone position. N Engl J Med 1993 (Aug 5);329:377–382.

56. Middlekauff HR, Stevenson WG, Saxon LA: Prognosis after syncope: Impact of left ventricular function. Am Heart J 1993 (Jan);125:121–127.

57. de Buitleir M, Grogan EW Jr, Picone MF, et al: Immediate reproducibility of the tilt-table test in adults with unexplained syncope. Am J Cardiol 1993 (Feb 1);71:304–307.

58. Müller G, Deal BJ, Strasburger JF, et al: Usefulness of metoprolol for unexplained syncope and positive response to tilt testing in young persons. Am J Cardiol 1993 (Mar 1):71:592–595.

59. Sra JS, Jazayeri MR, Avitall B, et al: Comparison of cardiac pacing with drug therapy in the treatment of neurocardiogenic (vasovagal) syncope with bradycardia or asystole. N Engl J Med 1993 (April 15);328:1085–1090.

60. Brooks R, Ruskin JN, Powell AC, et al: Prospective evaluation of day-to-day reproducibility of upright tilt-table testing in unexplained syncope. Am J Cardiol 1993 (Jun 1);71:1289–1292.

61. McIntosh SJ, Lawson J, Kenny RA: Clinical characteristics of vasodepressor, cardioinhibitory, and mixed carotid sinus syndrome in patients over 65 years of age. Am J Med 1993 (Aug 1993);95:203–208.

62. Morillo CA, Leitch JW, Yee R, et al: A placebo-controlled trial of intravenous and oral disopyramide for prevention of neurally mediated syncope induced by head-up tilt. J Am Coll Cardiol 1993 (Dec);22:1843–1848.

63. Hayes DL, Vlietstra RE: Pacemaker malfunction. Ann Intern Med 1993 (Oct 15);119:828–835.

64. Silka MJ, Kron J, Dunnigan A, et al: Sudden cardiac death and the use of implantable cardioverter-defibrillators in pediatric patients. Circulation 1993 (March);87:800–807.

65. Bardy GH, Hofer B, Johnson G, et al: Implantable transvenous cardioverter-defibrillators. Circulation 1993 (April);87:1152–1168.

66. Crandall BG, Morris CD, Cutler JE, et al: Implantable cardioverter-defibrillator therapy in survivors of out-of-hospital sudden cardiac death without inducible arrhythmias. J Am Coll Cardiol 1993 (April);21:1186–1192.

67. Bocker D, Block M, Isbruch F, et al: Do patients with an implantable defibrillator live longer? J Am Coll Cardiol 1993 (June);21:1638–1644.

68. Grimm W, Flores BT, Marchlinski FE: Shock occurrence and survival in 241 patients with implantable cardioverter-defibrillator therapy. Circulation 1993 (June);87:1880–1888.

69. Powell AC, Fuchs T, Finkelstein DM, et al: Influence of implantable cardioverter-defibrillators on the long-term prognosis of survivors of out-of-hospital cardiac arrest. Circulation 1993 (Sep);88:1083–1092.

70. Finch NJ, Leman RB, Kratz JM, et al: Driving safety among patients with automatic implantable cardioverter-defibrillators. JAMA 1993 (Oct 6);270:1587–1588.

71. Brooks R, Garan H, Torchiana D, et al: Determinants of successful nonthoracotomy cardioverter-defibrillator implantation: Experience in 101 patients using two different lead systems. J Am Coll Cardiol 1993 (Dec);22:1835–1842.

72. Kim SG, Maloney JD, Pinski SL, et al: Influence of left ventricular function on survival and mode of death after implantable defibrillator therapy (Cleveland Clinic Foundation and Montefiore Medical Center Experience). Am J Cardiol 1993 (Dec 1);72:1263–1267.

73. Garson A Jr, Dick M II, Fournier A, et al: The long QT syndrome in children. An international study of 287 patients. Circulation (June) 1993;87:1866–1872.

74. Walder LA, Spodick DH: Global T wave inversion: Long-term follow-up. J Am Coll Cardiol 1993 (June);21:1652–1656.

75. Wagshal AB, Schuger CD, Habbal B, et al: Invasive electrophysiologic evaluation in octogenarians: Is age a limiting factor? Am Heart J 1993 (Nov);126:1142–1146.

76. Krishnan R, Lu J, Zhu YY, et al: Myocardial perfusion scintigraphy in left bundle branch block: A perspective on the issue from image analysis in a clinical context. Am Heart J 1993 (Sep);126:578–586.

5

Systemic Hypertension

Prevalence in Framingham

Trends in hypertension prevalence are difficult to assess because of a massive increase in the prevalence of antihypertensive treatment. According to an investigation by Kannel and associates,[1] from Boston, Mass, and Bethesda, Md, over the past 3 decades, mean BP levels among the 5,209 members of the Framingham Study cohort have declined; and elevated BP is only one third as prevalent. However, if those receiving treatment who have normalized BPs are defined as hypertensive, in addition to those with elevated BP, the prevalence of hypertension has increased. No consistent secular trend in the incidence of hypertension was noted over 3 decades, but high BP eventually developed in two thirds of the study cohort. To determine whether untreated BP levels are changing over time, trends in mean BP were examined in normotensive subjects over 3 decades. Only a 1 mm Hg decline in mean systolic and diastolic BP over each 10-year interval was noted. Thus, BP in the normotensive segment of the population has been quite stable. Because the incidence of hypertension is very high and future hypertension arises from the upper end of the normal BP distribution, there is an urgent need for primary prevention. Preventive measures such as exercise, avoidance of salt and alcohol, and especially weight control deserve high priority.

Fifth Report of Joint National Committee on Detection, Evaluation, and Treatment

The Fifth Report on the Joint National Committee on Detection, Evaluation, and Treatment of High BP,[2] published on the 20th anniversary of the National High Blood Pressure Education Program, aims to contribute to progress in the primary prevention and control of high BP. Like its predecessors, this document builds on the available scientific evidence regarding the detection, evaluation, and treatment of systemic hypertension. This report guides practicing physicians and other health professionals in their care of hypertensive patients and health professionals participating in the many community high BP control programs. Several new features are in the report: (1) Prevalence, awareness, treatment, and control rates for high BP are reported from the 1988 to 1991 National Health and Nutrition Examination Survey (NHANES III) (Table 5-1). These are the first new data in more than a decade in this area. (2) A new classification schema of BP that includes systolic as well as diastolic levels is proposed to help convey the impact of high BP risk for cardiovascular disease. Many believe the previously used classification, particularly the term *mild hypertension*, sounded complacent and lacked sufficient emphasis and urgency (Table 5-2). (3) An expanded section on primary prevention translates a growing body of knowledge about preventing the disease into recommendations for action. (4) The list of agents that are suitable for initial monotherapy has been expanded— from diuretics, β-blockers, calcium antagonists, and angiotensin-converting enzyme inhibitors—to include the α_1 receptor blockers and the α-β-blocker. (5) Because diuretics and β-blockers are the only classes of drugs that have been used in long-term controlled clinical trials and shown to reduce morbidity and mortality, they are recommended as first-choice agents unless they are contraindicated or unacceptable, or unless there are special indications for other agents. (6) Information on special populations and situations has been expanded and now includes recommendations regarding hypertension in women, isolated systolic hypertension in older persons, cyclosporine, shock-wave lithotripsy, cocaine, and erythropoietin. (7) Pharmacologic tables have been updated and include new drugs, recommendations for reduced doses, drug-drug interactions, and drugs to be used in hypertensive crises. (8) The term *life-style modifications* is used, instead of *nonpharmacologic therapy*, as a treatment modality for prevention and management of high BP.

Table 5-1. Hypertension* Awareness, Treatment, and Control Rates. Reproduced with permission from Joint National Committee on Detection, Evaluation, and Treatment of High Blood Pressure.[2]

	1971-1972†	1974-1975†	1976-1980‡	1988-1991§
Aware: % of				
hypertensives told by physician	51	64	(54) 73	(65) 84
Treated: % of hypertensives taking medication	36	34	(33) 56	(49) 73
Controlled: % of hypertensives with blood pressure <160/95 mm Hg on 1 occasion and reported currently taking antihypertensive medications	16	20	(11) 34	(21) 55

*Defined as 160/95 mm Hg or more on one occasion or reported currently taking antihypertensive medication. Numbers in parentheses are percentages at 140/90 mm Hg or more.
†Source, National Health and Nutrition Examination Survey I.[1]
‡Source, National Health and Nutrition Examination Survey II.[2]
§Source: National Health and Nutrition Examination Survey III (unpublished data provided by the Centers for Disease Control, National Center for Health Statistics).

Table 5-2. Classification of Blood Pressure for Adults 18 Years and Older.* Reproduced with permission from Joint National Committee on Detection, Evaluation, and Treatment of High Blood Pressure.[2]

Category	Systolic, mm Hg	Diastolic, mm Hg
Normal†	<130	<85
High normal	130-139	85-89
Hypertension‡		
Stage 1 (mild)	140-159	90-99
Stage 2 (moderate)	160-179	100-109
Stage 3 (severe)	180-209	110-119
Stage 4 (very severe)	≥210	≥120

*Not taking antihypertensive drugs and not acutely ill. When systolic and diastolic pressures fall into different categories, the higher category should be selected to classify the individual's blood pressure status. For instance, 160/92 mm Hg should be classified as stage 2, and 180/120 mm Hg should be classified as stage 4. Isolated systolic hypertension is defined as a systolic blood pressure of 140 mm Hg or more and a diastolic blood pressure of less than 90 mm Hg and staged appropriately (eg, 170/85 mm Hg is defined as stage 2 isolated systolic hypertension).

In addition to classifying stages of hypertension on the basis of average blood pressure levels, the clinician should specify presence or absence of target-organ disease and additional risk factors. For example, a patient with diabetes and a blood pressure of 142/94 mm Hg, plus left ventricular hypertrophy should be classified as having "stage 1 hypertension with target-organ disease (left ventricular hypertrophy) and with another major risk factor (diabetes)." This specificity is important for risk classification and management.

†Optimal blood pressure with respect to cardiovascular risk is less than 120 mm Hg systolic and less than 80 mm Hg diastolic. However, unusually low readings should be evaluated for clinical significance.

‡Based on the average of two or more readings taken at each of two or more visits after an initial screening.

The National High Blood Pressure Education Program

The National High Blood Pressure Education Program (NHBPEP) was launched 20 years ago based on data from population studies and clinical trials that showed high BP was a major unsolved, but soluble, mass public health problem. Stamler and associates,[3] from Chicago, Ill, and Minneapolis, Minn, summarized recent data from US prospective population studies on BP and cardiovascular risk. The outcome variables included BP-related risks, primarily incidence and mortality from CAD, stroke, other and all cardiovascular diseases; cardiac abnormalities (roentgenographic, electrocardiographic, echocardiographic); and all-cause mortality and life expectancy. Data accrued during the past 20 years confirm that systolic BP and diastolic BP have continuous, graded, strong, independent, etiologically significant relationships to the outcome variables. These relationships are documented for young, middle-aged, and older men and for middle-aged and older women of varying socioeconomic backgrounds and ethnicity. Among persons aged ≥ 35, most have systolic BP/diastolic BP above optimal (<120/<80 mm Hg); hence, they are at increased cardiovascular disease risk (ie, the BP problem involves most of the population, not only the substantial minority with clinical high BP). For middle-aged and older persons, systolic BP relates even more strongly to risk than diastolic BP; at every diastolic BP level, higher systolic BP results in greater cardiovascular disease risk and curtailment of life expectancy. A great potential exists for improved health and increased longevity through control of the BP problem. Its realization requires a strategy combining populationwide and high-risk approaches, the former to prevent rise of BP with age and to achieve primary prevention of high BP by nutritional-hygienic means; the latter to enhance detection, treatment, and control of high BP. The newly expanded goals of the NHBPEP, aimed at implementing this broader strategy for the solution of the BP problem, merit active support from physicians and all health professionals.

Natural History of Borderline Isolated Systolic Elevation

Patients with isolated systolic hypertension are at increased risk for cardiovascular disease. Sagie and associates,[4] from Framingham and Boston, Mass, and Bethesda, Md, attempted to determine whether those with borderline isolated systolic systemic hypertension (systolic BP of 140 to 159 mm Hg and a diastolic BP < 90 mm Hg) have a greater risk of progression to definite (more severe) hypertension and of major morbid or fatal events than people with normal BP (<140/90 mm Hg) (Figures 5-1 and 5-2). A total of 2,767 of the original participants in the Framingham

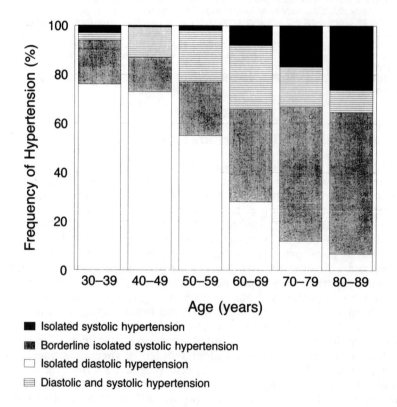

■ Isolated systolic hypertension

▨ Borderline isolated systolic hypertension

☐ Isolated diastolic hypertension

▤ Diastolic and systolic hypertension

Figure 5-1. Relative frequencies of untreated isolated systolic hypertension, borderline isolated systolic hypertension, isolated diastolic hypertension, and diastolic and systolic hypertension in men, according to age. The results are based on pooled data from biennial examinations 2 through 19. Reproduced with permission from Sagie et al.[4]

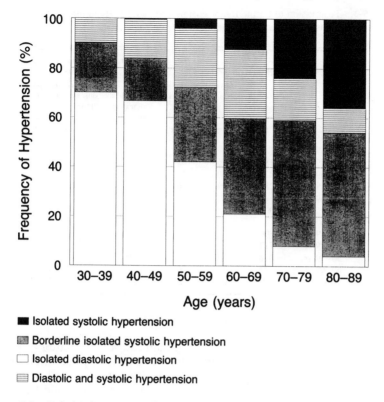

Figure 5-2. Relative frequencies of untreated isolated systolic hypertension, borderline isolated systolic hypertension, isolated diastolic hypertension, and diastolic and systolic hypertension in women, according to age. The results are based on pooled data from biennial examinations 2 through 19. Reproduced with permission from Sagie et al.[4]

Heart Study were monitored with biennial examinations for up to 34 years for the development of definite hypertension (defined as a systolic BP of ≥160 mm Hg, a diastolic BP of ≥90 mm Hg, or the initiation of antihypertensive therapy) and for major cardiovascular events. Borderline isolated systolic hypertension was the most common type of untreated hypertension among adults over the age of 60 (Table 5-3). After 20 years of follow-up, 80% of those with borderline isolated systolic hypertension had progression to definite hypertension, as compared with 45% of the normotensive participants. After adjustment for age, sex, and risk factors for cardiovascular disease, participants with borderline isolated systolic hypertension had an excess long-term risk of cardiovascular disease (hazard ratio, 1.47) and death from cardiovascular disease (1.57), as compared with normotensive participants. In an analysis of pooled data from biennial examinations to study short-term sequelae, subjects with borderline isolated systolic hypertension had an increased risk of progression to definite hypertension (odds ratio, 3.84) and of cardiovascular disease (odds ratio, 1.39). Thus, in the short term and the long term, subjects with borderline isolated systolic hypertension are at increased risk of progression to definite hypertension and the development of cardiovascular disease.

Table 5-3. Progression to Define Hypertension According to Hypertension Status at Baseline Examinations. Reproduced with permission from Sagie et al.[4]

GROUP	NORMAL BLOOD PRESSURE			BORDERLINE ISOLATED SYSTOLIC HYPERTENSION		
	NO. OF PARTICIPANTS	PROGRESSION BY 10 YR	PROGRESSION BY 20 YR	NO. OF PARTICIPANTS	PROGRESSION BY 10 YR	PROGRESSION BY 20 YR
		% of participants			% of participants	
Men						
30–39 yr	186	26	42	20	50	67
40–49 yr	422	30	45	33	77	90
50–59 yr	286	28	46	42	47	74
60–69 yr	112	22	47	35	51	76
Total	1006	28	45	130	61	80
Women						
30–39 yr	300	19	38	13	69	77
40–49 yr	710	26	43	52	56	80
50–59 yr	312	27	49	101	60	87
60–69 yr	88	36	59	55	55	80
Total	1410	26	45	221	59	81

Guidelines For Management of the Mild Form

A subcommittee of the World Health Organization/International Society of Hypertension presented a summary of the latest guidelines for the management of patients with mild systemic hypertension.[5] This subcommittee concluded that in both young and elderly people, mild hypertension is a risk factor for cardiovascular disease and should be treated. The article included several tables that are self explanatory (Tables 5-4, 5-5, and 5-6).

Relation of Birth Weight to Blood Pressure

To study the relation between birth weight and systolic BP in infancy and early childhood, Launer and associates,[6] from Rotterdam, The Netherlands, studied 476 Dutch infants born in 1980 to healthy women after uncomplicated pregnancies. Complete data were available on 392 infants. At 4 years of age, the relation between BP and birth weight appeared to be U shaped; low and high birth weight infants had raised BP. Current weight and previous BP were also positively associated with BP at that age. Low birth weight infants (birth weight <3,100 g) had a greater gain in BP and weight in early infancy. High birth weight infants (birth weight ≥3,700 g) had high BP at birth, and weight and BP tended to remain higher thereafter.

Relation of Well-Being to Blood Pressure

To examine the relation between systolic BP and self-perceived well-being in men aged 50 years, Rosengren and associates,[7] from Uppsala, Sweden, examined 776 men from a random sample population of 1,016 men aged 50 years. Low systolic BP was significantly related to impaired social well-being in four areas: work, home and family, financial situation, and housing. Of the items dealing with physical well-being, health,

Table 5-4. Management of Mild Hypertension (Diastolic Blood Pressure 9–105 mm Hg or Systolic Blood Pressure 140–180 mm Hg, or both). Reproduced with permission from Subcommittee of WHO/ISH Mild Hypertension Liaison Committee.[5]

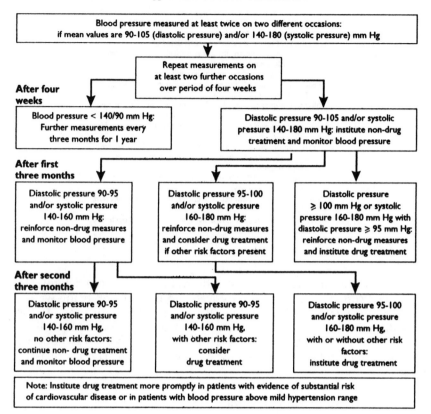

Table 5-5. Classification of Hypertension by Blood Pressure. Reproduced with permission from Subcommittee of WHO/ISH Mild Hypertension Liaison Committee.[5]

Classification	Systolic blood pressure (mm Hg)		Diastolic blood pressure (mm Hg)
Normal	<140	and	<90
Mild hypertension	140-180	and/or	90-105
Subgroup: borderline hypertension	140-160	and/or	90-95
Moderate and severe hypertension*	≥180	and/or	≥105
Isolated systolic hypertension	~140	and	~90
Subgroup: borderline isolated systolic hypertension	140-160	and	<90

*Risk to be indicated by reporting actual values of systolic and diastolic blood pressure.

memory, and appetite were significantly related to BP. As regards mental well-being, energy and self-confidence were significantly related to systolic BP. Diastolic BP was significantly related to housing, memory, energy, patience, and self-confidence. In multiple regression analyses

Table 5-6. Classification of Hypertension by Extent of Organ Damage. Reproduced with permission from Subcommittee of WHO/ISH Mild Hypertension Liaison Committee.[5]

Stage	Sign
I	No objective signs of organic changes
II	At least one of following signs of organ damage:
	left ventricular hypertrophy (*x* ray film, electrocardiogram, echocardiogram)
	generalised and focal narrowing of retinal arteries
	proteinuria or slightly raised plasma creatinine concentration (106-177 μmol/l), or both
	ultrasound or radiological evidence of atherosclerotic plaque (carotid arteries, aorta, iliac and femoral arteries)
III	Both symptoms and signs have appeared as result of organ damage, including
	heart—angina pectoris, myocardial infarction, heart failure
	brain—transient ischaemic attack, stroke, hypertensive encephalopathy
	optic fundi—retinal haemorrhages and exudates with or without papilloedema
	kidney—plasma creatinine concentration > 177 μmol/l, renal failure
	vessels—dissecting aneurysm, symptomatic arterial occlusive disease

that controlled for smoking, stress, physical activity, social activity, and emotional support, poor social, physical, and mental well-being were all significantly related to low systolic BP independently of other factors. Low diastolic BP was independently associated with poor physical and mental, but not social, well-being. Thus, low systolic BP was associated with poor perception of well-being in several areas. The cause is unclear.

Effect on Left Ventricular Filling

Kapuku and associates,[8] from Nagasaki, Japan, determined the effect of borderline hypertension on LV diastolic performance in 16 patients with borderline hypertension who did not have LV hypertrophy and in 16 age- and sex-matched patients with normotension of similar age and body-mass index. Pulsed Doppler echocardiography was used to record LV filling signals at rest and immediately after supine ergometer exercise. All individuals had normal LV structure and systolic function. At rest, the borderline hypertension group in comparison with the normotension group had a depressed peak velocity of early filling (44 ± 7 v 54 ± 10 cm/sec), no enhanced peak velocity of late filling (52 ± 8 v 50 ± 11 cm/sec), and a reduced early filling to late filling ratio (0.9 ± 0.2 v 1.1 ± 0.3). Atrial filling time and preejection period were similar in the two groups. The effect of exercise on LV filling velocity in patients with borderline hypertension resembled that in those with normotension. Percentages changes in early filling (+14% ± 12% v ±14% ± 13%) and late filling (+13% ± 8% v ±11% ± 12%) were equivalent, suggesting a preserved diastolic reserve for exercise in the borderline hypertension group. In conclusion, borderline hypertension appears to be predictive of early filling impairment, and a late filling compensatory mechanism is not yet apparent.

Abnormalities in LV structure and function have been shown in patients with diastolic hypertension and recently in subjects with isolated systolic hypertension. The purpose of this study by Sagie and associates,[9] from Framingham, Mass, was to determine whether abnormalities of cardiac structure or function are present in elderly subjects with borderline isolated systolic hypertension (defined as systolic BP between 140 and 159 mm Hg, and diastolic BP <90 mm Hg). Ninety-one subjects with a mean age of 77 years from the original Framingham Heart Study with untreated borderline isolated systolic hypertension, who were free of cardiovascular disease, were compared with 139 normotensive (BP <140/90 mm Hg) subjects (mean age, 76 years). Measurements included M-mode values for LV structure and six Doppler indexes of LV diastolic filling. Subjects with borderline isolated systolic hypertension and the control group differed in mean systolic (147 v 125 mm Hg) and diastolic (76 v 70 mm Hg) BP. Borderline systolic hypertension was the most frequent form of untreated hypertension in this elderly group. The sum of LV wall thicknesses (septum ± posterior wall) was significantly higher in borderline hypertensive subjects than in normotensive ones (21 v 20 mm). No difference was detected in LV internal dimension or systolic function. After adjustment for age and other clinical variables, comparisons between the groups revealed significant differences in indexes of Doppler diastolic filling. Peak velocity of early filling and the ratio of early to late peak velocities were lower in the hypertensive group (40 v 44 cm/s and 0.69 v 0.76, respectively). Healthy elderly subjects with borderline isolated systolic hypertension have similar LV systolic function, mildly increased LV wall thickness, and evidence of impaired Doppler diastolic filling compared with normotensive subjects.

Effect on Heart Rate Variability

Chakko and associates,[10] from Miami, Fla, and Oulu, Finland, elevated heart rate variability and its circadian rhythm in 22 patients with treated hypertension and LV hypertrophy in whom CAD was excluded by stress thallium or angiography. By using 24-hour Holter monitoring, heart rate variability and its spectral components were measured. Findings were compared with 11 age-matched normal controls. The difference between mean R-R intervals during sleep (11 PM to 7 AM) and while awake (9 AM to 9 PM) (73 ± 33 v 263 ± 63 ms) and the mean 24-hour standard deviation of the R-R intervals (55 ± 6.3 v 93 ± 11 ms) were lower among the hypertensive patients compared with controls. The percentage of difference between successive R-R intervals that exceeded 50 ms, a measure of parasympathetic tone, was also lower among the hypertensive patients (6.8 ± 7.1 v 14 ± 8.9 ms); it increased at night and decreased during the day among the controls, and this circadian rhythm was blunted among the patients. Spectral analysis showed that power in the high-frequency range (0.15 to 0.40 Hz) was lower among the hypertensive patients during 21 of 24 hours but that the difference was statistically significant only during 9 hours. Power in the low-frequency range (0.04 to 0.15 Hz) was lower at night, increased in the morning, and higher during the day among controls; this circadian rhythm was absent among hypertensive patients. Among hypertensive patients free of CAD, heart rate variability is decreased with a partial withdrawal of parasympathetic tone, and the circadian rhythm of sympathetic/parasympathetic tone is altered.

Left Ventricular Mass and Geometry

Høegholm and associates,[11] from Naestved, Denmark, designed a study to compare the cardiac mass and geometry in white coat hypertensive patients and established hypertensive patients through the prospective comparison of office BP, daytime ambulatory BP, and echocardiographically determined LV mass and cardiac geometry in consecutive patients. The authors studied 143 patients from general practice in an outpatient hypertension unit. The patients had newly diagnosed mild-to-moderate hypertension prior to the institution of pharmacological antihypertensive therapy. All patients had a diastolic office BP > 90 mm Hg; 90 had a consistently elevated diastolic BP (established hypertension), whereas 53 had an average daytime ambulatory BP < 90 mm Hg (white coat hypertension). LV mass index was significantly higher in the group with established hypertension, 102.4 ± 26.6 g/m^2 (mean $\pm$ SD) v 93.6 ± 23.5 g/m^2. Relative wall thickness was likewise significantly higher, 0.36 ± 0.07 v 0.33 ± 0.06. There was no significant difference in LA dimension. In a multiple regression model, the ambulatory measurements and not the office measurements were statistically significantly associated with the extent of cardiac hypertrophy. Further, 44/53 (83%) of the patients with white coat hypertension had normal LV dimensions v only 55/90 (61%) of the patients with established hypertension. Thus, white coat hypertensive patients display less cardiac involvement than patients with established hypertension, indicating that they should rather be treated as normotensives than as hypertensives, ie, not with pharmacological antihypertensive therapy.

Silent Myocardial Ischemia

Massie and associates,[12] from San Francisco, Calif, evaluated 226 asymptomatic men, aged 61 years, with essential hypertension and no clinical evidence of CAD to see if there was evidence of silent myocardial ischemia. Patients underwent a stress thallium-201 exercise test, 48-hour ambulatory electrocardiography, and echocardiography. Coronary angiography was performed in a subset (34 of 84 patients) with one or more positive test results. A positive thallium-201 scintigram was more common in the hypertensive group than in the control group (18% v 6%). This was also true for the exercise electrocardiogram (37% v 13%) and ambulatory ECG (15% v 0%). In the group undergoing coronary angiography, thallium-201 scintigraphy was 90% sensitive and 79% specific for epicardial atherosclerotic coronary disease. However, positive exercise and ambulatory ECGs occurred frequently in the absence of significant coronary stenoses. These authors concluded that the false positive ECGs and ambulatory ECGs occurred primarily because of the presence of a high frequency of LV hypertrophy. It appears that the thallium treadmill test has the ability to identify silent CAD disease among high-risk hypertensive patients, but the appropriate application of such screening remains to be determined.

Noctural Pressure After Cardiovascular Events

Verdecchia and associates,[13] from Perugia, Italy, studied 32 hypertensive patients with a first fatal or nonfatal major cardiovascular event who had off-therapy ambulatory BP monitoring 1 to 5 years earlier in the context of a registry of morbidity and mortality in hypertensive patients. Control subjects were 49 hypertensive patients free from cardiovascular events. The groups were matched with regard to date of baseline ambulatory BP monitoring, age, sex, clinic systolic and diastolic BP, and daytime ambulatory systolic and diastolic BP. At their baseline evaluation, cases and controls did not differ, in either sex, with respect to clinic BP, mean daytime ambulatory BP, age, sex, body weight, serum cholesterol, known duration and family history of hypertension, smoking habits, renal function, or prevalence of diabetes. Echocardiographic LV mass determined in a subset of patients was greater in cases than in controls in men. The time interval between baseline ambulatory BP monitoring and subsequent cardiovascular event or last contact with the study center did not differ between the groups. Nocturnal reductions of systolic and diastolic BP in men were 9% and 11%, respectively, in cases v 9% and 12%, respectively, in controls; whereas in women they were 3% and 8%, respectively, in cases v 11% and 16%, respectively, in controls (Figure 5-3). Thus, these data indicate that there is an association between the

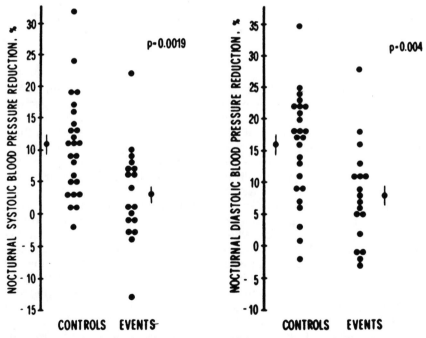

Figure 5-3. Individual values for the nocturnal fall in ambulatory systolic (left) and diastolic (right) blood pressure from daytime (6 AM to 10 PM) to nighttime (10 PM to 6 AM) hours in hypertensive women with future cardiovascular events (right columns) and control hypertensive women without events (left columns). Despite some overlap, there was a smaller nocturnal fall of ambulatory systolic and diastolic BP in case subjects compared with controls. Reproduced with permission from Verdecchia et al.[13]

reduction or absence of the usual nocturnal fall in BP and future cardiovascular events in white women with essential hypertension.

Psychological Predictors

To test the hypothesis that heightened anxiety, heightened anger intensity, and suppressed expression of anger increase the risk of systemic hypertension, Markovitz and associates,[14] from Birmingham, Ala, Pittsburgh, Pa, and Boston, Mass, followed a cohort of men and women from the Framingham Heart Study who had no evidence of systemic hypertension at baseline for 18 to 20 years. A total of 1,123 initially normotensive persons (497 men, 626 women) were included. Hypertension was defined as either taking medication for hypertension or BP > 160/95 mm Hg at a biennial examination. In univariate analyses, middle-aged men who went on to develop hypertension had greater baseline anxiety levels than men who remained normotensive. Older hypertensive men had fewer anger symptoms at baseline and were less likely to hold their anger in than normotensives. In multivariate Cox regression analysis including biological predictors, anxiety remained an independent predictor of hypertension in middle-aged men. Among older men, anger symptoms and anger-in did not remain significant predictors in the multivariate analysis. Further analysis showed that only middle-aged men with very high levels of anxiety were at increased risk. No psychological variable predicted hypertension in middle-aged or older women in either univariate or multivariate analyses. The results indicate that among middle-aged men, but not women, anxiety levels are predictive of later incidence of hypertension.

Serum Creatinine

To describe associations of past and current BP levels with serum creatinine levels and hypercreatinemia in the general population Perneger and associates,[15] from Baltimore, Md, and Geneva, Switzerland, studied 1,399 middle-aged residents of Washington, County, Md, who had their BP measured during a cancer screening campaign in 1974 ("Clue" Study) and had their BP and serum creatinine level measured in an atherosclerosis risk factors study from 1986 through 1989 (the Atherosclerosis Risk in Communities [ARIC] Study). The outcome variables were serum creatinine level and hypercreatinemia (serum creatinine >115 µmol/L in men; >97 µmol/L in women) measured from 1986 through 1989. Main predictors were 1986 to 1989 BP values (cross-sectional association) and 1974 BP values (longitudinal association). Gender-adjusted associations were assessed and compared by linear and logistic regression. Both serum creatinine and hypercreatinemia were better predicted by past than by current BP values. Creatinine values exhibited a gradual and statistically significant association with BP levels measured in 1974, even across "normal" values of BP and creatinine. The association with 1986 to 1989 BP measurements was weaker and nonsignificant. The odds of hypercreatinemia in 1986 through 1989 were increased 1.5-fold to 2-fold, with a 20 mm Hg increment in 1974 BP values, but the odds remained constant across 1986 to 1989 BP values. BP and creatinine level are associated in the general population. The observed association was stronger when a number of years had elapsed between the assessments of BP and creatinine level. These findings are consistent with the hypothesis that BP elevations, even below the hypertensive range, may induce renal damage.

Heart Failure With Normal Ejection Fraction

Previous studies have pointed out that CHF with normal EF presents a uniform clinical profile that is indistinguishable from heart failure with low EF. Iriarte and associates,[16] from Bilbao, Spain, studied 36 patients with systemic hypertension who had recently experienced CHF with normal EF and no clinical history of ischemic cardiomyopathy. The patients were divided into two groups according to degree of echocardiographic hypertrophy: group A (19 patients) with a ventricular mass/volume ratio >1.8 and group B (17 patients) with a ratio <1.8. Group A patients had a higher EF (67% v 57%), smaller ventricular diameters, and a lower thallium-201 positive rate at peak stress, with 8 of 10 showing severe coronary stenosis. Clinically, group A had a more frequent audible fourth sound, a low incidence of audible third sound, and a cardiothoracic ratio <0.5. The degree of radionuclide-detected resting diastolic dysfunction and exercise intolerance was similar in both groups. In conclusion, CHF with normal EF in hypertensive patients presents two different profiles: one characterized by severe hypertrophy and the other by a high rate of myocardial regional ischemia. Therapy should be aimed at pathophysiologic regression of the hypertrophy in the first case and at improvement of the ischemia in the second.

Intramural Coronary Arteries

Schwartzkopff and associates,[17] from Düsseldorf, Germany, studied 14 patients (10 men and 4 women) with arterial hypertension and 8 normotensive subjects to determine minimal coronary resistance and vasodilator reserve using dipyridarnole infusions after the angiographic exclusion of relevant CAD. Coronary reserve was depressed in hypertensive patients due to increased minimal coronary resistance (0.64 ± 0.3 v 0.24 ± 0.05 mm Hg/min/100 g/mL^{-1}). In right septal biopsies, mean external arteriolar diameter, mean arteriolar wall area, percent medial wall area, mean periarteriolar fibrosis area, and volume density of total interstitial fibrosis were increased in hypertensive patients compared with normotensive subjects. LV mass index and LV ventricular end-diastolic pressure did not correlate significantly with minimal coronary resistance. In multivariate analysis, fibrosis explained half of the variability of minimal coronary resistance. Thus, structural remodeling of the intramyocardial coronary arterioles and the accumulation of fibrillar collagen are important factors for the subsequent development of reduced coronary dilatory capacity in patients with arterial hypertension and angina in the absence of important CAD.

Impaired Endothelium-Mediated Relaxation

Treasure and associates,[18] from Atlanta, Ga, studied coronary microvascular responses in ten patients with LV hypertrophy secondary to essential hypertension. The mean arterial pressure at cardiac catheterization in these patients was 151/94 mm Hg, and their mean posterior LV wall thickness was 1.4 ± 0.1 cm. Nine control normal subjects with no history of hypertension and normal mean posterior LV wall thickness were also studied. An intracoronary Doppler catheter and quantitative coronary arteriography were used to assess changes in coronary blood flow. All patients had normal LVEFs. The endothelium-dependent vasodilator, acetylcholine, was infused at concentrations of 10^{-8} to 10^{-6} M and the endothelium-independent vasodilator adenosine at concentrations of 10^{-6} to 10^{-4} into the LAD. In response to acetylcholine, coronary blood flow increased only $32\% \pm 25\%$ in patients with hypertension, whereas it increased $192\% \pm 39\%$ in normal individuals. However, coronary blood flow increased $465\% \pm 93\%$ in patients with hypertension and $439\% \pm 41\%$ in normal control subjects in response to adenosine. Thus, endothelium-dependent vasodilation is impaired in the coronary microvessels of patients with hypertension and LV hypertrophy. Loss of this vasodilator mechanism may contribute to altered coronary flow patterns and symptoms in patients with hypertensive and hypertrophic heart disease.

Vascular endothelial function and dysfunction are proving to play an important role in a variety of clinical circumstances including CAD, CHF, and hypertension. Endothelial function has been previously shown to be impaired in patients with essential hypertension. Panza and associates,[19] from Bethesda, Md, studied 15 patients with essential hypertension before and after reduction of blood pressure with antihypertensive medications. The vascular responses to acetylcholine and sodium nitroprusside were evaluated. Patients were studied after withdrawal of medications when the BP had gone up and then back on appropriate antihypertensive medications. At control, the blood flow and vascular responses to acetylcholine were significantly reduced in the hypertensive patients. No significant differences between groups were observed to the responses to sodium nitroprusside. These responses were not modified by medical therapy. The time interval between the two studies averaged 4.8 months. They concluded that over this short time period clinically effective antihypertensive therapy does not restore impaired endothelial dependent vascular relaxation of patients with essential hypertension. It may be that endothelial dysfunction is either primary, becomes irreversible once the hypertensive process has become established, or requires a longer period of time to normalize.

Panza and associates,[20] from Bethesda, Md, investigated the role of endothelium-derived nitric oxide in the pathogenesis of systemic arterial hypertension by studying the vascular effect of the arginine analogue N^G-monomethyl-L-arginine, an inhibitor of the endothelial synthesis of nitric oxide, under baseline conditions and during infusion of acetylcholine, an endothelium-dependent vasodilator, and sodium nitroprusside, a direct smooth muscle dilator. Eleven hypertensive patients, including 7 men (mean age, 47 years), and 10 control subjects, including 7 men (mean age, 46 years), were evaluated. The drugs were infused into the brachial artery, and the response of the forearm vasculature was measured by strain-gauge plethysmography. Basal blood flow was similar in normal control subjects and hypertensive patients. The vasodilator response to acetylcholine was reduced in patients with hypertension compared with control subjects. N^G-monomethyl-L-arginine blunted the vasodilator response to acetylcholine in control subjects, but it did not significantly alter the response to acetylcholine in hypertensive patients. N^G-monomethyl-L-arginine did not modify the vasodilator response to sodium nitroprusside in either the controls or the hypertensive patients. These data indicate that patients with essential systemic arterial hypertension have a defect in the endothelium-derived nitric oxide system that may at least partly account for the increased vascular resistance under basal conditions and the impaired response to endothelium-dependent vasodilators.

Ambulatory Monitoring

To study the test-ordering behavior of practicing physicians regarding ambulatory monitoring of BP and to assess changes in patient management after this study, Grin and associates,[21] from Farmington, Conn, examined 237 consecutive patients referred by 65 community and hospital-based physicians. The main indications for ordering the test included borderline hypertension (27% of studies ordered), assessment of BP control during drug therapy (25%), evaluation for "white coat" or "office" hypertension (22%), and drug-resistant hypertension (16%). After the ambulatory BP study, only 13% of the patients had further testing (eg, echocardiography); the diagnosis was changed in 41% of the patients, and antihypertensive therapy was changed in 46%. In 122 patients for whom data were complete, office BP measured by the referring physician decreased from 161/96 ± 24/12 mm Hg before the ambulatory BP study to 151/86 ± 27/12 mm Hg 3 months after the study. One to 2 years after the study, office BP was 149/86 ± 24/12 mm Hg. Seventy-two percent of the patients had a lower office BP within 3 months of the ambulatory BP study. Practicing physicians use ambulatory BP recordings for appropriate indications, and data from the monitoring studies affected the management of patients with hypertension.

Accuracy of Measuring Devices

Appel and associates,[22] from Baltimore, Md, and Boston, Mass, reviewed published evidence on the use of ambulatory and self-measurement devices in the diagnosis and management of systemic hypertension. Studies that compared office, self-measured, and ambulatory BP have documented substantial, but nonsystematic, differences. Such findings have raised concern over the appropriateness of diagnosing hypertension and initiating drug therapy in individuals with high office BP but comparatively low self-measured or ambulatory BP ("office" or "white coat" hypertension). Evidence from a large number of cross-sectional studies and a single prospective study suggests that BP-related end-organ damage is more closely associated with ambulatory than with office BP. Less evidence supports self-measured BP in this regard, and data are insufficient to compare ambulatory and self-measured BP in terms of cardiovascular disease risk prediction. The estimated resource cost of an ambulatory BP test is approximately $120, whereas charges range from $100 to $450. The annualized resource cost of BP self-measurement is $50 or less. On a national level, the annual direct costs of ambulatory BP monitoring could be as high as $6 billion, if this technique were used routinely to diagnose and monitor hypertensive patients. The extent to which direct costs would be offset by savings from less frequent or more efficient treatment for hypertension cannot be estimated reliably. Several practical and technical issues also detract from the potential usefulness of ambulatory and self-measurement devices. Finally, there is some evidence that office BPs measured by well-trained nonphysicians may serve as an alternative to ambulatory and self-measurement techniques in estimating usual BP. Limited clinical applications of ambulatory BP monitoring and BP self-measurement in the diagnosis and management of hypertension appear to be warranted. Endorsement of these technologies for routine clinical use, however, will require more convincing evidence of their clinical effectiveness.

A position paper authored by Anne-Marie Audet[23] of the American College of Physicians was presented in the June 1, 1993 *Annals of Internal Medicine*. The recommendations were as follows: Self-measured BP and automated ambulatory BP monitoring devices may, in theory, have a specific role in the diagnosis, prognosis, and management of systemic hypertension. The evidence supporting the role of automated ambulatory BP measurement in the diagnosis and treatment of hypertension is, for the most part, indirect. The major studies showing the benefits of treatment in decreasing the morbidity and mortality risks associated with hypertension have used office-based BP measurements to make diagnoses and to treat and follow patients. Similar studies comparing treatment guided by self-measured BPs or automated ambulatory BPs to treatment guided by office-based BPs are required but have not been conducted. Therefore, the available evidence does not warrant widespread dissemination or routine use of automated ambulatory BP measurement at this time. On the other hand, the authors support a more circumspect use of such devices for research and for the care of subgroups of hypertensive patients with specific clinical problems. Self-measured BP devices are increasingly being used by patients, and this practice should be encouraged. However, it should also be clear that there has not been sufficient formal evaluation of this method to warrant managing patients solely using BP readings obtained with self-monitoring BP devices. On the other hand, when used as adjunct to physicians' and nonphysicians' office-based measurement, self-measured BPs are an invaluable source of information for the management of hypertension. Patients and physicians electing to use these devices should become knowledgeable about their optimal use. This will involve ensuring that patients are taught how to measure their BP and that they be given advice about when to measure it. The devices should also be checked regularly to ensure that measurements are accurate and reliable and that they correlate to BP readings obtained in the office.

TREATMENT

Vegetarian Diet

To determine the effects of a vegetarian diet on daytime ambulatory BP and heart rates, and to relate these to the estimated peak in plasma glucose, Sciarrone and associates[24] from Perth, Australia, studied 21 normotensive nonvegetarian male hospital workers who volunteered for the study. After 2 weeks of baseline measurement, the subjects followed an omnivorous or a lacto-ovovegetarian diet for 6 weeks. Twenty of the

21 subjects completed the study. Ambulatory systolic BP and heart rates were lower in the vegetarian group during the working day. The preprandial diastolic BP was attenuated on the vegetarian diet. There were no differences in plasma catecholamine, glucose, or insulin levels sampled after breakfast on the two dietary regimes. Thus, the BP-lowering effect of a lacto-ovovegetarian diet, which occurs throughout the working day, is associated with lower heart rates, suggesting a central nervous or cardiac mechanism.

In the Elderly

To estimate the incidence of newly treated systemic hypertension and to describe the patterns of antihypertensive medication used among persons aged 65 years and older, Psaty and associates,[25] from several US medical centers, used Medicare eligibility lists from four US communities to obtain a representative sample of 5,201 community dwelling elderly for the Cardiovascular Health Study, a prospective cohort study of risk factors for CAD and stroke. Participants were examined at baseline and again 1 year later. Among the 4,406 participants 1,613 used antihypertensive medications at both visits. Between the two visits, 144 started and 115 stopped antihypertensive therapy. Among nonusers at baseline, the annual incidence of newly treated hypertension was 5.2% in women and 5.6% in men. Due to the number of participants who stopped therapy, the overall prevalence of antihypertensive treatment increased only slightly, from 40.7% to 41.1% in women and from 37.1% to 38.2% in men, during 1 year of follow-up. After adjustment for age, systolic BP, number of antihypertensive drugs, diabetes, and cardiovascular disease, the newly treated hypertensives were about half as likely as the previously treated hypertensives to receive diuretics (odds ratio, 0.59) or β-blockers (0.52); and they were about twice as likely to receive calcium channel blockers (1.88) or angiotensin-converting enzyme inhibitors (2.40). A similar pattern of within-person changes over time was apparent among the continuous users. Between June 1990 and June 1991, physicians were increasingly prescribing angiotensin-converting enzyme inhibitors and calcium channel blockers in place of diuretics and β-blockers for the treatment of hypertension in elderly patients, especially for those just starting therapy.

Comparison of Six Antihypertensive Agents

Characteristics such as age and race are often cited as determinants of the response of BP to specific antihypertensive agents, but this clinically important issue has not been examined in sufficiently large trials, involving all standard treatments, to determine the effects of such factors. In a randomized, double-blind study at 15 clinics, Materson and associates,[26] for the Department of Veterans Affairs Cooperative Study Group on Antihypertensive Agents, assigned 1,292 men with diastolic BP of 95 to 109 mm/Hg, after a placebo washout period, to receive placebo or one of six drugs: hydrochlorothiazide (12.5 to 50 mg/day), atenolol (25 to 100 mg/day), captopril (25 to 100 mg/day), clonidine (0.2 to 0.6 mg/day), a sustained-release preparation of diltiazem (120 to 360 mg/day), or prazosin (4 to 20 mg/day). The drug doses were titrated to a goal of <90 mm Hg for maximal diastolic BP, and the patients continued to receive therapy for at least one year. The mean age of the randomized patients was 59 ± 10 years, and 48% were black. The average BP at baseline was 152 ± 14/99 ± 3 mm Hg. Diltiazem therapy had the highest rate of success: 59% of the treated patients had reached the BP goal at the end of the titration phase and had a diastolic BP of <95 mm Hg at one year (Figures 5-4, 5-5, and 5-6). Atenolol was successful by this definition in 51% of the patients, clonidine in 50%, hydrochlorothiazide in 46%, captopril in 42%, and prazosin in 42%; all these agents were superior to placebo (success rate, 25%). Diltiazem ranked first for young blacks (<60 years) and older blacks (>60 years), among whom the success rate was 64%; captopril ranked first for younger whites (success rate, 55%), and atenolol for older whites (68%). Drug intolerance was more frequent with clonidine (14%) and prazosin (12%) than with the other drugs. Among men, race and age have an important effect on the response to single-drug therapy for hypertension. In addition to cost and quality of life, these factors should be considered in the initial choice of a drug.

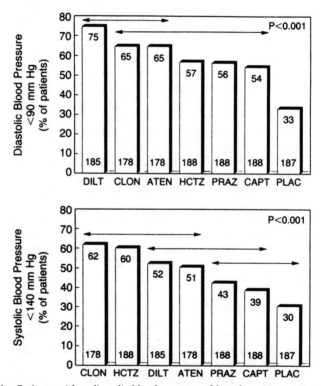

Figure 5-4. Patients with a diastolic blood pressure of less than 90 mm Hg or a systolic blood pressure of less than 140 mm Hg at the end of the titration phase. The P values were derived by a chi-square test comparing the treatments. On the basis of pairwise comparisons, the horizontal arrows group drugs the effects of which were not significantly different from one another but that were significantly different from the drugs not included under the arrow. ATEN denotes atenolol, CAPT captopril, CLON clonidine, DILT diltiazem, HCTZ hydrochlorothiazide, PRAX prazosin, and PLAC placebo. The numbers at the top of the bars indicate the percentage of patients with the response shown, and the numbers at the bottom of the bars indicate the number of patients in each group. Reproduced with permission from Materson et al.[26]

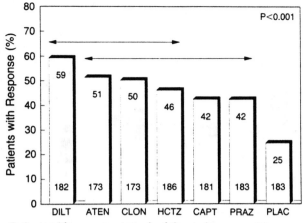

Figure 5-5. Patients with responses in each of the study groups. A response was defined as a diastolic blood pressure of less than 90 mm Hg at the end of the titration period and less than 95 mm Hg at the end of one year of treatment. The abbreviations and arrows are explained in the legend to Figure 5-1. Reproduced with permission from Materson et al.[26]

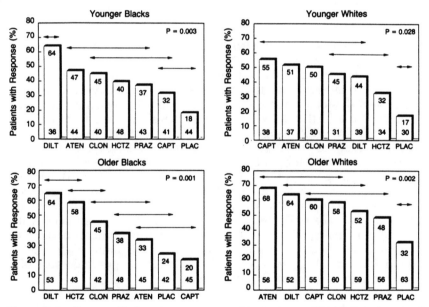

Figure 5-6. Younger black patients, younger white patients, older black patients, and older white patients with responses in each of the study groups. The abbreviations are explained in the legend to Figure 5-4. The arrows group the drugs whose effects do not differ from each other by more than 15%. Reproduced with permission from Materson et al.[26]

Doxazosin v Atenolol

The impact of treating hypertension on CAD has been less than anticipated from epidemiologic studies of cardiovascular risk factors. It has been suggested that adverse effects on lipids of traditional diuretic or

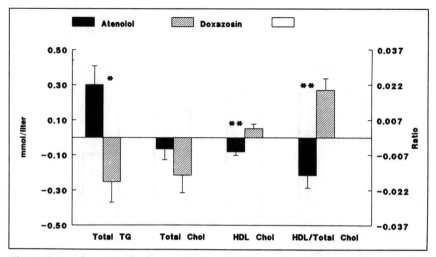

Figure 5-7. Changes in lipid concentrations between randomization and the conclusion of maintenance therapy for 24 weeks (mean + SEM). Chol = cholesterol; HDL Chol = high-density lipoprotein cholesterol (mmol/L); TG = triglyceride. HDL-cholesterol/total cholesterol (HDL/Total Chol) is expressed as a unitless ratio. $^*p <0.001$; $^{**}p <0.0001$. Reproduced with permission from Carruthers et al.[27]

β-blocker regimens may diminish the potential benefits of antihypertensive therapy. Carruthers and associates,[27] from Nova Scotia, Canada, randomly assigned patients with mild to moderate systemic hypertension and normal serum lipids to doxazosin or atenolol. After dose titration to goal diastolic blood pressure of ≤90 mm Hg, patients continued treatment for a further 24 weeks. The principal outcome measurement was overall CAD risk using the Framingham formula. Relative risk of CAD was reduced to 92% of baseline for evaluable patients taking atenolol and to 75% for patients taking doxazosin. In patients who met the strict Framingham criteria for age, total cholesterol, and HDL cholesterol, the relative risk of CAD for patients taking atenolol was reduced to 86% of baseline, and to 67% for patients taking doxazosin. Alpha blockade with doxazosin was more effective than β blockade with atenolol in reducing the risk of CAD in hypertensive patients because of the beneficial effects of doxazosin on HDL cholesterol (Figure 5-7). Overall withdrawal rate was greater in the α-blocker group because of a lower response rate and more adverse events.

Bisoprolol v Atenolol

Neutel and associates,[28] from multiple US medical centers, in a multicenter, double-blind, parallel group study, assessed the usefulness of ambulatory BP monitoring technique in differentiating between the once-daily administration of the β-blockers bisoprolol (10 to 20 mg) and atenolol (50 to 100 mg) in terms of efficacy and duration of action. The study population consisted of 659 patients with essential hypertension and an average office diastolic BP between 95 and 115 mm Hg after 4 weeks of placebo treatment. The office BP was recorded at the end of the 24-hour dosing interval. Ambulatory BP monitoring was performed in 11 of the

28 institutions participating in the study in a total of 203 patients. These procedures were performed at the end of the placebo phase and again after 8 weeks of active treatment. With the use of conventionally measured office BPs, the two drugs significantly decreased systolic and diastolic BPs to a similar extent. By 24-hour monitoring, bisoprolol demonstrated a 33% greater reduction in whole-day average diastolic BP than did atenolol (11.6 ± 0.7 mm Hg v 8.7 ± 0.8 mm Hg). Significant treatment differences in systolic and diastolic BPs were also noted for bisoprolol compared with atenolol during the final 4 hours of the dosing interval (-13.2 ± 1.5/-10.9 ± 1.0 mm Hg v -8.9 ± 1.6/-7.3 ± 1.1 mm Hg, respectively), and over the time period 6:00 AM to noon (-14.2 ± 1.3/ -11.5 ± 0.9 mm Hg v -9.9 ± 1.4/-7.7 ± 0.9 mm Hg). Whereas conventional BP measurements did not detect differences in the antihypertensive effects of the β-blockers bisoprolol and atenolol, ambulatory BP monitoring revealed significant treatment differences in both the efficacy and duration of action of these two agents. The findings indicate the power of this technique to discriminate potentially important differences between apparently similar antihypertensive drugs.

Enalapril

Hypertension in obese patients is associated with hyperinsulinemia and salt sensitivity. Very low-salt diets may exacerbate hyperinsulinemia, perhaps by activating the reninangiotensin system. Therefore, Egan and Stepniakowski,[29] from Milwaukee, Wis, studied the effects of a low-salt diet alone and with enalapril on BP and the insulin response to an oral glucose tolerance test in nine obese men with mild hypertension. Measurements were first obtained after a 2-week high-salt baseline period. The same measurements were repeated after 2 weeks on a low-salt diet and after 2 weeks on a low-salt diet with enalapril in random sequence. The insulin area under the curve increased from 13 mU-min/dL during high salt to 17 mU-min/dL. Plasma renin activity also increased with salt restriction from 1 to 3 ng/mL/hour. With addition of enalapril to the low sodium chloride diet, the insulin area under the curve was not significantly different from that during the high sodium chloride phase. Mean BP in the laboratory was 105 mm Hg with high salt versus 99 mm Hg with low salt. Addition of enalapril to the low-salt diet reduced mean BP to 87 mm Hg, largely by reducing total systemic resistance. Salt resistance decreases laboratory BP while raising insulin levels in obese men with mild hypertension. Enalapril diminishes the hyperinsulinemic effect and enhances the hypotensive action of the low-salt diet. These findings indicate that the hyperinsulinemic effect of severe salt restriction persists for ≥2 weeks. Moreover, activation of the resin-angiotensin system may contribute to impaired insulin metabolism during very low-salt diets.

Captopril v Enalapril

Testa and associates,[30] from Wellesley Hills and Boston, Mass, and the Quality-of-Life Hypertensive Group conducted a multicenter trial comparing two angiotensin-converting enzyme inhibitors to determine whether effects on quality of life during antihypertensive therapy are uniform within this pharmacologic class of agents and to relate the effects of the drugs on quality of life to objective adverse events, such as the loss of a job or the death of a spouse. After a 4-week washout period when they received placebo, 379 men with mild-to-moderately-severe hypertension were randomly assigned to receive captopril (25 to 50 mg twice daily, with or without hydrochlorothiazide) or enalapril (5 to 20 mg/day, with or without hydrochlorothiazide) for 24 weeks. BP, quality of life, and life events were monitored. Differences between treatments were evaluated by calibrating measures of quality of life with objective life events. Throughout the treatment period, no differences were found in BP, frequency of withdrawal of patients from the study, or major side effects. Patients treated with captopril had more favorable changes in overall quality of life, general perceived health, vitality, health status, sleep, and emotional control. The changes varied according to the quality of life at baseline; patients with a low quality of life at baseline remained stable or improved with either drug, whereas those with a higher quality of life remained stable with captopril but worsened with enalapril. The quality-of-life scales correlated with life events and symptom distress and calibration analysis indicated that differences between treatments were clinically important. Two angiotensin-converting enzyme inhibitors, captopril and enalapril, indistinguishable according to clinical assessments of efficacy and safety, had different effects on quality of life. Calibration with life events showed that drug-induced changes are substantial and that the different effects of these two agents on quality of life can be clinically meaningful.

References

1. Kannel WB, Garrison RJ, Dannenberg AL: Secular blood pressure trends in normotensive persons: The Framingham Study. Am Heart J 1993 (April); 125:1154–1158.

2. Joint National Committee on Detection, Evaluation, and Treatment of High Blood Pressure. The 50th Report of the Joint National Committee on Detection, Evaluation, and Treatment of High Blood Pressure (JNC V). Arch Intern Med 1993 (Jan 25);153:154–208.

3. Stamler J, Stamler R, Neaton JD: Blood pressure, systolic and diastolic, and cardiovascular risks. Arch Intern Med 1993 (March 8);153:598–615.

4. Sagie A, Larson MG, Levy D: The natural history of borderline isolated systolic hypertension. N Engl J Med 1993 (Dec 23);329:1912–1917.

5. Subcommittee of WHO/ISH Mild Hypertension Liaison Committee. Summary of 1993 World Health Organization-International Society of Hypertension guidelines for the management of mild systemic hypertension. Br Med J 1993 (Dec 11);307:1541–1546.

6. Launer LJ, Hofman A, Grobbee DE: Relation between birth weight and blood pressure in infants and children. Br Med J 1993 (Dec 4);307: 1451–1454.

7. Rosengren A, Tibblin G, Wilhelmsen L: Low systolic blood pressure and self-perceived well-being in middle-aged men. Br Med J 1993 (Jan 23);306: 243-246.

8. Kapuku GK, Seto S, Mori H, et al: Impaired left ventricular filling in borderline hypertensive patients without cardiac structural changes. Am Heart J 1993 (June);125:1710–1716.

9. Sagie A, Benjamin EJ, Galderisi M, et al: Echocardiographic assessment of left ventricular structure and diastolic filling in elderly subjects with borderline isolated systolic hypertension (the Framingham Heart Study). Am J Cardiol 1993 (Sep 15);72:662–665.

10. Chakko S, Mulingtapang RF, Huikuri HV, et al: Alterations in heart rate variability and its circadian rhythm in hypertensive patients with left ventricular hypertrophy free of coronary artery disease. Am Heart J 1993 (Dec);126:1364–1372.

11. Høegholm A, Kristensen KS, Bang LE, et al: Left ventricular mass and geometry in patients with established systemic hypertension and white coat hypertension. Am J Hypertens 1993 (April);6:282–286.

12. Massie BM, Szlachcic Y, Tubau JF, et al: Scintigraphic and electrocardiographic evidence of silent coronary artery disease in asymptomatic hypertension: A case-control study. J Am Coll Cardiol 1993 (Nov 15);22: 1598–1606.

13. Verdecchia P, Schillaci G, Gatteschi C, et al: Blunted nocturnal fall in blood pressure in hypertensive women with future cardiovascular morbid events. Circulation 1993 (Sep);88:986–992.

14. Markovitz JH, Matthews KA, Kannel WB, et al: Psychological predictors of hypertension in the Framingham Study. JAMA 1993 (Nov 24);270: 2439–2443.

15. Perneger TV, Nieto FJ, Whelton PK, et al: A prospective study of blood pressure and serum creatinine. JAMA 1993 (Jan 27);269:488–493.

16. Iriarte M, Murga N, Sagastagoitia D, et al: Congestive heart failure from left ventricular diastolic dysfunction in systemic hypertension. Am J Cardiol 1993 (Feb 1);71:308–312.

17. Schwartzkopff B, Motz W, Frenzel H, et al: Structural and functional alterations of the intramyocardial coronary arterioles in patients with arterial hypertension. Circulation 1993 (Sep);88:993–1003.

18. Treasure CB, Klein JL, Vita JA, et al: Hypertension and left ventricular hypertrophy are associated with impaired endothelium-mediated relaxation in human coronary resistance vessels. Circulation 1993 (Jan);87:86–93.

19. Panza JA, Quyyumi AA, Callahan TS, et al: Effect of antihypertensive treatment on endothelium-dependent vascular relaxation in patients with essential hypertension. J Am Coll Cardiol 1993 (April);21:1145–1151.

20. Panza JA, Casino PR, Kilcoyne CM, et al: Role of endothelium-derived nitric oxide in the abnormal endothelium-dependent vascular relaxation of patients with essential hypertension. Circulation 1993 (May);87: 1468–1474.

21. Grin JM, McCabe EJ, White WB: Management of systemic hypertension after ambulatory blood pressure monitoring. An Intern Med 1993 (June 1);118:833–837.

22. Appel LJ, Stason WB: Ambulatory blood pressure monitoring and blood pressure self-management in the diagnosis and management of hypertension. An Intern Med 1993(June 1);118:867–882.

23. American College of Physicians: Automated ambulatory blood pressure and self-measured blood pressure monitoring devices: Their role in the diagnosis and management of hypertension. An Intern Med 1993 (June 1);118: 889–892.

24. Sciarrone SEG, Strahan MT, Beilin LJ, et al: Ambulatory blood pressure and heart rate responses to vegetarian meals. J Hypertension 1993;11:277-285.

25. Psaty BM, Savage PJ, Tell GS, et al: Temporal patterns of antihypertensive medication use among elderly patients (The Cardiovascular Health Study). JAMA 1993 (Oct 20);270:1837–1841.

26. Materson BJ, Reda DJ, Cushman WC, et al: Comparison of six antihypertensive agents as a single-drug therapy for systemic hypertension in men. N Engl J Med 1993 (April 1);328:914–921.

27. Carruthers G, Dessain P, Fodor G, for the Alpha Beta Canada Trial Group: Comparative trial of doxazosin and atenolol on cardiovascular risk reduction in systemic hypertension. Am J Cardiol 1993 (March 1);71:575–581.
28. Neutel JM, Smith DHG, Ram CVS, et al: Application of ambulatory blood pressure monitoring in differentiating between bisoprolol and atenolol. Am J Med 1993 (Feb);94:181–187.
29. Egan BM, Stepniakowski K: Effects of enalapril on the hyperinsulinemic response to severe salt restriction in obese young men with mild systemic hypertension. Am J Cardiol 1993 (July 1);72:53–57.
30. Testa MA, Anderson RB, Nackley JF, et al, and the Quality-of-Life Hypertension Study Group: Comparison of captopril and enalapril for quality of life hypertensive therapy in men. N Engl J Med 1993 (April 1);328:907–913.

6

Valvular Heart Disease

MITRAL VALVE PROLAPSE

Effects of Hydration

Lax and associates,[1] from Tucson, Ariz, investigated the effect of hydration on MVP. Ten individuals with documented diagnosis of MVP were studied before and after oral hydration with 1 liter of fluid. Increased weight and cardiac output were present after hydration. Results showed that all ten individuals with diagnosis of MVP before hydration continued to have MVP after hydration; however, subtle changes were detected, especially on auscultation. Seven of nine individuals (with cardiac examination recorded before and after hydration) had auscultatory findings of MVP hefore hydration. No detectable auscultatory change after hydration was present in one individual; in six individuals, a loss of either a click or a murmur was detected after hydration. All individuals had echocardiographically detected MVP before hydration; evidence of MVP on two-dimensional or M-mode examination persisted after hydration in all ten individuals. Minor changes in the echocardiographic examination (M-mode n = 2, Doppler n = 1) were detected in three individuals. It was concluded that hydration of subjects with MVP did not alter the overall diagnosis; however, changes occurred, especially on auscultation. This suggests that alterations in hydration may affect auscultatory expression of MVP and could explain, in part, the variable auscultatory findings in patients with MVP.

MITRAL REGURGITATION

Mitral Valve Repair Results

David and associates,[2] from Toronto, Canada, analyzed 184 patients who had mitral valve repair for MR due to degenerative disease. The patients were operated on from June 1981 to August 1992. The mean age was 57 years, and 74% were men. One third of the patients were in AF, and 71% were in New York Heart Association classes III and IV. The MR was due to prolapse of the posterior leaflet in 97 patients (53%), prolapse of the anterior leaflet in 42 (23%), and prolapse of both leaflets in 45 (24%). The degree of myxomatous changes was assessed intraoperatively as mild in 125 patients (68%), moderate in 27 (15%), and severe in 32 (17%). Mitral valve repair was accomplished largely by techniques described by Carpentier. Ring annuloplasty was performed in 160 patients (66 with Carpentier ring and 94 with Duran ring). There was one operative death, and 5 patients experienced life-threatening complications. Patients were followed up from 5 to 132 months (mean, 41 months). The actuarial survival at 8 years was 88% ± 4% (Figure 6-1). The freedom from stroke at 8 years was 94% ± 2%, and freedom from transient ischemic attacks was 86% ± 6%. Age greater than 60 years was the only factor associated with higher risk of thromboembolic complications by logistic regression analysis. The actuarial freedom from reoperation at 8 years was 95% ± 2%. Advanced myxomatous changes in the leaflets of the mitral valve was the only significant factor associated with a higher risk of reoperation. Most patients were in New York Heart Association class I at the last follow-up. Late postoperative Doppler echocardiography revealed satisfactory mitral valve function in 96% of the patients. Mitral valve repair for MR due to degenerative disease provides excellent long-term results except in patients with advanced myxomatous changes in both leaflets, in whom there is a higher risk of recurrent MR and reoperation.

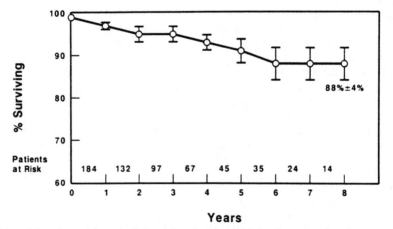

Figure 6-1. Actuarial survival. Reproduced with permission from David et al.[2]

MITRAL ANNULAR CALCIUM

Slowing of the Deposition by Nifedipine

Mitral annular calcium is a condition that often occurs in patients with systemic hypertension. To evaluate the effectiveness of nifedipine in preventing mitral annular calcium, Cacciapuoti and associates,[3] from Naples, Italy, selected 223 patients with systemic hypertension of recent onset and without mitral annular calcium and randomly enrolled the patients into three groups: group 1 (76 patients) received nifedipine; group 2 (72 patients) received enalapril; and group 3 (75 patients) received atenolol. After 5 years, these treatments significantly reduced systolic and diastolic BP in three treated groups. M-mode echocardiography revealed mitral annular calcium only in 2 patients in the nifedipine group (3%), in 13 in the enalapril group (18%), and in 15 in the atenolol group (20%). The degree of mitral annular calcium was mild in the 2 patients in group 1, in 5 of the 13 patients in group 2, and in 6 of the 15 patients in group 3, whereas it was severe in the remaining 8 patients in the enalapril group and in the other 9 patients in the atenolol group. There was also a significant correlation in the degree of mitral annular calcium, LA enlargement, and MR. In addition, AF and atrioventricular conduction defects were associated with severe mitral annular calcium. These results indicate that nifedipine is an effective drug both in the long-term management of systemic hypertension and in preventing or delaying mitral annular calcium.

MITRAL VALVE STENOSIS

Balloon Valvuloplasty

In an investigation performed by Patel and associates,[4] from Durban, South Africa, percutaneous balloon mitral valvotomy was attempted in severely symptomatic (New York Heart Association class III or IV) pregnant patients (mean age, 30 years) with tight MS. Nineteen patients were pregnant (mean gestation, 30 weeks; range, 26 to 34), and 1 patient was in the immediate postpartum period. All patients had undergone a trial of diuretic therapy and 16 were also taking atenolol. Percutaneous valvotomy was performed with the Inoue catheter (18 patients) or the Schneider-Medintag bifoil (2 x 19 mm) balloon catheter (2 patients). The fluoroscopy time was 9.2 ± 3.4 minutes. After percutaneous valvotomy, the mean mitral gradient decreased from 18 ± 6.2 to 5.9 ± 2.4 mm Hg. The mitral valve area (pressure half time) increased from 0.8 ± 0.2 to 1.7 ± 0.2 cm^2. These hemodynamic changes were accompanied by immediate symptomatic improvement by ≥1 New York Heart Association functional grade in all patients. Moderate MR developed in 1 patient. Eighteen patients had normal infants delivered vaginally at term without assistance, and 1 patient had a normal infant delivered by Cesarean section at 35 weeks of gestation. It was concluded that percutaneous balloon mitral valvotomy for pliable MS in pregnancy is safe for both the mother and fetus. It was also recommended that the procedure be performed in symptomatic patients with tight MS so as to avoid hemodynamic complications in the latter stages of pregnancy.

Ribeiro and associates,[5] from Riyadh, Saudi Arabia, and Loma Linda, Calif, studied the pulmonary vascular hemodynamics before and after mitral balloon valvotomy in 100 patients with severe MS. Before balloon valvotomy, 23 patients had a PA systolic pressure of <31 mm Hg (group 1), 54 patients had a PA systolic pressure between 31 and 50 mm Hg (group 2), and 23 patients had a PA systolic pressure of >50 mm Hg (group 3). After balloon valvotomy, the mean systolic PA pressure in group 1 decreased from 28 ± 3 to 26 ± 5 mm Hg. In group 2, the systolic PA pressure after balloon valvotomy decreased from 41 ± 5 to 33 ± 7 mm Hg and normalized to <31 mm Hg in 27 patients (50%). The mean LA pressure was abnormal (≥13 mm Hg) in 6 of 27 patients (22%) who had a systolic PA pressure of <31 mm Hg and in 6 of 27 patients (22%) who had a systolic PA pressure of ≥31 mm Hg. The pulmonary vascular resistance was abnormal in 36 of 54 patients (67%) after mitral balloon valvotomy; only 5 of 36 patients (14%) had a raised LA pressure (≥13 mm Hg). In group 3, the pulmonary vascular resistance was abnormal (>125 dynes/sec/cm^{-5}) in all 23 patients before and in 19 of 31 patients (91%) after balloon valvotomy. The mean systolic PA pressure decreased from 68 ± 14 to 46 ± 19 mm Hg, the mean PA pressure decreased from 42 ± 9 to 28 ± 11 mm Hg, and the LA pressure decreased from 21 ± 5 to 11 ± 4 mm Hg. After balloon valvotomy (group 3), the PA systolic pressure normalized (<31 mm Hg) in only 5 patients (24%). The LA pressure was normal (<13 mm Hg) in 9 of 16 patients and abnormal in 7 of 16 patients with persistent pulmonary hypertension (PA pressure ≥ 31 mm Hg). The mean pulmonary resistance decreased from 514 ± 255 to 388 ± 381 dynes/sec/cm^2. It was concluded that the PA pressure and pulmonary vascular resistance decreased without normalizing in the majority of patients with pulmonary hypertension immediately after mitral balloon valvotomy, even in patients with normal LA pressure.

Yasuda and associates,[6] from Osaka, Japan, investigated the LV diastolic pressure-volume response after percutaneous transvenous mitral commissurotomy to determine whether it was related to the baseline conditions of the LV. Left ventriculography was performed, and the measurements of LV pressure were obtained in 32 patients before and after transvenous mitral commissurotomy. Mitral valve area increased from 1.0 to 1.9 cm^2 after transvenous mitral commissurotomy, which caused a decrease in LA mean pressure (15 to 7 mm Hg). LV end-diastolic pressure increased in all patients 5 minutes after transvenous mitral commissurotomy. However, patients could be divided into two groups according to the following changes in LV end-diastolic pressure 20 minutes after transvenous mitral commissurotomy: in 22 patients, LV end-diastolic pressure returned to the near-baseline level 20 minutes after transvenous mitral commissurotomy with a significant increase in LV end-diastolic volume index and augmentation of LV stroke volume index. However, in the remaining 10 patients with a larger LV volume and reduced EF at baseline, LV end-diastolic pressure further increased 20 minutes after transvenous mitral commissurotomy without significant changes in LV volume. These findings suggest that the increase in LV end-diastolic pressure immediately after transvenous mitral commissurotomy increased LV volume with the augmentation of LV stroke volume and that this diastolic pressure-volume response was affected by the baseline LV condition.

Most reported studies of percutaneous balloon valvuloplasty in adults with acquired MS have used patients with severely stenosed valves. Herrmann and associates,[7] from Philadelphia, Pa, examined the risks and benefits of valvuloplasty in a multicenter registry of patients to determine whether balloon valvuloplasty can effectively dilate less severely obstructed valves and to clarify the role of this procedure in symptomatic patients with mild and moderate MS. The study groups were derived from the North American Inoue Balloon Valvuloplasty Registry. Full hemodynamic data were available in 264 patients; 45 with mild or moderate MS (mitral valve area ≥ 1.3 cm^2) were compared with the remaining 219 with severe MS (valve area <1.3 cm^2). Percutaneous balloon valvuloplasty was performed using the anterograde transseptal technique with an Inoue balloon. The mean age of patients with mild and moderate MS was 53 years, and all were symptomatic with a mean New York Heart Association functional class of 2.9. Balloon valvuloplasty resulted in an increase in calculated mitral valve area from 1.4 to 2.3 cm^2, and a final valve area ≥ 1.9 cm^2 was achieved in 37 patients (82%). There were no procedural deaths, but complications included RA perforation, transient ischemic attack, and emergency surgery for severe MR. One-year follow-up evaluation revealed symptomatic improvement in most patients. However, 2 patients needed repeat valvuloplasty for restenosis, and 5 had mitral-valve replacements. Patients with less severe stenosis had lower PA pressures and transmitral gradients, higher cardiac outputs, and lower total echocardiographic scores than did those with severe MS (Figure 6-2). A larger final valve area was achieved in patients with mild and moderate stenosis (2.3 v 1.7 cm^2).

To determine the rate of mitral restenosis and MR increase 1 year after mitral valvotomy using the Inoue balloon catheter, Ribeiro and associates,[8] from Riyadh, Saudi Arabia, studied 66 consecutive patients with severe pliable MS who had their mitral valve area calculated by two-dimensional echocardiography and Doppler before, immediately after balloon valvotomy, and at 1-year follow-up. Color Doppler studies were also done to detect small ASDs and MR. The mean age of the patients was 31 ± 12 years. Three patients were in New York Heart Association class II and 63 patients were in classes III to IV. After Inoue balloon valvotomy, the mitral valve area increased from 0.8 ± 0.2 to 1.9 ± 0.3 cm^2, and the Doppler mitral valve area increased from 0.8 ± 0.2 to 1.8 ± 0.3 cm^2. Detected were 4 of 66 cases (6%) with significant residual MS (mitral valve area <1.5 cm^2). MR increased in 14 of 66 patients (21%), but no patient developed severe MR. Fourteen of 66 patients (20%) had ASDs that were detected on color Doppler. At 1-year follow-up, the mean Doppler mitral valve area was maintained at 1.8 ± 0.4 cm^2, with 6 of 66 patients (9%) exhibiting significant mitral valve restenosis. The degree of MR was unchanged in 59 of 66 patients (90%); it increased in 5 of 66 patients (8%), being severe in 3 of 66 patients (5%) and decreased in 2 of 66 patients (2%). ASDs closed spontaneously in 9 of 14 patients (64%). At 1 year after Inoue mitral balloon valvotomy in a population of patients with severe pliable MS, mitral restenosis and the onset of severe MR jeopardized the initial favorable results in 14% of patients.

Balloon valvuloplasty is an important technique for treating rheumatic mitral stenosis. Herrmann and associates,[9] from Philadelphia,

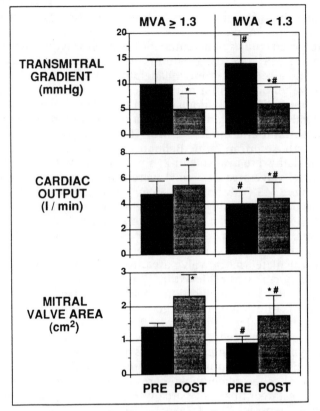

Figure 6-2. Hemodynamic results of percutaneous balloon valvuloplasty in patients with mild and moderate mitral stenosis compared with those with severe stenosis. MVA = mitral valve area; *p <0.05 before versus after; #p <0.05 mild/moderate versus severe. Reproduced with permission from Hermann et al.[7]

Pa, analyzed the incidence, mechanism, and outcome of severe MR induced by this technique using the Inoue balloon. In 280 patients in the North American Multicenter Registry, 21 patients developed either clinically significant or angiographically severe MR, giving an incidence of severe MR of 7.5%. The most common cause of MR (43%) was rupture of chordae tendineae to the anterior or posterior mitral leaflet. Tearing of a leaflet (usually the posterior one) occurred in 30% of patients; and no recognizable structural abnormality, with wide splitting of the commissures and a central regurgitant jet, was present in 5 patients (26%). All patients with definite posterior leaflet tears had heavily calcified leaflets. Patients who developed severe MR had fewer balloon inflations and a higher grade of preexisting MR, but were otherwise similar to the remaining patients without severe MR. During a 6 month follow-up, 71% of the patients with severe MR were treated surgically, the grade of MR decreased in 4 patients (19%), and 5 patients (24%) have not required mitral-valve replacement during 18 months of follow-up. These authors concluded that severe MR is a relatively infrequent complication of Inoue balloon valvuloplasty and results from disruption of valve integrity, including chordal rupture and leaflet tearing. Careful balloon positioning may help avoid chordal rupture, and heavily calcified posterior leaflets may be at greater risk of tearing. Most patients who develop severe MR will require nonemergency MVR.

Balloon Valvuloplasty v Closed Operative Valvotomy

Balloon mitral valvotomy constitutes an important alternative to surgical closed mitral valvotomy for the treatment of rheumatic MS. In an investigation by Arora and associates,[10] from New Delhi, India, to compare the immediate and long-term results of these procedures, 200 patients with rheumatic MS were randomly assigned to undergo either balloon mitral valvotomy (n = 100) or closed mitral valvotomy (n = 100). The age range was 10 to 30 years (mean, 19.4 ± 6.5). Both procedures resulted in significant and similar increases in mitral valve area (balloon mitral valvotomy 0.85 ± 26 to 2.39 ± 0.94 cm^2; closed mitral valvotomy 0.79 ± 0.21 to 2.2 ± 0.85 cm^2). MR developed in 14 patients after balloon mitral valvotomy and in 12 patients after closed mitral valvotomy. Eighty patients in each group have now been followed for a mean period of 22 ± 6.3 months (range, 6 to 38) by repeat echocardiographic study. Restenosis (defined as a loss of more than 50% of the achieved increase in mitral valve area) was seen in 4 patients (5%) after balloon mitral valvotomy and in 3 patients (4%) after closed mitral valvotomy. Symptomatic restenosis was seen in only 1 patient who at follow-up examination, 20 months after closed mitral valvotomy, had a mitral valve area of 0.8 cm^2 and underwent successful balloon valvotomy. It was concluded that the immediate and long-term results obtained with percutaneous balloon mitral valvotomy and surgical closed mitral commissurotomy are comparable.

Operative Commissurotomy

Scalia and associates,[11] from Padova, Italy, described results of mitral commissurotomy in 280 patients operated on for pure MS between January 1968 and December 1969. Closed commissurotomy was utilized in 134 patients, with a mean age of 38 ± 11 years and a mean valve area of 1.0 ± 0.29 cm^2. Open commissurotomy was performed in 146 older patients (mean age, 44 ± 11 years) with a mean valve area of 0.9 ± 0.3 cm^2. The perioperative mortality was 3% in closed procedures and 3.4% in open procedures. Surviving patients were evaluated by questionnaires or phone interviews, and 129 patients were examined by two-dimensional echocardiography with the purpose of analyzing long-term results. Follow-up was 95% complete (Grunkemeier-Starr method), with a median of 18 years in patients with closed commissurotomy and 6.6 years in patients with open commissurotomy. The actuarial survival at 21 years was 60.8% in patients having closed commissurotomies and 60.6% at 22 years in patients having open commissurotomies. The "effective palliation" rate, defined by clinical and echocardiographic criteria, was 47% at 15 years and 15% at 20 years. These authors concluded that mitral commissurotomy is the procedure of choice in pure mitral valve stenosis and should be applied early. When performed in patients aged <40 years, a 78% survival at 18 years and 67% "effective palliation" at 15 years were observed. The closed valvotomy results of the study support the present trend toward use of percutaneous balloon valvotomy.

Amiodarone for Atrial Fibrillation Conversion After Surgery

Skoularigis and associates,[12] from Johannesburg, South Africa, treated 30 consecutive patients with chronic rheumatic AF ≥3 months after successful mitral valve surgery and LA diameter <60 mm with oral amiodarone. Protocol included high loading dosages of amiodarone for 4 weeks; and if conversion to sinus rhythm was not achieved, then electrical cardioversion was performed. Patients converted to sinus rhythm were maintained on low-dose amiodarone for another 4 weeks when treatment was discontinued. Overall, 23 patients (77%) converted to sinus rhythm after 4 weeks of therapy: 12 (40%) taking amiodarone alone and 11 (37%) with the addition of electrical cardioversion. The duration of AF >48 months was an adverse factor in the ability to restore sinus rhythm. Sixteen patients (70%) remained in sinus rhythm at a mean follow-up of 17 months. The duration of AF ≥48 months alone or in combination with LA diameter ≥45 mm were the best predictors for long-term maintenance of sinus rhythm. Thus, short-term amiodarone with or without electrical cardioversion is effective and safe in the treatment of chronic rheumatic AF after mitral valve surgery. The duration of AF and LA size can be used to identify patients with successful outcome.

AORTIC VALVE STENOSIS

Predictors of Valve Structure

A number of reports have described the frequency of coronary arterial narrowing in patients with valvular AS. No published reports have examined the structure of the stenotic aortic valve in adults and related the valve structure to variables, including coronary arterial narrowing, useful in predicting that structure. Mautner and associates,[13] from Bethesda, Md, studied 188 patients having AVR for isolated valvular AS. All patients were >40 years of age at the time of aortic-valve replacement and all had coronary angiograms preoperatively. In 182 patients (97%), measurements of serum total cholesterol were obtained; and 184 (98%) had body-mass index calculated. The structure of the operatively excised valve was classified as unicuspid or bicuspid (congenitally malformed), or tricuspid aortic valve. A logistic regression model was developed that found four factors (age, serum total cholesterol, angiographic CAD, and body-mass index) to be predictive of aortic valve structure: (1) patients with at least three or all four factors high or present (i.e., age >65 years, serum total cholesterol >200 mg/dL, body-mass index >29 kg/m^2, and CAD) had a low probability (10% to 29%) of having a congenitally malformed valve; and (2) patients with at least three or all four factors low or absent (i.e., age <65 years, serum total cholesterol <200 mg/dL, body-mass index <29 kg/m2, and no CAD) had a high probability (72% to 90%) of having a congenitally malformed valve (Figure 6-3). Thus, the morphology of the operatively excised stenotic aortic valve can be predicted with knowledge of the age, serum total cholesterol, body-mass index, and coronary artery status of the patient.

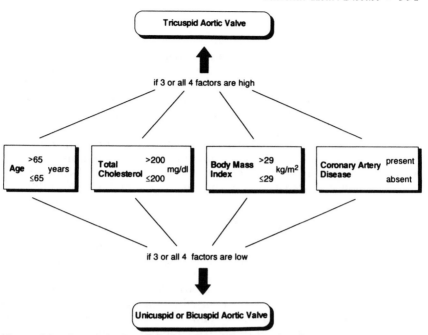

Figure 6-3. Summarization of the four factors that proved useful in predicting the aortic valve structure. Reproduced with permission from Mautner et al.[13]

AORTIC REGURGITATION

Nifedipine v Captopril

Röthlisberger and associates,[14] from Johannesburg, South Africa, compared the effects of a single dose of either nifedipine 20 mg (n = 10) or captopril 50 mg (n = 10) in 20 patients with symptomatic, chronic severe AR using angiography and micromanometer LV pressure measurements. At 90 minutes, mean arterial pressure was reduced comparably after both drugs (86 to 76 mm Hg for nifedipine v 95 to 77 mm Hg for captopril), as was wedge pressure (11 to 9 mm Hg v 13 to 9 mm Hg for captopril). Systemic vascular resistance was reduced more after nifedipine than after captopril. Heart rate declined after captopril (84 to 75/min) but not after nifedipine (78 to 80/min). Forward stroke volume increased after nifedipine (58 to 70 mL) but not after captopril (58 to 59 mL). Thus, cardiac output increased after nifedipine but decreased after captopril. Angiographic EF did not change significantly after either drug, nor did end-systolic wall stress. The ratio of end-systolic wall stress to end-systolic volume index was slightly reduced by both drugs. Thus, although both drugs comparably decreased arterial pressure in severe AR, only nifedipine increased forward stroke volume and cardiac output and decreased regurgitant fraction through a more potent vasodilation that offsets its reported negative inotropic effects.

The Marfan Syndrome

With effective surgical correction of vascular abnormalities, skeletal health is an important issue for patients with the Marfan syndrome. Osteopenia has been radiographically described, yet no systematic evaluation of bone status has been published. Kohlmeier and associates,[15] from Stanford and Palo Alto, Calif, determined the bone mineral density (BMD, g/cm^2) in 17 women with the Marfan syndrome. Their ages were 37 ± 7 years. Dual energy x-ray absorptiometry was used to measure BMD at the lumbar spine (L2-L4), proximal femur, and total body in all subjects. Scoliosis scores were assigned from 0 (no curvature) to 3 (severe curvature). Highly significant deficits in BMD were observed at the proximal femur as well as of the whole body (femoral neck BMD Z-score (mean ± SD) = −1.36 ± 0.94; trochanter Z = −1.07 ± 0.80; and intertrochanter Z = -1.44 ± 0.71; whole-body BMD Z-score = −0.48 ± 1.16). There was no significant association between BMD and scoliosis, nor between BMD and fracture history. To correct for bone size, the bone mineral apparent density (BMAD, g/cm^3) was calculated. The femoral neck BMAD values (mean ± SD) were significantly lower than predicted (0.125 ± 0.02 v 0.147 ± 0.001 g/cm^3, p<0.001). All subjects had normal menarche, and 15 reported regular menses. There was no history of nontraumatic fracture. Thus, women with the Marfan syndrome have bone deficits at the proximal femur as well as of the whole body. This deficit is not related to scoliosis and persists when corrected for bone size. Women with the Marfan syndrome may be at increased risk of proximal femoral fracture.

Ankylosing Spondylitis

Although cardiac involvement in the form of conduction abnormalities or AR occurs in 5% to 10% of patients with ankylosing spondylitis, few studies have assessed LV function. Crowley and associates,[16] in Dublin, Ireland, assessed the prevalence of both systolic and diastolic LV dysfunction and other cardiac abnormalities in patients with ankylosing spondylitis who had no clinical cardiac manifestations. Fifty-nine patients (49 men and 10 women) underwent full clinical examination; electrocardiography; 24-hour Holter monitoring; and two-dimensional, M-mode, and Doppler echocardiography. Mean disease duration was 17 years. Seventeen patients had evidence of noncardiac extra-articular manifestations. Precordial examination was normal in all. An age- and sex-matched control group of 44 healthy subjects was also studied. On echocardiography, abnormal LV diastolic function was detected in 12 patients (20%). Prolonged isovolumic relaxation time, prolonged deceleration time, reduced rate of descent of flow velocity in early diastole (EF slope), and reversal of the early and late peak transmitral diastolic flow velocities (E/A ratio) were noted in 9 patients. In 3 patients, there was an increased E/A ratio, reduced deceleration time, and increased EF slope. Mild AR and MR was seen in 1 and 3 patients, respectively. No abnormalities of LA size, LV systolic or diastolic dimensions, or wall thicknesses were noted. There was no correlation between the presence of LV diastolic dysfunction and age, disease severity, disease duration, or the presence of extra-articular manifestations. These investigators concluded that LV diastolic dysfunction occurs frequently in patients with ankylosing spondylitis, even in the absence of clinical cardiac involvement.

INFECTIVE ENDOCARDITIS

At a Large Community Hospital

Watanakunakorn and Burkert,[17] from Youngstown and Rootstown, Ohio, studied 210 episodes of infective endocarditis (IE) in 204 patients. The prevalence of this disease in our series ranged from 0.32 to 1.30 episodes (mean, 0.75) per 1000 admissions per year. There were 115 male and 89 female patients, whose ages ranged from newborn to 91 years (median, 60 to 70). One hundred forty-eight episodes involved host valves and another 33 episodes involved host valves and another 33 episodes occurred in intravenous drug users. There were 2 episodes of early and 27 episodes of late prosthetic valve endocarditis. *Staphylococcus aureus* accounted for 99 episodes (47.1%), alpha-hemolytic streptococci for 29 episodes (13.8%), IE for 11 episodes (5.2%), culture-negative endocarditis for 11 episodes (5.2%), and other organisms for 60 episodes (28.6%). Severe back pain was the chief complaint in 15 patients. Two-dimensional echocardiography was performed in 164 episodes, results in 67 (40.9%) of which were positive. Valve surgery was performed in 29 episodes (23 host valves and 6 prosthetic valves). The overall mortality was 21.4%. Autopsy was performed in 22 of the 45 patients who died (48.9%). The mortality rate increased with age, (10.1% and 31.5% for patients <60 years old and ≥60 years, respectively.

Involving Only the Mitral Valve

Although a number of clinicopathologic studies in patients with active infective endocarditis (IE) have been reported, none have focused on patients studied at necropsy with active IE isolated to the mitral valve. Fernicola and Roberts,[18] from Bethesda, Md, studied at necropsy 63 patients (aged 12 to 88 years [mean 50]; 44 males [70%]) with active IE limited to the native mitral valve. Twenty-one patients (33%) had pre-existing mitral valve disease (rheumatic in 9, MVP in 3, HC in 1, and mitral annular calcium in 9), and the other 42 patients (67%) had previously normal mitral valves. Of the latter 42 patients, 22 (52%) had recognized predisposing factors to IE: opiate addiction in 14, habitual alcoholism in 6, and/or chronic hemodialysis in 4. *Staphylococcus aureus* or *epidermidis* was the responsible organism in 32 patients (51%), and the active IE was associated with an infection elsewhere in the body in 31 patients (50%). The active IE caused rupture of mitral chordae tendineae in 11 patients (18%), perforation of the anterior mitral leaflet in 7 patients (11%), and mitral ring abscess in 10 patients (16%). Grossly visible systemic emboli were found in 44 patients (70%), and 33 (52%) had infarcts in one or more body organs. Thus, active IE isolated to the mitral valve in necropsied patients appears to be more common in males than females (2 to 1); the infection more commonly than not involves a preexisting anatomically normal valve rather than a preexisting abnormal one (2 to 1); the vegetations often do not cause or worsen valvular dysfunction; a predisposing factor is commonly present (2 to 3 patients); and the IE commonly is part of a generalized or systemic infection (1 of 2 patients).

Involving a Previously Stenotic v Nonstenotic Aortic Valve

No previous studies, either clinical or morphologic, have compared findings in patients with active infective endocarditis (IE) involving a previously stenotic versus a previously nonstenotic aortic valve. Consequently, Roberts and associates,[19] from Bethesda, Md, analyzed clinical and cardiac necropsy findings in 96 patients with active IE involving the aortic valve. Of the 96 patients, 25 (26%) had active IE superimposed on a previously stenotic aortic valve and 71 (74%) on a previously nonstenotic aortic valve. The patients with stenotic aortic valves had significantly higher mean ages (61 v 47 years), a higher percentage >60 years of age (52% v 24%), a higher percentage of men (92 vs 73%), a higher frequency of an absent or unknown predisposing factor to infection (68% v 38%), a lower frequency of a pericardial murmur of AR (44% v 79%), a lower percent with a long duration (>60 days) of signs and symptoms of active IE (4% v 23%), a larger mean heart weight (594 v 514 g), a higher percentage with aortic valve calcific deposits (100% v 24%), and a higher frequency of associated ring abscess (84% v 52%) (Table 6-1). Thus, active IE superimposed on a stenotic aortic valve differs in some features compared with active IE on a nonstenotic aortic valve. Because ring abscess is so common when active IE involves a stenotic aortic valve in adults, operative intervention at an early stage may be warranted.

Involving a Bioprosthetic Valve

When active infective endocarditis (IE) involves a bioprosthetic valve, the infective process may involve the cusps or sewing ring or both. Fernicola and Roberts,[20] from Bethesda, Md, studied 34 patients with infected bioprostheses to determine whether the infection involved the cusps or ring, or both, because these locations could affect prognosis. In the 5 patients in whom active IE began <60 days after operation, the infection involved the cusps only in 2, the ring only in 2, and both in 1. The 29 patients in whom signs and symptoms of active IE appeared >60 days after valve replacement were subdivided into three categories based on the valve or valves replaced. In the 16 patients with isolated AVR, the infection involved the cusps only in 6, the ring only in 4, and both in 6. In the 6 patients with isolated MVR, the infection involved the cusps only in 2, the ring only in 1, and both in 3. In the remaining 7 patients, 15 native valves were replaced with bioprostheses, and 10 of them were infected. The infection involved the cusps only in 7, and both the cusps and ring in 3. Of all 34 patients, 13 had operative excision of the infected bioprosthesis: 1 died within 60 days of the bioprosthetic excision, and 1 was lost to follow-up; of the remaining 11 patients, 4 died late (1.5, 3, 5, and 14 years), and the other 7 are alive 5 to 10 years after bioprosthetic excision (all in New York Heart Association functional class I or II). Thus, although infection limited to the bioprosthetic cusps may reasonably

Table 6-1. Comparison of Patients With Active Endocarditis Involving Stenoic and Nonstenoic Aortic Valves. Reproduced with permission from Roberts et al.[19]

	Stenotic (n = 25)	Nonstenotic (n = 71)	p Value
1. Age (year): range (mean)	21–86 (61)	17–81 (47)	0.002
≤ 30	2 (8%)	12 (17%)	0.278
31–60	10 (44%)	42 (59%)	0.098
> 60	13 (52%)	17 (24%)	0.009
2. Men: women	23 (92%): 2 (8%)	52 (73%): 19 (27%)	0.051
3. Diagnosis of AS in life	23 (92%)	—	—
4. Diagnosis of IE in life	20 (80%)	48 (68%)	0.241
5. Infecting organism			
Bacterium			
Staphylococcal	7 (28%)	20 (28%)	0.987
Streptococcal	9 (36%)	22 (31%)	0.645
Mixed	4 (16%)	10 (14%)	0.816
Fungus	0	2 (3%)	1.0
Unknown	5 (20%)	17 (24%)	0.687
6. Predisposing factor			
Alcoholism	5 (20%)	20 (28%)	0.424
Opiate addiction	0	11 (15%)	0.06
Dental procedure	2 (8%)	5 (7%)	0.874
Hemodialysis	1 (4%)	4 (6%)	0.752
Previous IE	0	4 (6%)	0.57
Unknown	17 (68%)	27 (38%)	0.010
7. Aortic regurgitation murmur	11 (44%)	56 (79%)	0.001
8. Duration of IE (days)			
≤ 60	20 (80%)	45 (63%)	0.126
> 60	1 (4%)	16 (23%)	0.037
Uncertain	4 (16%)	10 (14%)	0.816
9. Complete heart block	3 (12%)	4 (6%)	0.292
10. Pericardial effusion (> 50 ml)	6/15 (40%)	11/43 (26%)	0.446
11. Aortic valve replacement	3 (12%)	18 (26%)	0.165
12. Heart weight (g): range (mean)	315–920 (594)	240–980 (514)	0.013
Men (n = 62)	315–920 (604)	340–980 (549)	0.098
Women (n = 14)	490 and 500	240–570 (389)	—
13. Number of aortic valve cusps			
2	10 (40%)	21 (30%)	0.338
3	15 (60%)	47 (66%)	0.577
Uncertain	0	3 (4%)	0.533
14. Aortic valve calcium			
0–1+	2 (8%)	17 (24%)	0.0001
2+–3+	23 (92%)	0	0.0001
15. No. of cusps with vegetation			
Bicuspid aortic valves	10	21	—
1	0	4 (19%)	0.28
2	10 (100%)	15 (71%)	0.060
Uncertain	0	2 (10%)	0.548
Tricuspid aortic valve	15	47	—
1	2 (13%)	13 (28%)	0.471
2	4 (27%)	12 (26%)	0.930
3	8 (53%)	20 (42%)	0.465
Uncertain	1 (7%)	2 (4%)	—
16. Vegetation on mitral valve	6 (24%)	19 (22%)	0.787
17. Ring abscess	21 (84%)	37 (52%)	0.005
18. Mitral annular calcium	4 (16%)	6 (8%)	0.288
19. Coronary artery embolus	4 (16%)	5 (7%)	0.186
20. Acute myocardial infarct	4 (16%)	4 (6%)	0.107
21. Stroke	2 (8%)	5 (7%)	0.874

AS = aortic stenosis; IE = infective endocarditis.

allow a better outlook, reoperation with infection involving the annular ring (8 of 13 reoperation patients) does not prevent successful outcome.

Infective endocarditis involving mechanical prostheses or bioprotheses remains an infrequent but serious complication of cardiac valvular replacement. Sett and associates,[21] from Vancouver, Canada, diagnosed prosthetic valve endocarditis in 56 of 3,200 patients in whom one or more porcine bioprostheses were implanted between 1975 and 1988. Of the 56 patients with prosthetic valve endocarditis, there were 40 men and 16 women, with a mean age of 57 years at initial implantation (27 to 81 years). Of the 56 patients, 6 were initially treated for native valve endocarditis. There were 8 cases of early prosthetic valve endocarditis (defined as occurring 60 days after initial surgical intervention) and 48 cases of late prosthetic valve endocarditis (occurring after 60 days). The overall mortality rate of the 56 patients was 32% (18 patients). Of the 8 patients with early prosthetic valve endocarditis, 6 (75%) died. Of the 48 patients with late prosthetic valve endocarditis, 12 (25%) died. The predominant organisms were *Staphylococcus epidermidis* (12 cases), *Streptococcus viridans* (8 cases), and *Staphylococcus aureus* (7 cases). The presence of hemodynamic compromise, including CHF, septic embolism, persistent sepsis, and echocardiographic evidence of vegetations, dictated the mode and timing of the addition of surgical intervention to medical therapy. The survival rate for medically and surgically treated patients with late prosthetic valve endocarditis was 91% (20 patients); none of the patients with early prosthetic valve endocarditis survived (all had severe hemodynamic compromise). Eighteen factors were analyzed for the prediction of early and late death. The predictors of death by univariate analysis for both early and late prosthetic valve endocarditis were age, diagnosis time, renal status, sepsis, management mode, fever, dental procedures, and dental prophylaxis. The predictors by multivariate analysis were age, diagnosis time, renal status, and management mode for early prosthetic valve endocarditis, and only diagnosis time for late prosthetic valve endocarditis. Annular abscess formation occurred in 27% of the patients. There were no complex aortic or mitral reconstructions. There was 1 reoperation for recurrent and residual endocarditis. There was 1 late death as a result of recurrent prosthetic valve endocarditis. These authors advocate early diagnosis and aggressive combined medical and surgical treatment before the development of hemodynamic compromise and other characteristic signs when the culprit organisms are *Staphylococcus aureus*, gram-negative organisms, and *Candida albicans*.

To determine the incidence of endocarditis in bacteremic patients with prosthetic or bioprosthetic heart valves and the risks for and the effect of duration of antibiotic therapy on development of endocarditis in such patients, Fang and associates,[22] from six university teaching hospitals with high volume cardio-thoracic surgery, performed a prospective observational study involving 171 patients with prosthetic heart valves who developed bacteremia during hospitalization. The patients were evaluated when they were identified as having bacteremia and 1, 2, 6, and 12 months after its occurrence. Of the 171 patients, 74 (43%) developed endocarditis: 56 (33%) had prosthetic valve endocarditis at the time bacteremia was discovered ("endocarditis at outset"), whereas 18 (11%) developed endocarditis a mean of 45 days after bacteremia was discovered ("new endocarditis"). Mitral valve location and staphylococcal bacteremia (*Staphylococcus aureus* and *Staphylococcus epidermidis*) were significantly associated with the development of "new endocarditis." All 18 cases of new endocarditis were nosocomial; and in 6 of these cases (33%), bacteremia was acquired via intravascular devices. Twenty-one patients without evidence of endocarditis at the time of bacteremia received short-term antibiotic therapy (<14 days); 1 patient (5%) developed endocarditis. Eleven of 70 patients (16%) who received long-term antibiotic therapy (>14 days) developed endocarditis. Bacteremic patients with prosthetic heart valves were at notable risk for developing endocarditis, even when they received antibiotic therapy before endocarditis developed and regardless of the duration of such therapy. Intravascular devices were a common portal of entry.

VALVE REPLACEMENT

Transthoracic v Transesophageal Echocardiography Afterwards

Two-dimensional echocardiography is the diagnostic procedure of choice for evaluation of prosthetic valve abnormalities. However, transthoracic echocardiography may be limited owing to acoustic shadowing and poor acoustic windows. Some of these limitations may be overcome by transesophageal echocardiography. Daniel and associates,[23] from Hanover, Germany, studied 126 patients with 148 prosthetic valves (113 bioprostheses and 35 mechanical devices) by M-mode and two-dimensional transthoracic echocardiography and transesophageal echocardiography. Prosthetic valve morphology was confirmed by surgery or autopsy in all cases; 124 prostheses were classified as diseased (33 endocarditis, 8 thrombi, and 83 degeneration defined as leaflet thickening >3 mm with restricted motion) and 24 as normal. Prosthetic valve endocarditis and thrombi were correctly identified by transthoracic echocardiography in 12 of 33 (36%) and 1 of 8 (13%) prostheses, respectively, but could be diagnosed by transesophageal echocardiography in 27 of 33 (82%) and 8 of 8 (100%), respectively. Compared with transthoracic echocardiography, transesophageal echocardiography had a higher sensitivity for morphologic prosthetic valve abnormalities in patients with either bioprostheses or mechanical devices and in patients with a prosthesis in either the aortic (49 [77%] v 32 [50%] of 64) or mitral (58 [97%] v 39 [65%] of 60) position. Overall, sensitivity and specificity were 57% and 63%, respectively, for transthoracic echocardiography, and 86% and 88%, respectively, for transesophageal echocardiography. Transesophageal echocardiography is superior to transthoracic echocardiography in the correct identification of morphologic prosthetic valve abnormalities and should be used in patients with suspected prosthetic valve malfunction and negative transthoracic echocardiography.

In the Elderly

Davis and associates,[24] from Baltimore, Md, compared results of AVR and MVR in a large number of patients aged 70 or more to ascertain predictors of poor outcome. Because patients who had concomitant CABG were included (51% for AVR, 55% for MVR), patients who had isolated CABG were used as a comparison group. Between Jan 1, 1984, and June 30, 1991, 1,386 patients, aged 70 years and older, underwent CABG (n = 1,043), AVR (n = 245), or MVR (n = 98) (Table 6-2). The operative mortality rates were 5.3% for AVR, 20.4% for MVR, and 5.8% for CABG (Table 6-3). Late follow-up data for patients undergoing operation in 1984 and 1985 were available for 98% (231/237). Overall survival was comparable for all three groups through the first 5 years of follow-up (AVR, 68% ± 8%; MVR, 73% ± 8%; CABG, 78% ± 3%). After 5 years, survival for patients having AVR and MVR was less than that for those having CABG. Patient age, sex, New York Heart Association function class, concomitant CABG, prosthetic valve type, native valve pathology, and preoperative catheterization data were examined as possible predictors of outcome by multivariate logistic regression. Among MVR patients, New York Heart Association functional class, ischemic valvular pathology, and higher pulmonary artery wedge pressure were predictive of operative mortality; poor LV function was a predictor of poor long-term survival (17% v 100% at 7 years). Among AVR patients, only advanced functional class was associated with a poor outcome. Compared with MVR patients, AVR patients were older (76.5 ± 4.6 v 74.5 ± 3

Table 6-2. Valvular Pathology.[a] Reproduced with permission from Davis et al.[24]

Variable	Aortic (n = 245)	Mitral (n = 98)
Pure stenosis	208 (85)	16 (16)
Pure regurgitation	19 (8)	61 (62)
Mixed stenosis and regurgitation	18 (7)	21 (22)
Calcific	210 (86)	4 (4)
Ischemic	0 (0)	30 (31)
Rheumatic	6 (2)	35 (36)
Degenerative	5 (2)	17 (17)
Endocarditis	7 (3)	5 (5)
Other	17 (7)	7 (7)

[a] Numbers in parentheses are percentages.

Table 6-3. Thirty-Day and In-Hospital Mortality Rates.[a] Reproduced with permission from Davis et al.[24]

Mortality	AVR (n = 245)	MVR (n = 98)	CABG (n = 1,043)
30-Day	3.3%	14.3%	4.7%
	(1%–5.5%)	(7.2%–21.3^c)	(3.4%–6%)
In-hospital	5.3%	20.4%	5.8%
	(2.5%–8.1%)	(12.3%–28.5^c)	(4.3%–7.2%)

[a] Numbers in parentheses show 95% confidence interval.

AVR = aortic valve replacement; CABG = coronary artery bypass grafting; MVR = mitral valve replacement.

years), were more often male (55% v 39%), had a lower PA wedge pressure (18 ± 11 v 24 ± 10 mm Hg), and had fewer critically diseased vessels. These results suggest that AVR in the elderly has an operative mortality similar to that of isolated CABG. In contrast, MVR is less well tolerated, especially in patients with ischemic mitral disease. Survival 5 years postoperatively is similar among AVR, MVR, and CABG patients but becomes significantly worse thereafter for AVR and MVR patients.

Mechanical Prosthesis v Bioprosthesis

To compare the outcomes of patients who receive either mechanical heart valves or bioprosthetic valves, Hammermeister and associates,[25] for the Veterans Affairs Cooperative Study on Valvular Heart Disease from Denver, Colo, randomly assigned 575 men scheduled to undergo AVR or MVR to receive either a mechanical or a bioprosthetic valve. The primary endpoints were death from any cause and any valve-related complication. During an average follow-up of 11 years, there was no difference between the two groups in the probability of death from any cause or in the probability of any valve-related complication (Figure 6-4). There was a much higher rate of structural valve failure among patients who received bioprosthetic valves than among those who received mechanical valves. However, this difference was offset by a higher rate of bleeding complications among patients with mechanical valves than among those with bioprosthetic valves and by a greater frequency of periprosthetic valvular regurgitation among patients with mechanical mitral valves than among those with mitral bioprostheses. After 11 years, the rates of sur-

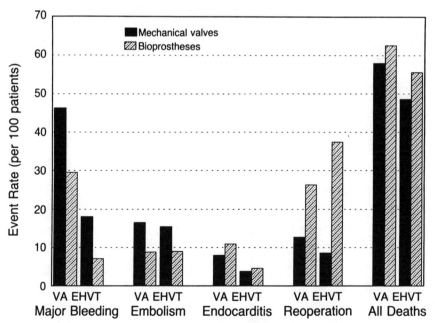

Figure 6-4. Event rates at 12 years in the Veterans Affairs Cooperative Study on Valvular Heart Disease (VA) and the Edinburgh Heart Valve Trial (EHVT). The 12-year event rates for the VA study were obtained from life-table analyses. Reproduced with permission from Hammermeister et al.[25]

vival and freedom from all valve-related complications were similar for patients who received mechanical heart valves and those who received bioprosthetic heart valves. However, structural failure was observed only with the bioprosthetic valves, whereas bleeding complications were more frequent among patients who received mechanical valves.

Double-Valve Replacement

Brown and associates,[26] from Bethesda, Md, did a study to determine if the combination of a mechanical and bioprosthetic valve in the aortic and mitral positions influences later morbidity and mortality when compared with patients who had dual mechanical or dual bioprosthetic valves inserted. The authors reviewed the course of 89 hospital survivors of combined AVR and MVR (Table 6-4). The mean postoperative follow-up interval was 6.6 years, with a total follow-up of 583 years (98% complete). At 12 months after operation, mean functional class decreased from 3.1 to 1.7, and mean cardiac index increased from 2.1 to 2.5 L · min^{-1} · m^{-2}. Actuarial survival for the 89 patients (exclusive of <30-day or in-hospital mortality, 14%) was 70%, 51%, and 33% at 5, 10, and 15 years, respectively (Figure 6-5). Freedom from re-operation was 93%, 78%, and 68%; and freedom from combined thromboembolism and anticoagulant-related hemorrhage was 82%, 60%, and 50%, respectively. These results show that there was no difference in overall survival in patients with dual mechanical valves, dual bioprosthetic valves, or a combination of both types at 15 years. There was, however, a lower reoperation rate in the group with dual mechanical valves as compared with the group with dual bioprosthetic valves or with a combination of valves. The higher the number of mechanical valves the higher the combined risk of thromboembolism and anticoagulant-related hemorrhage. Patients who received one or two Starr-Edwards prostheses had significantly higher rates of thromboembolism and anticoagulant-related hemorrhage and a lower survival than those who received other valve combinations. Patients who received two Hancock bioprostheses had significantly higher rates of re-operation and a decreased incidence of combined thromboembolic and anticoagulant-related hemorrhage. These authors concluded that combining a mechanical prosthesis and a bioprosthesis in the same patient is disadvantageous.

Table 6-4. Postoperative Data.[a] Reproduced with permission from Brown et al.[26]

Group	Substitute Valves (aortic-mitral)	Hospital Survivors	Total years FU (%)	Mean FC (0–4)	Mean PA s/d (mm Hg)	Mean CI (L · min^{-1} · m^{-2})	Warfarin Therapy	Total Mortality (%/y)	Reoperation (%/y)	TE (%/y) Fatal	TE (%/y) Total	ARH (%/y) Fatal	ARH (%/y) Total
1	SJM-SJM	10	20 (100%)	1.3 ± 0.1	31/14	2.3 ± 0.1	10 (100%)	0 (0.0%)	0 (0.0%)	0 (0.0%)	0 (0.0%)	0 (0.0%)	0 (0.0%)
2	SE-SE	34	259 (99%)	1.9 ± 0.0	43/18	2.6 ± 0.0	33 (97%)	26 (10.0%)	2 (0.7%)	5 (1.9%)	10 (3.8%)	1 (0.3%)	4 (1.5%)
3	SE-H	14	69 (90%)	1.9 ± 0.1	35/18	2.3 ± 0.1	12 (85%)	12 (17.3%)	2 (2.8%)	3 (4.3%)	5 (7.2%)	0 (0.0%)	0 (0.0%)
4	BS-H	12	109 (97%)	1.7 ± 0.1	45/21	2.3 ± 0.1	4 (21%)	6 (5.5%)	4 (3.6%)	1 (0.9%)	2 (1.8%)	1 (0.9%)	1 (0.9%)
5	H-H	19	125 (100%)	1.4 ± 0.0	36/16	2.5 ± 0.1	7 (37%)	10 (8.0%)	2 (1.6%)	0 (0.0%)	4 (3.2%)	0 (0.0%)	0 (0.0%)
A (1 + 2) Mechanical		44	279 (99%)	1.8 ± 0.1	31/14	2.6 ± 0.1	43 (98%)	26 (9.3%)	2 (0.7%)	5 (1.7%)	10 (3.5%)	1 (0.3%)	4 (1.4%)
B (3 + 4) Combined		26	178 (95%)	1.9 ± 0.1	43/18	2.3 ± 0.2	24 (92%)	18 (10.1%)	6 (3.4%)	4 (2.2%)	7 (3.9%)	1 (0.5%)	1 (0.5%)
C (5) Bioprosthetic		19	125 (100%)	1.3 ± 0.1	36/16	2.6 ± 0.2	4 (21%)	10 (8.0%)	2 (1.6%)	0 (0.0%)	4 (3.2%)	0 (0.0%)	0 (0.0%)
Total/mean		89	532 (98%)	1.7 ± 0.0	39/17	2.5 ± 0.0	69 (79%)	54 (9.3%)	10 (1.7%)	9 (1.5%)	21 (3.6%)	2 (0.3%)	5 (0.9%)
Range				1.0 ± 2.5	s, 15–75; d, 10–30	1.8–4.0							

[a] Values are shown as mean ± standard error of the mean.

ARH = anticoagulant-related hemorrhage;   BS = Björk-Shiley (tilting-disc);   CI = cardiac index;   FC = functional class;   H = Hancock;   PA = pulmonary artery pressure;   s/d = systolic/diastolic;   SE = Starr-Edwards;   SJM = St. Jude Medical;   TE = thromboembolism.

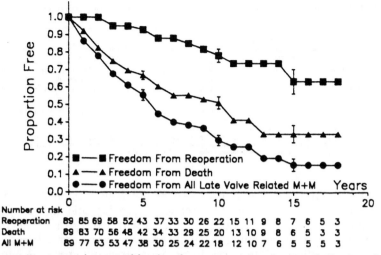

Figure 6-5. Actuarial curves of freedom from re-operation, death, and all valve-related late morbidity and mortality (M + M) in 89 hospital survivors of combined aortic- and mitral-valve replacement. Reproduced with permission from Brown et al.[26]

Triple-Valve Replacement

Brown and associates,[27] from Bethesda, Md, analyzed the effects of various combinations of mechanical and bioprosthetic valves in the aortic, mitral, and tricuspid positions on late morbidity and mortality of 40 hospital survivors of triple-valve replacement (Table 6-5). At operation the patients ranged in age from 27 to 69 years; 73% were women. The mean postoperative follow-up interval was 8.3 years, with a total follow-up of 331 years (100% complete). At 12 months after operation, functional class decreased from 3.3 to 1.6, cardiac index increased from 2.0 to 2.6 L · min^{-1} · m^{-2}, and pulmonary artery pressures decreased from 59/27 to 40/17 mm Hg. There were no differences in preoperative variables between groups. Actuarial survival for the 40 patients (exclusive of 30-day or in-hospital mortality, which was 31%) was 78% and 74% at 5 and 10 years (Table 6-6). At the same milestones, freedom from re-operation was 96% and 54%, freedom from combined throm-

Table 6-5. Preoperative Data. Reproduced with permission from Brown et al.[27]

Group	Substitute Valves AV	MV	TV	Hospital Survivors	Mean Age (y)	Sex (M/F)	History of: ARF	IE	AF	Mean FC	Mean PA (s/d; mm Hg)	Mean CI (L · min^{-1} · m^{-2})	MS AS TS	MS AS TR	MS AR TS	MS AR TR	MR AS TR	MR AR TR
1	MP	MP	MP	5	44	1/4	3	1	5	3.4	58/33	2.4	2	2	1	0	0	0
2	MP	MP	BP	5	54	0/5	3	0	5	2.8	67/26	1.9	1	2	2	0	0	0
3	MP	BP	BP	17	46	5/12	14	0	14	3.3	53/26	1.9	8	5	1	2	1	0
4	BP	BP	BP	13	52	5/8	8	1	12	3.3	62/31	2.0	1	4	3	2	1	2
Total/mean				40	49	11/29	28	2	36	3.3	59/27	2.0	12	13	7	4	2	2

AF = atrial fibrillation;   AR = aortic regurgitation;   ARF = acute rheumatic fever;   AS = aortic stenosis (with or without regurgitation);   AV = aortic valve;   BP = bioprosthesis;   CI = cardiac index;   F = female;   FC = functional class (New York Heart Association);   IE = infective endocarditis;   M = male;   MP = mechanical prosthesis;   MR = mitral regurgitation;   MS = mitral stenosis (with or without regurgitation); PA = pulmonary artery pressure;   s/d = peak systole/end-diastole;   TR = tricuspid regurgitation;   TS = tricuspid stensosis (with or without regurgitation);   TV = tricuspid valve.

Table 6-6. Postoperative Data. Reproduced with permission from Brown et al.[27]

Group	Substitute Valves AV	MV	TV	Hospital Survivors	Total Years FU[a]	Mean Years FU/pt	Mean FC	Mean PA (s/d; mm Hg)	Mean CI (L · min⁻¹ · m⁻²)	Warfarin Therapy	Total Mortality (%/y)	TE (%/y)	ARH (%/y)	Re-operation (%/y)
1	MP	MP	MP	5	39	7.9	1.7	40/18	2.6	5	3 (7.7)	2 (5.1)	0	0
2	MP	MP	BP	5	23	4.6	1.8	43/19	2.9	5	1 (4.3)	0	1 (4.3)	0
3	MP	BP	BP	17	168	9.9	1.5	37/16	2.5	17	13 (7.7)	9 (5.4)	5 (3.0)	9 (5.4)
4	BP	BP	BP	13	101	7.8	1.7	42/17	2.7	2	4 (4.0)	0	0	4 (4.0)
Total/mean				40	331	8.3	1.6	40/17	2.6	29 (73%)	21 (6.3)	11 (3.3)	6 (1.8)	13 (3.9)

[a] Actual follow-up was 100% of potential follow-up.

ARH = anticoagulant-related hemorrhage; AV = aortic valve; BP = bioprosthesis; CI = cardiac index; FC = functional class (New York Heart Association); FU = follow-up; MP = mechanical prosthesis; MV = mitral valve; PA = pulmonary artery pressure; pt = patient; s/d = peak systole/end-diastole; TE = thromboembolism; TV = tricuspid valve.

boembolism and anticoagulant-related hemorrhage was 68% and 56%, and freedom from all late valve-related morbidity and mortality was 64% and 25%. Comparison of the patients with two or more mechanical prostheses with the patients having two or more bioprostheses indicated no significant differences in actuarial freedom from late death, thromboembolic events, or anticoagulant-related hemorrhage. However the actuarial freedom from re-operation in the groups with two or more mechanical valves was lower than that of the groups with two or more bioprosthetic valves (0/10 v 13/30). Among 13 patients having re-operation, re-operation in 12 was prompted by degeneration of one or more bioprosthetic valves. Six of the patients who underwent re-operation died in the hospital, and 4 others died between 2 and 8 years after operation. These results support the view that mechanical prostheses provide better long-term results for triple-valve replacement than those produced using bioprostheses, primarily by reducing need for reoperation and its attendant complications.

Björk-Shiley Prosthesis

Orszulak and associates,[28] from Rochester, Minn, and Brussels, Belgium, described results of cardiac-valve replacement with use of only the Björk-Shiley prosthesis in 1,253 patients done between January 1973 and December 1982. There were 828 having AVR, 280 patients having MVR, and 145 patients having both AVR and MVR. Patient outcome was stratified according to multiple variables, including valve position and valve model (spherical v convexo-concave discs). No valve failure due to strut fraction was identified in 26 high-risk patients (MVR ≥29 mm implanted in patients ≤50 years of age) followed up for a mean of 10 years postoperatively. Fifteen patients had late thrombosis of their Björk-Shiley prosthesis (0.28 per 100 patient-years), but there was not significant difference in risk of valve thrombosis comparing the spherical and convexo-concave discs (0.27 per 100 patient-years v 0.27 per 100 patient-years). One hundred two patients had 128 thromboembolic episodes; rates of thromboembolism after AVR, MVR, and double-valve replacement were 2.1, 4,3, and 4.6 per 100 patient-years, respectively. Percentages of patients free from thromboemboli after AVR, MVR, and both AVR and MVR were 93% ± 1%, 86% ± 2%, and 89% ± 3% at 5 years postoperatively and 87% ± 2%, 79% ± 5%, and 77% ± 8% at 10 years postoperatively. There was no significant difference in the rates of thromboemboli for spherical and convexo-concave discs for all patients and for each of the subgroups. Ten-year actuarial survival estimates for patients dismissed alive from the hospital after AVR, MVR, and both AVR and MVR with the Björk-Shiley valve were 65% ± 4%, 63% ± 5%, and 55% ± 8%, respectively. Overall event-free survival (freedom from death, thromboembolism, anticoagulant-related bleeding, endocarditis, and re-operation) was similar for the three patient groups. Performance of the Björk-Shiley valve as judged by late patient follow-up is similar to other mechanical valves, and modifications in disc design do not appear to have reduced the threat of late valve thrombosis and thromboemboli. Evidence does not support elective explantation of this prosthesis.

St. Jude Medical Prosthesis

Kratz and associates,[29] from Charleston, SC, described results of isolated AVR (254 patients) or MVR (202 patients) with the St. Jude prosthesis inserted between Jan 1, 1979 and December 1990. The age ranged from 21 to 84 years (mean, 54 for AVR and 51 for MVR). Male sex predominated in the AVR group (66%) and female sex in the MVR group (64%). Ninety-two patients (20%) had associated CABG (AVR, 25%; MVR, 14%). There were 17 deaths (3.7%) occurring during the same hospitalization or within 30 days (AVR, 10/254 [3.9%]; MVR, 7/202 [3.5%]). Follow-up is 94.5% complete and ranges from 1.0 to 131 months (mean, 55 ± 37 months; total, 2,073 patient years). In the AVR group, 53 late deaths have occurred and actuarial survival is 80% ± 3% at 5 years and 47% ± 9% at 10 years. Twenty-one patients sustained thromboembolic episodes (1.8%/patient year), and the probability of remaining free of thromboembolism at 10 years was 67% ± 13%. The mean improvement in New York Heart Association functional class from preoperative to postoperative was 3.1 ± 0.76 to 1.6 ± 0.84. In the MVR group, there have been 41 late deaths; and the actuarial survival was 80% ± 3% at 5 years and 63% ± 5% at 10 years. Twenty-eight patients have sustained thromboembolic complications (2.9%/patient year), and the probability of remaining free of thromboembolism at 10 years was 77% ± 5%. The mean improvement in New York Heart Association functional class was from 3.4 ± 0.63 preoperatively to 1.8 ± 0.91 postoperatively. There were no mechanical failures, but 19 patients underwent 22 replacements of a previously implanted St. Jude prosthesis for endocarditis (14), paravalvular leak (4), thrombosis (2), and hemolysis (2). This intermediate-term follow-up confirms earlier impressions that in adults in whom valve repair is not possible, the St. Jude valve is a reliable, durable prosthesis with excellent hemodynamic function and a low rate of thrombosis/thromboembolism.

Omnicarbon Prosthesis

Misawa and associates,[30] from Tochigi, Japan, described results of implantation of Omnicarbon prosthetic heart valves in 124 patients (mean age, 53 ± 11 years); 66 of them had AVR, 40 had MVR, and 18 had both AVR and MVR. Preoperatively, 77% were in New York Heart Association class III or IV, and 85% were in class I or II after the operation. There were 6 (5%) early deaths and 7 late deaths. Survival was 85% ± 6% at 6 years in the AVR group, 94% ± 4% at 3 years in the MVR group, and 78% ± 11% at 4 years in the double-valve replacement group. Freedom from cardiac death was 89% ± 4% at 6 years (2.0% per patient-year) in the AVR group, 94% ± 4% at 3 years (1.8% per patient-year) in the MVR group, and 78% ± 11% at 4 years (6% per patient-year) in the double-valve replacement group. There were 6 valve-related complications. Freedom from valve-related complications was 92% ± 4% at 6 years (1.5% per patient-year) in the AVR group, and 97% ± 3% at 3 years (1.8% per patient-year) in the double-valve replacement group. Cerebral hemorrhage was seen in 2 patients in the AVR group. Freedom from all events was 80% ± 7% at 6 years in the AVR group, 88% ± 6% at 3 years in the MVR group, and 78% ± 11% at 4 years in the double-valve replacement group. Elevation of the postoperative serum lactate dehydrogenase levels was minimal in all groups. The maximum opening angle at rest was 60.0 ± 8.9 degrees in the aortic position and 54.1 ± 6.6 degrees in the mitral position. In conclusion, the Omnicarbon prothesis had excellent postoperative clinical status and negligible hemolysis.

Peter and associates,[31] from Basel, Switzerland, reviewed their experience from 1986 to 1990, in 172 patients aged 20 to 79 years who received 187 Omnicarbon valves (109 AVR, 48 MVR, and 15 MVR plus AVR). Patients were followed up for a median observation period of 2.5 years (range, 4 months to 5.2 years) by clinical and Doppler echocardiographic examination. Follow-up was complete in 98%. Operative mortality (death within 30 days) was 1.7%, and linearized late mortality was 2.6% per patient-year, corresponding to an actuarial survival rate for operative survivors of 89% after 4 years. The overall 4-year postoperative survival was 87% (93% for AVR, 77% for MVR). Compared with age- and sex-adjusted Swiss death rates, there was an excessive mortality of 5% after 4 years. Percentages of freedom from valve-related complications at 4 years are as follows: thromboembolism, 98% (98% for AVR, 96% for MVR); anticoagulant-related hemorrhage, 95%; valve endocarditis, 96%; reoperation, 96%; and permanent valve-related impairment, 99%. The overall 4-year event-free survival was 76% (80% for AVR, 69% for MVR). New York Heart Association class improved in 88% of the patients by one to three grades, and only 3% remained in class III after operation. For the most commonly used aortic valve (23 mm), Doppler echocardiography revealed a peak pressure gradient of 29 ± 10 mm Hg, a fractional shortening/peak pressure gradient ration of 1.34 ± 0.61, and a performance index of 0.35 ± 0.08. In the most commonly used mitral valve (27 mm), the mean pressure gradient was 4.0 ± 2.1 mm Hg. These authors concluded that excellent clinical and hemodynamic results can be obtained with the Omnicarbon prosthesis, in both the aortic and mitral positions.

Aortic Homograft

Cryopreserved aortic valve homografts have become an accepted aortic valve substitute, but long-term studies with echocardiographic assessment of valve function are essentially unavailable. Kirklin and associates,[32] from Birmingham, Ala, reviewed a total of 178 patients aged 9 months to 80 years (median, 46 years) who underwent implantation of a cryopreserved aortic valve homograft at their institution between 1981 through 1990. Serial two-dimensional Doppler echocardiographic studies were obtained in 149 patients. Overall survival was 91% at 1 year and 85% at 8 years. Survival of patients undergoing isolated primary infracoronary AVR was 99% at 1 month and 94% at 8 years. Twelve patients underwent homograft explantation. Freedom from explantation for leaflet degeneration was 95% at 8 years. Freedom from presumed leaflet failure (valve degeneration at explantation or AR grate 3/4 more without re-operation on echocardiography) was 94% at 5 years and 85% at 8 years. By multivariable analysis, younger recipient age was the only risk factor identified for leaflet failure. Ninety-five percent of patients followed up for 4 or more years were in New York Heart Association class I or II.

Anticoagulation Afterwards

Patients receiving long-term anticoagulant therapy may be subject to unnecessary risks of bleeding or thromboembolism because of variability in the commercial thromboplastins used to determine prothrombin time and consequent uncertainty about the actual intensity of anticoagulation. Eckman and associates,[33] from Boston, Mass, explored the effect of this uncertainty on the benefits and risks of anticoagulation in patients with prosthetic heart valves, using models of thromboembolic and hemorrhagic complications as a function of the intensity of anticoagulation, with quality-adjusted life expectancy and average variable costs used to describe outcomes. Anticoagulation provides a striking benefit for patients whose treatment is conducted within the recommended range of the international normalized ratio (INR) (i.e., 2.5 to 3.5); but if uncertainty about the laboratory results causes the intensity of anticoagulation to fall outside this range, the gain becomes smaller. Uncertainty about the true intensity of anticoagulation may reduce the potential gain in life expectancy, adjusted for quality of life, by more than half and may increase the ratio of costs to effectiveness to almost five times the optimal value. Variability in the intensity of anticoagulation is even greater if older recommendations advocating a higher level of anticoagulation are followed. Uncertainty about the sensitivies of the commercially available thromboplastins used in the US can have important clinical and economic effects. This problem could be eliminated if clinical laboratories uniformly reported the intensity of anticoagulation as the INR, by adjusting prothrombin-time ratios for variability in thromboplastins.

Aspirin + Warfarin v Warfarin Alone

Despite the use of warfarin, major systemic embolism remains an important complication in patients having heart-valve replacement. Although the addition of antiplatelet agents has the potential to reduce this complication, their efficacy and safety when given in combination with warfarin are uncertain. In a randomized, double-blind, placebo-controlled trial, Turpie and associates,[34] from Hamilton, London, and Montreal, Canada, assessed the efficacy and safety of adding aspiring (100 mg/day) to warfarin treatment (target international normalized ratio, 3.0 to 4.5) in 370 patients with mechanical heart valves or with tissue valves plus AF or a history of thromboembolism (Table 6-7). A total of 186 patients were randomly assigned to aspirin and 184 to placebo, and they were followed for up to 4 years (average, 2.5). Major systemic embolism or death from vascular causes occurred in 6 aspirin-treated patients (1.9%/year) and 24 placebo-treated patients (8.4%/year) (risk reduction

Table 6-7. Frequency of Major Systemic Embolism or Death from Vascular Causes in the Study Patients, According to Clinical Characteristics. Reproduced with permission from Turpie et al.[34]

CHARACTERISTIC	ASPIRIN	PLACEBO
	no. with event/no. in group (%)	
Valve position		
Aortic	2/87 (2.3)	7/85 (8.2)
Mitral	3/80 (3.8)	14/82 (17.1)
Multiple	1/19 (5.3)	3/17 (17.6)
Valve type		
Tissue	2/45 (4.4)	4/44 (9.1)
Mechanical	4/141 (2.8)	20/140 (14.3)
Preoperative rhythm		
Atrial fibrillation	2/83 (2.4)	15/83 (18.1)
Sinus or other	4/103 (3.9)	9/101 (8.9)
Left ventricular function		
Normal	2/93 (2.2)	11/101 (10.9)
Abnormal	4/68 (5.9)	9/62 (14.5)
Not assessed	0/25	4/21 (19.0)
Coronary arteries		
Normal	5/100 (5.0)	11/114 (9.6)
Abnormal	1/50 (2.0)	9/43 (20.9)
Not assessed	0/36	4/27 (14.8)
Concomitant bypass surgery		
Yes	1/32 (3.1)	5/32 (15.6)
No	5/154 (3.2)	19/152 (12.5)

with aspirin, 77%) (Table 6-8). Major systemic embolism, nonfatal intracranial hemorrhage, or death from hemorrhage or vascular causes occurred in 12 patients assigned to aspirin (3.9%/year) and 28 patients assigned to placebo (9.9%/year) (risk reduction, 61%); major systemic embolism or death from any cause occurred in 13 patients (4.2%) and 33 patients (11.7%), respectively (risk reduction, 65%); and death from all causes occurred in 9 patients (2.8%) and 22 patients (7.4%), respectively (risk reduction, 63%). Bleeding occurred in 71 patients in the aspirin group (35%) as compared with 49 patients in the placebo group (22%) (increase in risk, 55%); major bleeding occurred in 24 and 19 patients, respectively (increase in risk, 27%). In patients with mechanical heart valves and high-risk patients with prosthetic tissue valves, the addition of aspirin to warfarin therapy reduced mortality, particularly mortality from vascular causes, together with major systemic embolism. Although there was some increase in bleeding, the risk of the combined treatment was more than offset by the considerable benefit.

Thrombolysis for Thrombosed Prosthetic Valve

Silber and associates,[35] from Los Angeles, Calif, sought to determine the short- and long-term results of treating thrombosed St. Jude heart valves with thrombolytic therapy as the primary form of treatment. Between March 1978 and December 1991, 988 patients had St. Jude prosthetic valves implanted. All patients with thrombosed valves were identified prospectively. During this period, 17 patients, including 13 women and 4 men with a mean age of 67 years, developed prosthetic valve thrombosis. Prosthetic valve thrombosis occurred on 11 aortic and 6 mitral valves. In six patients, coumadin was stopped in preparation for elective

Table 6-8. Outcome Analysis. Reproduced with permission from Turpie et al.[34]

Outcome	Aspirin (N = 186)		Placebo (N = 184)		P Value	Observed Risk Reduction (95% CI)*
	No. of Events	Annualized Event Rate	No. of Events	Annualized Event Rate		
		%		%		%
Major systemic embolism or death from vascular causes	6	1.9	24	8.5	<0.001	77 (44–91)
Major systemic embolism, non-fatal intracranial hemorrhage, death from hemorrhage, or death from vascular causes	12	3.9	28	9.9	0.005	61 (24–80)
Major systemic embolism or death	13	4.2	33	11.6	<0.001	65 (33–82)
Death	9	2.8	22	7.4	0.01	63 (19–83)

*CI denotes confidence interval.

surgery. The clinical presentation of these patients was CHF in 13, syncope and fatigue in 2, and a cerebrovascular accident in 1. One patient was asymptomatic. The average duration of symptoms was 12 ± 12 days. Anticoagulation was subtherapeutic in all but 1 patient at the time of their clinical presentation. Cinefluoroscopy was the primary method used for diagnosis, and it was also used to follow the responses to therapy. Twelve patients were treated medically (including 10 with thrombolytic therapy and 2 with heparin), 3 were treated surgically, and 2 were diagnosed at autopsy. Of the 12 medically treated patients, 10 had marked improvement in leaflet motion and symptoms within 12 hours. Therefore, 10 of 12 patients (83%) had a good response to medical therapy alone. No medically treated patient died or had a major complication resulting in permanent damage. Nevertheless, 4 of the 12 medically treated patients had minor complications, including a transient episode of facial weakness in 1 patient, hematomas in 2, and epistaxis in 1. Late rethrombosis occurred in 2 patients in the medically treated group and was successfully treated with thrombolytic therapy. At 3 months, all of the patients are alive. Thus, thrombolytic therapy may be used to treat patients with thrombosed St. Jude valves with an excellent chance of success. In most instances, surgery can be reserved for patients who do not respond successfully to thrombolytic therapy.

Aortic Dissection Afterwards

Little information is available regarding the incidence of aortic dissection after previous AVR and factors associated with its development. Pieters and associates,[36] from Maastricht, The Netherlands, performed a meta-analysis of the literature and retrospectively studied a patient population. Data from published studies showed that 87% of 31 patients were men (mean age, 60 years), and 68% were known to have systemic hypertension. A dilated ascending aorta was observed at the time of AVR in 88% of patients. Aortic-valve replacement was performed because of pure AR in 55% of patients and combined AS and AR in 23%. More than 50% of patients did not survive dissection. The present series consisted of 7 patients. Four patients were known to the department before dissection occurred, and the other 3 were referred by other hospitals. Eighteen of 330 patients with previous aortic-valve replacement whose data were stored in an echocardiographic data base had an ascending aortic diameter >50 mm. Of these 18 patients, aortic dissection occurred in 4. Three of the remaining 14 patients underwent elective ascending aortic replacement. Characteristics including sex, age, severity of dilatation, presence of progression in diameter, LV function, and time interval after aortic-valve replacement were not helpful in determining a cumulative risk for developing dissection. Because dissection occurred in 4 of 18 patients (22%) with an ascending aorta diameter >50 mm, these investigators suggested consideration of replacement of the ascending aorta during AVR when a value of 50 mm is exceeded.

Left Ventricular Function Afterwards

To determine factors that influence survival and recovery of LV function in patients undergoing AVR in the current surgical era, Morris and associates,[37] from Rochester, Minn, analyzed baseline risk factors related to outcome in 1,012 patients undergoing AVR between 1983 and 1990. Forty-two percent of patients underwent concomitant CABG. Observed survival probabilities (expressed as 30-day/5-year) were 0.97/0.81 overall, 0.99/0.89 for patients aged less than 70 years, and 0.95/0.74 for patients aged 70 years or greater. Advanced age, decreased EF, extent of CAD, smaller prosthetic valve, and advanced New York Heart Association class were incremental risk factors for mortality. In patients with preoperative ventricular dysfunction (EF ≤0.45), EF measured 1.4 years after AVR improved in 72% and the mean increment in EF was 0.175. The increment in EF was greater in female patients than in male patients and greater in patients without CAD than with CAD. Female sex and lesser extent of CAD were independent predictors of change in EF. In all patients, early improvement in EF conveyed an independent subsequent survival benefit. The results of AVR in the current era are excellent, and most patients with ventricular dysfunction demonstrate significant improvement. Early improvement in EF, influenced by coexistent CAD and sex-associated factors, importantly affects subsequent survival.

Risk of Re-Operation

Cohn and associates,[38] from Boston, Mass, analyzed the risk of valve re-replacement in 640 patients re-operated on between 1980 and 1992. This represented 17% of total valve operations (640/3,764) during that period. A univariate and logistic multivariate analysis was carried out for four sequential periods for the 640 re-replacement patients to determine if changing methods of perfusion and myocardial protection affected recent results. There were 323 female and 317 male patients with a mean age of 58 years (range, 17 to 84 years). Ninety-seven (15%) had CABG, 135 (21%) were 70 years old or older, 377 (59%) were in New York Heart Association functional class III or less, and 263 (41%) were in functional class IV. The aortic valve was re-replaced in 245, the mitral valve in 289, and both aortic and mitral synchronously in 106. Four periods were

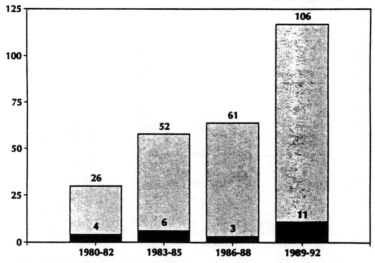

Figure 6-6. Patient number and mortality in aortic valve re-replacement in four periods. Reproduced with permission from Cohn et al.[38]

analyzed: 1980 through 1982, 1983 through 1985, 1986 through 1988, and 1989 through 1992. The overall operative mortality was 65 of 640 patients (10%), falling from 12/73 (16%) in 1980 through 1982 to 23/268 (8%) in 1989 through 1992. Univariate and multivariate logistic analysis documented that New York Heart Association functional class was highly significant for operative mortality; operative mortality was 4% for functional classes I through III, and 19% for functional class IV. The requirement for CABG was of borderline significance, and year of operation was also significant. Mortality for re-replacement of aortic valve fell from 15% to 10% (Figure 6-6), double valve from 20% to 9%

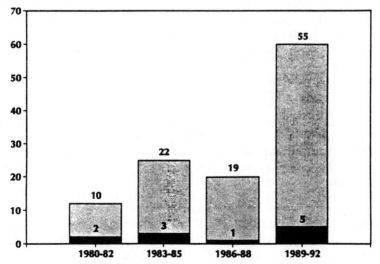

Figure 6-7. Patient number and mortality in aortic/mitral valve re-replacement in four periods. Reproduced with permission from Cohn et al.[38]

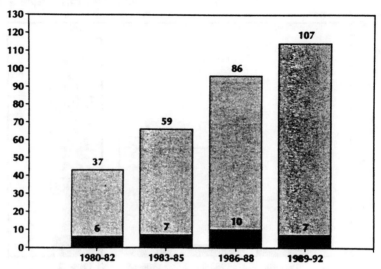

Figure 6-8. Patient number and mortality in mitral valve re-replacement in four periods. Reproduced with permission from Cohn et al.[38]

(Figure 6-7), and mitral valve from 16% to 6% (Figure 6-8). Postoperative nonfatal morbidity included rebleeding in 5.6%, stroke in 3.4%, low cardiac output in 7%, and AMI in 1.3%. With improvement in myocardial protection and cardiopulmonary bypass strategies, the operative risk in patients undergoing valve re-replacement has been markedly reduced.

MISCELLANEOUS TOPICS

Discontinuing Rheumatic Fever Prophylaxis

To assess the safety of discontinuing prophylaxis with antimicrobial agents in patients judged to be at relatively low risk for recurrence of acute rheumatic fever, Berrios and associates,[39] from Santiago, Chile, and Miami, Fla, studied 59 patients ranging in age at study entry from 15 to 44 years (mean, 25 years): 48 completed their prescribed period of prophylaxis and 11 refused or were allergic to intramuscular benzathine penicillin G and were not compliant with oral sulfadiazine. In patients who did not have carditis during their previous attacks, prophylaxis was discontinued after 5 years or at age 18, whichever was longer. In those with only mild MR or healed carditis, prophylaxis was stopped after 10 years or at age 25. Symptomatic intercurrent streptococcal throat infections were treated with antibiotics. During laboratory surveillance, at every 3 months during the study, significant increases in antibody titers were detected in 56 instances (28 per 100 patient-years), and 29 isolations of group A streptococci occurred (15 per 100 patient-years). The patients were followed for a total of 3,349 patient-months, during which time 2 acute rheumatic fever recurrences were observed (0.7 per 100 patient-years). No recurrences occurred during an outbreak of acute rheumatic fever in 52 patients in the study area in 1986. These and other data indicate that acute rheumatic fever prophylaxis can safely be discontinued in young adults judged to be at low risk for recurrence and who are maintained under careful prospective surveillance.

Doppler Assessment of Valvular Function

Enriquez-Sarano and associates,[40] from Rochester, Minn, determined the accuracy of quantitative Doppler and its ability to measure regurgitant volume in 120 patients, including 20 without AR, 19 with AR, and 81 with MR. In these patients, the stroke volume through the mitral annulus and LV outflow tract were measured using pulsed-wave Doppler with LV stroke volume calculated using LV volumes measured by two-dimensional echocardiography. Regurgitant volume and fraction were computed using Doppler or ventricular methods. In patients without valvular regurgitation, there were good correlations between Doppler and LV measurements of stroke volume. Doppler regurgitant volume and fraction were 4 ± 4 and 5 ± 5 mL, respectively. In patients with AR, there were good correlations between Doppler and LV measurements of stroke volume, regurgitant volume, and regurgitant fraction. In patients with MR, despite good correlations between Doppler and ventricular methods for stroke volume, regurgitant volume, and regurgitant fraction, these variables were overestimated by Doppler. However, in the last 54 patients compared with the first 27, overestimation significantly decreased for regurgitant volume and regurgitant fraction. These data indicate that quantitative Doppler may be performed in a large number of patients in a clinical laboratory. Its potential limitation is identified as overestimation of MR, which is diminished with increased experience. These techniques allow measurement not only of regurgitant fraction but also of regurgitant volume.

Carcinoid Heart Disease

Pellikka and associates,[41] from Rochester, Minn, studied 132 patients with carcinoid syndrome between 1980 and 1989 using echocardiography. The echocardiographic, Doppler, and clinical features of 74 patients (56%) with echocardiographic evidence of carcinoid heart disease were determined. Ninety-seven percent of patients had shortened, thickened tricuspid leaflets. Tricuspid regurgitation was present in all 69 patients with carcinoid heart disease who underwent Doppler examination, and it was of moderate to severe degree in 62 patients (90%). Severe TR was characterized by Doppler spectral profiles with an early peak pressure and rapid decline. The pressure halftime was prolonged consistent with associated tricuspid stenosis. The pulmonary valve appeared thickened and immobile in 36 patients (49%) and was diminutive to the extent of not being visualized in an additional 29 patients (39%). Among the 47 patients who underwent Doppler evaluation of the pulmonary valve, regurgitation was present in 81%, and stenosis was present in 53%. Left-sided valvular involvement was present in 5 patients (7%), 4 of whom had patent foramen ovales or carcinoid tumors involving the lung. Myocardial metastases were present in 3 patients (4%) and were confirmed by biopsy in each case. Small pericardial effusions were present in 10 patients (14%). Patients with and without echocardiographic evidence of carcinoid heart disease did not differ with regard to sex, age, location of the primary tumor, duration of diagnosis, or duration of symptoms of

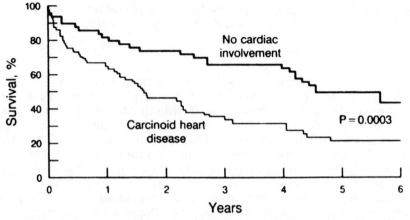

Figure 6-9. Curves compare the survival for 73 patients with echocardiographic evidence of carcinoid heart disease with that for 51 patients without cardiac involvement. Note the markedly improved 3- and 4-year survival of patients free of cardiac involvement. Reproduced with permission from Pellikka et al.[41]

carcinoid syndrome. However, the mean pretreatment level of urinary 5-hydroxyindoleacetic acid was higher in patients with carcinoid heart disease than in those without. Dyspnea was more prevalent among patients with carcinoid heart disease than in patients without. Treatment regimens and response to therapy were similar in the two groups. Survival of patients with echocardiographic evidence of carcinoid heart disease was reduced compared with those without cardiac involvement (Figure 6-9). Thus, the broad spectrum of carcinoid heart disease is described in this large series; and it includes not only right-sided valvular lesions but also left-sided involvement, pericardial effusion, and myocardial metastases.

References

1. Lax D, Eicher M, Goldberg SJ: Effects of hydration on mitral valve prolapse. Am Heart J 1993 (Aug);126:415–418.
2. David TE, Armstrong S, Sun Z, et al: Late results of mitral-valve repair for mitral regurgitation due to degenerative disease. Ann Thorac Surg 1993; 56:7–14.
3. Cacciapuoti F, Perrone N, Diaspro R, et al: Slowing of mitral valve annular calcium in systemic hypertension by nifedipine and comparisons with enalapril and atenolol. Am J Cardiol 1993 (Nov 1);72:1038–1042.
4. Patel JJ, Mitha AS, Hassen F, et al: Percutaneous balloon mitral valvotomy in pregnant patients with tight pliable mitral stenosis. Am Heart J 1993 (April);125:1106–1109.
5. Ribeiro PA, Al Zaibag M, Abdullah M: Pulmonary artery pressure and pulmonary vascular resistance before and after mitral balloon valvotomy in 100 patients with severe mitral valve stenosis. Am Heart J 1993 (April);125: 1110–1114.

6. Yasuda S, Nagata S, Tamai J, et al: Left ventricular diastolic pressure-volume response immediately after successful percutaneous transvenous mitral commissurotomy. Am J Cardiol 1993 (April 15);71:932–937.

7. Herrmann HC, Feldman T, Isner JM, et al, for the North American Inoue Balloon Investigators, Philadelphia, Pennsylvania: Comparison of results of percutaneous balloon valvuloplasty in patients with mild and moderate mitral stenosis to those with severe mitral stenosis. Am J Cardiol 1993 (June 1);71:1300–1303.

8. Ribeiro PA, Fawzy ME, Mimish L, et al: Mitral restenosis and mitral regurgitation 1 year after Inoue mitral balloon valvotomy in a population of patients with pliable mitral valve stenosis. Am Heart J 1993 (July);126: 136–140.

9. Herrmann HC, Lima JAC, Feldman T, et al, for the North American Inoue Balloon Investigators: Mechanisms and outcome of severe mitral regurgitation after Inoue balloon valvuloplasty. J Am Coll Cardiol 1993 (Sep);22: 783–789.

10. Arora R, Nair M, Kalra GS, et al: Immediate and long-term results of balloon and surgical closed mitral valvotomy: A randomized comparative study. Am Heart J 1993 (April);125:1091–1105.

11. Scalia D, Rizzoli G, Campanile F, et al: Long-term results of mitral commissurotomy. J Thorac Cardiovasc Surg 1993 (April);105:633–642.

12. Skoularigis J, Röthlisberger C, Skudicky D, et al: Effectiveness of amiodarone and electrical cardioversion for chronic rheumatic atrial fibrillation after mitral valve surgery. Am J Cardiol 1993 (Aug 15);72:423–427.

13. Mautner GC, Mautner SL, Cannon RO III, et al: Clinical factors useful in predicting aortic valve structure in patients >40 years of age with isolated valvular aortic stenosis. Am J Cardiol 1993 (July 15);72:194–198.

14. Rothlisberger C, Sareli P, Wisenbaugh T: Comparison of single-dose nifedipine and captopril for chronic severe aortic regurgitation. Am J Cardiol 1993 (Oct 1);72:799–804.

15. Kohlmeier L, Gasner C, Marcus R: Bone mineral status of women with the Marfan Syndrome. Am J Med 1993 (Dec);95:568–572.

16. Crowley JJ, Donnelly SM, Tobin M, et al: Doppler echocardiographic evidence of left ventricular diastolic dysfunction in ankylosing spondylitis. Am J Cardiol 1993 (June 1);71:1337–1340.

17. Watanakunakorn C, Burkert T: Infective endocarditis at a large community teaching hospital, 1980–1990. Medicine 1993;72:90–102.

18. Fernicola DJ, Roberts WC: Clinicopathologic features of active infective endocarditis isolated to the native mitral valve. Am J Cardiol 1993 (May 15);71:1186–1197.

19. Roberts WC, Oluwole BO, Fernicola DJ: Comparison of active infective endocarditis involving a previously stenotic versus a previously nonstenotic aortic valve. Am J Cardiol 1993 (May 1);71:1082–1088.

20. Fernicola DJ, Roberts WC: Frequency of ring abscess and cuspal infection in active infective endocarditis involving bioprosthetic valves. Am J Cardiol 1993 (Aug 1);72:314–323.

21. Sett SS, Hudon MPJ, Jamieson WRE, et al: Bioprosthetic valve endocarditis. J Thorac Cardiovasc Surg 1993 (March);105:428–434.

22. Fang G, Deys TF, Gentry LO, et al: Prosthetic valve endocarditis resulting from nosocomial bacteremia. Ann Intern Med 1993 (Oct 1);119:560–567.

23. Daniel WG, Mugge A, Grote J, et al: Comparison of transthoracic echocardiography for detection of abnormalities of prosthetic and bioprosthetic valves in the mitral and aortic positions. Am J Cardiol 1993 (Jan 15);71: 210–215.

24. Davis EA, Gardner TJ, Gillinov AM, et al: Valvular disease in the elderly. Ann Thorac Surg 1993;55:333–338.

25. Hammermeister KE, Sethi GK, Henderson WG, et al: A comparison of outcomes in men 11 years after heart-valve replacement with a mechanical valve or bioprosthesis. N Engl J Med 1993 (May 6);328:1289–1296.

26. Brown PS, Roberts CS, McIntosh CL, et al: Relation between choice of prostheses and late outcome in double-valve replacement. Ann Thorac Surg 1993 (June 15);55:631–640.

27. Brown PS, Roberts CS, McIntosh CL, et al: Late results after triple-valve replacement with various substitute valves. Ann Thorac Surg 1993;55:502–508.

28. Orszulak TA, Schaff HV, DeSmet JM, et al: Late results of valve replacement with the Björk-Shiley valve (1973-1982). J Thorac Cardiovasc Surg 1993 (Feb);105:302–312.

29. Kratz JM, Crawford FA Jr, Sade RM, et al: Effectiveness of St. Jude prosthesis for aortic and mitral-valve replacement. Ann Thorac Surg 1993;56:462–468.

30. Misawa Y, Hasegawa T, Kato M: Clinical experience with the Omnicarbon prosthetic heart valve. J Thorac Cardiovasc Surg 1993 (Jan);105:168–172.

31. Peter M, Weiss P, Jenzer H-R, et al. The Omnicarbon tilting-disc heart valve prosthesis. J Thorac Cardiovasc Surg 1993 (Oct);106:599–608.

32. Kirklin JK, Smith D, Novick W, et al: Long-term function of cryopreserved aortic homografts. J Thorac Cardiovasc Surg 1993 (July);106:154–166.

33. Eckman EH, Levine HJ, Pauker SG: Effect of laboratory variation in the prothrombin-time ratio on the results of oral anticoagulant therapy in patients with prosthetic heart valves. N Engl J Med 1993 (Sep 2);329:696–702.

34. Turpie AGG, Gent M, Laupacis A, et al: A comparison of aspirin with placebo in patients treated with warfarin after heart-valve replacement. N Engl J Med 1993 (Aug 19);329:524–529.

35. Silber H, Khan SS, Matloff JM, et al: The St. Jude valve: Thrombolysis as the first line of therapy for cardiac valve thrombosis. Circulation 1993 (Jan);87:30–37.

36. Pieters FAA, Widdershoven JW, Gerardy AC, et al: Risk of aortic dissection after aortic-valve replacement. Am J Cardiol 1993 (Nov 1);72:1043–1047.

37. Morris JJ, Schaff HV, Mullany CJ, et al: Determinants of survival and recovery of left ventricular function after aortic-valve replacement. Ann Thorac Surg 1993;56:22–30.

38. Cohn LH, Aranki SF, Rizzo RJ, et al: Operative risk of reoperative valve surgery. Ann Thorac Surg 1993;56:15–21.

39. Berrios X, Campo E, Guzman G, et al: Discontinuing rheumatic fever prophylaxis in selected adolescents and young adults. Ann Intern Med 1993 (March 15);118:401–406.

40. Enriquez-Sarano M, Bailey KR, Seward JB, et al: Quantitative Doppler assessment of valvular regurgitation. Circulation 1993 (March);87:841–848.

41. Pellikka PA, Tajik J, Khandheria BK, et al: Carcinoid heart disease: Clinical and echocardiographic spectrum in 74 patients. Circulation 1993 (April);87:1188–1196.

Myocardial Heart Disease

Distinguishing From Ischemic Dilated Cardiomyopathy

Thallium-201 scintigraphic defects are observed in most patients with ischemic cardiomyopathy and also can be found in idiopathic dilated cardiomyopathy. To determine the ability of qualitative and quantitative perfusion parameters to differentiate these entities, Tauberg and associates,[1] from Pittsburgh, Pa, performed thallium-201 exercise testing in 51 patients with coronary arteriography referred for evaluation of severe CHF. All patients had an LVEF <35%. Thirty-one ischemic patients had CAD >70% in ≥1 artery, and 20 idiopathic patients had no CAD or identifiable cause of heart disease. Similar exercise capacity, EF, and sex distribution were found in both groups. Ischemic patients more often had severe perfusion defects, large perfusion defects involving ≥40% of the LV contour, and increased thallium-201 lung uptake. Large severe defects were present in 90% of ischemic and only 5% of idiopathic patients. On quantitative analysis, the area of the thallium-201 curve less than normal was greater in ischemic than idiopathic patients. The degree and severity of redistribution were similar in both groups. Multivariate analysis identified the qualitative parameters of increased thallium-201 lung uptake, severe defects, and large severe defects as the only independent predictors of the presence of ischemic disease. The presence of large severe defects had a 97% predictive value for ischemic cardiomyopathy. The absence of severe defects had a 94% predictive value for idiopathic dilated cardiomyopathy. These investigators concluded that thallium-201 can reliably differentiate these two entities.

Discordant Ventricular Dilatation

There is considerable variability in the clinical course of individual patients with dilated cardiomyopathy. Although LV dilation is the distinguishing feature of this disease, the RV shows a more variable degree of variation in size. Lewis and associates,[2] from Washington, DC, evaluated the relative importance of the degree of dilation of LV and RV chambers on the clinical outcome of patients with dilated cardiomyopathy. Sixty-seven patients with dilated cardiomyopathy and no evidence of ischemic or primary valvular disease were followed. Thirty-eight patients were classified as having a relatively equal degree of LV and RV dilation, and 29 patients had disproportionate dilation of the LV. Patients with dilation of both ventricles showed more severe MR and TR than those in the group with primary LV dilation. Survival in the group of patients with primary LV dilation was significantly better than in the group with equal dilation of both chambers. They concluded that patients with a relatively smaller RV in dilated cardiomyopathy had a better overall survival and less MR and TR than patients with equal involvement of the two ventricles. Because this study was retrospective in design, it will need to be tested in a prospective manner.

Assessment of Left Ventricular Filling

In idiopathic dilated cardiomyopathy, an impaired LV filling as assessed by the Doppler echocardiographic mitral flow pattern is closely related to the severity of CHF. This study by Werner and associates,[3] from Goettingen, Federal Republic of Germany, examined the relation of LV filling and the clinical course of the disease in patients with a recent diagnostic procedure and initiation of medical therapy (group 1, n = 15) as compared with patients in a chronic stage of the disease (group 2, n = 24) with the diagnosis established >1 year before. All patients had to be in sinus rhythm to facilitate the Doppler echocardiographic evaluation of LV filing. The clinical status was assessed by the New York Heart Association classification and a heart failure score at baseline and after a period of 12 ± 7 months. At baseline the ratio of the peak early/atrial Doppler velocities was shifted toward the early diastole in group 1 as compared with group 2. Symptoms of CHF were more severe in group 1. During follow-up, the peak early/atrial Doppler velocities tended to decrease in group 1 and remained unchanged in group 2. In a subgroup of 10 patients who underwent repeat right-sided heart catheterization, the decrease of the peak early/atrial Doppler velocities coincided with a decrease of the PA wedge pressure. The changes of the clinical symptoms and the LV filling parameters during follow-up were concordant with a decrease of the peak early/atrial Doppler velocity in the case of a clinical improvement and an increase of the peak early/atrial Doppler velocity when the clinical course deteriorated. Medical therapy was comparable in both groups; however, duration of medical therapy was shorter in group 1. The serial evaluation of patients with idiopathic dilated cardiomyopathy showed a close association between the distribution of LV filling in early and late diastole and the clinical course of the disease.

Doppler echocardiography may serve as a tool for the monitoring of the beneficial effects of long-term medical therapy on LV diastolic function in such patients.

Signal Averaged Electrocardiogram

Mancini and associates,[4] in Philadelphia, Pa, determined whether an abnormal signal-averaged ECG could provide prognostic information in patients with nonischemic dilated cardiomyopathy. Signal average ECGs were evaluated in 114 patients with dilated nonischemic cardiomyopathy. Twelve-lead ECGs, LVEFs, hemodynamic measurements, and peak exercise oxygen consumption were measured. Signal averaged ECG was defined as abnormal by any of the three following criteria: filtered QRS duration >120 msec, root-mean-square voltage in the last 40 msec <20 µV, or duration <40 µV >38 msec at 40 Hz. Sixty-six patients had a normal signal averaged ECG, 20 patients had an abnormal signal averaged ECG, and 28 patients had bundle branch block. Mean follow-up was 10 ± 5 months. Age, LVEF, peak oxygen consumption, PA wedge pressure, and cardiac index were not different among the three groups. Use of antiarrhythmic drugs was similar among the groups, although patients with bilateral BBB had more implantable defibrillators. The incidence of previous atrial arrhythmias was similar for the three groups. Patients with abnormal signal averaged ECG or BBB had more past episodes of sustained VT and/or sudden death than patients with normal signal averaged ECGs (Figure 7-1). None of the 66 patients with normal signal averaged ECGs died suddenly or had sustained ventricular arrhythmias. Two deaths occurred from progressive CHF and three patients required urgent cardiac transplant. In 20 patients with an abnormal signal averaged ECG, 4 patients had sustained VT, 5 patients died suddenly, 2 patients died from progressive CHF, and 1 patient required urgent cardiac transplant. In the patients with bilateral BBB, 4 had sustained VT and 4 required urgent cardiac transplant. One-year event-free survival was 95% in patients with normal signal averaged ECGs, 88% in patients with bilateral BBB, and 39% in patients with an abnormal signal averaged ECG (Figure 7-2). Multivariate analysis demonstrated that the signal averaged ECG and New York Heart Association functional classification were independent predictors of survival. Thus, patients with nonischemic dilated cardiomyopathy and an abnormal signal averaged ECG have a statistically significant increase in risk of sustained ventricular arrhythmias and death.

Genetic Abnormality

Muntoni and associates,[5] from three medical centers in Italy, investigated a family with a severe form of x-linked dilated cardiomyopathy in which affected male family members had elevated serum levels of creatine kinase. The authors carried out a detailed study to confirm the possibility that this cardiomyopathy was caused by a genetic abnormality of dystrophin. The pedigree was constructed for the family (Figure 7-3). The proband (subject II-6) was a 23-year-old man of normal intelligence who was found to have dilated cardiomyopathy at the age of 13. The patient was found to have elevated levels of serum creatine kinase, type MM (Table 7-1). A muscle biopsy was performed, and he died of VF 2

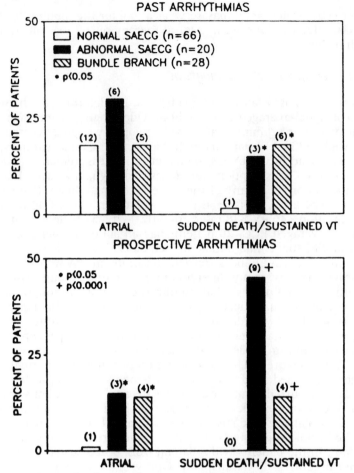

Figure 7-1. Bar graphs of past and prospective atrial and sustained ventricular arrhythmias in patients with normal signal-averaged ECGs (SAECG), abnormal SAECGs, or bundle branch block. VT, ventricular tachycardia. Reproduced with permission from Mancini et al.[4]

months later. Two maternal uncles had died of cardiomyopathy at ages 29 and 44 (Subjects I-2 and I-3, respectively, Figure 1). Three brothers of the proband (Subjects II-1, II-2, and II-5) had electrocardiographic abnormalities and echocardiographic signs indicative of dilated cardiomyopathy (Table 1). All the affected male family members had elevated creatine kinase levels (Table 7-1). The examination of these subjects, including manual muscle testing, did not reveal any muscle weakness. There was no muscle hypertrophy or wasting of any muscle groups. A needle biopsy of the vastus lateralis muscle was performed in the proband and studied according to standard techniques including immunocytochemistry. DNA was extracted from leukocytes by standard methods. DNA amplifications of the dystrophin exons were carried out with the multiplex polymerase chain reaction. Muscle biopsy revealed a mild variability in fiber size owing to the presence of hypertrophic and atrophic fibers. The numbers of internal nuclei were increased (18%;

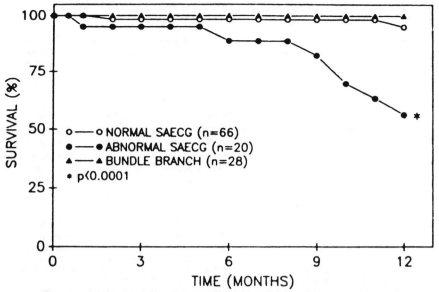

Figure 7-2. Survival curves comparing patients with normal signal-averaged ECGs (SAECG), abnormal SAECGs, or bundle branch block. The survival curve for patients with an abnormal SAECG is significantly reduced compared with patients with normal SAECG or bundle branch block (p <0.0001). Reproduced with permission from Mancini et al.[4]

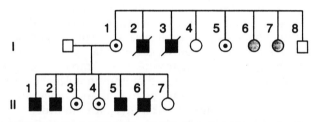

Figure 7-3. Pedigree of a family with x-linked dilated cardiomyopathy. Squares denote male family members; circles, female family members; open symbols, unaffected subjects; solid symbols, subjects; shaded symbols, subjects whose status was unknown; and circles with a dot, carriers. Deceased family members are indicated by a slash. Subject II-6 was the proband. Reproduced with permission from Muntoni et al.[5]

normal, <4%). No evidence of mitochondrial dysfunction was found. The immunohistochemical staining with antidystrophin antibodies was less intense in the muscle fibers from the proband than in the control muscle and thus suggestive of dystrophin abnormality. Staining of the dystrophin was clearly visible in the sarcolemma with all the antibodies used, indicating that the antibody-recognition epitopes were intact. All the exons investigated were present in the proband, whereas the muscle-promotor region showed a deletion. The first muscle exon was also found to be deleted, whereas the second exon and the brain promoter were successfully amplified. Identical deletions were documented in the other affected brothers (Subjects II-1, II-2, and II-5) whereas linkage analysis indicated that Subjects I-2, I-5, II-3, and II-4 were obligate carri-

Table 7-1. Selected Laboratory Findings in Various Family Members.* Reproduced with permission from Muntoni et al.[5]

Subject No.	Sex	Age	Serum CK	Serum CK-MB	Echocardiography			NYHA Class	ECG Results†	Zygosity for the Deletion
					FS	EDD	KINESIS			
		yr	U/liter		%	mm				
I-1	F	51	106	4	31	48	Normal	—	Normal	Homozygous
I-4	F	44	98	4	43	46	Normal	—	Normal	Hemizygous
I-5	F	39	71	5	28	50	Mild hypokinesia	I	Normal	Homozygous
I-8	M	27	112	3	41	45	Normal	—	Normal	Hemizygous
II-1	M	36	1368	40	20	66	Severe hypokinesia	II	Abnormal	Homozygous
II-2	M	30	1826	60	15	60	Severe hypokinesia	II	Abnormal	Homozygous
II-3	F	28	171	7	33	48	Normal	—	Normal	Homozygous
II-4	F	26	158	6	35	40	Normal	—	Normal	Homozygous
II-5	M	27	3312	37	18	59	Severe hypokinesia	II	Abnormal	Homozygous
II-6‡	M	23	3362	60	14	88	Severe hypokinesia	IV	Abnormal	Homozygous
II-7	F	18	90	3	43	44	Normal	—	Normal	Hemizygous

*CK denotes creatine kinase (normal level, <250 U per liter); CK-MB creatine kinase, MB isoform; FS fractional shortening; EDD left ventricular end-diastolic diameter; and NYHA New York Heart Association.[15]

†ECG denotes electrocardiographic. A finding of deep Q waves from lead V_4 to lead V_6 was considered abnormal.

‡Proband.

ers of the disorder. Thus, a deletion involving the first muscle exon containing the muscle promoter for the dystrophin gene was found in all affected members of a family with x-linked dilated cardiomyopathy. This mutation apparently involved the cardiac muscle in a specific way. No clinical evidence of skeletal-muscle weakness was found in 4 affected male family members (age 23 to 36 years); 2 more male family members, who died of dilated cardiomyopathy at the ages of 29 and 44, were also believed to be free from neuromuscular symptoms. On the basis of these results these authors proposed that immunohistochemical or Western blot analysis with various antidystrophin antibodies should be performed in families with x-linked cardiomyopathy in order to investigate a possible dystrophinopathy. The dystrophin gene, including the muscle-promoter region, should also be screened for mutations.

Antiheart Antibodies

It is presumed that autoimmune mechanisms may play a role in the pathogenesis of dilated cardiomyopathy. Latif and associates,[6] from Middlesex, United Kingdom, investigated the organ and disease specificity of antiheart antibodies in patients with dilated cardiomyopathy. An SDS-PAGE procedure followed by Western blotting was used to screen serum samples for antiheart antibodies of two immunoglobulin classes, IgM and IgG, from 52 patients with dilated cardiomyopathy and 48 patients with ischemic heart disease as controls. Strong IgG antiheart antibodies against myocardial proteins were detected in significantly more patients with dilated cardiomyopathy (46%) than with ischemic heart disease (17%). Patients with dilated cardiomyopathy showed a significantly greater frequency in reactivity of IgG antiheart antibodies against six myocardial proteins. These were identified as myosin light chain 1, tropomyosin, actin, heat shock protein, an unidentified protein, and myosin heavy chain, respectively. These authors concluded that this increased finding of antiheart antibodies in dilated cardiomyopathy supports the hypothesis of an immune involvement in dilated cardiomyopathy.

Metoprolol Therapy

Ishida and associates,[7] from Beppu, Japan, investigated the effect of the β-selective blocker, metoprolol, on the B-adrenergic receptor density of circulating lymphocytes in patients with dilated cardiomyopathy. Nine men in New York Heart Association functional classes II (6 patients) and III were given metoprolol for 6 months (mean dose, 46 ± 18 mg). Their cardiac function was assessed by echocardiography. Although there was no difference in the heart rate or pressure rate products, the end-systolic and end-diastolic dimensions significantly decreased in 6 patients after metoprolol treatment. The EF, fractional shortening, and mean LV circumferential shortening were significantly increased after the treatment. β-adrenoceptor densities of lymphocytes, examined by iodine 125-labeled iodocyanopindolol, were reduced in patients at entry but recovered to normal levels after the metoprolol treatment. The relation between β-adrenoceptor densities in lymphocytes and echocardiographic parameters showed a positive correlation with the plasma norepinephrine concentration. This study thus provides evidence that long-term metoprolol therapy for dilated cardiomyopathy is associated with β-receptor up-regulation, and the restoration of myocardial β-receptor density may be associated with the improved cardiac function as determined by echocardiography.

Several small studies have suggested beneficial effects of long-term β-blocker treatment in idiopathic dilated cardiomyopathy. Waagstein and associates, for the Metoprolol in Dilated Cardiomyopathy Trial Study Group,[8] randomly assigned 383 patients with CHF from idiopathic dilated cardiomyopathy (EF <0.40%) to either placebo or metoprolol. Of the 383 patients, 94% were in New York Heart Association functional classes II and III, and 80% were receiving other medications for CHF. A test dose of metoprolol (5 mg twice daily) was given for 2 to 7 days; those tolerating this dose (96%) entered randomization. Study medication was increased slowly from 10 mg to 100-150 mg daily. There were 34% fewer primary endpoints in the metoprolol than the placebo group; 2 and 19 patients, respectively, deteriorated to the point of needing transplantation; and 23 and 19 died. The change in EF from baseline to 12 months was significantly greater with metoprolol than with placebo (0.13 v 0.06). PA wedge pressure decreased more from baseline to 12 months with metoprolol than with placebo (5 v 2 mm Hg). Exercise time at 12 months was significantly greater in metoprolol-treated than in placebo-treated patients. Thus, in patients with idiopathic dilated cardiomyopathy, treatment with metoprolol prevented clinical deterioration, improved symptoms and cardiac function, and was well tolerated (Figure 7-4).

Nebivolol Therapy

Several β-blocking drugs have been reported to have a beneficial hemodynamic effect in patients with dilated cardiomyopathy. Few of these studies, however, have been placebo-controlled, randomized trials.

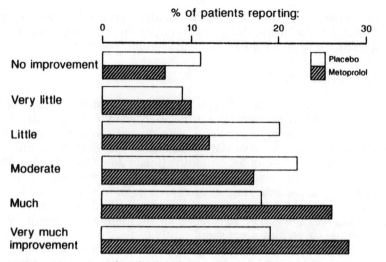

Figure 7-4. Assessment of quality of life in patients treated with placebo (n = 54) or metoprolol (n = 57) at 12 or 18 month follow-up. Reproduced with permission from Waagstein et al.[8]

Nebivolol is a new β-adrenergic blocking agent that also has peripheral vasodilating activity. Wisenbaugh and associates,[9] from Johannesburg, South Africa, studied 24 patients with idiopathic dilated (n = 22) or ischemic (n = 2) cardiomyopathy (EF 0.15 to 0.40) who were in stable New York Heart Association functional class II or III. In this double-blind, randomized trial of nebivolol, exercise time, invasive hemodynamic data, and ventricular function were examined at baseline and after 3 months of oral nebivolol (1 to 5 mg/day) (n = 11) or placebo (n = 13). The β-blocker decreased heart rate from 85 to 71 and increased stroke volume from 43 to 55. The decreases in systemic vascular resistance, systemic BP, wedge pressure, and PA pressure were not significantly different from placebo. EF increased from .23 to .33 in the nebivolol treated group and from .21 to .23 with placebo. Thus, nebivolol improved stroke volume, EF, and left ventricular end-diastolic pressure, not by reducing afterload or by a beneficial relaxing effect, but by improving systolic contractile performance. It is possible that this improved myocardial performance may be due to improved myocardial energetics, reduction of the toxic effects of high catecholamine levels on the myocardium, and/or increased β-receptor density. The vasodilating effects of the drug may help improve tolerability of the agent while the primary effects of improving contractility are occurring.

Endomyocardial Biopsy

The benefits of long-term β-blocker therapy in dilated cardiomyopathy remain uncertain. Yamada and associates,[10] from Osaka, Japan, evaluated several criteria in patients with dilated cardiomyopathy including histologic evaluation of endomyocardial biopsies in a retrospective study.

Eighteen patients showed improvement of at least one New York Heart Association class or an increase in EF of greater than .10, one year after drug administration. Twelve patients showed no such improvement. There were no significant differences between the two groups in age, gender, functional class, heart rate, BP, PA wedge pressure, cardiac index, LV end-diastolic dimension, and EF. However, on histologic examination of endomyocardial biopsies, percent fibrosis was significantly lower in the patients who responded (7.6%) than in those who did not respond (14.2%). When the type of fibrosis was classified as interfascicular and intercellular, there were 13 cases of interfascicular fibrosis in the good responders and 11 cases of intercellular fibrosis in the poor responders. These results suggest that patients with dilated cardiomyopathy are more likely to respond to β-blocker therapy if they have less myocardial fibrosis, with interfascicular fibrosis being the dominant type. A potential limitation of this study is the variability of fibrosis in different samples and the point counting method used to measure the percent fibrosis. It would be important to conduct a prospective trial before concluding that this is an important piece of information that should determine whether or not patients receive β-blocker therapy.

HYPERTROPHIC CARDIOMYOPATHY

Prognosis in a Clinic Population

Overall annual cardiac mortality in HC has been reported to be between 2% and 4%, although these numbers are primarily from retrospective studies of patients referred to large research institutions. Kofflard and associates,[11] from Rotterdam, The Netherlands, prospectively studied a clinic population of 113 patients with HC to assess cardiac mortality in the overall group and in selected subgroups commonly thought to be at high risk for sudden death. The mean age at diagnosis was 37 years. During follow-up, there were 11 cardiac and 2 noncardiac deaths. The annual cardiac mortality was 1%. Because of the small number of deaths, relative risk for cardiac death was not significantly different in the presence of young age (≤30 years), family history of HC and sudden death, history of syncope or previous cardiac arrest, or both, VT on 24-hour Holter monitoring, or septal myotomy/myectomy for refractory symptoms and outflow tract obstruction. These investigators concluded that HC has a relatively benign prognosis (1% annual cardiac mortality) that is two to four times less than that previously reported.

Obstruction to Right Ventricular Outflow

The mechanism by which obstruction to RV outflow occurs in patients with HC is not well understood. To clarify this issue, Maron and associates,[12] from Bethesda, Md, studied five severely symptomatic patients, aged 18 to 55 years (mean age, 30), with HC and marked subpulmonic obstruction (basal peak systolic pressure gradient 60 to 118 mm Hg). Four patients also had obstruction to LV outflow (maximal basal or provocable pressure gradient 12 to 110 mm Hg). The RV outflow obstruction in each patient resulted from greatly hypertrophied musculature comprised of crista supraventricularis, moderator band, or trabeculae. Operative resection of portions of this muscle resulted in abolition or substantial reduction of the RV outflow gradient (to 0–11 mm Hg) in the three patients with both preoperative and postoperative hemodynamic studies. The LV wall and ventricular septum also were massively thickened (32 to 40 mm) in each patient. These findings support the view that marked RV outflow tract obstruction in patients with HC is due to greatly hypertrophied RV muscle and that operative resection will relieve the outflow gradients and normalize RV systolic pressure. The muscular RV hypertrophy causing obstruction appeared to constitute a primary and excessive hypertrophic process involving both ventricles.

Comparison of Mitral Valve Dimensions to Aortic Valve Stenosis and Aortic Regurgitation

To assess the effect of LV dilatation on MV size, Mautner and associates,[13] from Bethesda, Md, compared the dimensions of the mitral valve in patients with aortic valve disease and HC. A total of 216 valves, removed at operation or necropsy, were analyzed by quantitative morphometric methods from (1) two patient groups with dilated LV cavities (17 patients with dilated valvular AS and 31 with pure AR), (2) two patient groups without dilated LV cavities (29 patients with nondilated AS and 9 with HC), and (3) 45 control subjects without heart disease (Table 7-2). Mean mitral leaflet areas in patients with AS with dilated LV cavities and AR were significantly greater than in control subjects (Figure 7-5). Mean mitral leaflet areas in patients with AS without dilated LV cavities were similar to those of normal valves. However, mean mitral leaflet area in patients with HC, in whom LV cavities were also nondilated, was significantly greater than in those with nondilated AS and in normal subjects. Therefore, increased mitral leaflet area (1) is often present in patients with aortic valve disease with dilated LV in whom it appears to be secondary to LV chamber dilatation; and (2) cannot be attributed to LV cavity dilatation in patients with HC, because their cavities were of normal or small size. Thus, increased mitral leaflet area in HC, which is considered to be a primary myocardial and not valvular disease, may be due to a primary effect on the mitral valve.

Table 7-2. Clinical, Hemodynamic, and Morphometric Data in Patients with Aortic Stances, Aortic Regurgitation and Hypertrophic Cardiomyopathy, and in Normal Control Subjects. Reproduced with permission from Mautner et al.[13]

	Control Subjects	Aortic Stenosis Without Dilatation	Aortic Stenosis With Dilatation	Aortic Regurgitation	Hypertrophic Cardiomyopathy
No. of patients	45	29	17	31	94
Age (years)	45 ± 17	55 ± 9*	52 ± 9	48 ± 16	43 ± 15
Men:women	24:21	17:12	16:1*†	28:3*†	49:45
LV-SA psg (mm Hg)	0	90 ± 34*	87 ± 33*	0	56 ± 47*†
Heart weight (g)	271 ± 47	530 ± 113*	760 ± 152*†	745 ± 185*†	597 ± 164*
Mitral valve measurements					
Areas (cm²)					
Anterior leaflet	4.3 ± 1.0	5.1 ± 1.3	7.3 ± 1.4*†	6.7 ± 2.7*†	5.9 ± 1.7*
Posterior leaflet	1.7 ± 0.5	2.1 ± 0.7	1.9 ± 0.3	1.9 ± 0.4	2.6 ± 1.1*
Total leaflets	8.7 ± 2.0	9.8 ± 2.0	13.1 ± 3.0*†	12.0 ± 3.6*†	12.8 ± 3.7*†
Circumference (cm)	8.2 ± 0.8	8.3 ± 1.1	9.7 ± 1.5*†	10.0 ± 1.4*†	8.5 ± 1.7‡
Lengths (cm)					
Anterior leaflet	1.8 ± 0.3	1.9 ± 0.3	2.3 ± 0.4*†	2.4 ± 0.6*†	2.2 ± 0.5*†
Posterior leaflet	1.1 ± 0.2	1.2 ± 0.2	1.3 ± 0.3	1.4 ± 0.4*†	1.4 ± 0.4†
Weight (g)	1.0 ± 0.3	1.5 ± 0.5*	2.1 ± 0.9*†	2.0 ± 0.9*†	2.0 ± 0.5*†

*Significantly greater compared with normal control subjects (p <0.001); †significantly greater than in patients with aortic stenosis without left ventricular dilatation (p <0.001); ‡significantly smaller than in patients with aortic stenosis with dilatation, and aortic regurgitation (p <0.001).
LV = left ventricular; psg = peak systolic gradient; SA = systemic arterial.

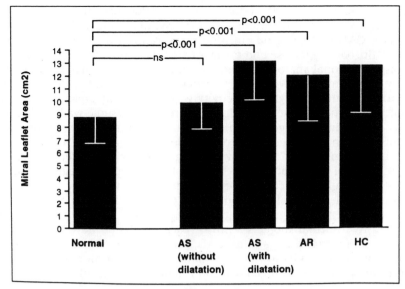

Figure 7-5. Total mitral leaflet area in five subgroups of patients: normal controls, aortic stenosis (AS) without left ventricular dilatations, AS with left ventricular dilatation, aortic regurgitation (AR), and hypertrophic cardiomyopathy (HC). In addition to the statistical comparisons shown, total mitral leaflet area was significantly smaller in AS without left ventricular dilatation than in AS with left ventricular dilatation, AR, and HC. Reproduced with permission from Mautner et al.[13]

Systolic Function, Myocardial Blood Flow, and Glucose Uptake

Nienaber and associates,[14] from Hamburg, Germany, used positron emission tomography to study 13 symptomatic patients with HC-making myocardial blood flow and glucose utilization measurements with intravenous N-13 ammonia and F-18 deoxyglucose at rest and, in 4 patients, again during supine bicycle exercise. At rest, blood flow was significantly lower in hypertrophied than in normal myocardium, whereas rates of glucose utilization were similar. With exercise, blood flow and glucose utilization failed to increase in hypertrophic and normal segments but became more heterogeneous throughout the LV myocardium. Blood flow-metabolism mismatches indicative of myocardial ischemia were noted in three patients at rest and in three of the four patients during exercise and were due to reduced flow in the presence of maintained glucose uptake. The discordance between flow and glucose metabolism in hypertrophied myocardium was more prominent in younger than older individuals. Thus, the normal or elevated rates of glucose utilization and diminished blood flow in hypertrophied myocardium in patients with HC suggest the presence of myocardial ischemia in some patients with symptomatic HC.

Decreased ^{18}flurodeoxyglucose uptake and blood flow at rest in the ventricular septum, as compared with the lateral wall, have been reported in mildly symptomatic patients with HC. To assess whether regional metabolic heterogeneity in patients with HC is related to heterogeneous regional systolic function, Perrone-Filardi and associates,[15] from Bethesda, Md, studied ten symptomatic patients with HC and no CAD with positron emission tomography with oxygen-15-water and [18]flurodeoxyglucose and nuclear magnetic resonance imaging at rest to assess regional anatomy and systolic function. Regional absolute blood flow was similar between the ventricular septum and lateral wall. In contrast, [18]flurodeoxyglucose activity was significantly greater in the lateral wall than in the septum. However, regional systolic wall thickening was also significantly greater in the lateral wall than in the septum. Patients were then divided into group A with similar regional wall thickening in the septum and lateral wall and group B with greater thickening in the lateral wall than in the septum. In both groups, regional blood flow was similar between the septum and lateral wall. However, the regional septal-to-lateral [18]flurodeoxyglucose activity ratio was 0.97 in group A and 0.74 in group B; the ratio in group A did not differ from that in five normal subjects. Thus, myocardial blood flow is normal at rest in patients with HC and no CAD; the heterogeneity in regional glucose uptake is parallel to that of regional systolic function and does not necessarily represent a metabolic abnormality at the cellular level.

Coronary Flow Velocity

Tomochika and associates,[16] from Ube, Japan, assessed the flow velocity profiles of the LAD in seven patients with nonobstructive HC and in six normal subjects by transesophageal pulsed Doppler echocardiography and evaluated their characteristics and the hemodynamic determinants. Systolic peak flow velocity of the LAD was significantly lower in patients with HC than in normal subjects, and there was a significant inverse correlation between systolic peak flow velocity and the thickness of the ventricular septum. In two cases of HC with ventricular septal thickness of >20 mm, a remarkable systolic reverse flow was observed in the LAD. However, there was no significant difference in diastolic peak flow velocity between HC and normal subjects. During early diastole, the acceleration time of LAD flow velocity was significantly prolonged and the acceleration rate was significantly decreased in patients with HC. The time constant of the LV pressure decay was significantly prolonged in patients with HC compared with normal subjects. In HC, increased intramural perivascular pressure of the thickened ventricular septum during systole may be attributed to systolic LAD flow pattern. However, the early and mid-diastolic LAD flow pattern may be affected by impaired LV relaxation.

Genetics

Yu and associates,[17] from Houston, Tex, and Denver, Colo, evaluated β-myosin heavy chain gene alterations in patients with familial obstructive HC. Their aim in this study was to demonstrate whether a common mutation for β-myosin heavy chain is expressed in patients with HC, expressed in both cardiac muscle messenger RNA and skeletal muscle RNA (mRNA). Biopsies were obtained of skeletal muscle from a proband with HC known to have the missense mutation in exon 13 of the β-myosin heavy chain gene. RNA was extracted from skeletal muscle and lymphocytes. Polymerase chain reaction was performed to amplify the segment encompassing exon 13. In this proband, skeletal muscle and lymphocytes showed four DNA fragments resulting from mutations in exon 13. These data indicate that the mutation in the cardiac muscle in affected individuals is also expressed in the mRNA of skeletal muscle and lymphocytes. Whether the β-myosin heavy chain mutation expressed in skeletal muscle has a physiologic consequence is not yet clear. However, these data indicate that skeletal muscle may be used as a readily accessible source of mRNA for expression studies and purification of the β-myosin heavy chain protein.

Marian and associates,[18] from Houston, Tex, determined the distribution frequency of angiotensin converting enzyme polymorphism in 100 patients with HC and 106 of their unaffected siblings and offspring. The distribution of angiotensin converting enzyme genotypes was different in the two groups: allele D frequency of 0.69 in patients and 0.57 in relatives. The frequency of allele D was also higher in HC families with a high incidence of sudden cardiac death than those with a low incidence (0.74 v 0.55). In 25 HC patients with a strong family history of sudden cardiac death, the frequency of allele D was 0.82.

In Nonhuman Animals

Liu and associates,[19] from New York, NY, and Bethesda, Md, compared morphologic features of spontaneously occurring HC in 38 humans, 51 cats, and 10 dogs. Asymmetric hypertrophy of the ventricular septum, marked disorganization of cardiac muscle cells, abnormal intramural coronary arteries, and myocardial fibrosis were each present in the ventricular septum of human, feline, and canine forms of HC; these abnormalities were generally more severe and most frequently identified in humans. Asymmetric LV hypertrophy (based on the calculated septal-to-free wall thickness ratio) was most frequently identified in humans (31 of 38 [81%]) and dogs (8 of 10 [80%]), as compared with cats (16 of 51 [31%]) with HC; in all three species, hypertrophy was often diffuse, involving substantial portions of the anterolateral and posterior free walls, and the ventricular septum. Marked septal disorganization (≥5% of the tissue section) was present in 35 patients (92%) but in only 14 cats (27%) and 2 dogs (20%). Abnormal intramural coronary arteries occurred with similar frequency in the ventricular septum of patients, cats, and dogs. Moderate-to-severe septal fibrosis was identified more commonly in humans (15 of 38 [39%]) than in animals (13 of 61 [21%]). In all three species, abnormal intramural coronary arteries were most commonly observed within or at the margins of areas of fibrous tissue. These morphologic findings describe spontaneously occurring models of HC in cats and dogs with substantial structural similarities to the well-recognized disease entity in humans.

Disopyramide

In an investigation carried out by Kimball and associates,[20] from Toronto, Canada, to evaluate the acute hemodynamic effects of intravenous disopyramide in obstructive HC, 25 patients (12 men, 13 women) with an average age of 40 years (range, 18 to 70 years) were evaluated while undergoing cardiac catheterization-angiography. Biplane LV angiography was performed with standard intracardiac-systemic hemodynamics, including resting and provoked (after VPC) outflow tract gradients, by using simultaneous LV and aortic pressures as disopyramide was being administered (total dose 100 mg; bolus 10 mg every 3 minutes). Average baseline thermodilution cardiac output equalled 4.5 ± 1.2 L/min, with all 25 patients demonstrating systolic anterior motion of the mitral apparatus (mild, 3; moderate, 8; severe, 14). Although heart rate originally slowed during disopyramide administration, average heart rate increased during the final stages (before 78 ± 15 v after 82 ± 13 beats/min). Systemic aortic pressures increased during intravenous disopyramide (before 107 ± 21/71 ± 19 mm Hg v after 120 ± 28/81 ± 13 mm Hg), with a decline in LV end-diastolic pressure (before 19 ± 7 v after 16 ± 6 mm Hg). Maximum LV systolic pressures decreased (before 193 ± 32 v after 146 ± 29 mm Hg), with a substantial reduction in resting LV outflow tract gradients (before 86 ± 34 v after 27 ± 20 mm Hg) in conjunction with less inducible obstruction (before 124 ± 33 v after 64 ± 33 mm Hg). Only minor electrocardiographic changes were seen during disopyramide infusion. Therefore, intravenous disopyramide favorably alters acute hemodynamics in obstructive HC; there were substantial reductions in both resting and provoked (after VPC) LV outflow tract obstruction with minimal electrocardiographic changes.

Nadolol and Verapamil

Both β-blockers and calcium antagonists have been used to treat patients with HC. Gilligan and associates,[21] from London, United Kingdom, evaluated verapamil and nadolol versus placebo for periods of 4 weeks each in 18 patients with mild or moderately symptomatic HC in a double-blind crossover trial. Two patients withdrew from the trial due to symptomatic sinus bradycardia during nadolol therapy. Neither drug improved maximal oxygen consumption. Peak exercise workload was reduced in 81% of patients during nadolol therapy and 25% during verapamil therapy. Despite these apparent adverse effects on exercise capacity, 81% of patients preferred drug treatment (8 verapamil, 5 nadolol) over placebo. Verapamil improved reported performance at work compared with nadolol and tended to improve other measures of health related behavior and symptoms compared with nadolol and placebo. These authors concluded that in patients with mild or moderate symptomatic HC, exercise capacity was not improved by nadolol or verapamil, and individuals were more often impaired by nadolol than with verapamil. Nevertheless, many patients derived symptomatic benefit from drug therapy, especially with verapamil. No controlled trial of therapy has yet been carried out relative to the prognosis of patients with HC.

Transaortic Myectomy

Schulte and associates,[22] from Düsseldorf and Dortmund, Germany, reported results in 364 patients with HC operated on in 1963 to 1991 (217 male, 146 female; aged 5 months to 76 years [mean, 40 years]). Transaortic subvalvular myectomy was performed in 272 patients (hospital mortality, 2.9%), and 92 patients needed additional cardiac procedures simultaneously (hospital mortality, 10.9%). A complete follow-up study (100%) included 346 patients who survived the operation. The shortest follow-up time was 2 months and the longest 25.2 years (mean,

8.2 years). Most of the patients improved clinically by 1 to 3 classes (New York Heart Association). During the observation period, 38 patients (10.4%) died. The death of 17 patients was closely related to the original disease (4.9%). Other causes, unrelated to obstructive HC, were responsible for the death of 21 patients (5.8%). In consideration of these data, the yearly total death rate was 2.2%; in close relation to HC, it was about 0.6%. The cumulative survivals were 88% after 10 years and 72% after 20 years. In our long-term clinical experience, it is increasingly evident, despite the restrictions of a retrospective study, that patients with symptomatic HC and failing medical therapy benefit from transthoracic subvalvular myectomy.

Cardiac Transplantation

Shirani and associates,[23] from Bethesda, Md, reviewed clinical records, electrocardiographic, echocardiographic, hemodynamic, and radionuclide data, and the operatively excised hearts in 10 patients, aged 19 to 46 years (mean, 35), who had cardiac transplantation for HC. Severe CHF unassociated with outflow obstruction was the indication for transplantation in 9 patients. During a pretransplantation period ranging from 45 to 312 months (mean, 137) in these 9 patients, PA wedge pressure increased from 19 ± 9 to 27 ± 7 mm Hg, LVEF decreased from $51 \pm 11\%$ to $41 \pm 1\%$, LV end-diastolic dimension increased from 42 ± 6 to 48 ± 4 mm, and total 12-lead QRS voltage decreased from 209 ± 50 to 156 ± 41 mm. In these 9 patients, the explanted hearts had dilated LV cavities, and 8 had LV scars without significant narrowing of the epicardial coronary arteries. The tenth patient had a nondilated LV cavity and had transplantation because of recurrent, refractory syncope. Of the 10 patients, 3 died within the first month and another died 8 months after transplantation. The remaining 6 patients have survived 20 to 54 months (mean, 39) after transplantation and are in functional class I or II.

IDIOPATHIC MYOCARDITIS

From January 1985 through December 1990, 534 patients underwent endomyocardial biopsy for suspected myocardities at The Johns Hopkins Hospital. These findings were reviewed by Herskowitz and associates,[24] from Baltimore, Md. One hundred thirty-eight (26%) biopsy specimens were diagnosed histologically by two cardiac pathologists as either active (16%) or borderline (10%) myocarditis. Of the 138 patients, 60 were excluded based on either specific concurrent clinical conditions or noncongestive heart failure presentations. Immunohistochemical staining for common leukocyte antigen infiltrating cells performed on the remaining 78 specimens confirmed the presence of focal or multifocal inflammatory infiltrates in 58, of which 49 had histologic evidence of active myocarditis. All 49 patients presented with CHF and LVEF of <40%. Compared with patients with either idiopathic dilated cardiomyopathy (207) or ischemic cardiomyopathy (44), these patients with myocarditis had a less striking male predominance and were younger. Racial distributions were similar. A recent history of a discrete flu-like illness was obtained in 52%, two thirds of which were clustered between the months of December and

March. Onset of CHF peaked between December and April and was low between May through September. A peak in the proportion of patients found to have active myocarditis on biopsy occurred in 1986. In conclusion, patients presenting clinically with idiopathic dilated cardiomyopathy with histologic evidence of active myocarditis confirmed by immunohistochemical staining accounted for 9% of all patients undergoing endomyocardial biopsy. Both seasonal and yearly variations in the proportion of such patients with biopsy-proven myocarditis appear significant.

ASSOCIATION WITH A CONDITION AFFECTING PRIMARILY A NONCARDIAC STRUCTURE(S)

Human Immunodeficiency Virus

Herskowitz and associates,[25] from Baltimore, Md, examined the prevalence and incidence of LV dysfunction in patients infected with the human immunodeficiency virus. Sixty-nine randomly selected patients diagnosed with immunodeficiency virus infection who were followed in the clinics were prospectively evaluated by two-dimensional echocardiography. Mean follow-up duration was 11 months. Additionally, 39 consecutive immunodeficiency virus infected patients referred to the Cardiomyopathy Service and found to have LV dysfunction by two-dimensional echocardiography were also studied. Of the 39 referred patients, 34 (87%) were referred for recent onset, unexplained, CHF. During this time, the immunodeficiency virus clinic population comprised 1,819 alive and actively followed patients; the 39 cardiomyopathy referrals therefore constituted a crude rate of 2% for this population. Of the 69 prospectively studied patients without clinical heart disease, a 15% prevalence of global LV hypokinesia and an incidence of 18%/patient-year were found. During a maximal 18-month follow-up period, 4 prospective patients (6%) developed symptoms of CHF. A greater proportion of prospective and referred patients with LV dysfunction had CD4 counts <100/mm^3 than did that of those without LV dysfunction. In conclusion, the high rate of unexpected LV dysfunction in this immunodeficiency virus-infected population suggests that early cardiac contractile abnormalities may involve a significant number of patients, most of whom have low CD4 counts. A subgroup of these patients appears to progress to symptomatic CHF.

Duchenne Muscular Dystrophy

X-linked cardiomyopathy is a rapidly progressive primary myocardial disorder presenting in teenage males as CHF. Manifesting female carriers have later onset, often 5th decade, and slower progression in development of CHF. In this study, the x-linked cardiomyopathy gene locus was sought in two families using molecular genetic analyses. Towbin and associates,[26] in Houston, Tex, performed linkage analysis using 60 X-chromosome-specific DNA markers in a previously reported large XLC pedigree and a smaller new pedigree. Two-point and multipoint linkage were calculated using the LINKAGE computer program package. Deletion analysis included multiplex polymerase chain reaction. Dystrophin protein was evaluated by Western blotting with N-terminal and C-terminal dystrophin antibody. Linkage of XLC to the centromeric portion of the dystrophin or Duchenne muscular dystrophy locus at Xp21 was demonstrated with combined maximum logarithm of the scores of +4.33. Abnormalities of cardiac dystrophin were shown by Western blotting with N-terminal dystrophin antibody, whereas skeletal muscle dystrophin was normal, suggesting primary involvement of the Duchenne muscular dystrophy gene with preferential involvement of heart muscle. Therefore, XLC is due to an abnormality within the centromeric half of the dystrophin genomic region in the heart. This abnormality could be due to (1) a point mutation, (2) a cardiac-specific promoter mutation, (3) splicing abnormalities, or (4) deletion mutants.

Acromegaly

Heart muscle disease in acromegaly manifests usually as cardiac hypertrophy. Based on a retrospective analysis, it was suggested that cardiac hypertrophy is slowly reversible after normalization of plasma growth hormone levels. The reversibility of acromegalic heart muscle disease during and after treatment of acromegaly was studied prospectively by Hradec and associates,[27] from Prague, Czech Republic. A cohort of 78 patients was examined echocardiographically in 1981, and 38 survivors of this group were reexamined 10 years later. Patients were classified according to original hormonal activity in 1981 and change in hormonal activity during follow-up into the following four groups: group I, hormonally inactive for entire follow-up (10 patients); group II, hormonally active for entire follow-up (11 patients); group III, initially hormonally inactive with later resurgence (6 patients); and group IV, initially hormonally active with later normalization of growth hormone levels (11 patients). No significant echocardiographic changes occurred during follow-up in group I. LV posterior wall and septal diastolic thickness, and LV mass increased significantly in group II. LV posterior wall thickness, mass, and diastolic volume increased significantly in group III. On the contrary, there were significant decreases in LV mass and both diastolic and systolic LV volumes in group IV. These investigators concluded that both hypertrophy and dilatation of the LV in acromegaly are slowly reversible after successful treatment. On the contrary, continuing or relapsed hyperproduction of growth hormone causes further deterioration of acromegalic heart disease.

Ifosfamide Toxicity

To determine the incidence and characterize the occurrence of cardiac toxicity with high-dose ifosfamide, Quezado and associates,[28] from Bethesda, Md, studied 52 consecutive patients with advanced lymphoma or carcinoma enrolled in phase I trials of high-dose ifosfamide as part of combination chemotherapy with autologous bone marrow transplantation. The patients were given escalating doses (10 to 18 g/m^2) of ifosfamide in combination with carboplatin and etoposide or with lomustine and vinblastine. Nine patients treated with ifosfamide developed CHF (17%). Eight of these patients, experiencing dyspnea, tachycardia, weight gain, and signs of pulmonary edema, required admission to an intensive care unit. LV contractility was found to be depressed when evaluated by radionuclide cineangiography, echocardiography, or both. Most patients responded to diuretic, vasodilator, and inotropic therapies. Two patients developed malignant ventricular arrhythmias. One patient died of intractable cardiogenic shock. Five patients died of multiorgan failure, despite showing improvement in LVEF. Three patients survived and regained baseline LVEF. High-dose ifosfamide is associated with severe but usually reversible myocardial depression and malignant arrhythmias.

MISCELLANEOUS TOPICS

Subepicardial Myocardial Lesions

Subepicardial myocardial lesions are rarely seen at necropsy, and a description of them and their causes has not been reported. During an 11-year period, Shirani and Roberts,[29] from Bethesda, Md, studied 22 patients with subepicardial myocardial lesions at necropsy. They ranged in age from 14 to 73 years (mean, 47), and 20 were men. The lesions were associated with atherosclerotic CAD in 6 patients, sarcoidosis in 5, idiopathic dilated cardiomyopathy in 4, lymphocytic myocarditis in 2, and hypoplastic right and LC coronary arteries in 1. In 4 patients the cause was unclear. In the patients with atherosclerotic CAD, the subepicardial myocardial lesions were small, few in number, and located in the LV posterior wall. In patients with sarcoidosis or myocarditis, the subepicardial lesions were extensive and commonly associated with transmural left and RV lesions. The RV half of the ventricular septum also was frequently affected. In the remaining 9 patients, the subepicardial lesions were small and unassociated with transmural LV lesions. Thus, subepicardial myocardial lesions occur in a variety of cardiac diseases.

Myocardial Contusion

Paone and associates,[30] from El Paso, Tex, sought the frequency of myocardial contusion in 147 patients, studied prospectively with blunt chest trauma resulting from motor vehicle accidents in 132 patients (90%), crush injury in 9 patients (6%), fall in 4 patients, and all-terrain vehicle accidents in 2 patients. Of the 147 patients, 97 were male and 50 were female. They ranged in age from 2 to 97 years (mean, 39). There were 5 deaths, none of cardiac origin. Total lactate dehydrogenase values were elevated in 115 patients (78%); total creatine phosphokinase values were elevated in 100 patients (68%). Cardiac isoenzyme patterns were consistent with myocardial contusion in 18 patients (12%). Seventy-five patients had abnormal electrocardiograms, and 10 of these had ectopic rhythms. Two-dimensional echocardiograms were completed in 58 cases; 12 of these (21%) were abnormal. Nineteen patients (25%) with abnormal rhythms had elevated lactate dehydrogenase values, and 26 (35%) had elevated creatine phosphokinase values. One patient (10%) with ectopy had an abnormal echocardiogram. Two patients (11%) with abnormal isoenzyme patterns experienced dysrhythmias. Costs for hospitalization and studies amounted to $1,886 per patient. Given the poor predictive value of laboratory testing in patients with significant (ie, symptomatic) cardiac contusion, observation alone with electrocardiographic monitoring and treatment of symptomatic dysrhythmias is an adequate and cost-conscious treatment.

References

1. Tauberg SG, Orie JE, Bartlett BE, et al: Usefulness of thallium-201 for distinction of ischemic from idiopathic dilated cardiomyopathy. Am J Cardiol 1993 (March 15);71:674–680.
2. Lewis JF, Webber JD, Sutton LL, et al: Discordance in degree of right and left ventricular dilation in patients with dilated cardiomyopathy: Recognition and clinical implications. J Am Coll Cardiol 1993 (March 1);21:649–654.
3. Werner GS, Schaefer C, Dirks R, et al: Doppler echocardiographic assessment of left ventricular filling in idiopathic dilated cardiomyopathy during a one-year follow-up: Relation to the clinical course of disease. Am Heart J l993 (Dec);126:1408–1416.
4. Mancini DM, Wong KL, Simson MB: Prognostic value of an abnormal signal-averaged electrocardiogram in patients with nonischemic congestive cardiomyopathy. Circulation 1993 (April);87:1083–1092.
5. Muntoni F, Cau M, Ganau A, et al: Deletion of the dystrophin muscle-promoter region associated with x-linked dilated cardiomyopathy. N Eng J Med 1993 (Sep 23);329:921–925.
6. Latif N, Baker CS, Dunn MJ, et al: Frequency and specificity of antiheart antibodies in patients with dilated cardiomyopathy detected using SDS-PAGE and western blotting. J Am Coll Cardiol 1993;(Nov 1);22:1378–1384.
7. Ishida S, Makino N, Masutomo K, et al: Effect of metoprolol on the β-adrenoceptor density of lymphocytes in patients with dilated cardiomyopathy. Am Heart J 1993 (May);125:1311–1315.
8. Waagstein F, Bristow MR, Swedberg K, et al: Effects of metoprolol in idiopathic dilated cardiomyopathy. Lancet 1993 (Dec 11);342:1441–1446.
9. Wisenbaugh T, Katz I, Davis J, et al: Long-term (3-month) effects of a new beta blocker (nebivolol) on cardiac performance in dilated cardiomyopathy. J Am Coll Cardiol 1993 (April);21:1094–1100.
10. Yamada T, Fukunami M, Ohmori M, et al: Which subgroup of patients with dilated cardiomyopathy would benefit from long-term beta-blocker therapy? A histologic viewpoint. J Am Coll Cardiol 1993 (March 1);21:628–633.
11. Kofflard MJ, Waldstein DJ, Vos J, et al: Prognosis in hypertrophic cardiomyopathy observed in a large clinic population. Am J Cardiol 1993 (Oct 15);72:939–943.
12. Maron BJ, McIntosh CL, Klues HG, et al: Morphologic basis for obstruction to right ventricular outflow in hypertrophic cardiomyopathy. Am J Cardiol 1993 (May 1);71:1089–1094.
13. Mautner SL, Klues HG, Mautner GC, et al: Comparison of mitral valve dimensions in adults with valvular aortic stenosis, pure aortic regurgitation and hypertrophic cardiomyopathy. Am J Cardiol 1993 (April 15);71:949–953.
14. Nienaber CA, Gambhir SS, Vaghaiwalla F, et al: Regional myocardial blood flow and glucose utilization in symptomatic patients with hypertrophic cardiomyopathy. Circulation 1993 (May);87:1580–1590.
15. Perrone-Filardi P, Bacharach SL, Dilsizian V, et al: Regional systolic function myocardial blood flow and glucose uptake at rest in hypertrophic cardiomyopathy. Am J Cardiol 1993 (July 15);72:199–204.

16. Tomochika Y, Tanaka N, Wasaki Y, et al: Assessment of flow profile of left anterior descending coronary artery in hypertrophic cardiomyopathy by transesophageal pulsed doppler echocardiography. Am J Cardiol 1993 (Dec 15);72:1425–1430.

17. Yu Q-T, Ifegwu J, Marlan AJ, et al: Hypertrophic cardiomyopathy mutation is expressed in messenger RNA of skeletal as well as cardiac muscle. Circulation 1993 (Feb);87:406–412.

18. Marian AJ, YU Q, Workman R, et al: Angiotensin-converting enzyme polymorphism in hypertrophic cardiomyopathy and sudden cardiac death. Lancet 1993 (Oct 30);342:1085–1086.

19. Liu S-K, Roberts WC, Maron BJ: Comparison of morphologic findings in spontaneously occurring hypertrophic cardiomyopathy in humans, cats and dogs. Am J Cardiol 1993 (Oct 15);72:944–951.

20. Kimball BP, Bui S, Wigle ED: Acute dose-response effects of intravenous disopyramide in hypertrophic obstructive cardiomyopathy. Am Heart J 1993 (June);125:1691–1697.

21. Gilligan DM, Chan WL, Joshi J, et al: A double-blind, placebo-controlled crossover trial of nadolol and verapamil in mild and moderately symptomatic hypertrophic cardiomyopathy. J Am Coll Cardiol 1993 (June);21:1672–1679.

22. Schulte HD, Bircks WH, Loesse B, et al: Late results of transaortic myectomy for hypertrophic cardiomyopathy. J Thorac Cardiovasc Surg 1993 (Oct);106:709–717.

23. Shirani J, Maron BJ, Cannon RO III, et al: Clinicopathologic features of hypertrophic cardiomyopathy managed by cardiac transplantation. Am J Cardiol 1993 (Aug 15);72:434–440.

24. Herskowitz A, Campbell S, Deckers J, et al: Demographic features and prevalence of idiopathic myocarditis in patients undergoing endomyocardial biopsy. Am J Cardiol 1993 (April 15);71:982–986.

25. Herskowitz A, Vlahov D, Willoughby S, et al: Prevalence and incidence of left ventricular dysfunction in patients with Human Immunodeficiency Virus infection. Am J Cardiol 1993 (April 15);71:955–958.

26. Towbin JA, Hejtmancik JF, Brink P, et al: X-linked dilated cardiomyopathy: Molecular genetic evidence of linkage to the Duchenne muscular dystrophy (dystrophin) gene at the Xp21 locus. Circulation 1993 (June);87:1854–1865.

27. Hradec J, Marek J, Kral J, et al: Long-term echocardiographic follow-up of acromegalic heart disease. Am J Cardiol 1993 (July 15);72:205–210.

28. Quezado ZMN, Wilson WH, Cunnion RE, et al: High-dose ifosfamide is associated with severe, reversible cardiac dysfunction. Ann Intern Med 1993 (Jan 1);118:31–36.

29. Shirani J, Roberts WC: Subepicardial myocardial lesions. Am Heart J 1993 (May);125:1346–1352.

30. Paone RF, Peacock JB, Smith DLT: Diagnosis of myocardial contusion secondary to blunt chest trauma. Southern Med J 1993 (Aug);86:867–870.

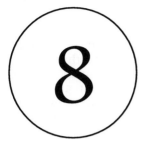

Congenital Heart Disease

Detection by Echocardiography

In an investigation by Wu and associates,[1] from Taipei, Taiwan, to define the prevalence rate of left-to-right interatrial shunt through patent foramen ovale in adults with symptomatic left-sided cardiac lesions, 56 patients were examined with transthoracic and transesophageal echocardiography and cardiac catheterization. By transesophageal echocardiography, 15 patients (group A) were found to have left-to-right interatrial shunt through patent foramen ovale, constituting a prevalence rate of 27%. In group A, transthoracic echocardiography detected the interatrial shunt in 2 patients, and catheterization detected it in only 1. The remaining 41 patients (group B) had no shunt demonstrated by either echocardiographic or catheterization examinations. In another 44 patients (group C) with no significant left-sided cardiac lesions, no interatrial shunt could be found by transesophageal echocardiography even though some of them had a patent foramen ovale. All patients with such shunt had LA size >34 mm (45.1 ± 6.0 mm), LA pressure >13 mm Hg (23 ± 7.6 mm Hg), and pressure gradient between left and right atria >10 mm Hg (19 ± 5.2 mm Hg). These findings support the concept that in the presence of a patent foramen ovale any left-sided cardiac lesion increasing LA size and pressure may induce left-to-right interatrial shunt through this channel and that the prevalence rate is much higher than generally acknowledged.

In an investigation by Konstantinides and associates,[2] from Freiburg, Germany, the occurrence of a RA negative contrast effect as an indicator of left-to-right shunt was studied in 101 patients with ASD by peripheral venous contrast injection during transthoracic and transesophageal echocardiography. Confirmation of the diagnosis was provided by cardiac catheterization or by autopsy in 72 patients (72%). The defect could be visualized directly in 57 patients (57%) during the transthoracic and in 93 patients (93%) during the transesophageal examination. A negative RA echo contrast effect was observed in 53 of 92 patients (58%) from the transthoracic and in 86 of 92 patients (93%) from the transesophageal approach. Among these were 7 patients (7%) with an aneurysmal interatrial septum but no directly visible defect during conventional transesophageal imaging. Appearance of contrast in the left atrium indicating right-to-left shunting was seen in 70 of 92 patients (76%) from the transthoracic and in 91 of 92 patients (99%) from the transesophageal approach. Contrast injection during transesophageal imaging also helped identify additional malformations in 12 patients (12%). Thus, transesophageal echocardiography with echo contrast injection is a very reliable diagnostic method in patients with suspected ASD.

Late Outcome After Operative Closure

Meijboom and associates,[3] from Rotterdam, The Netherlands, assessed the long-term cardiac status after surgical closure of ASD of 104 of 135 children who consecutively underwent surgery at ages 0 to 14 years at one institution between 1968 and 1980. Mean follow-up was 14.5 ± 3 years and most patients (87%) believed their health to be good or very good. Sinus rhythm was present in 89% and echocardiography showed that RV dilatation was present in 27 patients (26%) of whom 2 had a residual ASD. Bicycle ergometry revealed that 88% had a normal exercise capacity. Both supraventricular and ventricular arrhythmias were observed in 67% of patients by 24-hour ambulatory ECG, but only 3% had received antiarrhythmic medication and 4% had needed a pacemaker. In the group of patients with RV dilatation, the exercise capacity and prevalence of arrhythmias did not differ from those with a normal sized right ventricle. In addition, there was no difference in outcome between secundum ASD versus sinus venosus ASD. These authors indicated good long-term functional cardiac status after surgical closure of an ASD with persisting RV dilatation in a significant number of patients that did not appear to be related to whether or not surgery was undertaken before or after 3 years of age.

Follow-Up After Closure by Double Umbrella Device

Boutin and associates,[4] from Toronto, Canada, evaluated the medium-term results of ASD device occlusion and factors influencing residual shunting. Transesophageal echocardiograms in 49 patients immediately following surgical closure revealed residual shunting in 2% compared with 91% after device occlusion. This proportion decreased to 53% after a mean follow-up of 10 months in patients with device occlusion, and actuarial analysis indicates a progressive resolution of shunting with time. Residual shunting was not influenced by dimension, location, or position with relation to the device as assessed by transesophageal echocardiography, location of the defect, or device size relative to the stretched dimension of the defect. In 15 patients, a poor correlation between transesophageal and transthoracic echocardiographic findings was observed. Variability in serial transthoracic echocardiographic findings was observed in 14 patients. RV dimension, heart size, and the presence of a murmur at follow-up did not correlate with the presence or size of residual shunting after device occlusion. These authors showed residual shunting in a significant number of patients after ASD closure. They did indicate that heart size returned to normal on the x-ray, although echocardiographic dimensions of the right ventricle did not change significantly in this rather short follow-up. Further data on RV size and function, as well as overall heart size, would have been of interest. Although the device appears to have been hemodynamically successful, residual shunting remains a problem and hopefully can be minimized in future studies to make this procedure comparable to surgery in terms of complete closure in those defects amenable to interventional treatment.

ATRIOVENTRICULAR SEPTAL DEFECT

Repair in Infancy

Hanley and associates,[5] from Boston, Mass, reviewed data from 301 patients with complete atrioventricular canal defect presenting in infancy between January 1972 and January 1992. A retrospective analysis examined 46 patient-related, morphologic, procedure-related, and postoperative variables for association with perioperative death and re-operation. Operative mortality decreased significantly over the period of the study from 25% before 1976 to 3% after 1987. A number of the 46 variables examined showed trends over time that were similar to that for mortality. Palliative procedures decreased and re-operation for most residual lesions also decreased. The exception to this was re-operation for postoperative left AV regurgitation, which also decreased but remained at 7% in recent years. Both technical and support-related procedural variables showed no trends over time with the exception of the performance of left AV annuloplasty, which increased. Closure of the left-sided cleft was performed in 61% of patients with no trend over time. Annuloplasty and cleft closure were not associated with less postoperative left AV regurgitation, fewer re-operations, or lower mortality. Multivariate logistic regression analysis identified only earlier year of operation, the presence of double-orifice left AV, and postoperative residual regurgitation of the left AV as risk factors for death. These authors presented a great deal of data regarding repair of this defect. They did not shed any light on when to perform two ventricular repairs and when to resort to a single ventricle type of approach for patients with minor degrees of RV dominance and LV hypoplasia.

VENTRICULAR SEPTAL DEFECT

Taussig-Bing Anomaly

Kawashima and associates,[6] from Osaka, Japan, reviewed 41 patients with Taussig-Bing anomaly who underwent intracardiac repair with 10 patients treated by intraventricular rerouting. The ages at operation ranged from 1 month to 8 years with an average of 2-1/4 years. Primary repair was done in 4 at an average age of 2-1/2 years, and repair was done after PA banding in 6 at an average age of 2 years. The relationship of the great arteries was side-by-side in 9 patients and oblique in 1. After extensive resection of the infundibular septum, a distance of 8 to 18 mm from tricuspid ring or chordae to the pulmonary valve was obtained, which was equal to 24% to 71% of the total circumference for the subaortic route. The subaortic route was created to obtain an internal diameter of at least equal to that of the aortic root. Tricuspid chordal or papillary muscle reattachment was performed in 2 patients, and there were no early or late deaths. Follow-up ranged from 1 to 22 years, with an average of 5-1/2 years, and re-operation was required in 1 patient for residual pulmonary stenosis. The intraoperative pressure gradient between the left ventricle and aorta was 0 to 24 mm Hg with an average of 10 mm Hg, and postoperative study showed the gradients to be <19 mm Hg in 8. The age at operation, LV-aortic pressure gradient, and postoperative TR were not significantly affected by the presence of severe hypertrophy of the infundibular septum. These results indicate that intraventricular rerouting may be feasible in most patients who have a Taussig-Bing anomaly, and age and conal anatomic variations do not appear to be significant limiting factors.

Lui and associates,[7] from Ontario, Canada, reported use of the Damus-Kaye-Stansel procedure in 9 children with double outlet right ventricle (DORV) and 38 with univentricular heart plus subaortic stenosis. There were 38 survivors (81%) and 3 late deaths during a mean follow-up of 3 years with a 5-year survival of 72%. All 6 children surviving a Damus-Kaye-Stansel and biventricular repair of DORV have required conduit replacement at a mean interval of 46 months. In the children with univentricular heart, relief of subaortic stenosis was successful in all except 2. The late function of the semilunar valves is of concern, as 36% of the aortic and 52% of the pulmonary valves have some degree of incompetence. This operation is useful for a number of children who develop subaortic stenosis or as an adjunct to the repair of those with DORV with a Taussig-Bing anomaly. More data on long-term survival and semilunar valve function are needed in this group of patients.

PULMONIC VALVE STENOSIS

Natural History

Hayes and associates,[8] from New York, NY, and the Natural History Study Group, reviewed follow-up data from 580 of 592 patients with PS who were alive at the completion of Natural History Study #1. New data were obtained in 464 (78.4%) of the original cohort. Probability of 25-year survival was 96% with survival less (80%) in a subgroup of patients entering the Natural History Study at age >12 years with cardiomegaly. Valvotomy was required in <20% of patients managed medically during Natural History Study #1, and only 4% of operated patients required a second operation. Bacterial endocarditis was extremely rare, and 95% were asymptomatic. There was a small but higher-than-normal prevalence of serious arrhythmias. Most patients, whether managed medically or surgically, had low Doppler maximum gradients, and final clinical status was excellent or good in 83%. Probability of survival is similar to that of the general population, and the vast majority of patients are asymptomatic. If valvotomy or valvuloplasty is required in a child, re-operation is rarely necessary. Patients with gradients <25 mm Hg do not experience an increase in gradient, and patients with a gradient ≥50 mm Hg should have valvotomy or valvuloplasty. There continues to be a choice of management for patients with gradients of 40 to 49 mm Hg with no consensus for optimal care. Patients with PS generally do well if they do not have critical stenosis as newborns and if severe stenosis is relieved relatively early in life. Valvuloplasty has proven to be a very satisfactory form of treatment for nearly all patients who do not have dysplastic valves.

Valvuloplasty

In this report by Kaul and associates[9] from New Delhi, India, percutaneous balloon pulmonary valvuloplasty for congenital pulmonary valve stenosis was performed in 40 adult patients (aged 18 to 56 years). The duration of follow-up was 25 ± 12 months. The peak systolic pressure gradient from the right ventricle to the PA decreased from 107 ± 29 to 37 ± 25 mm Hg immediately after the procedure. On follow-up, the gradient obtained either by cardiac catheterization or Doppler echocardiography was 31 ± 13 mm Hg. In 8 patients with residual gradient after valvuloplasty of 50 mm Hg, the mean peak systolic gradient decreased from 75 ± 18 to 34 ± 14 mm Hg on follow-up. Thus, balloon pulmonary valvuloplasty is a safe and effective procedure for the treatment of adult patients with pulmonic stenosis; there is a tendency for high residual gradients to regress on follow-up.

TETRALOGY OF FALLOT

Long-Term Outcome After "Repair"

Although corrective surgery for TF has been available for more than 30 years, the occurrence of late sudden death in patients in whom surgery was apparently successful remains worrisome. Murphy and associates,[10] from Rochester, Minn, studied long-term survival among 163 patients who survived 30 days after complete repair of TF, by examining follow-up hospital records and death certificates when relevant (Table 8-1). The overall 32-year actuarial survival rate among all patients who survived surgery was 86%, as compared with an expected rate of 96% in a control

Table 8-1. Surgical Variables in 163 Patients Undergoing Complete Repair of Tetralogy of Fallot. Reproduced with permission from Murphy et al.[10]

VARIABLE	NO. OF PATIENTS (%)
Previous palliative shunt procedure, with closure at the time of complete repair*	
No previous shunt	125 (77)
Blalock–Taussig shunt	27 (17)
Waterston or Potts shunt†	11 (7)
Pulmonary-outflow patch	
No patch	84 (52)
Patch through annulus‡	62 (38)
Patch up to annulus	17 (10)
Site of pulmonary stenosis	
Infundibulum	73 (45)
Pulmonary valve and infundibulum	90 (55)

*The mean (±SD) age at the time of palliative surgery was 6±5 years (Blalock–Taussig shunt, 6±5 years; Waterston or Potts shunt, 7±2 years). The mean interval from palliative surgery to complete surgical repair was 7±3 years (Blalock–Taussig shunt, 8±3 years; Waterston or Potts shunt, 7±3 years). Because of rounding, percentages do not total 100.

†The Waterston shunt involves anastomosis of the ascending aorta to the right pulmonary artery, and the Potts shunt anastomosis of the descending aorta to the left pulmonary artery.

‡Fifteen patients (56 percent) with a Blalock–Taussig shunt had a patch through the pulmonary annulus at the time of definitive repair. Three patients (27 percent) with a Waterston or Potts shunt had a patch through the pulmonary annulus, of whom two died within two years after surgery.

population matched for age and sex (Figure 8-1). Thirty-year actuarial survival rates were calculated for the patient subgroups. The survival rates among patients <5 years old, 5 to 7 years old, and 8 to 11 years old were 90%, 93%, and 91%, respectively—slightly less than the expected rates. Among patients 12 years old or older at the time of surgery, the

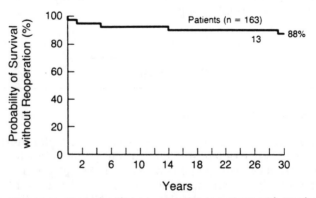

Figure 8-1. Long-term survival without re-operation in patients with tetralogy of Fallot who underwent complete repair. The value under the curve is the number of surviving patients who have completed the period of actuarial follow-up at this writing and have not undergone re-operation. Reproduced with permission from Murphy et al.[10]

survival rate was 76%, as compared with an expected rate of 93%. The performance of a palliative Blalock-Taussig shunt procedure before repair, unlike the performance of Waterston or Potts shunt procedures, was not associated with reduced long-term survival, nor was the need for a transannular patch at the time of surgery. Independent predictors of long-term survival were older age at operation and a higher ratio of RV to LV systolic pressure after surgery. Late sudden death from cardiac causes occurred in 10 patients during the 32-year period. Among patients with surgically repaired TF, the rate of long-term survival after the postoperative period is excellent but remains lower than that in the general population. The risk of late sudden death is small. This article was followed from an editorial by Amnon Rosenthal,[11] from Ann Arbor, Mich, entitled "Adults with tetralogy of Fallot—repaired, yes; cured, no."

Late Pulmonic Regurgitation

Rebergen and associates,[12] from Leiden, The Netherlands, studied forward and regurgitant flow using magnetic resonance velocity mapping in 18 patients aged 17 ± 7 years at a mean time of 13 ± 5 years after repair of TF. Pulmonary regurgitation volumes were compared with the differences between the corresponding RV and LV stroke volumes with volumes measured with a multisection gradient magnetic resonance method. Measurement of pulmonary regurgitant volume with magnetic resonance velocity mapping closely corresponded with the tomographically determined volumes. Forward pulmonary volume was nearly identical to RV volume, and pulmonary regurgitant volume was significantly correlated with end-diastolic volume, end-systolic volume, and stroke volume but not with RV ejection fraction. This method may prove useful for assessment of RV performance in patients with significant pulmonary regurgitation following surgical reparative operations. The question of when to intervene in such patients continues to be a difficult one for all physicians who deal with these patients.

Restoration of Pulmonic Valve After Earlier "Repair"

Warner and associates,[13] from Boston, Mass, studied 16 patients with symptoms of diminished exercise tolerance and echocardiographic evidence of progressive pulmonary regurgitation with severe RV dilatation who underwent placement of allografts in the RV outflow tract at a median age of 12 years (10 years after TF repair). Abnormal exercise tolerance tests were documented in 10 patients. Additional surgical procedures included PA augmentation in 6, closure of residual left-to-right shunt in 3, and subendocardial resection for monomorphic VT in 1. Preoperative or postoperative balloon dilatations of PA stenoses were performed in 6, and all patients had symptomatic improvement. At a mean follow-up of 26 months, the severity of pulmonary regurgitation improved in all but 1 patient. In 12 patients (group 1), conduit regurgitation was either trace in 11 or mild in 1. Four patients (group 2) had moderate conduit regurgitation. PA diameters and cross-sectional areas were significantly smaller in the group 1 patients when compared with the group 2 patients. With the exception of 1 patient, RV end-diastolic diameter fell after allograft insertion in each patient, and the reduction in diameter was significantly greater in group 1 than in group 2. These authors showed good early results for this treatment. When to intervene in this situation remains an unresolved question.

With Coronary Anomaly

Carvalho and associates,[14] from London, United Kingdom, performed both a retrospective and prospective of the use of angiography for diagnosing anomalous coronary artery passing anterior to the RV outflow tract in TF. Standard angiographic views were used in 295 patients, which were reviewed, and 10 of these had a coronary vessel traversing the RV outflow tract. The diagnosis was not suspected before operation in 9 of 10 patients. A prospective study was then performed in 30 patients with TF (range, from 1 month to 12 years of age). An aortogram was performed with ≥45° caudocranial and 20° to 30° left anterior oblique angulation. The RV outflow tract lay in the left and anterior (seen as superior) position in relation to the aortic root. Paired left anterior descending coronary artery were found with a large vessel originating from the right coronary and passing across the left RV outflow tract. This procedure shows great promise in making this diagnosis prior to surgery. Although echocardiography is useful, it may not be diagnostic in all patients.

PULMONIC VALVE ATRESIA

Management Evolution With Intact Ventricular Septum

Leung and associates,[15] from Hong Kong, examined the impact on survival and clinical course of incorporating the morphologic classification of the right ventricle into the evolving management, for infants with pulmonary atresia and intact septum. The surgical results and follow-up status for the first 62 consecutive patients managed between 1979 and 1990 were reviewed. Before 1984, all 23 patients underwent primary RV outflow reconstruction irrespective of RV morphology and size (group I). Since 1984, depending on morphology and size, 39 babies had either closed transventricular pulmonary valvotomy (n = 31) or a shunt operation (n = 8) (group II). There were 10 hospital and 2 late deaths (mortality, 52%) in group I patients, and 3 of 11 long-term survivors had cyanosis at rest; but none had any residual pulmonary stenosis. Group II patients had 6 hospital and 4 late deaths (mortality, 26%). Of the 29 long-term survivors, 9 had a second-stage RV outflow tract reconstruction, 8 had balloon valvuloplasty, and 2 had successful Fontan operation. At the latest follow-up, 5 children from this group have cyanosis at rest, 1 has a residual 55 mm Hg gradient, and 3 have RV dysfunction. The hospital and total mortality for patients in group II was significantly lower than that in group I. These data indicate that tailoring of the treatment to the RV anatomy results in a lower overall mortality although long-term hemodynamic abnormalities were observed in both groups. Most centers have recognized the futility of attempting biventricular repair in infants who have either severe coronary abnormalities or extremely small right ventricles, which can be assessed most easily by tricuspid valve size. Those with severe coronary abnormalities are probably only candidates for transplantation, and patients with small tricuspid valves and small right ventricles are candidates for Fontan repair or transplantation.

Influence of Right Ventricular Size on Outcome

Giglia and associates,[16] from Boston, Mass, used echocardiography to assess the influence of right heart size on outcome independent of the presence of RV dependent coronary circulation in 37 neonates with pulmonary atresia and intact ventricular septum. Coronary artery anatomy was adequately assessed by angiography in 36. RV volume and tricuspid valve were significantly smaller in patients with RV dependent coronary circulation than in those without. There was no statistically significant association between RV volume or tricuspid valve diameter and survival among patients with or without RV dependent coronary circulation. Among 29 patients without RV dependent coronary circulation, 23 of 24 (96%) who achieved RV decompression are alive compared with 1 of 5 (20%) who did not achieve RV decompression. Of the 23 survivors, 21 have a complete two-ventricle physiology with low right atrial pressure. Among 7 patients with RV dependent coronary circulation, 2 patients who underwent RV decompression died early of LV failure, whereas 4 of 5 who did not undergo RV decompression have survived single ventricle palliation. Small right heart size is associated with RV dependent coronary circulation but is not associated with survival in pulmonary atresia-intact ventricular septum. These are good results from early RV decompression in patients without RV dependent coronary circulation independent of RV or tricuspid valve size. It is important that each patient have complete assessment of whether or not they have RV dependent coronary circulation as such patients will probably only be candidates for single ventricle palliation.

With Ventricular Septal Defect

Rome and associates,[17] from Boston, Mass, reported a 14-year experience in the treatment of patients with TF, pulmonary atresia, and diminutive PAs. There were 91 patients between 1978 and 1988 who had adequate evaluation of their PA anatomy before any surgical management. Diminutive PAs (38 to 104 mm^2/m^2) were present in 48 of these patients with pulmonary flow from aortopulmonary collaterals. There were four different management strategies, including primary repair in 9 with 7 dying early and 2 survivors with poor hemodynamic outcome. There were 9 patients with conservative management with no intervention before 5 years of age with 4 dying and only 1 having a satisfactory hemodynamic result. There were 10 shunted patients with 3 deaths and 3 with satisfactory repairs. Since 1984, rehabilitation of PAs has been performed with RV to PA surgical graft, balloon dilation of residual PA stenoses, embolization of collateral vessels, and surgical closure of VSD and repair of remaining obstructions. Of 20 patients so managed, 7 died after various stages, but 10 of 20 had complete repair. All repaired patients with subsystemic RV pressures had at least one successful PA dilation. These authors make a case for combined catheter-surgery approach at an early age in patients with TF, pulmonary atresia, and diminutive PAs. This is a difficult group, and the plan to begin treatment at an early age seems like a reasonable approach.

Effects of Right Ventricular Decompression on Left Ventricular Function

Gentles and associates,[18] from Boston, Mass, studied the effect of RV decompression on LV function using preoperative cineangiograms and preoperative and postoperative echocardiograms to analyze global and regional LV function. Preoperative cineangiograms demonstrated fistulas with and without one coronary artery stenosis in 12 of 24 patients, aged 2 days to 33 months at the time of RV decompression. One infant with fistulas involving two coronary arteries and stenosis of the right coronary artery died from severe global LV dysfunction after RV decompression. Despite this, mean LV end-diastolic volume and mean LV ejection fraction were similar in patients with and without coronary arterial abnormalities before and after RV decompression. Before RV decompression, regional LV dysfunction was seen in 8 of 132 (6%) regions in those with coronary artery abnormalities and in 3 of 132 (2%) in those without coronary artery abnormalities. After RV decompression, there were 16 of 132 (12%) abnormal regions in those with coronary artery abnormalities and 1 of 132 (<1%) in those without coronary anomalies. In regions with normal wall motion before RV decompression, the presence of coronary artery abnormalities were related to regional LV dysfunction. In this study, only patients who did not have obstruction on the multiple coronary arteries were included and all had reduction in RV pressure to <2/3 of systemic blood pressure. Regional abnormalities in LV function, both before and after RV decompression, were rare in patients without angiographically demonstrated coronary anomalies. In those with coronary anomalies, none of whom have obstruction to more than 1 coronary artery, regional LV dysfunction was common; but severe global LV dysfunction was rare. Dependence of the myocardium on high RV pressure for adequate perfusion appears to be less than expected in patients with coronary fistulae; those with lesser RV dependence seem to survive RV decompression but manifest localized areas of LV dysfunction that are probably due to ischemia. The long-term outlook for these patients is unclear.

Bidirectional Cavopulmonary Anastomosis + Biventricular Repair

Muster and associates,[19] from Chicago, Ill, report five patients with hypoplastic right ventricle with severe outlet obstruction or atresia and a small tricuspid valve who had ASD closure at the time of biventricular repair. The right ventricle had a mean diastolic volume of 48% of normal and a mean stroke volume of 40% of predicted. A bidirectional cavopulmonary anastomosis supplemented the biventricular repair in four patients, and these had no evidence of RA or superior vena cava hypertension postoperatively. One patient had atypical TF with tricuspid stenosis and developed recurrent pericardial tamponade and marked hepatomegaly following conventional repair with ASD closure. These complications were controlled after a bidirectional cavopulmonary anastomosis. These authors demonstrated a new use for the bidirectional Glenn shunt as an adjunct to a biventricular repair. It should gain wider acceptance for this select group of patients.

TRANSPOSITION OF THE GREAT ARTERIES

With Intact Ventricular Septum

Davis and associates,[20] from Melbourne, Australia, presented data on arterial switch for infants with simple TGA who were over 21 days of age at the time of repair. There were 18 patients (range, from 21 to 118 days old; mean, 38 days). There was echocardiographic or catheter evidence (or both) of low LV pressure in 14 of 18 at the time of operation. None of the patients had preliminary PA banding. Mortality was 5.6% (1 of 18, CL 0.8% to 17%) for the older group versus 0% for 100 patients who had operations during a similar time period and were <21 days of age. The single death occurred in a 22 day old, 1.8 kg baby. One patient required a LV assist device for two days after operation in the older patient group. These authors concluded that arterial switch can be carried out as a primary procedure for patients up to the age of 1 month and probably up to the age of 2 months. These authors presented interesting data about arterial switch repair in older patients. Although the data do suggest that patients had low LV pressure at the time of repair, catheterization data at the time of surgery were available in only a few patients. These are encouraging reports for use of this operation in older patients, but getting a successful result in most centers will probably be difficult for patients who are beyond 3 weeks of age who have documented low LV pressure.

With Ventricular Septal Defect

Planche and associates,[21] from Paris, France, reported 40 patients who underwent anatomic repair of TGA, VSD, and aortic arch obstruction. In group 1, 26 patients underwent repair in a two-stage procedure with phase A including repair of the aortic obstruction with (16) or without (10) PA banding through a left thoracotomy at a mean age of 19 ± 23 days. Phase B included arterial switch operation with closure of the VSD at a mean age of 96 ± 122 days. In group 1, there were 8 early and 2 late deaths, with 11 patients requiring re-operation. The mean stay in the intensive care unit was 25 ± 20 days. Follow-up at a mean of 5 years revealed all but 1 were asymptomatic. Actuarial survival and rate of freedom from re-operation at 5 years were 58% and 50%, respectively. In group 2, 14 patients had a one-stage procedure through midsternotomy: arterial switch operation with closure of VSD and repair of the arch obstruction at a mean age of 10 ± 6 days. There were 2 early deaths and 1 late death after re-operation for overlooked multiple VSDs. Two patients required re-operation and the mean stay in intensive care unit was 12 ± 3 days. Mean follow-up at 22 months revealed all were asymptomatic, without medication. Actuarial survival rate and rate of freedom from re-operation at 3 years were 79% and 82%, respectively. The one-stage procedure allowed complete repair in neonates without the need for multiple operations. This approach may decrease the mortality rates (14% v 31%), reduce the re-operation rate and cumulative stay in the intensive care unit, and significantly decrease the overall morbidity. These authors presented outstanding results from this difficult problem. Hopefully, other centers can match these outstanding results.

Senning Procedure

Dihmiss and associates,[22] from Bristol, United Kingdom, studied all 34 patients who had the Senning operation between March 1983 and December 1986. There were 2 operative deaths and 1 sudden late death with 31 survivors. There was no clinical evidence of obstructed venous pathways and no re-operation required. The average mean pressure gradient at the junction of the SVC and systemic venous atrium was 2 mm Hg although 2 patients had gradients of 7 mm Hg. The average gradient was .7 mm Hg in the IVC and 1.4 mm Hg between the mean pulmonary arterial wedge and pulmonary venous atrial pressures. Only the 2 patients with gradients of 7 mm Hg at the junction of the SVC and the systemic venous atrium had considerable narrowing of the pathway and retrograde flow in the azygous vein. These authors showed excellent results for the systemic and pulmonary venous pathway of the commonly seen baffle obstruction in patients following Mustard repair.

Arterial Switch in Infancy

Hourihan and associates,[23] from Boston, Mass, investigated the size and growth potential of the neoaortic root and aortic anastomosis using serial echocardiogram on 50 patients with D-TGA who underwent arterial switch operation in infancy. Before surgery, the native pulmonary root (future neoaortic root) was 1.6 SD larger and the native pulmonary annulus (future neoaortic annulus) was 1.4 SD larger in infants with D-TGA than the aortic root and annulus of control patients. At a mean of 22 months (12 months to 6.5 years) after surgery, the diameter of the aorta at the anastomosis was .45 SD smaller, the neoaortic root was 2.9 SD larger, and the neoaortic annulus was 1.6 SD larger than the comparable structures in the control population. Growth of the aortic anastomosis was commensurate with somatic growth, but the dilation of the neoaortic root appeared to be progressive over time. The neoaortic root was significantly more dilated in patients with a history of PA banding and in patients with neoaortic regurgitation. This study emphasized the importance of continued acquisition and examination of data regarding long-term outcome after arterial switch operation.

TRUNCUS ARTERIOSUS

Repair in the Neonate

Hanley and associates,[24] from Boston, Mass, reported 63 patients with truncus arteriosus who underwent surgical repair between September 1986 and December 1991. According to both univariate and multivariate techniques, severe truncal valve regurgitation, interrupted aortic arch, coronary artery anomalies, and age >100 days at repair were important risk factors for perioperative death. In the 33 patients without these risk factors, early survival was 100%. In the 30 patients with one or more risk factors, survival was 63%. Pulmonary hypertensive episodes were fewer and duration of ventilator dependence and PA pressure were significantly less in patients undergoing operation before 30 days of age. Re-operation for RV outflow tract obstruction at a mean follow-up time of 23 months was carried out in 7 patients with no deaths. These authors showed excellent results for the relatively uncomplicated truncus patient. The anomalies listed continue to be problems although recent reports indicate the feasibility of successful repair of truncus associated with interrupted arch in neonates.

Coronary Anatomy

Bogers and associates,[25] from Rotterdam and Leiden, The Netherlands, studied coronary anatomy in 44 postmortem specimens of hearts with common arterial trunk. In 38 hearts, the normal distribution of left and right coronaries were found. The coronary orifices were abnormal, however, with 5 being pinpoint and 3 showing a double orifice. The left coronary orifice was positioned in the posterior part of the truncus; the right coronary orifice was positioned in the right anterior and lateral part. In 19 hearts, coronary orifices were found above sinus level, with left coronary orifices more often than right coronary orifices. The truncal valve was bicuspid in 11, tricuspid in 25, and quadricuspid in 8. Malformations of the coronary artery were found in 28 hearts (64%). In 27 hearts (61)%, the coronary anatomy might have had clinical consequences, including 9 hearts in which the coronary orifices were at risk for damage at the time of excision of the PAs from the common arterial trunk.

AORTIC VALVE STENOSIS

Incidence in Liverpool

Kitchiner and associates,[26] from Liverpool, United Kingdom, identified 239 patients born with AS between 1960 and 1990 and provided follow-up to assess the severity. Congenital AS occurred in 5.7% of patients with congenital heart disease born in this area with a median age at present of 16 months (range, 0 to 20 years). Stenosis was mild at presentation in 145 patients, moderate in 33, severe in 1, and critical in 21. Bicuspid aortic valve without stenosis was diagnosed in 39. Additional cardiac lesions were significantly more common in children presenting under 1 year of age and in those with critical stenosis. Coarctation, PDA, and VSD were the most common associated lesions. The median duration of follow-up was 9.2 years (range, 1 to 28 years). Only 7 patients were lost to follow-up. There were 81 operations in 60 patients. The re-operation rate was 28% after a median duration of 9 years. Only 15% of patients presenting with mild stenosis subsequently required operation compared with 67% of those with moderate stenosis. There were no sudden unexpected deaths and no deaths after simple valvotomy except in those presenting with critical stenosis. Overall mortality was 17%, but patients presenting with critical AS had a much worse prognosis. SBE occurred in 3 patients (1.3 per 1,000 patient-years of follow-up). These authors were able to capture most of the patients born with this condition in their area. The progression of moderate stenosis, defined as a Doppler velocity of from 3 to 4.5 mm/sec to severe stenosis, is common. Five- and 20-year survivals for 72% and 45%, respectively, for the moderate group and 98% and 94%, respectively, for the mild group. Over a 10-year follow-up, only 25% of mild patients progressed to moderate stenosis. An accurate clinical and echocardiographic diagnosis of severity at presentation provides a good guide to prognosis in early adult life.

Rapidity of Progression of Stenosis With Bicuspid Valve

The rapidity of progression of AS in patients with congenital bicuspid aortic valves and its relation to aging and valve anatomy are not well known. To elucidate these aspects, Beppu and associates,[27] from Osaka, Japan, examined 75 patients (aged 15 to 76 years) by echocardiography. Aortic valve sclerosis began from the second decade, the sclerotic index progressing with age. Aortic valve calcium was noted from the fourth decade. Aortic valve pressure gradient increased approximately 18 mm Hg each decade, concomitant with progression of valve sclerosis. Progression of cusp sclerosis was faster in patients with anteroposteriorly located cusps than in those with right-left-located cusps and was faster in those with eccentric cusps than in those with symmetric cusps. In patients with eccentric and anteroposteriorly located cusps, aortic valve pressure gradient increased 27 mm Hg per decade. In patients with congenital bicuspid aortic valves, the progression of AS is rapid, and the rapidity depends to some extent on the position and eccentricity of the cusps.

DISCRETE SUBAORTIC STENOSIS

Operative Age and Gradient as Predictors of Late Aortic Regurgitation

Rizzoli and associates,[28] from Padova, Italy, described 100 patients operated on for discrete subaortic stenosis between 1969 and 1990. There were three deaths in the perioperative period. Patients with intrinsic lesions, prosthetic valve replacement, or extensive operative remodeling of the aortic valve were excluded from analysis. The 67 remaining patients had a median follow-up of 62 months. Preoperatively, 8 patients had no AR, 51 had mild AR, and 8 had moderate AR. At follow-up, mild AR persisted in 27 patients and moderate AR in 6 patients. In 1 patient, AR worsened from none to mild and in another from mild to moderate. The probability of AR at follow-up was significantly and simultaneously related to older age at operation, higher preoperative gradient, preoperative cardiomegaly, and surgical myectomy. The data from this study support early operation for moderate gradients. The decision to operate obviously has to be an individual one, and gradients in the mild range can probably be delayed in the young child without increasing the prevalence of severe AR postoperatively.

AORTIC VALVE ATRESIA

Cardiac Transplantation

Ruiz and associates,[29] from Loma Linda, Calif, reported five infants with hypoplastic left heart syndrome who underwent stenting of the ductus arteriosus as a bridge to cardiac transplantation. All patients had successful stents placed with marked increase in diameter of ductus and abolition of any pressure gradient across the ductus. Four of the five subsequently underwent successful orthotopic cardiac transplantation, and one died of an unrelated problem prior to transplant. Histopathological exam of the ductus in all patients showed a patent, endothelialized stent without clot. This new technique has appeal for providing stable hemodynamics without the use of prostaglandin E_1.

To determine whether cardiac transplantation improves the natural history of infants with hypoplastic left-heart syndrome and to examine differences in outcome as a function of the pretransplant period, Chiavarelli and associates,[30] from Loma Linda, Calif, analyzed 111 infants with hypoplastic left-heart syndrome who entered and completed a protocol leading to transplantation from Nov 19, 1985, to Dec 31, 1991. Infants who died while waiting for transplantation were included. Transplantation procedures were performed in 84 infants (76%) (range, from 3 hours to 151 days old). Twenty-seven infants who were registered for transplantation died while awaiting a donor heart. Operative mortality was 13%, and 69 patients were late survivors (62% of the study group and 82% of the transplant recipients). Overall 5-year survival was 81% (Figure 8-2). Freedom from re-operation was 89% at 5 years. Thus, cardiac transplantation for hypoplastic left-heart syndrome has a significant positive impact on the natural history of this uniformly lethal lesion.

STENOTIC OR INTERRUPTED AORTIC ARCH

Bove and associates,[31] from Ann Arbor, Mich, reported results from surgery on seven patients with aortic arch obstruction, subaortic stenosis resulting from posterior deviation of the infundibular septum, and VSD. There were seven patients with coarctation in four and interrupted arch in three. Primary repair was performed with a technique that included transatrial resection of the infundibular septum. Patients ranged in age from 5 to 63 days and weights from 1.3 to 5.4 kg with a mean of 3.1 kg. Systolic and diastolic ratios of the diameter of the LV outflow tract to that of the descending aorta were .53 ± .09 and .73 ± .11 mm, respectively. At operation, the displaced infundibular septum was partially re-

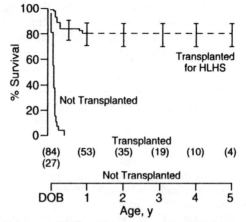

Figure 8-2. Survival curves (Kaplan–Meier estimate) in 111 infants with hypoplastic left-heart syndrome (HLHS) completing a protocol of cardiac transplantation. The lower curve displays survival of the 27 patients who died while waiting for a donor (Not Transplanted). Transplanted patients (n = 84) had a 5-year survival of 81% (Transplanted for HLHS). The numbers in parentheses indicate patients at risk beyond that time; the horizontal dashed line, traced event-free patients; the bars, 95% confidence intervals; and DOB, date of birth. Reproduced with permission from Chiavarelli et al.[30]

moved through a right atrial approach by resecting the superior margin of the VSD up to the aortic annulus. The resulting enlarged VSD was then closed with a patch to widen the subaortic area and the arch was repaired by direct anastomosis. All patients survived operation; there was one death from noncardiac causes at 3 months. The survivors remain well from 3 to 14 months (mean, 8 months) after repair and one patient underwent successful balloon dilatation of a residual aortic arch obstruction. No patient has significant residual subaortic stenosis, although one has valvar AS. These authors presented outstanding results for a very difficult group of patients.

AORTIC ISTHMIC COARCTATION

Late (20 to 44 Years) Results After "Repair"

Stewart and associates,[32] from London, United Kingdom, examined the health and lifestyle of a group of patients who had repair of coarctation of the aorta 20 to 44 years ago. There were 149 operations performed and 70 of the 106 patients presumed to be alive were traced. Information was obtained by questionnaire in 62, and 42 of these 62 were examined. Cardiovascular disorder was present in 69%, but there was no evidence of previously unrecognized major recoarctation. Hypertension was present in 46% of patients at follow-up with enlargement of the aortic root or arch in 16%. Aortic valve abnormalities were present in 36%. There was no evidence of cerebrovascular accidents. The good news in these adult patients is that recoarctation is rare when repair is performed after growth is completed and that cerebrovascular accidents are relatively rare in this group. The bad news is that there is considerable cardiovascular morbidity in this group with only 31% free of evidence of any cardiovascular problems. These patients need continued surveillance for hypertension, aortic valve abnormalities, and aortic root enlargement with potential for aortic aneurysms. A subsequent report from this cohort of patients who died revealed 6 patients who died after aortic rupture with 5 of the 6 having been operated on when they were more than 10 years old, with a mean age at operation of 20 years. It is hoped that the current practice of early operation may reduce the likelihood of long-term development of aortic aneurysm.

Left Ventricular Function After "Repair"

Krogmann and associates,[33] from Dusseldorf, Germany, and Zurich, Switzerland, studied 12 patients, 3 to 12 years after successful repair of coarctation. There were 8 patients who were normotensive, and 4 had borderline hypertension. Data at rest and after nitroprusside infusion were evaluated and compared with 12 control subjects. Systolic ventricular function including EF-end systolic wall stress relationships were normal in all patients. However, LV muscle mass, right atrial pressure, and LV end-diastolic pressure were significantly higher in patients than in control subjects. There was a linear relationship between muscle mass and LV end-diastolic or right atrial pressure. LV relaxation and myocardial stiffness were normal. There was an upward shift of the diastolic pressure-volume curve when compared with control values, but this shift was reversed by nitroprusside. These authors showed interesting late abnormalities after successful coarctation repair. It appears that the hypertrophy per se causes an abnormal diastolic pressure-volume relationship, which was persistent despite relief of hypertension in most patients.

Magnetic Resonance Imaging v Angiography After Balloon Angioplasty

In a study by Fawzy and associates,[34] from Riyadh, Saudi Arabia, between July 1986 and December 1990, 24 consecutive adult patients (aged 15 to 55 years [mean, 25]) with native coarctation of the aorta underwent balloon dilatation. Dissection of the aorta developed in 1 patient. The remaining 23 patients were restudied by catheterization and magnetic resonance imaging 8 to 60 months (mean, 21) after dilatation. Both studies were performed between 1 and 180 days (mean, 40) of each other. The diameter of the aorta at the site of previous coarctation was measured on angiogram and magnetic resonance imaging by two independent observers. The data were compared by means of linear regression analysis. The gradient across the previous coarctation site ranged from 0 to 20 mm Hg (mean, 7 ± 7.3). The diameter of the aorta at the site of previous coarctation measured on angiogram was 14 ± 3.7 mm, and on magnetic resonance imaging it measured 14 ± 3.7 mm with excellent correlation. Two patients had small aneurysms, 2 cm in diameter, demonstrated by angiography and magnetic resonance imaging; and 2 patients developed restenosis, diagnosed correctly by both cardiac catheterization and magnetic resonance imaging. This study demonstrated that magnetic resonance imaging provides excellent visualization of the anatomy of the aorta and is a good noninvasive method for follow-up of patients undergoing balloon coarctation angioplasty.

Angioplasty v Operation

Shaddy and associates,[35] from Salt Lake City, Utah, reviewed data from 36 patients who were prospectively randomized to either angioplasty in 20 or surgery in 16. Reduction in peak systolic gradient across the coarctation was similar (86%) immediately after both balloon angioplasty and surgery. On follow-up, aneurysms were seen only in the angioplasty group in 20%. No aneurysms have shown progression or required surgery. The incidence of other complications was similar in both groups, although 2 patients experienced neurological complications after surgery. Although not statistically different, the prevalence of restenosis, defined as a gradient ≥20 mm Hg, tended to be greater in the angioplasty group (25%) than in the surgery group (6%). Restenosis after angioplasty occurred more frequently in patients with an aortic isthmus/descending aorta diameter <.65 and was associated with an immediate catheterization residual peak gradient across the coarctation ≥12 mm Hg. These authors showed good immediate gradient reduction in unoperated coarctation with the use of balloon angioplasty. The risk of small aneurysm formation and possible restenosis may be higher than after surgery, although risks of other complications were similar. Balloon angioplasty for coarctation may provide an effective initial alternative to surgical repair of unoperated coarctation of children beyond infancy, particularly in patients with a well-developed isthmus. Follow-up is necessary to determine the long-term risks of postangioplasty aneurysms.

PATENT DUCTUS ARTERIOSUS

Transcatheter v Operative Closure

Transcatheter implantation of the Rashkind PDA occluder is an alternative to conventional surgical closure of isolated PDA. Neither the clinical outcomes nor the costs of these procedures have been formally compared. Gray and associates,[36] for the Patent Ductus Arteriosus Closure Comparative Study Group, performed a retrospective cohort study to evaluate the clinical outcomes within a 7-month period for comparable patients with PDA who underwent either placement of an occluder or surgical closure. The patients were treated between 1982 and 1987 at 14 major North American centers where PDA was closed predominantly by a surgical procedure or by the occluder technique. To estimate inpatient and follow-up costs, the authors multiplied the observed use of resources by 1989 unit costs based on hospital-accounting and physician-reimbursement data. On the basis of cardiac auscultation at follow-up, the initial procedure resulted in closure of the ductus arteriosus in 77.3% of 185 patients in whom the occluder was implanted and 99.8% of 446 surgical patients. Second procedures increased the percentage of successful closures to 87.6% and 100% for patients in the occluder and surgical groups, respectively. There were no deaths. Major complications occurred in 2.7% of the patients in whom the occluder was implanted and 0.2% of the patients who underwent surgery; moderate complications in 16.8% and 15.0%, respectively; and minor complications in 11.4% and 24.9%. Including the cost of follow-up care, the mean estimated cost per case treated surgically was $8,838 (in 1989 US dollars), as compared with $11,466 per case treated with the occluder technique. Sensitivity analyses based on our data identified no plausible situations in which the costs of surgery and of implantation of the occluder would be equal. The more effective and less costly surgical procedure was superior to transcatheter placement of the occluder for closure of isolated PDA. Consequently, these results do not support the widespread dissemination of the occluder procedure for the management of this common congenital lesion.

Transcatheter Occlusion

Rao and associates,[37] from Madison, Wis, Amarillo, Tex, Riberao Preto, Brazil, Lille Cedex, France, and Berlin, Germany, reported initial results of 14 patients who underwent transcatheter closure of PDA with an adjustable button device delivered via a 7F sheath. Patients were aged 15 months to 8 years and weighed 7.2 to 19 kg. The PDA measured from 2 to 7.5 mm with a median of 3 mm at the narrowest diameter. It was occluded with devices measuring 15 to 20 mm. The ratio of pulmonary to systemic flow decreased from $1.9 \pm .6$ to $1.05 \pm .1$. The murmur typical of PDA appeared in 13 of 14 patients with small residual shunts by color Doppler were found in 4 of 14. All patients were followed for 1 to 24 months with the device intact in all. No shunts were seen in 12 of 14 on follow-up, and minute residual shunts were seen in 2 children. There were no major complications. This report represents another device for transcatheter ductal closure. It is unclear as to which device will be most useful long-term, and studies continue with several different prostheses.

Lloyd and associates,[38] from Ann Arbor, Mich, and Tucson, Ariz, attempted PDA closure with Gianturco coils in 24 consecutive patients aged 8 months to 30 years with a mean ductus diameter of 1.5 ± 8 mm. There were two coil embolizations in the first 4 patients with successful coil retrieval. Based on this experience, coils were successfully implanted using a coil helical diameter twice or more the minimum ductus diameter with coil length sufficient for three or more loops. With these recommendations, coils were successfully implanted in the subsequent 20 patients. There were 22 patients with successful coil implantation with 15 (68%) showing no residual shunting, and 7 had trace residual shunting by angiography. The continuous murmur was abolished in all patients, and there were no significant complications. Patients were discharged within 24 hours of implantation. These authors showed excellent results in patients with ductus diameters up to 3.3 mm. This may provide a relatively low cost method for closure of small PDAs.

MITRAL STENOSIS

Barbero-Marcial and associates,[39] from Sao Paulo, Brazil, reported an LV apical approach for surgical treatment of MS in patients aged 2 to 74 months, with nine patients <24 months. All patients had severe or moderately severe symptoms, and parachute-type MS was found in nine.

Associated anomalies were present in every patient, and five had undergone previous operation. Repair of the MS was done through an apical left ventriculotomy. Removal of mitral obstruction starts from below; the papillary muscle was split and the chordae were divided or fenestrated. The commissurotomies were performed from the ventricular aspect of the mitral valve. Associated anomalies were corrected simultaneously, including VSD closure, resection of subaortic stenosis, and coarctation repair. There was no operative mortality and only one late death, which was unrelated to cardiovascular status. Echocardiographic studies up to 52 months postoperatively showed no significant residual MS and normal global and regional function of the LV in all but one patient.

CORONARY ARTERIAL ANOMALY

Intramural Coronary Artery

Pasquini and associates,[40] from Boston, Mass, studied all infants with d-TGA who underwent echocardiography and surgical repair from January 1987 to June 1992 to attempt to identify those with an intramural coronary artery. Among 435 infants, 29 were diagnosed as having an intramural coronary artery. In 27 cases, the diagnosis was confirmed at surgery or autopsy, and there were 2 false-positive echocardiographic diagnoses (specificity, 99.5%). An intramural coronary artery was correctly diagnosed prospectively by echocardiography in 20 or 27 infants (sensitivity, 75%), including 17 of 23 infants with an intramural left coronary artery or left anterior descending coronary artery and 3 of 4 infants with an intramural right coronary artery. Two primary diagnostic criteria were identified: a major coronary artery arising from the contralateral septal sinus near the usually intercoronary commissure and a course for this vessel within the posterior aortic wall between the great arteries creating a "double-border" appearance. Retrospective review using these criteria identified 26 of the 27 intramural arteries with no false-positive diagnoses. This report indicated that echocardiography is a promising technique for defining coronary anatomy in patients with d-TGA and intramural coronary arteries. This diagnosis is extremely important to make because of the higher risk for arterial switch and the need for considering optional surgical procedures.

Role of Transesophageal Echocardiography

Fernandes and associates,[41] from Detroit, Mich, used transesophageal echocardiography with color flow Doppler to study nine patients with angiographically confirmed anomalous coronary arteries. The abnormal origins of the anomalous coronary arteries was confirmed by transesophageal echocardiography in all nine patients. The LM coronary artery originated from right sinus of Valsalva. Transesophageal echocardiography demonstrated the course of the anomalous LM coronary artery between the aorta and PA better than angiography. Other anomalies visualized included two patients with origin of the right coronary artery from the left aortic sinus, one patient with origin of the LAD from the right sinus, one patient with origin of the circumflex from the right sinus, and one patient with origin of the LM coronary artery from the pulmonary artery. Thus, transesophageal echocardiography is a useful noninvasive test for diagnosing anomalous origin of the coronary arteries. It is a valuable adjunct to angiography in demonstrating the abnormal course of the LM coronary artery interposed between the aorta and the PA, a potentially life-threatening entity.

Solitary Coronary Ostium

Ogden JA and Goodyer AVN published in the *Yale Journal of Biology and Medicine* in 1970 an article entitled "Patterns of distribution of the single coronary artery," and in that article, classified "single coronary artery" into 14 basic distribution patterns. Since then, other patterns of distribution of single coronary artery have been recognized. Distinction has also been made between the cases with and without other major congenital cardiovascular anomalies or coronary artery atresia and those without these additional abnormalities. Single coronary artery has been generally considered to be a benign clinical entity. Shirani and Roberts,[42] from Bethesda, Md, described 10 cases of single coronary artery at necropsy and reviewed 87 previously reported cases, 35 diagnosed at necropsy and 52 by coronary angiography. These authors classified single coronary artery into 20 categories on the basis of the location of the solitary coronary ostium, the presence or absence of an aberrant-coursing coronary artery, and the course taken by the aberrant-coursing coronary artery (Figure 8-3, Table 8-2). When atherosclerotic CAD was absent, 15% (8 of 53) of the patients reviewed with single coronary artery had myocardial ischemia as a direct consequence of the coronary anomaly. The anatomic classification presented is useful from both clinical and surgical viewpoints. This comprehensive classification of this rare anomaly facilitates description of the various distribution patterns of single coronary artery and their clinical significance.

FONTAN OPERATION

DiDonato and associates,[43] from Rome, Italy, treated 23 patients between 1986 and 1989 with ventricular hypertrophy, complex cardiac anomalies with unrestricted pulmonary blood flow, and subaortic stenosis. Surgery consisted of combining a main PA-ascending aorta anastomosis with bidirectional cavopulmonary anastomosis. The average age of the patients was 57 ± 36 months (7 to 155 months). Single ventricle with TGA was present in 9, and the other 14 had more complex cardiac anomalies unsuitable for biventricular repair. Subaortic obstruction was defined by a hemodynamic criterion in 6 and by a morphologic criterion in 17. There were 5 hospital deaths (22%); all 3 patients older than 7 years of age died. Follow-up averaged 28 ± 21 months (range, 1 to 58). Among the 18 hospital survivors, 1- and 5-year survival were 78% and 63%, respectively. Postoperative catheterization in 11 patients showed no or trivial subaortic gradient, a mean cavopulmonary pressure of 10 ± 3 mm Hg and a mean arterial oxygen saturation of 83%. A secondary

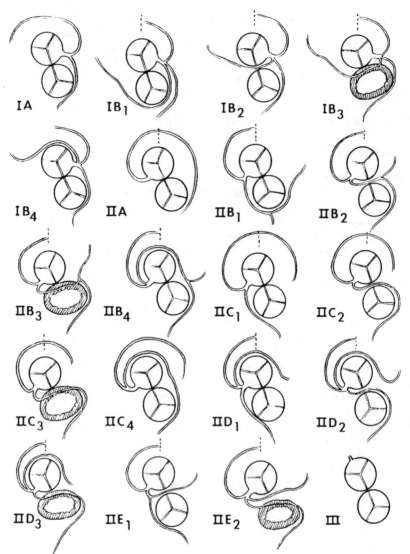

Figure 8-3. The origin and pattern of distribution of various types of solitary coronary ostium in the aorta. Reproduced with permission from Shirani et al.[42]

Fontan repair was performed in 9 patients 21 ± 4 months after palliation with no deaths. One other patient died elsewhere 3.7 years after palliation during attempted Fontan operation, for an overall mortality at repair of 10%. The other 8 patients are awaiting Fontan operation. This staged approach reduces both pressure and volume overload and provides adequate oxygenation before the Fontan operation. It can be useful in selected patients with complicated anomalies.

Michielon and associates,[44] from Rochester, Minn, reported patients with anomalies of systemic and/or pulmonary venous connection who underwent a modified Fontan operation at a mean age of 10 ± 6 years. Isolated anomalies of the systemic venous connection were present in 46 patients, isolated pulmonary venous anomalies in 4 patients, and a com-

Table 8-2. Solitary Coronary Ostium in the Aorta. Reproduced with permission from Shirani et al.[42]

I. Solitary ostium in (or immediately cephalad to) the *left* aortic sinus
  A. Unassociated with an aberrant-coursing coronary artery (anatomic single coronary artery) (1–11,21,29–38)
  B. Associated with an aberrant-coursing right coronary artery (RCA); RCA arising from the left main coronary artery (LMCA) or from the left anterior descending coronary artery (LADCA) and coursing to the right atrioventricular sulcus:
    1. *anterior* to the right ventricle (type *a*) (6,39–42)
    2. *between* the pulmonary trunk and the ascending aorta (type *b*) (12,30,43–45)
    3. in the *crista* supraventricularis (type *c*) (13,46)
    4. *dorsal* to the ascending aorta (type *d*) (30)

II. Solitary ostium in (or immediately cephalad to) the *right* aortic sinus
  A. Unassociated with an aberrant-coursing coronary artery (anatomic single coronary artery) (14–16,48)
  B. Associated with an aberrant-coursing LMCA. LMCA arising from the RCA and coursing to the left side (to divide into the LADCA and the left circumflex coronary artery [LCCA]):
    1. *anterior* to the right ventricle (type *a*) (17,30,43,49–52)
    2. *between* the pulmonary trunk and the ascending aorta (type *b*) (15,18,30,53–55)
    3. in the *crista* supraventricularis (type *c*) (15,19,20,56)
    4. *dorsal* to the ascending aorta (type *d*) (11,21,30,54,57–60)
  C. Associated with an aberrant-coursing LADCA. RCA courses in the atrioventricular groove, past the crux, to form the LCCA. LADCA arises from the RCA and courses to the left side:
    1. *anterior* to the right ventricle (type *a*) (61)
    2. *between* the pulmonary trunk and the ascending aorta (type *b*) (23)
    3. in the *crista* supraventricularis (type *c*) (24,25)
    4. *dorsal* to the ascending aorta (type *d*)*
  D. Associated with aberrant coursing of both the LADCA and the LCCA. LCCA arising from the RCA and coursing to the left side dorsal to ascending aorta. LADCA arising from the RCA and coursing to the left side:
    1. *anterior* to the right ventricle (type *a*)*
    2. *between* the pulmonary trunk and ascending aorta (type *b*) (54,62)
    3. in the *crista* supraventricularis (type *c*) (26–28)
  E. Associated with aberrant coursing of both the LADCA and LCCA. LCCA arising from the RCA and coursing to the left side between the pulmonary trunk and the ascending aorta. LADCA arising from the RCA and coursing to the left side:
    1. *anterior* to right ventricle (type *a*)*
    2. in the *crista* supraventricular (type *c*)*

III. Solitary ostium in (or immediately cephalad to) the *posterior* aortic sinus*

---

*No reported example of this anomaly.

bination of the 2 in 54 patients. Previous palliative operations had been performed in 93 patients. Surgical repair was accomplished by atrial septation or placement of an intra-atrial conduit combined with cavopulmonary anastomosis if required. Survival, including operative mortality, was 56% at 10 years, not significantly different from the overall survival of the Fontan population. Insufficiency of the systemic AV valve, preoperative mean pulmonary pressure >15 mm Hg, and PA resistance >4 U · m² were associated with higher mortality. These authors showed good early results with this complicated group (Figures 8-4, 8-5, 8-6, and 8-7).

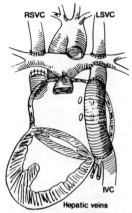

Figure 8-4. Corrective procedures for isolated anomalies. Left: A lateral tunnel is preferred in the presence of a single atrioventricular valve or atresia of the left atrioventricular valve. A cavopulmonary connection completes the procedure. SVC indicates superiod vena cava; IVC, inferior vena cava; CS, coronary sinus; RPV, right pulmonary veins; IPV, left pulmonary veins; LSVC, left superior vena cava; Ao, aorta; RPA, right pulmonary artery; and LPA, left pulmonary artery. Middle and right: When the pulmonary venous connection interferes with the construction of a lateral tunnel, an intra-atrial conduit is preferred. Reproduced with permission from Michielon et al.[44]

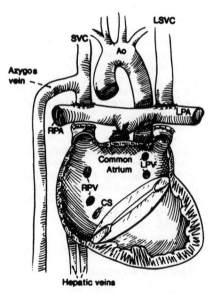

Figure 8-5. Direct cavopulmonary anastomosis. A total cavopulmonary connection is preferred in the presence of interruption of the inferior vena cava with azygous/hemiazygous continuation. As suggested by Kawashima et al,[6] the hepatic veins are left free to drain toward the systemic circulation. SVC indicates superior vena cava; Ao, aorta; LSVC, left superior vena cava; RPA, right pulmonary artery; LPA, left pulmonary artery; RPV, right pulmonary veins; LPV, left pulmonary veins; and CS, coronary sinus. Reproduced with permission from Michielon et al.[44]

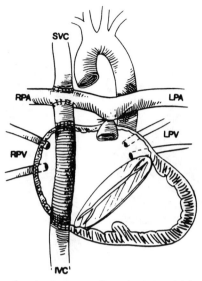

Figure 8-6. Rerouting of systemic venous flow. An intra-atrial conduit is selected in the case of connection of left and right pulmonary veins (LPV and RPV, respectively) to opposite sides of the common atrium. This avoids the potential for obstruction of both the systemic and pulmonary venous flow. SVC indicates superior vena cava; IVC, inferior vena cava; RPA, right pulmonary artery; and LPA, left pulmonary artery. Reproduced with permission from Michielon et al.[44]

Long-term morbidity and mortality continue to be a troublesome future of this group of patients.

Cromme-Dijkhuis and associates,[45] from Rotterdam and Groningen, The Netherlands, evaluated 66 patients 1 to 14 years after a Fontan-type operation. Clinical condition was reported by 51 patients, and 15 patients had symptoms and were restricted in their daily life. Bicycle exercise capacity was tested in 41 patients and ranged from 50% to 110% of predicted value with a mean of 85%. In 16 patients, a decreased capacity (<85%) was related to arrhythmias and the presence of protein-losing enteropathy. A 24-hour ambulatory ECG was available in 56 patients and found to be normal in only 57%. Arrhythmias were present in 21 patients, 6 of whom had symptoms; and 3 patients had previous pacemaker implantation. One or more abnormalities in liver enzyme and function tests were present in 40 patients (61%) and in coagulation in 46 patients (69%). The most pronounced abnormality was a protein C deficiency, a known thrombotic risk factor, present in 41 patients. The occurrence of arrhythmias increased with time of follow-up, and the occurrence of protein C deficiency decreased with time. The occurrence of abnormal liver enzyme and function tests was not related to follow-up time. With regard to age at operation, arrhythmias did not occur in patients who underwent operation at a mean age of 4 ± 2 years in contrast to patients who underwent operation at a mean age of 8 ± 4 years. Liver abnormalities or coagulation disorders were not related to age at operation. There was a higher prevalence of arrhythmias in patients with valved right atrium to PA connections than in patients with nonvalved or direct right atrium to PA connections. Even patients with apparently

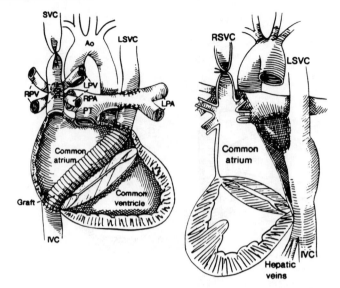

Figure 8-7. Left: Diagram shows isolation technique for correction of total anomalous pulmonary venous connection (TAPVC) to the superior vena cava (SVC). The right SVC is ligated above the entrance of the right and left pulmonary veins (RVC and LVC, respectively). This creates malalignment between the inferior vena cava (IVC) and the left superior vena cava (LSVC). An intra-atrial conduit is selected to reroute the systemic venous flow, preventing the potential for obstruction. Ao indicates aorta; RPA, right pulmonary artery; and LPA, left pulmonary artery. Right: Diagram shows isolation of a TAPVC to one SVC (the right SVC [RSVC]) by ligation of the cava above the entrance of the pulmonary veins, creating alignment between the left SVC (LSVC) and IVC. A lateral tunnel can be constructed. Reproduced with permission from Michielon et al.[44]

good clinical condition are at risk for arrhythmias, abnormal liver enzyme and function tests, and coagulation factor abnormalities. Serial follow-up of these patients is recommended.

Pridjian and associates,[46] from New Orleans, La, used echocardiographic follow-up studies to determine the degree of valvular regurgitation in 40 patients who had the right AV valve taken down to improve exposure for VSD repair. On the basis of the area of the color flow jet, valvular regurgitations was graded as none in 22 patients and trivial in 10 patients. There was no heart block and no deaths. These authors concluded that takedown and resuspension of the AV valve is a safe and effective technique that improves exposure for VSD repair and does not adversely affect valve competence.

MISCELLANEOUS TOPICS

Vascular Rings

van Son and associates,[47] from Rochester, Minn, reviewed results in 37 patients who underwent operation for the relief of tracheoesophageal obstruction that resulted from vascular rings and related entities at the

Table 8-3. Distribution of Vascular Anomalies in 37 Mayo Patients with Vascular Rings.*
Reproduced with permission from van Son et al.[47]

	Patients		Age (yr)	
Anomaly	No.	%	Range	Mean
Double aortic arch	18	49	4 wk-25	3.9
With both arches patent and L ductus				
or ligamentum arteriosum	10			
With atresia of L arch distal to origin of				
L subclavian artery and L ligamentum				
arteriosum	8			
R aortic arch with aberrant L subclavian				
artery and L ductus or ligamentum arteriosum	11	30	16 wk-34	6.7
L aortic arch with aberrant R subclavian artery	4	11	32 wk-60	32.0
Pulmonary artery sling	2	5	16-24 wk	20 wk
R aortic arch with mirror-image branching				
and L ligamentum arteriosum	1	3	...	16 wk
L aortic arch with R descending aorta and				
R ductus arteriosus	1	3	...	2.0
Total	37			6.5

*L = left; R = right.

Mayo Clinic from 1947 to 1992 (Table 8-3). Of the 37 patients, 18 had a double aortic arch; 11 had a right aortic arch with an aberrant left subclavian artery; 4 had a left aortic arch with an aberrant right subclavian artery; 2 had a pulmonary artery sling; 1 had a right aortic arch with mirror-image branching and a left ligamentum arteriosum; and 1 had a left aortic arch, a right descending aorta, and a right ductus arteriosus (Figure 8-8). Symptoms consisted of stridor, recurrent respiratory infections, and dysphagia. The anomaly was approached through a left thoracotomy in 31 patients, through a right thoracotomy in 4, and through a median sternotomy in 2. Only 1 early postoperative death (3%) and no late deaths occurred. At long-term follow-up (maximal duration, 45 years), 3 patients had residual symptomatic tracheomalacia, 1 of whom required right middle and lower lobectomy for recurrent pneumonia. Magnetic resonance imaging is the imaging technique of choice for accurate delineation of the vascular and tracheal anatomy. When patients are symptomatic, vascular ring should be repaired. The surgical risk is minimal, and the long-term results are excellent.

Cardiopulmonary Responses to Exercise in Aortic Stenosis, Pulmonic Stenosis, or Ventricular Septal Defect

Driscoll and associates,[48] from Rochester, Minn, and the Natural History Study, performed exercise testing on 134 of 235 Natural History Study 2 participants with AS, 195 of 331 with PS and 324 of 594 with SD. A Bruce treadmill exercise was used; and mean exercise duration for patients with AS, PS, and VSD was 87%, 94%, and 91% of predicted, respectively. For patients with AS, there was a direct relation between echocardiographic Doppler maximum transaortic gradient and ST-segment change during exercise. ST-segment change during exercise was very uncommon for patients with PS. For patients with VSD, there was

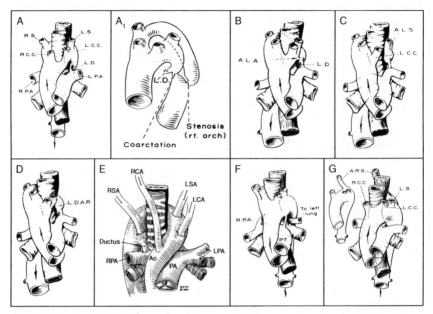

Figure 8-8. Seven types of vascular ring present in the current series of patients: A, double aortic arch with both arches patent; A_1, double aortic arch associated with coarctation of aorta; B, double aortic arch with atretic zone in left arch distal to origin of left subclavian artery; C, right aortic arch with aberrant left subclavian artery and left ductus or ligamentum arteriosum; D, right aortic arch with mirror-image branching and left ligamentum arteriosum; E, left aortic arch, right descending aorta, and right ductus arteriosus; F, anomalous left pulmonary artery (pulmonary artery sling); and G, left aortic arch with aberrant right subclavian artery. ALA indicates atretic left arch; ALS, aberrant left subclavian artery; Ao, right ascending aorta; ARS, aberrant right subclavian artery; LCA and LCC, left common carotid artery; LD, left ductus arteriosus; LDAR, left dorsal aortic root; LPA, left pulmonary artery; LS and LSA, left subclavian artery; PA and PT, pulmonary artery trunk; RCA and RCC, right common carotid artery; RPA, right pulmonary artery; RS and RSA, right subclavian artery; rt, right. (A through D, F, and G from Stewart and associates.[32] By permission of Charles C Thomas, Publisher.) Reproduced with permission from van Son et al.[47]

an association between arrhythmia noted during exercise and the presence of associated AR. Patients with AS who required aortic valve replacement had more serious arrhythmias than patients with AS who had not required operation. Although exercise capacity was reasonably well-preserved in patients with each of these three lesions, nonetheless it was subnormal. Exercise capacity was less well preserved in patients with AS than in those with VSD or PS. These data indicate mildly subnormal treadmill responses in a number of patients although exercise duration was reasonably well preserved in most.

Infective Endocarditis in Aortic Stenosis, Pulmonic Stenosis, or Ventricular Septal Defect

Gersony and associates,[49] from New York, NY, and the Natural History Study Group, assessed the prevalence of infective endocarditis for patients admitted to the First Natural History between 1958 and 1965, and who were eligible for the Second Natural History Study. Most patients with severe defects were managed surgically, and most with mild defects were managed medically. Final examination in the first study was carried out 8 years after admission. The 2,401 patients admitted to Natural History Study have been followed for a total of 40,855 person years for an average of 17 ± 8 person years of follow-up per patient. For AS, the prevalence rate of infective endocarditis was 27 per 10,000 person years with an incidence of 15.7 for those managed medically and 40.9 for those managed surgically. Most patients managed surgically had severe AS, and severity was more important to the risk of infective endocarditis than the method of management. For PS, only 1 of 592 patients experienced infective endocarditis. For VSD, the incidence was 14.5 per 10,000 person years, and size of VSD was not associated with risk. The risk of infective endocarditis before VSD closure was more than twice that after surgery. The prevalence rate of SBE was nearly 35-fold the population based rate. The presence of AR in patients with AS did not increase the risk of developing infective endocarditis.

Double Outlet Right Ventricle

Serraf and associates,[50] from Le Plessis-Robinson, France, reported 30 patients, aged 15 days to 15 years, who underwent repair of double outlet right ventricle (DORV) with associated subaortic stenosis. Eighteen patients had a palliative procedure before complete repair. The VSD was subaortic in 15, doubly committed in 1, noncommitted in 9, and subpulmonary in 5. The subaortic obstruction was the result of a restrictive VSD in 29 patients and of double straddling of mitral and tricuspid valves in 1 patient. The preoperative peak systolic pressure gradient between the left ventricle and aorta was 69 ± 23 mm Hg. Reconstruction of the LV outflow tract comprised a ventral enlargement of the VSD in subaortic, double committed, and those subpulmonary VSDs scheduled for an arterial switch operation or a conal resection in noncommitted or other subpulmonary forms. Reconstruction of the RV outflow tract included primary closure of the right ventricle in 12, an infundibular patch in 9, transannular patch in 4, and insertion of a RV to pulmonary valve conduit in 5. There were 2 early deaths (6.6%) and 2 late (7.1%) deaths. Re-operation was required in 3 patients. A mean follow-up of 60 ± 47 months was achieved in all the survivors. They were all without symptoms or with mild symptoms and in sinus rhythm. At last follow-up, the mean LV-aortic gradient was 8 ± 6 mm Hg, and LV function indices were within normal range. Actuarial survival and freedom from re-operation rates at 8 years were 87% and 87%, respectively. These authors showed outstanding results from dealing with this very difficult problem.

Sinus of Valsalva Aneurysm

Echocardiographic and Doppler data of 62 patients with aneurysm of the sinus of Valsalva were examined in this investigation by Dev and associates,[51] from New Delhi, India. Catheterization and angiography were performed in 38 cases and surgery in 25 of the 38. The origin of these aneurysms was the right coronary sinus in 56 cases, noncoronary sinus in 5, and left coronary sinus in 1 case. Seven had unruptured aneurysms (6 rising from the right coronary sinus dissected into the ventricular septum) producing heart block in 4, AR in 5, and MR in 1; 1 aneurysm rising from the left coronary sinus was asymptomatic. In other cases (n = 55), the aneurysm had ruptured into one of the cardiac chambers. Thirty-two of the 50 right coronary sinus aneurysms ruptured into the RV outflow tract, 13 into the RV cavity, 2 into the right atrium, and 3 into the left ventricle. Of the 5 noncoronary sinus aneurysms, 3 ruptured into the right atrium, 1 into the right ventricle, and 1 into both the right atrium and right ventricle. Associated VSD was identified in 16 (26%) of 62 cases. All of these patients had right coronary sinus aneurysms that ruptured into the RV outflow tract. Echocardiography missed VSD in 3 cases that at surgery were found to have VSD. AR was found in 34 of 62 cases. Echocardiography identified discrete subaortic stenosis in 2 cases but missed subvalvar pulmonic stenosis in 2 of the 3 cases. A detailed echocardiographic study (two-dimensional, Doppler, and color flow imaging) is accurate in the diagnosis of aneurysm of the sinus of Valsalva, in the identification of its site of origin and rupture, and in the evaluation of the associated defects; in the vast majority of cases, it can totally supplant the need for angiography.

Amrinone in Children

Robinson and associates,[52] from Miami, Fla, studied 19 patients, aged 2 months to 8 years, with catheterization measurements before and 10 minutes after administration of a bolus injection of amrinone. In 5 patients with normal PA pressure and resistance, amrinone significantly reduced mean PA pressure by 19%, mean left atrial pressure by 39%, and systemic resistance by 17%. In 7 patients with PA hypertension and normal pulmonary vascular resistance, amrinone significantly reduced the PA pressure by 27%, systolic arterial pressure by 5%, mean aortic pressure by 12%, pulmonary arteriolar resistance by 36%, and total pulmonary vascular resistance by 26%. In 7 patients with pulmonary hypertension and elevated pulmonary vascular resistance, amrinone significantly reduced the pulmonary arteriolar resistance by 49%, total pulmonary resistance by 47%, and pulmonary arteriolar/systemic vascular resistance ratio by 45%. These authors showed marked pulmonary vasodilator effects with amrinone. This drug may be effective in children for treatment of pulmonary hypertension without causing systemic hypotension.

Stents

O'Laughlin and associates,[53] from Houston, Tex, and Boston, Mass, reported results in 85 patients who underwent placement of 121 stents for PA stenosis in 58, conduit or outflow tract stenosis in 9, and venous stenoses or narrowed Fontan anastomoses in 21. These procedures resulted in a gradient reduction from 55 ± 33 to 14 ± 14 mm Hg in PAs, from 41 ± 26 to 21 ± 17 in conduits or outflow tracts, and from 10 ± 7 to 2 ± 3 in venous stenoses or Fontan anastomoses. Diameter of narrowing increased from 5 ± 2 to 11 ± 3 mm in the PA, from 9 ± 4 to 13 ± 3 mm in conduits, and from 4 ± 3 to 11 ± 3 mm in venous stenoses. Follow-up has shown stent fracture in 1 patient, restenosis in 1, and sudden death in 1. Recatheterization has been done in 38 patients an average of 9 months after stent installation. Compared with immediately postimplant data, there were no significant changes in luminal diameter or pressure gradient. Redilation was performed in 14 patients (17 stents) 1 week to 24 months after implantation with a small but significant increase in stenosis diameter. These authors showed outstanding short-term results for stent placement in patients whose lesions previously had not been amenable to interventional therapy.

Bidirectional Cavopulmonary Shunt

Chang and associates,[54] from Boston, Mass, reported 17 consecutive infants, aged 4 to 6.5 months, who underwent bidirectional cavopulmonary shunts. The diagnoses were hypoplastic left heart syndrome in 7, single right ventricle in 5, and single left ventricle in 5. Prior surgery had been performed in 15 of 17. The bidirectional cavopulmonary shunt was performed early on an elective basis in 9 patients; of the remaining patients, 6 had progressive cyanosis, 1 had severe ventricular failure, and 1 had coexisting restrictive bulboventricular ventricular foramen. The median preoperative PA pressure and pulmonary vascular resistance were 15 mm Hg and 2.3 U $\cdot$ m^2, respectively. One patient died; overall hospital survival was 94%. The most common postoperative problem was transient systemic hypotension, observed in 14 (88%) of 16 survivors. Systemic arterial oxygen saturation increased from a median of 75% to a median of 85%. The median hospital stay was 6 days, and there were no late deaths during follow-up (mean, 12 months). At postoperative cardiac catheterization performed in 9 of 16 survivors, there was no evidence of severe hypoxemia, shunt narrowing, or pulmonary arteriovenous fistulas. Of the 16 survivors, 6 have had a subsequent Fontan operation at a mean age of 2 years, and there were 5 survivors. The end-diastolic pressure of the systemic ventricle was >10 mm Hg in 4 patients, mean PA pressure >15 mm Hg in 6 patients, and pulmonary vascular resistance >4 U $\cdot$ m^2 in 3 patients. These authors showed excellent results for this interim operation in young patients and in patients with significant risk factors for early Fontan repair. It remains unclear as to the role of this operation versus a fenestrated Fontan or regular Fontan in infants and young children with good or only slightly increased risk factors.

Lasers in Valve Atresia

Rosenthal and associates,[55] from London, United Kingdom, studied the efficacy and safety for transcatheter laser-assisted valve dilatation for atretic valves in 11 children, aged 1 day to 11 years, with atresia of pulmonary or tricuspid valve. After delineating the atretic valve by angiography and/or echocardiography, a 0.018 inch "hot tip" laser wire was used to perforate the atretic valve. Subsequently, the valve was dilated with conventional balloon dilatation catheters up to the valve annulus diameter. Dilation was successfully accomplished in 9 children. In 2 neonates with pulmonary atresia and intact ventricular septum, the procedure resulted in cardiac tamponade; 1 died immediately and 1 later at surgery. During a follow-up of 1 to 17 months, 2 infants with pulmonary valve atresia and intact septum died (one with CHF). The remainder are either well palliated and do not require further procedures or are awaiting further transcatheter or surgical procedures because of associated defects. These authors showed promising data in using laser-assisted valve dilatation. This requires considerable expertise with interventional procedures by more than one physician. Whether or not it will be widely applicable to a number of centers awaits further reports.

Aortic Valve Allografts

Clarke and associates,[56] from Denver, Colo, provided follow-up on 47 children (aged 3 years or older in 33 and <3 years in 14 at age of operation) who underwent aortic root replacement with cryopreserved aortic valve allografts. In the older patient group, there were 3 (9%) hospital deaths, and 1 child underwent cardiac transplantation 30 hours after aortic root replacement because of LV failure. Clinical follow-up of the 29 surviving older children is from 4 months to 6.6 years with a mean of 3 years, and 1 patient was lost to follow-up. Re-operation has been required in 2 children (7%), but primary allograft degeneration was not observed. In the younger patient group, there were 3 (21%) hospital deaths; and follow-up ranged from 2.5 months to 4.7 years with a mean of 2.3 years. Among 11 operative survivors, 1 late death resulted from a pulmonary embolus. Progressive allograft calcification or insufficiency was found in 7 of 10 of the remaining allograft recipients. Re-operation has been required in 6 of these 7 to explant the allograft, and 1 child is currently receiving cyclosporine therapy with the original valve allograft. The cause of allograft failure is possibly immunologic. The prevalence of early aortic valve allograft degeneration has prompted consideration of nonviable allografts or xenografts, pulmonary autografts, or minimal immunosuppression as alternatives when LV outflow tract reconstruction is necessary in children <3 years of age. These are disturbing findings for these patients with aortic valve allografts of LV outflow obstruction. Although problems with degeneration have occurred with the use of this type of graft in the pulmonary position, the prevalence has not been nearly as high. Further data are needed to determine what alternate strategy might be most useful in these patients.

Hypothermic Circulatory Arrest v Low-Flow Cardiopulmonary Bypass

Newburger and associates,[57] from Boston, Mass, compared the prevalence of perioperative brain injury after deep hypothermia and support consisting predominantly of total circulatory arrest with the incidence after deep hypothermia and support consisting predominantly of low-flow cardiopulmonary bypass in a randomized, single-center trial. There were 171 patients with dTGA; 129 had intact ventricular septum, and 42 had a VSD. After adjustment for diagnosis, assignment to circulatory arrest as compared with low-flow bypass was associated with a higher risk of clinical seizures, a tendency to a higher risk of ictal activity on continuous EEG monitoring during the first 48 hours after surgery, a longer recovery time to the first reappearance of EEG activity, and greater release of the brain isoenzyme of creatine kinase in the first six hours after surgery. Analysis comparing duration of circulatory arrest produced results similar to those of analysis comparing treatments. These authors showed definite changes in terms of early seizures in the circulatory arrest group. A large portion of infants in both groups and categories had neurological examinations that were possibly (31%) or definitely (28%) abnormal. Differences between treatment groups were not apparent. The significance of these studies awaits further reports of long-term neurological outcome.

Pulmonary Hypertension After Cardiopulmonary Bypass

Wessel and associates,[58] from Boston, Mass, infused the endothelium-dependent vasodilator acetylcholine into the pulmonary circulation of pulmonary hypertensive children with congenital heart disease either before (n = 12) or after (n = 22) surgical repair using cardiopulmonary bypass. The dose response to acetylcholine was recorded for hemodynamic variables, and 9 additional postoperative patients were studied with acetylcholine followed by inhalation of 80 ppm nitric oxide, an endothelium-independent smooth muscle relaxant. Plasma levels of cyclic GMP were measured before and after acetylcholine and nitric oxide administration. Pulmonary vasodilation with acetylcholine was seen in all preoperative patients but was markedly attenuated in postoperative patients. Baseline pulmonary vascular resistance of 5.6 ± 1 U $\cdot$ m^2 fell 46% $\pm$ 5% in preoperative patients but declined only 11% $\pm$ 4% from baseline in postoperative patients. Inhalation of 80 ppm nitric oxide after acetylcholine infusion in postoperative patients, however, lowered pulmonary vascular resistance by 33% $\pm$ 4% with minimal effects on the systemic circulation. This finding suggests that the capacity for smooth muscle relaxation and pulmonary vasodilation was present in postoperative patients but could not be induced by acetylcholine. Plasma level of cyclic GMP in postoperative patients were unchanged after acetylcholine but rose more than three-fold during vasodilation with nitric oxide. These data have important diagnostic and therapeutic implications in patients with congenital heart disease. Nitric oxide may prove to be a valuable therapeutic aid for children with pulmonary vascular disease.

Heart Transplantation

Bailey and associates,[59] from Loma Linda, Calif, reported 140 consecutive orthotopic transplantation procedures in 139 infants (aged 3 hours to 12 months). Indications for transplant included hypoplastic left heart syndrome in 63%, other complex anomalies in 29%, myopathy in 7%, and tumors in 2%. Most recipients had ductus-dependent circulation and received continuous infusion of prostaglandin E$_1$. Heart donors were usually victims of trauma, sudden death, or birth asphyxia. A donor-recipient weight ratio of 4 or less was found to be acceptable, and graft cold ischemic time ranged from 64 to 576 minutes. Procurement was facilitated by a single dose of cold crystalloid cardioplegic solution and cold immersion transport. Profound hypothermic circulatory arrest was used for graft implantation. There were 124 recipients (89%) who survived transplantation and were discharged from the hospital. There were 9 late deaths with an 83% overall survival. The overall 5-year actuarial survival is 80%, with newborn recipient survival of 84%. Chronic immunomodulation was cyclosporine-based and steroid-free. Surveillance was noninvasive and relied heavily on echocardiography, electrocardiography, and clinical intuition. There was 1 documented late lethal infection, and coronary occlusive disease was known to exist in only 1 long-term survivor. There were no tumors in this experience. These authors showed outstanding results from transplantation in infants. It is possible that younger children will fare better in terms of immunosuppression and lack of complications thereof, although this is yet to be proven.

References

1. Wu C-C, Chen W-J, Chen M-F, et al: Left-to-right shunt through patent foramen ovale in adult patients with left-sided cardiac lesions: A transesophageal echocardiographic study. Am Heart J 1993 (May);125: 1369–1374.

2. Konstantinides S, Kasper W, Geibel A, et al: Detection of left-to-right shunt in atrial septal defect by negative contrast echocardiography: A comparison of transthoracic and transesophageal approach. Am Heart J 1993 (Oct);126: 909–917.

3. Meijboom F, Hess J, Szatmari A, et al: Long-term follow-up (9 to 20 years) after surgical closure of atrial septal defect at a young age. Am J Cardiol 1993 (Dec 15);72:1431–1434.

4. Boutin C, Musawe NM, Smallhorn JF, et al: Echocardiographic follow-up of atrial septal defect after catheter closure by double-umbrella device. Circulation 1993 (Aug);88:621–627.

5. Hanley FL, Fentor, KN, Jonas RA, et al: Surgical repair of complete atrioventricular canal defects in infancy. J Thorac Cardiovasc Surg 1993 (Sep);106:387–397.

6. Kawashima Y, Matsuda H, Yagihara T, et al: Intraventricular repair for Taussig-Bing anomaly. J Thorac Cardiovasc Surg 1993 (April);105:531–597.

7. Lui RC, Williams WG, Trusler GA, et al: Experience with the Damus-Kaye-Stansel procedure for children with Taussig-Bing hearts or univentricular hearts with subaortic stenosis. Circulation 1993 (Nov);88[part 2]:170–176.

8. Hayes CJ, Gersony WM, Driscoll GJ, et al, for the Second Natural History Study of Congenital Heart Defects: Results of treatment of patients with pulmonary valvar stenosis. Circulation 1993 (June);(suppl I):I-28–I-37.

9. Kaul UA, Singh B, Tyagi S, et al: Long-term results after balloon pulmonary valvuloplasty in adults. Am Heart J 1993 (Nov);126:1152–1155.

10. Murphy JG, Gersh BJ, Mair DD, et al: Long-term outcome in patients undergoing surgical repair of tetralogy of fallot. N Engl J Med 1993 (Aug 26);329:593–599.

11. Rosenthal A: Adults with tetralogy of fallot—repaired, yes; cured, no. N Engl J Med 1993 (Aug 26);329:655–656.

12. Rebergen SA, Chin JGJ, Ottenkamp J, et al: Pulmonary regurgitation in the late postoperative follow-up of tetralogy of Fallot. Volumetric quantitation by nuclear magnetic resonance velocity mapping. Circulation 1993 (Nov);88[part 1]:2257–2266.

13. Warner KG, Anderson JE, Fulton DR, et al: Restoration of the pulmonary valve reduces right ventricular volume overload after previous repair of tetralogy of Fallot. Circulation 1993 (Nov);88[part 2]:189–197.

14. Carvalho JS, Siiva CMC, Rigby ML, et al: Angiographic diagnosis of anomalous coronary artery in tetralogy of Fallot. Br Heart J 1993 (July);70: 75–78.

15. Leung MP, Mok C, Lee J, et al: Management evolution of pulmonary atresia and intact ventricular septum. Am J Cardiol 1993 (June 1);71: 1331–1336.

16. Giglia TM, Jenkins KJ, Matitiau A, et al: Influence of right heart size on outcome in pulmonary atresia with intact ventricular septum. Circulation 1993 (Nov);88[part 1]:2248–2256.

17. Rome JJ, Mayar JE, Castanada AR, et al: Tetralogy of Fallot with pulmonary atresia: Rehabilitation of diminutive pulmonary arteries. Circulation 1993 (Oct);88[part 1]:1691–1698.

18. Gentles TL, Colan SD, Giglia TM, et al: Right ventricular decompression and left ventricular function in pulmonary atresia with intact ventricular septum: The influence of less extensive coronary anomalies. Circulation 1993 (Nov);88[part 2]:183–188.

19. Muster AJ, Zales VR, Ilbawi MN, et al: Biventricular repair of hypoplastic right ventricle assisted by pulsatile bidirectional cavopulmonary anastomosis. J Thorac Cardiovasc Surg 1993 (Jan);105:112–119.

20. Davis AM, Wilkinson JL, Karl TR, et al: Transposition of the great arteries with intact ventricular septum. J Thorac Cardiovasc Surg 1993 (July); 106:111–115.

21. Planche C, Serraf A, Comas JV, et al: Anatomic repair of transposition of great arteries with ventricular septal defect and aortic arch obstruction: One-stage versus two-stage procedure. J Thorac Cardiovasc Surg 1993 (May);105:925–933.

22. Dihmiss WC, Hutter JA, Joffe HS, et al: Medium-term clinical results after Senning procedure with haemodynamic and angiographic evaluation of the venous pathways. Br Heart J 1993 (May);69:436–444.

23. Hourihan M, Colan SD, Wernovsky G, et al: Growth of the aortic anastomosis, annulus, and root after the arterial switch procedure performed in infancy. Circulation 1993 (Aug);615–620.

24. Hanley FL, Heinemann MK, Jonas RA, et al: Repair of truncus arteriosus in the neonate. J Thorac Cardiovasc Surg 1993 (June);105:1047–1056.

25. Bogers AJJC, Bartelings MM, Bokenkamp R, et al: Common arterial trunk, uncommon coronary arterial anatomy. J Thorac Cardiovasc Surg 1993 (Dec);106:1133–1137.

26. Kitchiner DJ, Jackson M, Walsh K, et al: Incidence of prognosis of congenital aortic valve stenosis in Liverpool (1960–1990). Br Heart J 1993 (Jan); 69:71–79.

27. Beppu S, Suzuki S, Matsuda H, et al: Rapidity of progression of aortic stenosis in patients with congenital bicuspid aortic valves. Am J Cardiol 1993 (Feb 1);71:322–327.

28. Rizzoli G, Riso E, Mazzucco A, et al: Discrete subaortic stenosis: Operative age and gradient as predictors of late aortic valve incompetence. J Thorac Cardiovasc Surg 1993 (July);106:95–104.

29. Ruiz CE, Gamra H, Zhang HP, et al: Brief report: Stenting of the ductus arteriosus as a bridge to cardiac transplantation in infants with the hypoplastic left heart syndrome. N Engl J Med 1993 (June 3);328:1605–1608.

30. Chiavarelli M, Gundry SR, Razzouk AJ, et al: Cardiac transplantation for infants with hypoplastic left-heart syndrome. JAMA 1993 (Dec 22/29);270: 2944–2947.

31. Bove EL, Minich L, Pridjian AK, et al: The management of severe subaortic stenosis, ventricular septa, defect, and aortic arch obstruction in the neonate. J Thorac Cardiovasc Surg 1993 (Feb);105:289–296.

32. Stewart AB, Ahmed R, Travill CM, et al: Coarctation of the aorta life and health 20–44 years after surgical repair. Br Heart J 1993 (Jan);69:65–70.

33. Krogmann ON, Rammos S, Jakob M, et al: Left ventricular diastolic dysfunction late after coarctation repair in childhood: Influence of left ventricular hypertrophy. J Am Coll Cardiol 1993 (May);21:1454–1460.

34. Fawzy NE, von Sinner W, Rifai A, et al: Magnetic resonance imaging compared with angiography in the evaluation of intermediate-term result of coarctation balloon angioplasty. Am Heart J 1993 (Dec);l26:1380–1384.

35. Shaddy RE, Boucek MM, Sturtevant JE, et al: Comparison of angioplasty and surgery for unoperated coarctation of the aorta. Circulation 1993 (March);87:793–799.

36. Gray DT, Flyer DC, Walker AM, et al: Clinical outcomes and costs of transcatheter as compared with surgical closure of patent ductus arteriosus. N Engl J Med 1993 (Nov 18);329:1517–1523.

37. Rao PS, Sideris EB, Haddad J, et al: Transcatheter occlusion of patent ductus arteriosus with adjustable buttoned device: Initial clinical experience. Circulation 1993 (Sep);88:1119–1126.

38. Lloyd TR, Fedderly R, Mendelsohn AM, et al: Transcatheter occlusion of patent ductus arteriosus with Gianturco coils. Circulation 1993 (Oct);88 [part 1]:1412–1420.

39. Barbero-Marcial M, Riso A, DeAlbuquerque AT, et al: Left ventricular apical approach for the surgical treatment of congenital mitral stenosis. J Thorac Cardiovasc Surg 1993 (July);106:105–110.

40. Pasquini L, Parness IA, Colan SD, et al: Diagnosis of intramural coronary arteries using two-dimensional echocardiography. Circulation 1993 (Sep);88:1136–1141.

41. Fernandes F, Alam M, Smith S, et al: The role of transesophageal echocardiography in identifying anomalous coronary arteries. Circulation 1993 (Dec);88:2532–2540.

42. Shirani J, Roberts WC: Solitary coronary ostium in the aorta in the absence of other major congenital cardiovascular anomalies. J Am Coll Cardiol 1993 (Jan);21:137–143.

43. DiDonato RM, Amodeo A, diCarlo DD, et al: Staged Fontan operation for complex cardiac anomalies with subaortic obstruction. J Thorac Cardiovasc Surg 1993 (March);105:398–405.

44. Michielon G, Gharagozloo F, Julsrud PR, et al: Modified Fontan operation in the presence of anomalies of systemic and pulmonary venous connection. Circulation 1993 (Nov);88[part 2]:141–148.

45. Cromme-Dijkhuis AH, Hess J, Hahlen K, et al: Specific sequelae after Fontan operation at mid- and long-term follow-up: Arrhythmia, liver dysfunction, and coagulation disorders. J Thorac Cardiovasc Surg 1993 (Dec);106:1126–1132.

46. Pridjian AK, Pearce FB, Culpepper WS, et al: Atrioventricular valve competence after takedown to improve exposure during ventricular septal defect repair. J Thorac Cardiovasc Surg 1993 (Dec);106:1122–1125.

47. van Son JAM, Julsrud PR, Hagler DJ, et al: Surgical treatment of vascular rings. Mayo Clin Proc 1993 (Nov);68:1056–1063.

48. Driscoll DJ, Wolfe RR, Gersony WM, et al: Cardiorespiratory responses to exercise of patients with aortic stenosis, pulmonary stenosis, and ventricular septal defect. Circulation 1993 (Feb);87(suppl I):I-102–I-113.

49. Gersony WM, Hayes CJ, Driscoll DJ, et al: Bacterial endocarditis in patients with aortic stenosis, pulmonary stenosis, or ventricular septal defect. Circulation 1993 (Feb);67(suppl I):I-121–I-126.

50. Serraf A, Lacour-Gayet F, Houyel L, et al: Subaortic obstruction in double outlet right ventricles: Surgical considerations for anatomic repair. Circulation 1993 (Nov);88[part 2]:177–182.

51. Dev V, Goswami KC, Shrivastava S, et al: Echocardiographic diagnosis of aneurysm of the sinus of Valsalva. Am Heart J 1993 (Oct);126:930–936.

52. Robinson BW, Gelband H, Mas MS: Selective pulmonary and systemic vasodilator effects of amrinone in children: New therapeutic implications. J Am Coll Cardiol 1993 (May);21:1461–1465.

53. O'Laughlin MP, Slack MC, Grifka RG, et al: Implantation and intermediate-term follow-up of stents in congenital heart disease. Circulation 1993 (Aug);88:605–614.

54. Chang AC, Hanley FL, Wernovsky G, et al: Early bidirectional cavopulmonary shunt in young infants: Postoperative course and early results. Circulation 1993 (Nov);88[part 2];149–158.

55. Rosenthal E, Qureshi SA, Kakadekar AP, et al: Technique of percutaneous laser-assisted valve dilatation for valvar atresia in congenital heart disease. Br Heart J 1993 (June);69:556–562.

56. Clarke DR, Campbell DN, Hayward AR, et al: Degeneration of valve allografts in young recipients. J Thorac Cardiovasc Surg 1993 (March); 105:934–942.

57. Newburger JW, Jonas RA, Wernovsky G, et al: A comparison of the perioperative neurologic effects of hypothermic circulatory arrest versus low-flow cardiopulmonary bypass in infant heart surgery. N Engl J Med 1993 (Oct 7);329:1057–1064.

58. Wessel DL, Adatia I, Gigla TM, et al: Use of inhaled nitric oxide and acetylcholine in the evaluation of pulmonary hypertension and endothelial function after cardiopulmonary bypass. Circulation 1993 (Nov);88[part 1]:2128–2138.

59. Bailey LL, Gundry SR, Razouk AJ, et al, for the Loma Linda University Pediatric Transplant Group: Bless the babies: One hundred fifteen late survivors of heart transplantation during the first year of life. J Thorac Cardiovasc Surg 1993 (May);105:805–815.

9

Congestive Heart Failure

Incidence and Prevalence in Rochester, Minn

Although CHF is a fairly common clinical syndrome and the societal costs associated with its care are high, relatively little is known about the incidence or prevalence of the condition in the community. Using the resources of the Rochester Epidemiology Project, Rodeheffer and associates,[1] from Rochester, Minn, identified all 46 persons aged 0 to 74 years who had a new diagnosis of CHF during 1981 and all 113 persons with a prevalent diagnosis on Jan 1, 1982, in the city of Rochester, Minn. After confirming the diagnosis in the medical record by using criteria similar to those in the Framingham study, these authors found the annual incidence of CHF to be 110 per 100,000 after adjusting for age (Figure 9-1). Incidence rates were higher among male than among female study subjects (157 v 71 per 100,000). In both male and female subjects, the incidence generally increased with advancing age, reaching 1,618 per 100,000 and 981 per 100,000, respectively (Table 9-1). Prevalence rates on Jan 1, 1982, demonstrated similar patterns (Table 9-2). Overall, the prevalence of CHF was higher among male than among female subjects (327 v 214 per 100,000) and increased exponentially with advancing age, reaching almost 3% of both sexes. Survival after a diagnosis of CHF was extremely poor, with only 80% alive at 3 months and 66% at 1 year. These data underscore the effect of CHF in the community and provide estimates of the number of persons who might benefit from early intervention.

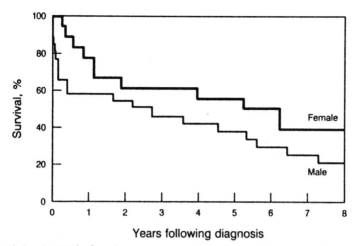

Figure 9-1. Survival after diagnosis of congestive heart failure in incidence cohort, Rochester, Minn, 1981, stratified by sex. Reproduced with permission from Rodeheffer et al.[1]

Table 9-1. Incidence* of Congestive Heart Failure: Comparison of Framingham, Mass, and Swedish Cohorts with Population of Rochester, Minn. Reproduced with permission from Rodeheffer et al.[1]

Age (yr)	Framingham†		Rochester	
	Men	Women	Men	Women
45-54	200	100	80	0
55-64	400	300	402	128
65-74	800	500	1,319	724
	Swedish men born in 1913‡		Rochester (men)	
50-54	150		86	
55-60	430		402	
61-67	1,020		1,618	

*Rates per 100,000 person-years.
†Data based on 34 years of follow-up experience.[16]
‡Data based on 17 years of follow-up experience.[14]

Triage Practice Guideline

Decisions regarding the appropriate timing for transfer of patients hospitalized with CHF from the coronary care unit to the medical ward are often not based on well-founded medical data. Weingarten and associates,[2] from Los Angeles, Calif, investigated the potential safety and effectiveness of a practice guideline recommending early "step-down" transfer to low-risk patients with CHF. These authors studied the use of a practice guideline for 384 patients hospitalized with CHF in a hypothetic experiment. The guideline stated that patients without any of the following conditions may be suitable for transfer to a nonmonitored bed 24

Table 9-2. Prevalence of Congestive Heart Failure in Rochester, Minn, Jan 1, 1981, through Dec 31, 1981. Reproduced with permission from Rodeheffer et al.[1]

Age (yr)	Female subjects		Male subjects	
	No.	Rate*	No.	Rate*
0-4	0	0	2	86.1
5-9	0	0	1	48.7
10-44	0	0	0	0
45-49	1	72.6	1	74.4
50-54	3	225.6	1	84.5
55-59	4	323.8	8	730.9
60-64	8	716.8	11	1,203.5
65-69	12	1,134.8	18	2,595.5
70-74	28	2,743.8	15	2,765.0
0-74†	56	213.6 (28.8)	57	327.3 (43.8)
0-74‡		265.8 (25.2)		

*Rate per 100,000 person-years.
†Rates per 100,000 person-years, adjusted to age distribution of US whites, 1980 (standard error).
‡Rate per 100,000 person-years, adjusted to age and sex distribution of US whites, 1980 (standard error).

hours after admission: AMI or ischemia, complications, active or planned cardiac interventions, unstable comorbidity, worsening clinical status, or lack of response to diuretic therapy. Patients with any of the above conditions were classified as higher risk and potentially not suitable for early transfer. Life-threatening complications were 15.2 times more likely and death 14.5 times more likely if the patient was classified as "high risk" rather than "low risk" by the guideline. The negative predictive value and sensitivity of the practice guideline for detecting patients who had life-threatening complications were 99.2% and 96.4%, respectively. Thirty-one percent of patients with CHF hospitalized in either the coronary care unit or intermediate care unit were at low risk and potentially suitable for transfer to a nonmonitored bed 24 hours after admission. Use of the guideline would have reduced intermediate care unit lengths of stay from 2.91 days to 2.22 days and coronary care unit length of stay from 2.06 to 2.04 days had it been used to triage patients with CHF. This reduction in length of stay would have resulted in 172 more intermediate care unit bed-days available per year to accommodate additional patients. On initial review, at least one cardiologist reviewer judged that use of the guideline may have adversely affected quality of care for 4% of patients. After a consensus among the cardiologist reviewers, it was judged that the guideline may have adversely affected care for only 0.8% of patients, and that no patient would have had an unexpected life-threatening complication because of the guideline. Use of a practice guideline has the potential to reduce the intermediate care unit length of stay for selected low-risk patients with CHF.

Physical Findings

Although the physical signs of acute CHF have been shown to correlate relatively well with cardiac hemodynamics, their reliability in estimating hemodynamics in patients with chronic heart failure has been questioned. Butman and associates,[3] from Tucson, Ariz, evaluated the sensitivity, specificity, and utility of the cardiovascular examination in predicting cardiac hemodynamics in patients with advanced chronic CHF. In 52 patients with chronic CHF undergoing in-hospital evaluation for possible heart transplantation, a variety of physical signs at the bedside and hemodynamic measurements were obtained. Pulmonary rales, a LV third heart sound, jugular venous distension, and the abdominojugular test, when positive, indicated higher right heart pressures and lower measures of cardiac performance. The presence of jugular venous distension, at rest or inducible, had the best combination of sensitivity (81%), specificity (80%), and predictive accuracy (81%) for elevation of the PA wedge pressure (>18 mm Hg). Furthermore, in this population sample, the probability of an elevated wedge pressure was 0.86 when either variable was present. These authors concluded that the bedside cardiovascular examination is extremely useful in identifying patients with elevation of right and left heart pressures. Examination for jugular venous distension at rest or by the abdominojugular test is simple and highly sensitive and specific in assessing left-sided heart pressures in these patients.

Cyclic Breathing Pattern

Cheyne-Stokes respiration has been noted to occur in patients with severely decompensated CHF and in those with primary neurological dysfunction. Normalization of this pattern has been noted to occur after effective medical therapy of decompensated CHF. Feld and Priest,[4] from Brooklyn, NY, evaluated the breathing pattern of patients with poor LV systolic function but compensated CHF. These included 36 consecutive patients with an EF <40%. Measurements were made with a computerized expiratory gas analyzer. Nine of the 36 patients demonstrated a cyclic breathing pattern with a cycle length of 132 seconds. At the peak of the cycle, minute ventilation was 16.7 L/min, and at the nadir of the cycle, minute ventilation was 9.5 L/min. Respiratory rate was 27 breaths/min at peak and 4 breaths/min at nadir. Patients with a cyclic respiratory pattern had a significantly lower EF (15%) compared with patients without cyclic respirations (26%). There was no relationship to origin of heart failure, clinical status, or exercise performance between the two groups. These authors concluded that a cyclic respiratory pattern occurs commonly in patients with mild to moderate heart failure. It is commonly found in patients with EFs <25% and consists of a variation in tidal volume only. Respiratory rate is relatively constant and true apnea does not occur.

Syncope

Mortality remains high in the management of advanced CHF despite the availability of vasodilators, which have been shown to prolong life. Middlekauff and associates,[5] from Los Angeles, Calif, analyzed the potential importance of syncope as a warning sign for sudden death in advanced CHF. They determined the relative importance of both cardiac syncope and syncope from other causes. In 491 patients who were functional class 3 or 4 with a mean ejection fraction of 20%, 60 had a history of

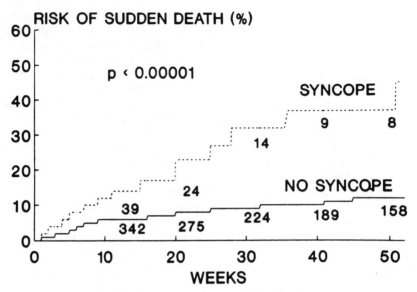

Figure 9-2. Reproduced with permission from Middlekauff et al.[5]

syncope; about half had a cardiac origin and half were due to other causes. The etiology of CHF was split about evenly between CAD and dilated cardiomyopathy. During a mean follow-up of 1 year, 69 patients died suddenly, and 66 patients died of progressive CHF (Figure 9-2). The incidence of sudden death by 1 year was significantly greater in patients with (45%) than in those without (12%) syncope. The risk of sudden death was the same in patients with either cardiac syncope or syncope from other causes. This study concluded that syncope was an adverse marker for the risk of sudden death in patients with advanced CHF, regardless of the mechanism of syncope.

Skeletal Muscle Dysfunction

Wilson and associates,[6] from Philadelphia, Pa, determined whether there is a subpopulation of patients with CHF who develop exertional fatigue due to skeletal muscle dysfunction rather than to reduced muscle blood flow. Thirty-four patients were evaluated and 6 normal subjects were also studied to define normal leg flow and femoral venous lactate responses to exercise. Patients with peak exercise leg flow levels within the normal mean flow ± 2 standard error of the mean were considered to have normal skeletal muscle blood flow during exercise. Nine of the 34 patients with CHF had normal leg blood flows during exercise. All of these patients terminated exercise due to leg fatigue, and all exhibited abnormal increases in femoral venous lactate concentrations. There were no significant differences between patients with normal leg flows and those with reduced flows with regard to age, LVEF, and resting hemodynamic measurements. However, those patients with normal flows exhibited more normal cardiac output responses to exercise and tended to have a higher peak exercise oxygen consumption. Thus, a significant number of patients with chronic CHF develop exertional fatigue due to skeletal muscle dysfunction rather than to reduced skeletal muscle blood flow. In these patients, therapeutic interventions should probably be directed at improving skeletal muscle abnormalities rather than at increasing blood flow.

Atrial Natriuretic Peptide

Early identification of patients with symptomless LV dysfunction and early pharmacologic intervention may have an impact on the outlook of patients with CHF. Atrial natriuretic peptide (ANP) is a cardiac hormone that is released as a C-terminal peptide (C-ANP) and an N-terminal peptide (N-ANP). Since N-ANP has reduced clearance rates compared with C-ANP, N-ANP circulates at higher concentrations. Based on the known increased concentration of C-ANP in symptomatic CHF, Lerman and associates,[7] from Rochester, Minn, evaluated prospectively the N-ANP profile and LV function in 180 subjects with symptomless and symptomatic CHF, and the role of plasma N-ANP as a marker for early identification of patients with CHF. Blood was taken for measurement of C-ANP and N-ANP before angiography. Patients were grouped according to New York Heart Association CHF classification and LV function. Mean plasma N-ANP concentration in patients with symptomless LV dysfunction was 243 pmol/L and was higher than in 25 control subjects. A plasma N-ANP concentration above 54 pmol/L had a sensitivity of 90% and a specificity of 92% for detection of patients with symptomless LV dysfunction. These authors showed that plasma N-ANP concentrations are significantly increased in patients with symptomless LV dysfunction and that this peptide can serve as a marker for diagnosis of such patients.

β-Adrenergic Receptors

Ungerer and associates,[8] from Munich, Germany, investigated the expression of β-adrenergic receptor kinase and β-adrenergic receptor numbers in LV samples of patients with idiopathic dilated cardiomyopathy or ischemic cardiomyopathy and from nonfailing control ventricles. Contractile responses to β-receptor stimulation were decreased in the failing hearts compared with the control hearts, whereas those to forskolin and calcium remained unchanged. The messenger RNA levels of β-adrenergic receptor kinase, and β_1- and β_2-receptors were determined using polymerase chain reactions. β-adrenergic receptor kinase enzyme activity assays were also performed and the levels of β_1- and β_2-receptors determined by radioligand binding. β-adrenergic receptor kinase messenger RNA levels were increased almost 3-fold in both forms of CHF, and β-adrenergic receptor kinase activity was enhanced. However, β_1-receptor messenger RNA levels and β_1-receptor numbers were decreased by about 50% in both heart failure groups, whereas these levels were unchanged for β_2-receptors. There were no differences between dilated and ischemic cardiomyopathy for any of these variables. Thus, diminished responses to β-receptor agonists in patients with severe CHF may be related to the combined effects of enhanced expression of β-adrenergic receptor kinase and reduced expression of β_1-receptor numbers.

To determine the effect of angiotensin converting enzyme inhibitor therapy on lymphocyte β-adrenoceptor function and density, as well as the in vivo myocardial response to β-agonist stimulation, Townend and associates,[9] from Birmingham, United Kingdom, studied 12 patients with chronic severe CHF before and after 16 weeks of treatment with quinapril. Lymphocyte β-adrenoceptor function was studied as a surrogate tissue for myocardium, and increased significantly after quinapril. Lymphocyte β-adrenoceptor density (6 patients) measured by radionuclide iodocyanopindolol binding, increased from 242 ± 72 to 884 ± 17 receptors/cell. Changes in functional myocardial β-adrenoceptor status were determined by measuring changes in hemodynamic responses to exercise and to incremental dobutamine infusion. Following quinapril, there were significant improvements in cardiac index, stroke volume, and cardiac power output during submaximal exercise testing and dobutamine infusion; stroke work index in response to dobutamine (but not exercise) improved significantly. Angiotensin converting enzyme inhibitors cause lymphocyte β-adrenoceptor upregulation in CHF, which is associated with an improved cardiac pumping capacity in response to β-agonist stimulation.

Angiotensin-Converting Enzyme DD Genotype

Polymorphism in the angiotensin-converting enzyme gene has been shown to correlate with circulating angiotensin-converting enzyme concentrations and also to be an independent risk factor for the development of AMI, particularly in men thought to be at low risk by standard criteria. Raynolds and associates,[10] from Denver, Colo, determined the genotypes of individuals with end-stage CHF due to either ischemic dilated cardiomyopathy (102 patients) or idiopathic dilated cardiomyopathy (112 patients) and compared these with organ donors with normally functioning hearts (79 patients). Genotypes were determined by the polymerase chain reaction with oligonucleotide primers flanking the polymorphic region in intron 16 of the angiotensin-converting enzyme gene to amplify template DNA isolated from patients. Compared with the DD frequency in the control population, the frequency of the angiotensin-converting enzyme DD genotype was 48% higher in individuals with idiopathic dilated cardiomyopathy and 63% higher in subjects with ischemic cardiomyopathy, suggesting that an angiotensin-converting enzyme gene variant may contribute to the pathogenesis of both types of cardiomyopathy.

Physical Activity

Exercise intolerance is a major limiting symptom in patients with CHF. Skeletal muscle hypoperfusion has been implicated in this problem. Arteriolar vasodilators that have improved cardiac output do not immediately increase exercise capacity, suggesting that intrinsic abnormalities of skeletal muscle also play a role. Adamopoulos and associates,[11] from Oxford, United Kingdom, used phosphorous-31 NMR spectroscopy to study muscle metabolism during exercise in 12 patients with stable ischemic CHF undergoing 8 weeks of home-based bicycle exercise training in a randomized crossover controlled trial. The results were compared with those in 15 age-matched control subjects who performed a single study only. Before the training, phosphocreatine depletion, muscle pH, and an increase in ADP during the first four minutes of exercise were all increased compared with values in control subjects. Training produced an increase in plantar flexion exercise tolerance. Phosphocreatine depletion and the increase in ADP during exercise were reduced significantly at all submaximal work loads. There was, however, no significant change in the response of muscle pH to exercise. After training, changes in ADP were not significantly different from those of control subjects, although phosphocreatine depletion was still greater in trained patients than in control subjects. Thus, these authors concluded that a substantial correction of the impaired oxidative capacity of skeletal muscle in chronic heart failure can be achieved by exercise training. Mechanisms may include improvement in biochemical pathways and hypertrophy due to exercise. Other mechanisms may also be playing a role. Whatever the mechanism, however, this data supports the view that modest exercise training may benefit patients with CHF.

To determine the level of daily physical activity routinely performed by patients with CHF and the ability of clinical and laboratory assessments of function to predict peak daily activity levels, Oka and associates,[12] from San Francisco, Calif, evaluated 45 patients with CHF in the laboratory and during two days of usual activity. Subjects performed symptom-limited treadmill exercise tests with respiratory gas analysis and wore a Vitalog activity monitor with continuous measurement of heart rate and body motion. Mean maximal oxygen uptake for this sample was 17 mL/kg/min. Peak daily physical activity involved walking on a flat surface (44%), or general activities (housework/yardwork, 42%). Most subjects were asymptomatic (49%) during daily physical activity, 22% noted dyspnea, 16% fatigue, and 13% sore muscles/joints. Perceived intensity of peak daily physical activity was similar to perceived exertion reported at ventilatory threshold measured during treadmill exercise testing. Subjects may control their peak daily physical activity to minimize symptoms experienced. It was further observed that current methods of assessing functional capacity in these patients were inadequate for estimating the peak level of daily activity. In conclusion, daily physical activity levels are low in patients with CHF, and a gap exists between exercise capacity and actual performance of daily physical activity.

Kestin and associates,[13] from Worcester, Mass, used a whole blood flow cytometric method to study platelet activation state and reactivity of 12 physically active and 12 sedentary individuals before and after standardized treadmill exercise testing. A panel of fluorescent-labeled monoclonal antibodies was used to monitor activation-dependent platelet surface changes, including downregulation of glycoprotein Ib and upregulation of GMP-140, the GPIIb-IIa complex, and GPIV. In samples obtained before exercise, platelets not exposed to thrombin showed no evidence of in vitro activation. In the sedentary subjects, exercise caused a consistent and significant increase in platelet activation state and reactivity. Exercise increased the binding of the GPIIb-IIIa complex at a single thrombin concentration. In the physically active subjects, exercise failed to cause a consistent alteration in either platelet activation state or reactivity. No significant differences were found among the 12 male and 12 female volunteers. Thus, strenuous exercise in sedentary subjects, but not in physically active subjects, results in both platelet activation and platelet hyperactivity.

Incidence of Stroke

The current study by Katz and associates,[14] from Bronx, New York, was undertaken to determine prospectively the risk of cerebral thromboembolism and the prognostic significance of LV thrombus in ambulatory patients with chronic CHF. A total of 264 ambulatory patients (mean age, 62 years; mean LVEF, 27%) were followed prospectively for 24 ± 9 months to determine the incidence of nonhemorrhagic stroke, transient ischemic attack, and mortality. Two-dimensional echocardiographic studies, performed for clinical indications other than previous systemic thromboembolism in 109 patients, were analyzed to relate the presence of LV thrombus to subsequent outcome. Nine cerebral thromboembolic events occurred in 264 patients during the 2-year mean follow-up period, yielding a rate of 1.7 thromboembolic events per 100 patient-years of follow-up. Known risk factors for stroke (hypertension, diabetes mellitus, and/or AF) were present in all 9 patients with cerebral thromboembolic events. The 109 patients with echocardiographic studies had more severe CHF than patients without echocardiographic studies (functional class 2.6 v 2.1), greater risk of a thromboembolic event (2.4 v 1.4 events per 100 patient-years of follow-up), and higher mortality (21 v 5.5 deaths per 100 patient-years). LV thrombus, detected in 54 (50%) of these patients, was associated with a greater risk of thromboembolism in a univariate model and was an independent predictor of mortality in Cox analysis. Thromboembolic stroke and transient ischemic attack occurred infrequently in ambulatory patients with CHF during a 2-year follow-up period. In selected patients with echocardiographic studies, LV thrombus was associated with increased mortality.

Endothelial-Dependent Responses

Katz and associates,[15] from Bronx, New York, evaluated the vasodilator response to intra-arterial administration of acetylcholine in patients with CHF compared with that of normal subjects. Thirty-one patients with CHF (New York Heart Association functional class II and III) and five age-matched normal subjects were studied. Regional vascular responses in the forearm to infusions of acetylcholine, an endothelium-dependent vasodilator (10^{-7} to 10^{-5} mol/L), and nitroglycerin, an endothelium-independent vasodilator (10^{-6} mol/L), in the brachial artery were determined with venous occlusion plethysmography before and after regional α-adrenergic blockade with intra-arterial phentolamine and systemic cyclooxygenase inhibition with oral indomethacin (50 mg). Administration of phentolamine significantly increased resting baseline forearm blood flow in 11 patients with CHF and normal subjects. Before administration of phentolamine, intra-arterial infusions of acetylcholine increased forearm blood flow in patients with CHF and to an even greater degree in normal subjects. After administration of phentolamine, the vasodilator responses to intra-arterial infusions of acetylcholine and nitroglycerin did not change in the patients with CHF or normal subjects. Administration of indomethacin did not alter resting forearm blood flow in 15 patients with CHF or normal subjects. Administration of indomethacin significantly increased the vasodilator response to infusions of acetylcholine by an average of 39% in patients with CHF but did not change the vasodilator response to acetylcholine in normal individuals. In patients with CHF, baseline forearm blood flow and the vasodilator response to intra-arterial infusions of acetylcholine and nitroglycerin were less than those in normal subjects both before and after the administration of phentolamine and indomethacin. Thus, the reduced vasodilator response to intra-arterial infusion of acetylcholine in patients with CHF is probably the result of coexistent abnormalities in peripheral vascular function, including abnormal production of cyclooxygenase dependent vasoconstricting factor, impaired endothelial release of nitric oxide, and decreased vascular smooth muscle responsiveness to cyclic GMP-mediated vasodilation.

Defective PA endothelium-dependent responses have been observed in chronic CHF models in animals. Porter and associates,[16] from Richmond, Va, and Boston, Mass, studied PA endothelial responses in humans with CHF. Twenty-two patients with chronic treated CHF (12 with secondary PA hypertension and 10 with normal pulmonary artery pressure) and 8 control patients constituted the study groups. Intravascular ultrasound measurements of PA area were evaluated in response to increasing doses of acetylcholine from 10^{-6} to 10^{-4} mol/L. The 10^{-6} mol/L infusion was repeated after methylene blue infusion. Indomethacin (5 µg/mL) was sequentially added to this combination in 17 patients. There were no significant differences among the three groups in vascular area response to the 10^{-6} to 10^{-5} mol/L acetylcholine. The 10^{-4} mol/L infusion resulted in significant constriction in the patients with secondary PA hypertension. Pretreatment with methylene blue in this group also resulted in significant PA vasoconstriction. The addition of indomethacin resulted in reversal of the constriction in these patients. These authors concluded that the PA endothelium may play a significant role in inhibiting vasoconstriction in patients with CHF who maintain normal PA pressures.

Quality of Life (SOLVD)

The improvement of aspects of a patient's quality of life may be as important as prolonging survival in evaluating clinical trials of CHF. Gorkin and associates,[17] from Providence, RI, designed a study to analyze the psychometric properties of the baseline measures from the quality-of-life substudy from the Studies of Left Ventricular Dysfunction (SOLVD) trial. The measures included the six-minute walk test, dyspnea scale, living with heart failure, physical limitations, psychologic distress, and health perceptions, as reported by both patients and staff. Cognitive functioning, such as vocabulary, digit span, and trails making, was also assessed. Patients were classified as New York Heart Association class I (n = 158) versus II or III (n = 150). The internal consistencies of the self-report measures were high, except for the Health Perceptions of Class II or III patients. Reliability of the quality-of-life battery was confirmed by significantly better life quality among New York Heart Association class I patients versus class II or III patients combined on the walk test, physical limitations, dyspnea, living with CHF, psychologic distress, and staff perceptions of patient health. In accordance with prior studies, the measures were uncorrelated with LVEF. By demonstrating strong internal consistencies, reliability based on physician reports, and independence of EF levels, use of this quality-of-life assessment battery in this and other clinical trials of compromised ventricular functioning is supported.

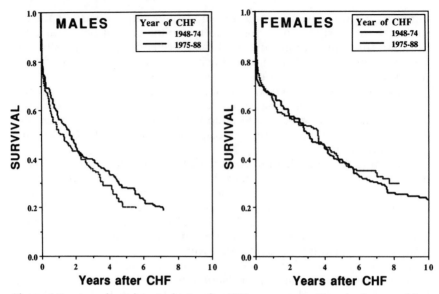

Figure 9-3. Age-adjusted survival rates after CHF was recognized by calendar year of first diagnosis of CHF for men and women developing CHF during the calendar years 1948 to 1988. Reproduced with permission from Ho et al.[18]

Survival (Framingham Study)

Ho and associates,[18] from Framingham, Mass, used proportional hazards models to evaluate the effects of selected clinical variables on survival after the onset of CHF in 652 members of the Framingham Heart Study. Fifty-one percent of these patients were men (mean age, 70 ± 11 years). The individuals studied developed CHF between 1948 and 1988. The subjects were older at the time of diagnosis of CHF in the later decades of the study. Median survival after the onset of CHF was 2 years in men and 3 years in women. Overall, 1-year and 5-year survival rates were 57% and 25% in men and 64% and 38% in women, respectively. Survival was better in women than in men, but mortality increased with advancing age in both sexes (Figure 9-3). Adjusting for age, there was no significant temporal change in the prognosis of CHF during the 40 years of observation. Thus, CHF remains a highly lethal disease with slightly better prognosis in women and younger individuals.

Prognostic Predictors

Saxon and associates,[19] from Los Angeles, Calif, retrospectively reviewed data on 528 consecutive patients hospitalized for treatment of advanced CHF (LVEF 0.2) and cardiac transplant evaluation, who were stabilized with medical therapy and discharged home. Predictors of CHF death or rehospitalization for urgent transplantation were identified using the Cox proportional hazards model. Within 1 year, 59 patients (11%) died suddenly and 70 (13%) died of CHF or required urgent transplantation. A serum sodium ≤134 mEq/L, PA diastolic pressure >19 mm Hg, LV diastolic dimension index >44 mm/m², peak oxygen consumption during exercise testing <11 mL/kg/min, and the presence of a permanent pace-maker were independent predictors of hemodynamic deterioration. In the absence of these risk factors, the risk of hemodynamic deterioration within 1 year from this study was only 2%. This risk increased to >50% in the presence of hyponatremia and any two additional risk factors. Thus, patients with advanced CHF at highest risk for progressive hemo-dynamic deterioration can be identified from clinical variables that could aid in triaging such patients to earlier cardiac transplantation.

Bittner and associates,[20] for the SOLVD investigators, studied the po-tential usefulness of the six-minute walk test, a self-paced submaximal exercise test, as a prognostic indicator in patients with LV dysfunction. Twenty tertiary care hospitals in the United States, Canada, and Belgium participated in the study. The participants in the study included a strati-fied random sample of 898 patients from the SOLVD Registry who had either radiologic evidence of CHF and/or an EF of 0.45 or less. The pa-tients were followed up for a mean of 242 days. During follow-up, 52 walk-test participants (6.2%) died and 252 (30.3%) were hospitalized. Hospitalization for CHF occurred in 78 participants (9.4%), and the com-bined endpoint of death or hospitalization for CHF occurred in 114 walk-test participants (13.7%). Compared with the highest performance level, patients in the lowest performance level had a significant greater chance of dying (10.23% v 2.99%), of being hospitalized (40.91% v 19.90%), and of being hospitalized for CHF (22.16% v 1.99%). In a logistic regres-sion model, EF and distance walked were equally strong and indepen-dent predictors of mortality and CHF hospitalization rates during follow-up. The six-minute walk test is a safe and simple clinical tool that strongly and independently predicts morbidity and mortality in patients with LV dysfunction.

TREATMENT

Digoxin + Diuretic

Although digoxin is a traditional therapy in CHF, there is still uncer-tainty regarding its efficacy in patients in sinus rhythm. Uretsky and associates,[21] from Pittsburgh, Pa, conducted a digoxin or placebo with-drawal study in a prospective randomized double-blind multicenter trial of patients with chronic stable, mild to moderate CHF secondary to left ventricular dysfunction. All patients were in normal sinus rhythm and were receiving long-term treatment with diuretic drugs and digoxin. Pa-tients withdrawn from digoxin showed worsened maximal exercise ca-pacity compared with that of patients who continued to receive digoxin. Patients withdrawn from digoxin therapy showed an increased incidence of treatment failures (39% v 19%) and a decreased time to treatment failure. In addition, patients who continued to receive digoxin had a lower body weight and heart rate and a higher LVEF. These data provide strong evidence for the clinical efficacy of digoxin in patients with nor-mal sinus rhythm and mild to moderate chronic CHF secondary to sys-tolic dysfunction who are treated with diuretics.

Ibopamine + Digoxin

Van Veldhuisen and associates[22] evaluated the effects of ibopamine and digoxin in patients with mild to moderate CHF. They studied 161 patients with mild to moderate CHF (80% in New York Heart Association function class II and 20% in class III) who were treated with ibopamine (n = 53), digoxin (n = 55), or placebo (n = 55) for 6 months. Background therapy consisted of furosemide, but all other drugs for CHF were excluded. Eighty percent of the patients completed the study. Compared with placebo, digoxin, but not ibopamine, significantly increased exercise time after 6 months. Ibopamine was only effective in patients with relatively preserved LV function. No patient receiving digoxin withdrew from the study because of progression of CHF compared with 6 patients receiving ibopamine and 2 receiving placebo. At 6 months, plasma norepinephrine was decreased with digoxin and ibopamine therapy but increased with placebo administration. Total mortality and ambulatory arrhythmias were not significantly affected by the two drugs. These authors concluded that ibopamine and digoxin both inhibit neurohumoral activation in patients with mild to moderate chronic CHF. However, digoxin was a more effective drug in improving exercise time, although ibopamine was helpful in patients with relatively preserved LV function. It is unclear from this study whether ibopamine has a role in the management of patients with CHF.

Captopril + Furosemide

McLay and associates,[23] from Dundee, Aberdeen, and Edinburgh, Scotland, examined the effects of conventional doses of oral captopril on the renal responses to oral furosemide in ambulant patients with stable chronic CHF. Twenty-five men (mean age, 63 years) were randomized to one of two groups. Group 1 received placebo on days 1 and 2 before furosemide. Group 2 received placebo on day 1 before furosemide and captopril thereafter (captopril before furosemide on day 2). Urine was collected after either placebo or captopril and after furosemide (taken after placebo or captopril pretreatment). Captopril by itself did not affect renal function. Captopril did, however, significantly affect the renal response to furosemide. The increase in urine flow rate after furosemide in group 2 was decreased from 225% with placebo to 128% with captopril. The increase in sodium excretion after furosemide was decreased from 623% with placebo to 242% with captopril. Pretreatment with captopril abolished the increase in creatinine clearance after furosemide. The increase in urinary albumin excretion (used as a marker of glomerular function) after furosemide was also significantly blunted by captopril. Conventional doses of captopril acutely inhibit the natriuretic and diuretic responses to furosemide at the glomerular level in ambulant patients with stable chronic heart failure.

Enalapril

Pouleur and associates[24] used LV function data and RV volumes obtained at baseline and after an average follow-up for 12 months in 42 patients with an LVEF of 35% or less. After baseline measurements, the patients were randomized to placebo (n = 16) or enalapril. In the placebo group, the changes in LV function were characterized by increases in end-diastolic and end-systolic volumes accompanied by a downward and rightward shift of the diastolic BP volume relation. Decrease in end-diastolic and end-systolic volumes accompanied by a slight upward and leftward shift of the diastolic pressure-volume relations were noted in the enalapril group. These changes in LV volumes were different between groups but were not attended by changes in LV end-diastolic BP. The changes in chamber stiffness constant β between baseline and follow-up were significantly different between placebo and enalapril group. Another index of chamber compliance also confirmed the presence of opposite changes in LV chamber compliance in the placebo group and in the enalapril group. The mean diastolic wall stress increased with placebo but not with enalapril, whereas LV mass and the indexes of LV sphericity tended to improve in the enalapril group. The changes in plasma levels of norepinephrine, atrial natriuretic peptide, and arginine vasopressin were, however, comparable in both groups. The data indicate that in patients with severe systolic LV dysfunction, the progressive LV dilatation was accompanied by a decrease in LV chamber stiffness. Enalapril therapy prevents or partially reverses these changes and reduces LV mass and LV sphericity.

Lisinopril

Gilbert and associates[25] evaluated the effects of an angiotensin converting enzyme inhibitor, lisinopril, on cardiac adrenergic drive in subjects with CHF. In a placebo-controlled, double-blind crossover study of 14 patients, they measured cardiac and systemic adrenergic drive, myocardial and lymphocyte β-adrenergic receptors, and hemodynamic changes at baseline and after 12 weeks of therapy. Relative to placebo, lisinopril therapy was associated with minimal, statistically insignificant changes in hemodynamics, a significant increase in myocardial β-adrenergic receptor density, no change in cardiac or systemic adrenergic drive, and no detectable change in lymphocyte β-receptor density. When subjects were rank ordered into groups with the highest and lowest coronary sinus norepinephrine levels, those with the highest norepinephrine values demonstrated significant decreases in central venous norepinephrine, coronary sinus norepinephrine, and an increase in myocardial β-receptor density relative to changes in placebo or relative to baseline values. Subjects with lower cardiac adrenergic drive exhibited no significant change in coronary sinus or systemic norepinephrine levels or in myocardial β-adrenergic receptor density. Therefore, the angiotensin converting enzyme inhibitor, lisinopril, lowered cardiac adrenergic drive and increased β-receptor density in subjects with increased cardiac adrenergic drive but had no effects on these variables in patients with normal cardiac adrenergic drive. The data indicate that cardiac antiadrenergic properties contribute to the efficacy of angiotensin converting enzyme inhibitors in patients with CHF.

Quinapril

ACE inhibitors have emerged as premier therapy in the management of patients with CHF. Pflugfelder and associates,[26] from London, United Kingdom, and Ottawa, Canada, reported on a multicenter trial designed to evaluate the efficacy, safety, and clinical consequences of abrupt cessation of quinapril in a placebo-controlled randomized double-blind withdrawal trial. After 10 or more weeks of single-blind quinapril therapy, 224 patients with New York Heart Association class II or III CHF were randomized in double-blind fashion to continue quinapril (n = 114) or to receive placebo (n = 110) for 16 weeks. Patients withdrawn to placebo had a significant deterioration in exercise tolerance versus quinapril. New York Heart Association functional class and quality of life were improved, and signs and symptoms of CHF were lessened in those remaining on quinapril therapy compared with those receiving placebo. Eighteen patients were withdrawn from the placebo group because of worsening CHF compared with 5 patients withdrawn from the quinapril treatment. Withdrawal from quinapril was associated with steady worsening of CHF beginning 4 to 6 weeks after randomization to placebo. These authors concluded that quinapril is an effective and safe drug for maintaining clinical stability in patients with moderate CHF. Withdrawal of quinapril resulted in a slow progressive decline in clinical status. This data supports the concept that the class of ACE inhibitors are similar in terms of their beneficial effects in CHF.

Losartan

Gottlieb and associates,[27] from Baltimore, Md; Rogaland, Norway; Berlin, Germany; New Brunswick, NJ; Detroit, Mich; Bronx, NY; and Brussels, Belgium, used losartan, a new specific angiotensin II receptor antagonist with no agonist properties, to study the consequences of angiotensin II blockade in patients with CHF. Patients were randomized to receive a single dose of placebo or varying doses of losartan in a double-blind sequential fashion. Hemodynamic and neurohormonal variables were measured periodically for 24 hours. Losartan caused vasodilatation in a dose-dependent manner. The reduction in mean arterial pressure and systemic vascular resistance increased up to a dose of 25 mg, but the higher 75 and 150 mg doses did not produce additional vasodilatation. In response to losartan, there were compensatory increases in both angiotensin II concentrations and plasma renin activity, which were greatest at the highest doses. Aldosterone concentrations were significantly lowered with losartan. Blockade of the angiotensin II receptor with the antagonist, losartan, causes vasodilator and neurohormonal effects in patients with CHF. Lack of additional vasodilator response with doses >25 mg suggests that neurohormonal activation might limit the efficacy of high doses of losartan.

Enoximone

Few options are available for patients with severe CHF that is unresponsive to therapy with digoxin, diuretics, and vasodilators. In an investigation by Dec and associates,[28] from Boston, Mass, clinical responses and predictors of survival were studied in 41 consecutive patients with New York Heart Association class IV CHF during long-term oral enoximone therapy (mean dose, 232 ± 15 mg/day). The mean age was 60 ± 1 years, and the initial LVEF was 0.19 ± 0.01. The cause of CHF was either CAD (n = 23) or dilated cardiomyopathy (n = 18). Symptomatic improvement occurred in the majority (83%) of patients; 24% improved ≥2 New York

Heart Association classes. Although the 12-month mortality rate for the entire group was high (54% ± 8%), a subgroup of patients with dilated cardiomyopathy achieved a sustained benefit with a decrease in symptoms >1 New York Heart Association class, fewer hospitalizations, and a survival rate at 24 months of 60%. Multivariate analysis identified the cause of CHF, LVEF, and clinical improvement within 60 days of enoximone therapy as predictors of a favorable long-term outcome. The presence of CAD was most predictive of early mortality, with only 5% of patients surviving >18 months compared with 66% of those with dilated cardiomyopathy. Median survival rates were 132 ± 31 and 921 ± 214 days for the CAD and dilated cardiomyopathy populations, respectively. Oral enoximone can provide symptomatic improvement and a palliative option for the majority of patients with refractory CHF resulting from cardiomyopathy.

Milrinone

Brecker and associates,[29] from London, United Kingdom, used M-mode echocardiography and Doppler to assess the effects of phosphodiesterase inhibition on subendocardial function in dilated cardiomyopathy, and in particular, to study interactions with both systolic and diastolic LV function. Twelve adult patients with dilated cardiomyopathy were studied (6 ischemic in origin and 6 idiopathic), 7 of whom were being considered for cardiac transplantation. Cardiac index increased without significant change in heart rate or BP. Longitudinal mitral ring motion, which had been uniformly reduced, increased markedly after intravenous milrinone. LV cavity size decreased, and shortening fraction, posterior wall thickness, and rates of posterior wall thickening and thinning increased markedly. LA pressure decreased, and isovolumic relaxation time increased. However, the peak velocity and duration of the transmitral E wave increased, with no change in the A wave. Improved longitudinal (subendocardial) function was reflected by improved posterior wall dynamics, and early filling, possibly by augmentation of restoring forces. Thus, severely reduced subendocardial function in dilated cardiomyopathy is potentially reversible, with marked effects on systolic and diastolic function. These previously unrecognized actions of milrinone provide further evidence to justify its short-term use in supporting the severely depressed myocardium.

Flosequinan

Flosequinan is a vasodilator and inotropic agent that has a distinctive mechanism. It works by inhibiting the inositol-triphosphate/protein kinase C pathway, which is an important mechanism of vasoconstriction. Packer and associates,[30] from New York, NY, evaluated 193 patients with CHF (New York Heart Association functional class 2 or 3 and LV EF <40%) receiving digoxin and diuretic drugs. These patients were randomly assigned in a double-blind manner to receive either 100 mg flosequinan daily or placebo in the REFLECT Study. After 12 weeks, maximal treadmill exercise time increased by 96 seconds in the flosequinan group but by only 47 seconds in the placebo group (p = .02). Symptomatically, 55% of patients receiving flosequinan benefitted as compared with 36% in the placebo group. Fewer patients in the flosequinan treated group required a change in medication or withdrawal from the study. By intention to treat, 7 patients died in the flosequinan treated group compared with 2 patients in the placebo treated group. These authors concluded that flosequinan appeared to be helpful in the short-time therapy of patients with CHF. A subsequent as yet unpublished study with flosequinan in a mortality trial, showed that flosequinan increased mortality at a dose of 100 mg, and the drug was subsequently withdrawn from the market. It is unclear, however, whether lower doses of the drug might have had hemodynamic benefit without adverse effects on mortality.

Massie and associates,[31] from San Francisco, Calif, determined whether oral flosequinan, a new direct-acting arterial and venous vasodilator with possible dose-dependent positive inotropic effects, improves exercise tolerance and quality of life. In a randomized, double-blind multicenter trial, 322 patients with predominantly New York Heart Association class II or III CHF and LVEFs of 35% or less stabilized on a diuretic, angiotensin converting enzyme inhibitor and digoxin were treated with 100 mg flosequinan once daily, 75 mg flosequinan twice daily, or matching placebo. Efficacy was determined with serial measurements of treadmill exercise time, responses to the Minnesota Living With Heart Failure Questionnaire, and clinical assessments during a baseline phase and increment in median exercise time compared with placebo. Flosequinan (100 mg once daily) given for 16 weeks improved the Living With Heart Failure criteria significantly compared with placebo. Flosequinan (100 mg) increased median exercise time. Most clinical assessments tended to improve on active therapy. These results indicate that additional symptomatic benefit can be attained by adding flosequinan to a therapeutic regimen already including a converting enzyme inhibitor and digoxin. Because most patients may fall into this category in the future, flosequinan is a potential adjunctive agent in the management of severe CHF.

Propranolol v Metoprolol

Haber and associates,[32] from Charlottesville, Va, evaluated the acute hemodynamic effects of β-adrenergic blockade on systolic and diastolic LV function and ventriculo-arterial coupling in patients with CHF. Isolated myocardium from patients with CHF is known to show a downregulation of β_2-receptors, and these authors hypothesized that nonselective β-adrenergic blockade would have greater negative inotropic effects than β_1 blockade in patients with CHF. Patients with clinical evidence of CHF (n = 24) and control patients without CHF (n = 24) were given either the nonselective β-blocker, propranolol, or the β-selective blocker, metoprolol. LV pressure-volume relations were obtained before and after the administration of intravenous β-blocker, and measures of LV systolic and diastolic function were examined. Patients with CHF had a deterioration of LV systolic function with a fall in LV systolic pressure, cardiac index, dP/dt, and end-systolic elastance. There was deterioration of active LV relaxation but no change in passive LV diastolic function. Control patients had no change in these same variables. The effects of propranolol as compared with metoprolol on these hemodynamic variables in patients with CHF were similar. Therefore, these data do not support a greater in vivo physiologic role of the myocardial β_2-receptor in CHF.

The preservation of passive diastolic function and ventriculo-arterial coupling provide possible explanations for why β-adrenergic blockade is tolerated by patients with CHF.

Magnesium Chloride

Magnesium deficiency frequently develops in patients with CHF and may increase susceptibility to lethal arrhythmias and sudden death via multiple pathophysiologic mechanisms. Bashir and associates,[33] from London, United Kingdom, investigated the effects of peroral magnesium supplementation in a randomized, double-blind, crossover trial involving 21 patients with stable CHF secondary to CAD. All were receiving long-term loop diuretics and had normal renal function and low or normal serum magnesium concentrations. Subjects alternately received enteric-coated magnesium chloride (16 mmol magnesium per day) and placebo for 6 weeks. Magnesium therapy increased serum magnesium from 0.87 to 0.92 mmol/L, serum potassium from 4.0 to 4.3 mmol/L, and urinary magnesium excretion from 2.8 to 4.7 mmol/24 hours. There was no significant change in heart rate or Doppler cardiac index, but mean arterial pressure decreased from 91 to 87 mm Hg and systemic vascular resistance from 1,698 to 1,613 dynes s cm^{-5}. The frequency of isolated VPCs was reduced by 23%, couplets by 52%, and nonsustained VT episodes by 24%. Plasma epinephrine decreased from 447 to 184 pg/mL, but there was no corresponding change in plasma norepinephrine or heart rate variability. Gastrointestinal adverse effects were reported by 6 patients, necessitating withdrawal in 2 cases. In conclusion, magnesium supplementation reduced the frequency of asymptomatic ventricular arrhythmias, possibly due to secondary changes in potassium homeostasis, and produced a minor degree of vasodilation.

References

1. Rodeheffer RJ, Jacobsen SJ, Gersh BJ, et al: The incidence and prevalence of congestive heart failure in Rochester, Minnesota. Mayo Clin Proc 1993 (Dec);68:1143–1150.
2. Weingarten SR, Riedinger MS, Shinbane J, et al: Triage practice guideline for patients hospitalized with congestive heart failure. Am J Med 1993 (May);94:483–490.
3. Butman SM, Gordon AE, Standen JR, et al: Bedside cardiovascular examination in patients with severe chronic heart failure: Importance of rest or inducible jugular venous distension. J Am Coll Cardiol 1993 (Oct);22:968–974.
4. Feld H, Priest S: A cyclic breathing pattern in patients with poor left ventricular function and compensated heart failure: A mild form of cheyne-stokes respiration? J Am Coll Cardiol 1993 (March 15);21:971–974.
5. Middlekauff HR, Stevenson WG, Stevenson LW, et al: Syncope in advanced heart failure: High risk of sudden death regardless of origin of syncope. J Am Coll Cardiol 1993 (Jan);21:110–116.
6. Wilson JR, Mancini DM, Dunkman WB: Exertional fatigue due to skeletal muscle dysfunction in patients with heart failure. Circulation 1993 (Feb); 87:470–475.

7. Lerman A, Gibbons RJ, Rodeheffer RJ, et al: Circulating N-terminal atrial natriuretic peptide as a marker for symptomless left-ventricular dysfunction. Lancet 1993 (May 1);341:1105–1109.

8. Ungerer M, Böhm M, Elce JS, et al: Altered expression of β-adrenergic receptor kinase and $β_1$-adrenergic receptors in the failing human heart. Circulation 1993 (Feb);87:454–463.

9. Townend JN, Virk SJS, Qiang FX, et al: Lymphocyte beta adrenoceptor upregulation and improved cardiac response to adrenergic stimulation following converting enzyme inhibition in congestive heart failure. Euro Heart J 1993 (Feb);14:243–250.

10. Raynolds MV, Bristow MR, Bush EW, et al: Angiotensin-converting enzyme DD genotype in patients with ischemic cardiomyopathy or idiopathic dilated cardiomyopathy. Lancet 1993 (Oct 30);342:1073–1075.

11. Adamopoulos S, Coats AJS, Urunotte F, et al: Physical training improves skeletal muscle metabolism in patients with chronic heart failure. J Am Coll Cardiol 1993 (April);21:1101–1106.

12. Oka RK, Stotts NA, Dae MW, et al: Daily physical activity levels in congestive heart failure. Am J Cardiol 1993 (April 15);71:921–925.

13. Kestin AS, Ellis PA, Barnard MR, et al: Effect of strenuous exercise on platelet activation state and reactivity. Circulation 1993 (Oct);88[part 1]:1502–1511.

14. Katz SD, Marantz PR, Biasucoi L, et al: Low incidence of stroke in ambulatory patients with heart failure: A prospective study. Am Heart J 1993 (July);126:141–146.

15. Katz SD, Schwarz M, Yuen J, et al: Impaired acetylcholine-mediated vasodilation in patients with congestive heart failure. Role of endothelium-derived vasodilating and vasoconstricting factors. Circulation 1993 (July);88:55–61.

16. Porter TR, Taylor DO, Cycan A, et al: Endothelium-dependent pulmonary artery responses in chronic heart failure: Influence of pulmonary hypertension. J Am Coll Cardiol 1993 (Nov 1);22:1418–1424.

17. Gorkin L, Norvell NK, Rosen RC, et al, for the SOLVD Investigators: Assessment of quality of life as observed from the baseline data of the studies of left ventricular dysfunction (SOLVD) trial quality-of-life substudy. Am J Cardiol 1993 (May 1);71:1069–1073.

18. Ho KKL, Anderson KM, Kannel WB, et al: Survival after the onset of congestive heart failure in Framingham Heart Study subjects. Circulation 1993 (July);88:107–115.

19. Saxon LA, Stevenson WG, Middlekauff HR, et al: Predicting death from progressive heart failure secondary to ischemic or idiopathic dilated cardiomyopathy. Am J Cardiol 1993 (July 1);72:62–65.

20. Bittner V, Weiner DH, Yusuf S, et al: Prediction of mortality and morbidity with a 6-minute walk test in patients with congestive heart failure. JAMA 1993 (Oct 13);270:1702–1707.

21. Uretsky BF, Young JB, Shahidi E, et al, on behalf of the PROVED Investigative Group: Randomized study assessing the effect of digoxin withdrawal in patients with mild to moderate chronic congestive heart failure: Results of the PROVED trial. J Am Coll Cardiol 1993 (Oct);22:955–962.

22. Van Veldhuisen DJ, Veld AJM, Dunselman PHJM, et al, on behalf of the DIMT Study Group: Double-blind placebo-controlled study of ibopamine and digoxin in patients with mild to moderate heart failure: Results of the Dutch ibopamine multicenter trial (DMIT). J Am Coll Cardiol 1993 (Nov 15);22:1564–1573.

23. McLay JS, McMurray JJ, Bridges AB, et al: Acute effects of captopril on the renal actions of furosemide in patients with chronic heart failure. Am Heart J 1993 (Oct);126:879–886.

24. Pouleur H, Rousseau MF, van Eyll C, et al, for the SOLVD Investigators: Effects of long-term enalapril therapy on left ventricular diastolic properties in

patients with depressed ejection fraction. Circulation 1993 (Aug);88:481–491.

25. Gilbert EM, Sandoval A, Larrabee P, et al: Lisinopril lowers cardiac adrenergic drive and increases β-receptor density in the failing human heart. Circulation 1993 (Aug);88:472–480.

26. Pflugfelder PW, Baird MG, Tonkon MJ, et al, for the Quinapril Heart Failure Trial Investigators: Clinical consequences of angiotensin converting enzyme inhibitor withdrawal in chronic heart failure: A double-blind, placebo-controlled study of quinapril. J Am Coll Cardiol 1993 (Nov 15);22:1557–1563.

27. Gottlieb SS, Dickstein K, Fleck E, et al: Hemodynamic and neurohormonal effects of the angiotensin II antagonist losartan in patients with congestive heart failure. Circulation 1993 (Oct);88[part 1]:1602–1609.

28. Dec GW, Fifer MA, Herrmann HC, et al: Long-term outcome of enoximone therapy in patients with refractory heart failure. Am Heart J 1993 (Feb); 125:423–429.

29. Brecker SJD, Xiao HB, Mbaissouroum M, et al: Effects of intravenous milrinone on left ventricular function in ischemic and idiopathic dilated cardiomyopathy. Am J Cardiol 1993 (Jan 15);71:203–209.

30. Packer M, Narahara KA, Elkayam U, et al, and the principal investigators of the REFLECT study: Double-blind, placebo-controlled study of the efficacy of flosequinan in patients with chronic heart failure. J Am Coll Cardiol 1993 (July);22:65–72.

31. Massie BM, Berk MR, Brozena SC, et al, for the FACET investigators: Can further benefit be achieved by adding flosequinan to patients with congestive heart failure who remain symptomatic on diuretic, digoxin, and an angiotensin converting enzyme inhibitor? Results of the Flosequinan-ACE Inhibitor Trial (FACET). Circulation 1993 (Aug);88:492–501.

32. Haber HL, Simek CL, Gimple LW, et al: Why do patients with congestive heart failure tolerate the initiation of β-blocker therapy? Circulation 1993 (Oct);88[part 1]:1610–1619.

33. Bashir Y, Sneddon JF, Staunton HA, et al: Effects of long-term oral magnesium chloride replacement in congestive heart failure secondary to coronary artery disease. Am J Cardiol 1993 (Nov 15);12:1156–1162.

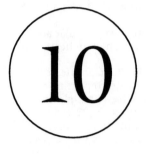

Miscellaneous Topics

Etiology of Effusions

To determine the effectiveness of the preoperative evaluation and over-all diagnostic efficacy of subxiphoid pericardial biopsy with fluid drainage in patients with new, large pericardial effusions, Corey and associates,[1] from Durham, NC, studied 57 of 75 consecutive patients hospitalized with new, large pericardial effusions studied over a 20-month period. Each patient was assessed by a comprehensive preoperative evaluation followed by subxiphoid pericardiotomy. The patients' tissue and fluid samples were studied pathologically and cultured for aerobic and anaerobic bacteria, fungi, mycobacteria, mycoplasmas, and viruses. A diagnosis was made in 53 patients (93%). The principal diagnoses consisted of malignancy in 13 patients (23%); viral infection in 8 patients (14%); radiation-induced inflammation in 8 patients (14%); collagen-vascular disease in 7 patients (12%); and uremia in 7 patients (12%) (Table 10-1). No diagnosis was made in 4 patients (7%). A variety of un-expected organisms were cultured from either pericardial fluid or tissue: cytomegalovirus (3 patients), *Mycoplasma pneumoniae* (2 patients), herpes simplex virus (1 patient), *Mycobacterium avium-intracellulare* (1 patient), and *Mycobacterium chelonei* (1 patient). The pericardial fluid yielded a diagnosis in 15 patients (26%), 11 of whom had malignant effusions. The examination of pericardial tissue was useful in the diagnosis of 13 patients (23%), 8 of whom had an infectious agent cultured. Of the 57 patients undergoing surgery, the combined diagnostic yield from both fluid and tissue was 19 patients (33%). Therefore, a systematic preoperative

Table 10-1. Primary Diagnoses. Reproduced with permission from Corey et al.[1]

Etiology	Definite	Probable	Possible	Total	% of 57 Patients
Malignancy	11	0	2	13	23
Viral	4	4	0	8	14
Radiation	0	5	3	8	14
Collagen-vascular disease	4	3	0	7	12
Uremic	0	7	0	7	12
Mycobacterial	2	0	2	4	7
Mycoplasma	2	0	0	2	4
Bacterial	0	1	0	1	2
Idiopathic	0	0	0	4	7
Other[†]	0	3	2	5	9
Total	23	23	9	59*	104

*Two patients had two definite diagnoses.
†Drug-induced and sympathetic.

evaluation in conjunction with fluid and tissue analysis following subxiphoid pericardiotomy yields a diagnosis in most patients with large pericardial effusions. This approach may also result in the culturing of "unusual" infectious organisms from pericardial tissue and fluid.

Percutaneous Balloon Pericardiotomy

Pericardial effusion and tamponade are complications of malignant disease. Generally such patients are poor candidates for surgical pericardiotomy because their life expectancy may be limited, and they are frequently quite ill. Ziskind and associates[2] described a percutaneous balloon pericardiotomy technique in 50 patients as part of a multicenter registry. Thirty-six patients had cardiac tamponade, and 14 patients had a moderate to large pericardial effusion. The technique involved entering the pericardium from a standard subxiphoid approach with an 18-gauge pericardial needle following appropriate local anesthesia. A .035 inch J tip guide wire was advanced into the pericardial space and the needle removed. Following dilation with an 8 French dilator, an 8 French pigtail or straight side hole catheter was advanced into the pericardial space. Pressures were measured and fluid removed for appropriate studies. Dye (20 mL) was then injected and an extra stiff J tip guide wire advanced into the pericardial space so that it was looped. The pericardial catheter was removed and the track dilated with a 10 French dilator. Following this a 20 mm wide, 3 cm long dilating balloon (Mansfield) containing radiographic contrast medium was advanced over the guide wire to straddle the pericardial border. Gentle inflation of the balloon was used to locate the pericardial margin. After this, the balloon was inflated to create the window. After dilation the balloon was removed and the pericardial catheter replaced over the wire. The procedure was considered successful in 46 out of 50 patients with a mean follow-up of 3½ months. Complications included the necessity for an operation in 2, bleeding from a pericardial vessel in 1, and persistent pericardial catheter drainage in 1. Two patients required a late operation for recurrent tamponade. Minor complications occurred in 6 of the first 37 patients who had fever.

Subsequently, prophylactic antibiotics were instituted. Thoracentesis or chest tube placement were required in 8, and a small resolving pneumothorax occurred in 2 patients. Despite short-term success, the long-term prognosis of the 44 patients with malignant disease was poor with a mean survival time of 3 1/3 months. Because life expectancy is limited in these patients with malignant disease, a less invasive procedure such as percutaneous balloon pericardiotomy may be better than surgery. More experience, however, and a longer follow-up is required to further clarify the role of this new technique.

Constriction

Patients with constrictive pericarditis usually require pericardiectomy to relieve their symptoms. In some patients, however, constrictive pericarditis may resolve spontaneously or with medical treatment. Oh and associates,[3] from Rochester, Minn, described 4 patients with transient constrictive pericarditis. Although the cause of pericarditis differed, all patients had a small to large amount of pericardial effusion, followed by symptoms, signs, and Doppler features typical of constrictive pericarditis. Symptomatic improvement occurred after treatment with some combination of nonsteroidal anti-inflammatory agents, corticosteroids, and antibiotics. The resolution of the symptoms paralleled the normalization of characteristic respiratory changes in Doppler flow velocities. The condition of the patients most likely was related to a transient inflammation (or thickening) of the pericardium due to viral, bacterial, or immunologically mediated pericarditis. Resolution of the thickened pericardium was documented by magnetic resonance imaging in one patient. Awareness of the possible transient nature of constrictive pericarditis in a subgroup of patients with constriction has important clinical implications when pericardiectomy is considered. The resolution of constrictive pericarditis can be documented by serial Doppler echocardiographic examination.

CARDIAC AND/OR PULMONARY TRANSPLANTATION

Trends in Patient Selection

Heart transplantation is a well-established treatment for patients with end-stage heart failure. The 5-year survival rate for heart transplant recipients is approximately 70% to 80% in contrast to the 20% to 30% survival rate for a comparable group of patients with severe heart failure. In a single center, Kubo and associates,[4] from Minneapolis, Minn, reviewed specific outcomes of patient referrals and the utility of selection criteria for heart transplantation, and assessed these trends over a 5-year period. They retrospectively reviewed 511 consecutive referrals of adult patients with heart failure from Jan 1, 1987 to Dec 31, 1991. Patients were followed up to one of five endpoints: (1) acceptance onto the transplant waiting list, (2) rejection from the transplant waiting list, (3) death, (4) referral to another program, and (5) still pending evaluation. Of the 511 referred patients, 43% were accepted onto the waiting list, 43% were rejected, 8% died before the evaluation was completed, 3% were referred to another program, and 3% were still pending evaluation. There were no consistent trends in the acceptance/rejection ratio over the 5-year period. Of the 221 patients accepted onto the waiting list, 52% underwent transplantation, 22% died, 5% were removed from the list because of clinical improvement, 4% were referred to another program, and 16% were still on the waiting list. The progressive shortage of donor organs resulted in an increase in the size of the waiting list from 12.6 patients in 1987 to 36.5 in 1991. There was also an increase in the time on the waiting list before transplantation. Over 5 years, 50 patients were considered "too well" for transplantation. Of these 50 patients, 86% were alive, and 7 were lost to follow-up during a mean period of 29 months. All 12 patients taken off the active transplant list because of improvement in symptoms, EF, or exercise, were alive with a mean follow-up period of 28 months. These authors confirmed that transplant referrals are a selected group of patients with a high mortality rate. Eight percent died before evaluation could be completed, and 22% died waiting for a suitable donor organ. Furthermore, patient selection criteria can identify a small subset of patients with a low mortality risk who have a reasonably good prognosis. These data also highlight the implications of decreasing donor hearts and a longer waiting list for transplant.

Transesophageal Echocardiography in Donor Screening

Transthoracic echocardiography has played a useful role in the screening of cardiac transplant donors. However, transthoracic echocardiograms may be suboptimal in many patients on ventilators. The role of transesophageal echocardiography in cardiac donor screening is unknown. Therefore, Stoddard and Longaker,[5] from Louisville, Ky, compared the potential benefit of transesophageal echocardiography combined with transthoracic echocardiography in 24 (16 men and 8 women) consecutive brain-dead patients with a mean age of 29 ± 9 years (range, 16 to 44 years), who were being considered as cardiac transplant donors. Transthoracic echocardiography was performed immediately before or after transesophageal echocardiography. Transthoracic echocardiography was technically difficult in 7 of 24 patients (29%). Results of transesophageal echocardiography were abnormal in 5 of the 7 patients and demonstrated LV (n = 4) and RV (n = 3) wall-motion abnormalities and concentric LV hypertrophy (n = 2). The 4 patients with wall-motion abnormalities were eliminated as potential donors. In 16 of 17 patients with technically adequate transthoracic echocardiograms, transesophageal and transthoracic echocardiographic findings agreed and demonstrated normal hearts in 13 patients, LV (n = 2) and RV (n = 1) ventricular wall-motion abnormalities in 2 patients, and isolated concentric LV hypertrophy in 1 patient. In 1 of the 17 patients with a technically adequate transthoracic echocardiographic study, a bicuspid aortic valve was demonstrated by transesophageal echocardiography but not diagnosed by transthoracic echocardiography. Overall, 7 patients were eliminated as cardiac donors on the basis of transesophageal echocardiograms (n = 7), transthoracic echocardiograms (n = 2), or both. The yield of abnormal echocardiographic studies was higher with transesophageal echocardiography (9 of 24 patients) as compared with transthoracic echocardiography (3 of 24 patients). Direct surgical inspection, postmortem examination, or both confirmed the transesophageal echocardiographic findings. Fourteen of

17 cardiac recipients (82%) survived surgery and were discharged. Two cardiac recipients died intraoperatively, and 1 patient died postoperatively. Transesophageal echocardiography is a useful adjunct to transthoracic echocardiography in the screening of potential cardiac donors and may eliminate the need for alternative methods such as cardiac catheterization or direct surgical inspection when transthoracic echocardiograms are technically inadequate.

Effects of Pulmonary Arterial Pressure on Operative Survival

In an investigation by Murali and associates,[6] from Pittsburgh, Pa, the influence of preoperative transpulmonary pressure gradient and pulmonary vascular resistance on early post-transplant mortality was evaluated in 425 orthotopic transplant recipients. The overall 30-day post-transplant mortality rate was 13%; the majority of the deaths (53%) were due to primary allograft failure. The 0 to 2 day mortality rate was 3-fold higher in patients with severe preoperative pulmonary hypertension (transpulmonary pressure gradient ≥15 mm Hg), whereas the 3 to 7 day and 8 to 30 day mortality rates were similar. Early post-transplant mortality (0 to 2 days and 8 to 30 days) was also significantly higher (16% v 3.9% and 9.9% v 2.8%, respectively) in women compared with men. Women with severe preoperative pulmonary hypertension had higher 0 to 2 day post-transplant mortality than comparable men. According to univariate analysis, recipients with preoperative transpulmonary pressure gradient ≥15 mm Hg had a significantly higher 30-day postoperative mortality rate, irrespective of their level of pulmonary vascular resistance. Furthermore, patients with severe preoperative pulmonary hypertension who underwent transplantation between 1980 and 1987 had a higher 0 to 2 day post-transplant mortality rate compared with patients operated on after that time. Multiple logistic regression analysis identified female recipient sex and preoperative transpulmonary pressure gradient but not preoperative pulmonary vascular resistance, era of transplantation, or recipient age as significant independent predictors of early post-transplant mortality.

Lung and Heart-Lung Transplantation

Griffith and associates,[7] from Pittsburgh, Pa, reviewed their experience with lung transplantation at the University of Pittsburgh from March 1982 to December 1992, including heart-lung, double lung, and single lung. Heart-lung was the most commonly performed operation followed by double lung and single lung. Major indications included primary pulmonary hypertension, obstructive lung disease, Eisenmenger's syndrome, cystic fibrosis, and retransplantation. Since May 1991, 115 procedures have been performed and heart-lung transplantation has decreased from 61% to 15% of the cases with a corresponding doubling in double lung from 24% to 43% and single lung from 15% to 42%. The 1-, 2-, and 5-year survival rates in all 232 recipients were 61%, 55%, and 44%, respectively. The actuarial survival rate was significantly better for those 107 recent recipients compared with the 125 early recipients (70% v 61%). Overall, the 63 single (70%) and 74 double (65%) lung procedures were more successful than heart-lung transplantation (53%).

Table 10-2. 106 Deaths Among 232 Lung Transplants (May 1982 to December 1992). Reproduced with permission from Griffith et al.[7]

Infection	40
Allograft dysfunction	23
Obliterative bronchiolitis	13
Bleeding	10
Technical	6
Lymphoma	4
Acute rejection	3
Diaphragm paralysis	2
Multisystem failure	2
Stroke	2
Liver failure	1
Airway dehiscence	1

Recently, however, lung transplantation has been associated with an improvement in the survival rate from 48% to 72%. The survival rate has also improved from 53% to 77% for single lung transplant recipients. The causes of death in 106 recipients included infection, early allograft dysfunction, obliterative bronchiolitis, and inoperative bleeding (Table 10-2). Poor outcomes also included technical problems, lymphoma, acute rejection, diaphragmatic paralysis, multisystem organ failure, liver failure, and airway dehiscence. These authors concluded that the long-term outlook for lung transplant recipients has improved. There appears to be significant conservation of organs with single lung and double lung transplantation, finding greater acceptance for diseases once exclusively treated by heart-lung transplantation alone. The improved long-term outlook will be dependent upon better treatment for chronic rejection of the airways that histologically is defined by obliterative bronchiolitis.

Coronary Arteries Afterwards and Effects of Diltiazem

In an investigation carried out by Pflugfelder and associates,[8] from London, Canada, intracoronary ultrasonographic imaging was performed in 60 patients 0.3 to 9 years (mean, 2.9 ± 1.9) after heart transplantation. By using a 1.8 mm intravascular ultrasonographic catheter, 192 (80%) of 240 angiographically visualized major epicardial coronary arteries (right, LM, LAD, and LC) were imaged by ultrasonography. Coronary luminal irregularities were detected in 15% of arteries by angiography compared with 34% by ultrasonography. The typical abnormality detected by ultrasonography consisted of crescentic and/or concentric intimal and medial thickening. Calcification in vascular lesions was rare (<1% of arteries studied). Although the prevalence of angiographic abnormalities tended to be time dependent, ultrasonographic abnormalities were more strongly associated with donor age (normal, 22 ± 8 years v abnormal, 33 ± 10 years). Cardiac allograft CAD is significantly underestimated by contrast angiography. Intravascular ultrasonography provides a useful adjunct for identification and serial follow-up of this significant problem.

Percutaneous coronary angioscopy and intravascular ultrasound are sensitive intravascular imaging methods for detecting early changes in coronary morphology in cardiac transplant recipients. To compare the two imaging modalities, Ventura and associates,[9] from New Orleans, La, studied 29 consecutive cardiac transplant recipients with percutaneous coronary angioscopy and intravascular ultrasound during annual coronary angiography. Surface morphology, presence of plaque, and percent area stenosis were determined with each procedure. Percutaneous coronary angioscopy was more sensitive in detecting the presence of plaque and stenosis than was coronary angiography (plaque, 79% v 10%; stenosis, 24% v 3%). Intravascular ultrasound was also more sensitive in detecting plaque (76% v 10%) and stenosis (45% v 3%) than was coronary angiography. Although both angioscopy and ultrasound identified atherosclerotic plaque, only percutaneous coronary angioscopy could show luminal surface morphology and pigmentation of the plaque. Conversely, ultrasound could detect calcification and presence of intimal thickening and was more accurate in assessing the severity of stenosis (45% v 24%). In conclusion, percutaneous coronary angioscopy and intravascular ultrasound, in conjunction, provide information not only regarding the appearance of the luminal surface but also quantitative information regarding the structure and extent of the disease in the coronary artery wall.

Accelerated CAD is a major cause of late morbidity and mortality among heart transplant recipients. Because calcium antagonist can suppress diet-induced atherosclerosis in laboratory animals, Schroeder and associates,[10] from Stanford, Calif, assessed the efficacy of diltiazem in preventing CAD in transplanted hearts. Consecutive eligible cardiac transplant recipients were randomly assigned to receive diltiazem (n = 52) or no calcium antagonist (n = 54). Coronary angiograms obtained early after cardiac transplantation and annually thereafter were used for the visual assessment of the extent of CAD. The average diameters of identical coronary artery segments were measured on the angiograms obtained at baseline at the first and second follow-up examinations. In the 57 patients who had all three angiograms, the average coronary artery diameter (± SD) decreased in the group that received no calcium-channel blocker from 2.41 ± 0.3 mm at baseline to 2.2 ± 0.3 mm at one year and to 2.2 ± 0.3 mm at 2 years (P <0.001 for both years). The average diameter of the diltiazem group changed little from the baseline value of 2.3 ± 0.2 mm (2.3 ± 0.3 mm at one year and 2.4 ± 0.2 mm at 2 years). The average change in the diameter of the segment differed significantly between the two treatment groups, and the estimated effect of treatment changed only negligibly after adjustment for other relevant clinical variables. New angiographic evidence of CAD developed in 14 patients not given diltiazem, as compared with 5 diltiazem-treated patients (Figure 10-1). Coronary stenoses >50% of the luminal diameter developed in 7 patients not given diltiazem, as compared with 2 patients given diltiazem; death due to CAD or retransplantation occurred in 5 patients in the group that did not receive calcium-channel blockers and in none of those who received diltiazem. These authors preliminary results suggest that diltiazem can prevent the usual reduction in the diameter of the coronary artery in cardiac transplant recipients.

Immunosuppression Without Prednisone

Livi and associates,[11] from Padova, Italy, analyzed results of 112 operative survivors of heart transplantation between January 1987 and September

1991, and all patients were treated initially only with cyclosporin A and azathioprine without prednisone. Eighty-eight patients (79%) remained on a regimen of double therapy for a mean follow-up of 25 ± 15 months (range, 1 to 54 months), whereas 24 patients (21%) had oral prednisone, 5 mg/day, added to maintenance therapy for persistent or repeated rejection. There were 5 early deaths (4%) because of acute rejection (4 patients) or infection (1 patient). Only 1 patient died late after heart transplantation of chronic rejection. Actuarial survival was 95% ± 2% and 94% ± 3% at 12 and 48 months, respectively. Mean rate of acute rejection was 1.7 ± 1.0 episodes per patient, with a 5% ± 2% freedom from rejection at 48 months. Ten patients (9%) required in-hospital treatment for infection; the actuarial freedom from infectious episodes was 85% ± 4% at 48 months. Actuarial freedom from hypertension was 43% ± 7% at 48 months. At annual catheterization, mean LVEF was 0.64 ± 0.08 and 0.62 ± 0.05 at 1 year and 4 years, respectively, with evidence of coronary lesions in 9 patients (8%). Thus, steroid-free immunosuppression after heart transplantation is associated with a high incidence of acute rejection. However, the excellent medium-term survival and the

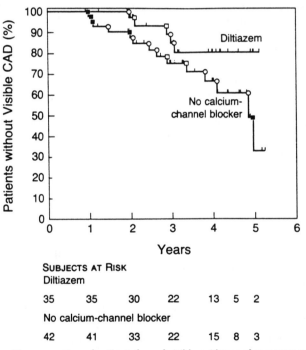

Figure 10-1. The proportion of patients free of visible evidence of coronary artery disease (CAD) after transplantation. The P value for the chi-square statistic derived from a Mantel-Haenszel log-rank test for the equality of survival curves is 0.082. Patients in whom any new evidence of coronary artery disease appeared without the development of stenosis of >50% are represented by open circles; patients with initial evidence of coronary artery disease in whom stenosis of >50% subsequently developed without death or retransplantation, open squares; and patients with initial stenosis of >50% and later death or retransplantation due to coronary artery disease, solid squares. The numbers at the bottom of the figure are the numbers of patients at risk in each group. Reproduced with permission from Schroeder et al.[10]

low incidence of both infection and chronic rejection seem to justify a wider use of such treatment.

Gastrointestinal Cytomegalovirus Infection Afterwards

Cytomegalovirus (CMV) infection of the upper gastrointestinal tract is a major cause of morbidity in heart transplant recipients. Arabia and associates,[12] from Tucson, Ariz, analyzed data since April 1985 on 201 patients who had undergone heart transplantation at their institution. Immunosuppressive therapy was with a triple drug regimen of cyclosporin A, prednisone, and azathioprine. Fifty-three of these patients had upper gastrointestinal symptoms, which primarily consisted of abdominal pain or nausea and vomiting despite prophylactic treatment with antacids, H_2 blockers, or both. A total of 79 esophagogastroduodenoscopies were performed in this group; 15 patients required more than one esophagogastroduodenoscopy for recurrent symptoms. Of these 53 patients with persistent gastrointestinal symptoms, 16 (30.2%) had diffuse erythema or ulceration of the gastric mucosa (14), esophagus (1), and duodenum (1) with biopsy results that were positive for CMV on viral cultures (incidence, 8%). All patients with positive biopsy results were treated with intravenous ganciclovir at a dose of 10 mg · kg^{-1} · day^{-1} in two divided doses for a period of 2 weeks. Recurrence developed in 6 patients (37.5%) and necessitated repeat therapy with ganciclovir. None of the 16 patients died as a result of gastrointestinal CMV infection. Patients who were seronegative for CMV and received a seropositive heart experienced earlier clinical manifestation of CMV infection. Infection of the upper gastrointestinal tract with CMV is a major cause of morbidity in cardiac transplant patients that may progress to a life-threatening complication if left untreated. Early diagnosis with esophagogastroduodenoscopy and biopsy for viral cultures is essential for documentation and proper management.

Non-Hodgkin's Lymphoma Afterwards

Organ transplant recipients receive immunosuppressive drugs to prevent graft rejection. This treatment has been associated with higher rates of non-Hodgkin lymphoma than in the general population. Opelz and Henderson,[13] for the Collaborative Transplant study, assessed the incidence of non-Hodgkin lymphoma in a multicenter study of 45,141 kidney transplant patients and 7,634 heart transplant recipients. The non-Hodgkin lymphoma rate was especially high during the first post-transplant year among both kidney transplant (101 cases v 2.7 expected in general population; 224 per 10^5) and heart transplant recipients (93 v 0.6 expected; 1,218 per 10^5). The incidence was lower in subsequent years (43 and 371 per 10^5 in kidney and heart transplant recipients). During the first year, the non-Hodgkin lymphoma incidence was higher in North America than in Europe (relative risk, 1.12). There were also significant increases in risk for patients who received rejection prophylaxis with antilymphocyte antibodies (1.80 [1.31–2.46]) and in those who received both cyclosporin and azathioprine rather than another immunosuppressive combination (1.47 [1.03–2.08]). This study quantified the risk of non-Hodgkin lymphoma after kidney or heart transplantation. It suggests that the risk of non-Hodgkin lymphoma is related to the aggressiveness of the immunosuppressive regimen.

Osteoporosis Afterwards

Shane and associates,[14] from New York, NY, determined the prevalence of osteopenia and fractures in 40 adult patients that had received a cardiac transplant between 1982 and 1990 and who were receiving immunosuppressive therapy with prednisone and cyclosporine A. Bone densitometric measurements by dual-energy x-ray absorptiometry of the lumbar spine and femoral neck and radiographs of the thoracic and lumbar spine were obtained for all patients. Routine serum and urine biochemical values as well as more specialized biochemical analyses (intact parathyroid hormone, metabolites of vitamin D, and osteocalcin) were obtained. Osteopenia was present in 28% of the patients at the lumbar spine and 20% of the patients at the femoral neck. Vertebral fractures were present in 35% of patients. In contrast to other patients receiving glucocorticoids, serum osteocalcin, a marker of bone formation, was elevated in 60% of patients. Thus, osteopenia and vertebral fractures are common in patients after cardiac transplantation. The presence of elevated osteocalcin levels suggests that the pathogenesis of the osteoporosis in these patients differs from that of glucocorticoid-induced osteoporosis.

AORTIC DISEASE

Transesophageal Echocardiography in Dissection

Erbel and associates,[15] from Hannover, Germany; Rotterdam, The Netherlands; Naples, Pisa, Triest, Italy; and Vichy, France, studied 168 patients in eight centers (124 men and 44 women) ranging in age from 23 to 84 years with proven aortic dissection by transesophageal echocardiography in the acute phase, after initiating medical and/or surgical therapy, and during follow-up at a mean of 10 months. Analyses were performed prospectively according to a study protocol. Patients were subdivided by transesophageal echocardiography according to a modified DeBakey classification. Type I aortic dissection was found in 35% of patients, type II aortic dissection in 17%, type III aortic dissection in 48%. Preoperative mortality was 3%, 7%, and 2%, and survival rates were 52%, 69%, and 70%, respectively. Type III aortic dissections could be subdivided into those with communication and antegrade dissection (50%), with communication and retrograde dissection limited to the descending aorta (10%), with dissection extended to the aortic arch and ascending aorta (27%), and with noncommunicating aortic dissection (13%). An open false lumen with no thrombus formation was present in types I, II, and III in 17%, 21%, and 39%, respectively. During follow-up in patients who survived, thrombus was demonstrated in the false lumen in 80% of type I aortic dissections and 81% of type III. Open false channel was seen in type II aortic dissections in 18%. Spontaneous healing occurred in 4% with type II and 4% with type III aortic dissections. Patients with fluid extravasation, pleural effusion, pericardial tamponade, and periaortic effusion as well as mediastinal hematoma had a mortality of 52%. Re-operations were necessary in 12% to 29%, with the highest rate in patients with type III aortic dissection. Thrombus formation in the false lumen appears to be a good prognostic sign. Surgery is only a first step in the treatment of aortic dissection. Second surgery or closure of entry sites based on intraoperative echocardiography may help induce thrombus formation and reduce aortic wall stress.

Detection of Aortic Plaque By Transesophageal Echocardiography

Nihoyannopoulos and associates,[16] from London, United Kingdom, performed transesophageal echocardiographic studies in 152 consecutive patients older than age 40 years referred for assessment of the prevalence of atherosclerosis in the thoracic aorta and related this to a history of systemic embolization. Forty-four patients (29%) had at least one atherosclerotic lesion in the thoracic aorta. This was associated with a higher prevalence of CAD (78%), carotid artery disease (88%), and peripheral vascular disease. Forty-two of all patients (28%) had systemic emboli, 20 of whom had at least one atheromatous lesion in the thoracic aorta. Conversely, only 24 of 110 patients without previous systemic emboli had atheromatous lesions. These investigators concluded that atherosclerotic lesions in the thoracic aorta can readily be identified with transesophageal echocardiography. The detection of atherosclerotic plaques of the aorta represents a marker of diffuse atherosclerotic disease, often associated with carotid, coronary, and peripheral vascular disease and with the occurrence of systemic emboli. Transesophageal echocardiography may be used serially to investigate whether dietary or pharmacologic maneuvers, or both, can shrink established atherosclerotic plaques in the thoracic aorta.

Ascending Aneurysms

Aneurysms of the ascending aorta are often unsuspected, yet they can quickly lead to death from aortic rupture or dissection. To examine the clinical spectrum of patients with aneurysms of the ascending aorta, Eisenberg and associates,[17] from San Francisco, Calif, searched the University of California, San Francisco, Echocardiography Data Base for all patients with aneurysms of the ascending aorta (≥5.0 cm in diameter) seen over a 7-year period. The echocardiograms and clinical courses of these patients were then reviewed. Identified were 15 patients with aneurysms of the ascending aorta: 5 had aneurysms >7 cm in diameter, 3 had aneurysms 6.0 to 6.9 cm, and 7 had aneurysms 5.0 to 5.9 cm in diameter. Among the 5 patients <50 years of age, 4 had Marfan's syndrome; and among the 10 patients ≥50 years of age, 8 had evidence of atherosclerotic vascular disease. At presentation, 13 patients had nonspecific symptoms, and 2 were asymptomatic. Echocardiography demonstrated that 12 patients had at least mild AR and that 5 had aortic dissections. One of the 7 patients who underwent surgical resection died of an intraoperative cardiac arrest, and 2 of the 8 patients treated medically died within 1 week of presentation. It was concluded that the clinical spectrum of patients with aneurysms of the ascending aorta is wide. Because these aneurysms are often unsuspected, physicians should have a low threshold for imaging the ascending aorta in patients with the Marfan syndrome or atherosclerotic vascular disease, particularly when AR is present.

Cost-Effectiveness of Screening For Abdominal Aneurysm

To evaluate the cost-effectiveness of screening by physical examination or abdominal ultrasonography for abdominal aortic aneurysm (AAA) in men aged 60 to 80 years, Frame and associates,[18] from Rochester, NY, Madison, Wis, and Hamilton, Canada, reviewed published English language studies that present data relevant to screening for AAA. Using the "most probable" values for the simulation parameters, a single screening procedure of abdominal palpation followed by abdominal ultrasound scan for patients with positive screening results was estimated to gain 20 life-years at a cost of nearly $29,000 per life-year. A single ultrasound screen gains 57 life-years at a cost of nearly $42,000 per life-year. A repeated ultrasound screen after 5 years gained 1 additional life-year at a cost of nearly $907,000. Thus, a single screen for AAA by abdominal palpating in men aged 60 to 80 years might be considered cost-effective but of small benefit. A single screen with ultrasonography is at the high end of the cost-per-life-year range that might be considered cost-effective and also is of modest benefit. Repeated screening is not cost-effective.

Abdominal Aneurysm Resection

During 8 years of an ultrasound screening program for abdominal aortic aneurysm (AAA), Scott and associates,[19] from Chichester, United Kingdom, scanned 8,944 people aged 65 to 80 years: 356 (4%) had AAA ≥3 cm in diameter (Table 10-3). Under their criteria, repair was indicated if the aortic diameter reached 6 cm, if expansion reached 1 cm per year, or if the AAA caused symptoms; 124 patients met these criteria (Table 10-4). Among the 8,820 screened patients who did not meet the criteria, 1 death (0.4%) was attributed to ruptured aneurysm, although the retroperitoneal hematoma had developed within 5 days of surgery for a colon tumor. The risk of aortic rupture in patients with AAA <6 cm in diameter with these criteria (0.4%) was lower than that for elective surgery (1% to 8%). Surgical repair is unnecessary and possibly detrimental in such patients, according to the authors, provided ultrasound surveillance is undertaken.

Table 10-3. Distribution of Aortic Diameter in 356 Patients found to have AAA. Reproduced with permission from Scott et al.[19]

	No of people with aortic diameter (cm) of:				
	3·0–3·9	4·0–4·9	5·0–5·9	≥6·0	Total
Men	184	62	22	26	294
Women	47	7	6	2	62
Total	231	69	28	28	356

Table 10-4. Screened Subjects who Satisfied Criteria for Surgery. Reproduced with permission from Scott et al.[19]

	Men	Women	Total
AAA ≥ 6 cm at initial screening	26	2	28
AAA reached 6 cm during follow-up	24	3	27
Expansion ≥ 1 cm per year	84	11	95
Symptoms of AAA	1	0	1
Total	111	13	124

PERIPHERAL ARTERIAL DISEASE

Effects on Skeletal Muscle

Regensteiner and associates,[20] from Cleveland, Ohio, determined whether peripheral arterial disease is associated with an impairment in muscle histology, metabolism, and function. Twenty-six patients with peripheral arterial disease and six age-matched control subjects were studied. Ten of the peripheral arterial disease patients had unilateral disease, which permitted paired comparisons between their diseased and nonsymptomatic legs. All peripheral arterial disease patients had a lower peak treadmill walking time and peak oxygen consumption than controls. Vascular disease was associated with decreased calf muscle strength compared with control values. In patients with unilateral disease, the diseased legs had a greater percentage of angular fibers indicating chronic denervation and a decreased type II fiber cross-sectional area compared with nonsymptomatic, control legs. In diseased legs, gastrocnemius muscle strength was correlated with the total calf cross-sectional area and type II fiber cross-sectional area. Activities of citrate synthase, phosphofructokinase, and lactate dehydrogenase in all 26 patients with peripheral arterial disease did not differ from control values. Despite a wide range in citrate synthase activity in the patients with peripheral arterial disease, activity of the enzyme was not correlated with muscle strength or treadmill exercise performance. Thus, these data indicate that patients with peripheral arterial disease have gastrocnemius muscle weakness associated with muscle fiber denervation and decreased type II fiber cross-sectional area. However, the peripheral arterial disease patients displayed heterogeneity in muscle enzyme activities that was not associated with exercise performance. Denervation and type II fiber atrophy may contribute to the muscle dysfunction in patients with peripheral arterial disease and further confirm that the pathophysiology of chronic peripheral arterial disease extends beyond arterial obstruction.

Variation in Use of Procedures

To examine associations between demographic characteristics and use of interventional procedures in patients with peripheral arterial disease, Tunis and associates,[21] from Baltimore, Md, studied 7,080 patients having angioplasty, bypass surgery, or amputation for lower-extremity peripheral arterial disease in 1988 through 1989. A total of 1,185 angioplasties, 4,005 bypass operations, and 1,890 amputations were identified. Population-based annual rates showed that angioplasty use peaked at about 70 per 100,000 at the age of 65 to 74 years, bypass surgery use peaked at more than 250 per 100,000 at 75 to 84 years of age, and amputation use peaked at about 225 per 100,000 at 85 years of age and older. The age-adjusted likelihood of having a procedure for peripheral arterial disease was 1.7 times higher in men than in women and 1.6 times higher in blacks than in whites. Compared with patients who had angioplasty or bypass surgery, patients who had amputations were more likely to be more than 65 years old, to be black (odds ratio, 2.5), to have Medicaid or no insurance (odds ratio, 1.7), to have diabetes mellitus (3.0), and not to have systemic hypertension (3.1). Compared with patients who had bypass surgery, patients who had angioplasty were more likely to be under 65 years old, to be white (1.7), and not to have diabetes mellitus (1.3). Patient race is associated with differences in the frequency with which angioplasty, bypass surgery, and amputation are performed for peripheral arterial disease, and insurance status is associated with the likelihood of having amputation.

Exercise Therapy

Ernst and Fialka,[22] from Vienna, Austria, did a computerized literature search to identify all controlled trials of the usefulness of exercise therapy in patients with intermittent claudication. Without exception, all 5 studies reviewed from 1966 through 1989 showed that exercise can prolong the pain-free walking distance of claudicants. The studies, however, showed quite a variability of increase in walking ability. The optimal exercise program should be supervised, performed regularly, and be of high intensity.

Percutaneous Peripheral Ultrasound Angioplasty

A number of new devices have been tried for both coronary and peripheral angioplasty. Siegel and associates,[23] from California and United Kingdom, performed percutaneous ultrasound angioplasty on 50 arterial lesions in 45 patients. The ablation system had a frequency of 19.5 kHz. A fixed wire probe with 2 mm or 3 mm ball tips and a 3 mm over-the-wire probe were used to treat 40 femoral, 7 popliteal, and 3 tibioperoneal lesions. Thirty-four percent of the lesions were calcific. Eighty-six percent of 35 occluded segments were recanalized. In the 45 patient arteries, the stenosis decreased from 94% to 55% after ultrasound angioplasty and to 12% after balloon angioplasty. Mechanical arterial dissections (n = 4) and perforations (n = 4) occurred only with the fixed non-over-the-wire probes. No evidence of embolism or vasospasm was detected. There were no clinical manifestations of acute reocclusion. Six- to 12-month clinical and ankle-brachial index follow-up data for 35 patients treated with ultrasound and adjunctive balloon angioplasty were indicative of restenosis in 7 patients. These authors concluded that percutaneous peripheral ultrasound angioplasty can be useful for recanalization of fibrous calcific and thrombotic arterial occlusions. It reduces arterial stenoses and improves flow. More data will be needed to fully assess the role of this new technique in the management of peripheral vascular disease.

Venodilation in Raynaud's Disease

The pathogenesis of Raynaud's disease remains unclear. An enhanced response to catecholamines has been hypothesized to contribute to this vasospastic disorder. Impaired endothelium-dependent dilation occurs in other diseases associated with vasospasm, such as coronary atherosclerosis. Bedarida and associates,[24] from Stanford and Palo Alto, Calif, investigated both endothelium-dependent and endothelium-independent venodilatory function in Raynaud's disease using the hand-vein compliance technique. Full dose-response curves to noradrenaline were constructed in ten subjects with primary Raynaud's disease and 10 age- and sex-matched control subjects. The two groups did not have a different response to noradrenaline. Mean (SD) long values of ED_{50}s (the dose producing half maximum response) were 1.00 (0.59) (geometric mean, 10 ng/min) in Raynaud's disease compared with 1.29 (0.66) (20 ng/min) in control subjects. The efficacy of noradrenaline as a venoconstrictor was similar in the two groups: mean maximum dilation (E_{max}) to noradrenaline was 81 (14%) in the Raynaud's group and 89 (8%) in the control group. Full dose-response curves to the endothelium-dependent dilator bradykinin were constructed. E_{max} to bradykinin was significantly lower in the Raynaud's group than in the control group (65 [21%] v 91 [29%]). ED_{50} values (doses producing half maximum response) for bradykinin were similar in the two groups. Maximum dilation with nitroprusside, a direct releaser of the vasodilator nitric oxide, was not diminished in the Raynaud's group (94 [23%] v 102 [15%] in controls). These results suggest that endothelium-dependent venodilation is impaired in peripheral vessels in Raynaud's disease, possibly due to diminished release of nitric oxide, and may contribute to the pathogenesis of the disorder.

Aspirin for Carotid Arterial Narrowing

Ranke and associates,[25] from Hannover, Germany, investigated the effects of aspirin on the initial stages of carotid atherosclerosis. Patients were recruited from a prospective, randomized, double-blind clinical trial to compare two doses of aspirin, including 900 mg versus 50 mg daily with a regard to restenoses after lower limb angioplasty. Among the 383 patients admitted to the angioplasty trial, 27 patients with 104 small carotid atheroma with <50% lumen narrowing were examined at entry and after 1 year of aspirin treatment with the use of a high resolution ultrasound duplex system. Disease progression and regression were defined by a change of maximal plaque area of more than 2 SDs of the method. The change in plaque area was significantly different for the treatment groups: average plaque size remained unchanged after treatment with 900 mg of aspirin daily but increased markedly after treatment with 50 mg of aspirin daily. There were more lesions in the 50 mg group showing progression than in the 900 mg group plaques. Ultrasonic disappearance of a lesion was observed only in the 900 mg group in 9 cases who had seven soft plaques and 2 ulcerative plaques. The 6 patients on 50 mg of aspirin who continued smoking during the study showed significantly more progression compared with the other 7 nonsmokers in the 50 mg group. The results of this study indicate that aspirin treatment slows carotid plaque growth in a dose-dependent manner with a dose of 900 mg being more effective than a dose of 50 mg.

Carotid Endarterectomy

The efficacy of carotid endarterectomy in patients with asymptomatic carotid stenosis has not been confirmed in randomized clinical trials, despite the widespread use of operative intervention in such patients. Hobson and associates,[26] from the Veterans Affairs Cooperative Study Group from 11 Veterans Affairs medical centers, conducted a multicenter clinical trial to determine the influence of carotid endarterectomy on the combined incidence of transient ischemic attack, transient monocular blindness, and stroke. These authors studied 444 men with asymptomatic carotid stenosis shown arteriographically to reduce the diameter of the arterial lumen by 50% or more. The patients were randomly assigned to optimal medical treatment including antiplatelet medication (aspirin) plus carotid endarterectomy (the surgical group, 211 patients) or optimal medical treatment alone (the medical group, 233 patients). All the patients at each center were followed independently by a vascular surgeon and a neurologist for a mean of 48 months. The combined incidence of ipsilateral neurologic events was 8.0% in the surgical group and 20.6% in the medical group (Table 10-5), giving a relative risk (for the surgical group v the medical group) of 0.38. The incidence of ipsilateral stroke alone was 4.7% in the surgical group and 9.4% in the medical group. An analysis of stroke and death combined within the first 30 postoperative days showed no significant differences. Nor were there significant differences between groups in an analysis of all strokes and deaths (surgical, 41.2%; medical, 44.2%; relative risk, 0.92). Overall mortality, including postoperative deaths, was primarily due to coronary atherosclerosis. Carotid endarterectomy reduced the overall incidence of

Table 10-5. Incidence of Stroke, Deaths from Stroke, and All Other Deaths. Reproduced with permission from Hobson et al.[26]

END POINT	SURGICAL GROUP (N = 211)	MEDICAL GROUP (N = 233)
	no. (%) of patients	
Stroke		
Nonfatal	17 (8.1)	25 (10.7)
Fatal	1 (0.5)	4 (1.7)
Other deaths		
MI, cardiac causes, sudden death*	44 (20.9)	47 (20.2)
Other medical causes	19 (9.0)	17 (7.3)
Unknown cause	6 (2.8)	10 (4.3)
All†	87 (41.2)	103 (44.2)

*Includes four perioperative deaths. MI denotes myocardial infarction.

†P not significant for the comparison between groups (relative risk, 0.92; 95 percent confidence interval, 0.69 to 1.22).

ipsilateral neurologic events in a selected group of male patients with asymptomatic carotid stenosis. Thus, these authors did not find a significant influence of carotid endarterectomy on the combined incidence of stroke and death.

COCAINE

Effect on Platelets

Kugelmass and associates,[27] from Boston, Mass, determined whether cocaine activates human platelets using flow cytometric analysis of whole blood to which cocaine was added. Activated platelets were detected by "two-color" flow cytometric analysis of the binding of fluorescently labeled antibodies directed against either platelet-associated fibrinogen or P-selectin found on the surface of platelets after stimulation. Platelets were distinguished from other constituents of whole blood by their ability to bind an antiglycoprotein Ib antibody bound to both activated and resting platelets. Incubation of whole blood with cocaine, in concentrations of 10 μm to 13 μm, induced significant increases in both platelet-associated fibrinogen and P-selectin expression. In platelets suspended in either buffer or plasma, however, P-selectin expression was detected only at the highest cocaine concentration. Neither aspirin nor the ADP scavenger, apyrase, inhibited cocaine-induced P-selectin expression. Cocaine inhibited the uptake of ^{14}C-radiolabeled serotonin by platelets. P-selectin expression and fibrinogen binding were found after the addition of cocaine alone to blood taken from some but not all donors. However, platelet activation in response to submaximal concentrations of the agonists, ADP or epinephrine, was enhanced by a low concentration of cocaine added to blood from every donor. Therefore, these data indicate that cocaine, in concentrations similar to those found clinically, induces activation of platelets studied in whole blood from some but not all donors, and platelet response to physiologic agonists is also enhanced. Cocaine-induced platelet activation may contribute to thrombosis following cocaine ingestion.

Effects on Left Ventricular Function

Cocaine-induced cardiac complications are responsible for a growing number of deaths in young people. Eisenberg and associates,[28] from San Francisco, Calif, tested the hypothesis that intravenous cocaine in doses commonly self-administered in nonmedical settings can cause myocardial ischemia and LV dysfunction. Quantitative echocardiograms and 12-lead electrocardiograms were obtained in 20 subjects before and after single intravenous doses of high dose cocaine (1.2 mg/kg body weight), low dose cocaine (0.6 mg/kg), and placebo. The rate/pressure product was increased significantly for either dose compared with placebo. Echocardiography showed that the frequency of hyperdynamic LV wall segments doubled after high dose cocaine compared with placebo. There was no change in either LVEF or wall motion score index, both of which were normal. These authors concluded that intravenous cocaine in doses commonly self-administered does not cause myocardial ischemia or LV dysfunction. It may be that idiosyncratic coronary artery vasospasm with exceptionally high doses, or cocaine induced coronary artery thrombosis, may be responsible for the AMI and sudden death associated with this drug.

ODDS AND ENDS

Nuclear Cardiology Review

Zaret and Wackers,[29] from New Haven, Conn, provided a thorough review of present day nuclear cardiology.

Hearts Aged 90 Years and Older

Roberts,[30] from Bethesda, Md, described observations in 93 patients aged 90 years or greater at necropsy. The clinical findings are summarized in Table 10-6 and the necropsy findings in Table 10-7.

Massive Fatty Deposits in the Atrial Septum

Large deposits of adipose tissue in the atrial septum were first described in 1964 and have been referred to as "lipomatous hypertrophy" of the atrial septum. A relation between these fatty deposits and atrial arrhythmias has been suggested. Shirani and Roberts,[31] from Bethesda, Md, studied at necropsy 91 patients in whom the maximal thickness of the

Table 10-6. Clinical Findings in 93 Patients ≥ 90 Years of Age. Reproduced with permission from Roberts.[30]

Variable	Number (%)
1. Age (year) (mean)	90–103 (93)
2. Men:women	51 (55%):42 (45%)
3. Black:white:Asian	33 (35%):59 (63%):1 (1%)
4. Systemic hypertension	50 (54%)
5. Diabetes mellitus	8 (9%)
6. Atrial fibrillation	21/56 (38%)
7. Bundle branch block	18/51 (35%)
Right = 7	
Left = 9	
Both = 2	
8. Clinical evidence of myocardial ischemia	20 (21%)
Angina pectoris only = 3	
Acute myocardial infarction only = 16	
Both angina and acute infarction = 1	
9. Chronic congestive heart failure	21 (23%)
10. Cause of death	
Cardiac	29 (31%)
Vascular, noncardiac	17 (18%)
Noncardiac, nonvascular	47 (51%)

Table 10-7. Cardiac Necropsy Findings in 93 Patients 90 Years of Age. Reproduced with permission from Roberts.[30]

Variable	Number (%)
1. Heart weight (g) (mean)	220–660 (418)
Men 260–660 (436)	
Women 220–630 (397)	
2. Increased heart weight	51 (55%)
(>400 g—men) 29/51 (57%)	
(>350 g—women) 22/42 (52%)	
3. ≥1 major coronary artery narrowed >75% in cross-sectional area by plaque	59 (63%)
Men 33/51 (65%)	
Women 26/42 (62%)	
4. Numbers of 4 major coronary arteries in the 93 patients narrowed >75% in cross-sectional area by plaque	107/372 (29%)
Men 57/204 (28%)	
Women 50/168 (30%)	
5. Myocardial infarct	35 (38%)
Acute only = 10 (posterior = 4)	
Healed only = 21 (posterior = 14)	
Both = 4	
6. Calcium in:	
Coronary arteries	88 (95%)
Mitral valve annulus	39 (42%)
1+ = 20/39 (51%)	
2+ = 8/39 (21%)	
3+ = 11/39 (28%)	
Aortic valve cusps	59 (63%)
1+ = 43/59 (73%)	
2+ = 10/59 (17%)	
3+ = 6/59 (10%)	
Papillary muscles	22/25 (88%)
7. Dilated cardiac ventricle	21/53 (40%)
Right ventricle only = 3/53 (6%)	
Left ventricle only = 1/53 (2%)	
Both = 17/53 (32%)	
8. Cardiac amyloidosis	16 (17%)
Causing cardiac dysfunction = 9/16 (56%)	
Not causing cardiac dysfunction = 7/16 (44%)	
9. Fibrous obliterative pericardial disease	5 (5%)
Idiopathic = 4	
Iatrogenic = 1	

atrial septum cephalad to the fossa ovalis ranged from 1.5 to 6 cm including 80 patients in whom this thickness was ≥2 cm (Table 10-8). The thickness of the septum in the 80 patients correlated with body weight and the thickness of the adipose tissue in the AV groove and that covering the RV. In 53 patients (67%), one or more of the four major epicardial coronary arteries were narrowed >75% in cross-sectional area by atherosclerotic plaque. Atrial arrhythmias were present in 31 patients (40%). Patients with larger deposits of fat (atrial septal thickness ≥3 cm) had a higher frequency of atrial arrhythmias (60% v 34%) (Table 10-9). The atrial septum was significantly thicker in patients with atrial arrhythmia compared with those without atrial arrhythmias (2.9 v 2.3 cm). Of the 28 patients with available electrocardiograms, 20 (71%)

Table 10-8. Clinical and Morphologic Findings in 80 Patients with Massive Fatty Deposits in the Atrial Septum. Reproduced with permission from Shirani et al.[31]

	All Patients (n = 80)	Men (n = 52)	Women (n = 28)
Age (yr), range (mean)	48–91 (69 ± 9)	48–91 (68 ± 9)	53–86 (71 ± 9)
White/black	72/8	47/5	25/3
Heart disease in life	47/77 (61%)	30/49 (61%)	17 (61%)
Angina pectoris	19/77 (25%)	16/49 (33%)	3 (11%)
Myocardial infarction	20/77 (26%)	14/49 (29%)	6 (32%)
Congestive heart failure	21/77 (27%)	11/49 (22%)*	10 (36%)*
Sudden death	26/79 (33%)	21/51 (41%)*	5 (18%)*
Arrhythmias			
Supraventricular	31/77 (40%)	18/49 (37%)	13/28 (48%)
Ventricular	6/78 (8%)	6/50 (12%)	0 (0%)
Systemic hypertension	46/77 (60%)	31/49 (63%)	15 (54%)
Habitual alcoholism	10/76 (13%)	9/48 (19%)	1 (4%)
Diabetes mellitus	19/77 (25%)	15/49 (31%)	4 (14%)
Corticosteroid therapy	10/76 (13%)	6/48 (13%)	4 (14%)
Cancer			
All	28/78 (36%)	17/50 (34%)	11 (39%)
Fatal	22/28 (79%)	15/17 (88%)	7/11 (64%)
Body weight (kg), range (mean)†	55–125 (79 ± 14)	57–118 (82 ± 13)	55–125 (75 ± 16)
Height (cm), range (mean)†	145–193 (168 ± 12)	150–193 (173 ± 10)*	145–193 (162 ± 12)*
Cause of death			
Cardiac	37 (46%)	27 (52%)	10 (36%)
Vascular	10 (13%)	6 (11%)	4 (14%)
Noncardiovascular	33 (41%)	19 (37%)	14 (50%)
Death outside hospital	13/75 (17%)	10/47 (21%)	3 (9%)
Heart weight (g), range (mean)	300–915 (545 ± 125)	345–915 (566 ± 118)	300–880 (505 ± 134)
Heart floats in water	52/69 (75%)	35/48 (73%)	17/21 (81%)
No. of coronary arteries with >75% ↓ in CSA by plaque			
4	3 (4%)	2 (4%)	1 (4%)
3	13 (16%)	9 (18%)	4 (14%)
2	18 (23%) ⎱ 53 (67%)	16 (31%) ⎱ 41 (80%)*	2 (7%) ⎱ 12 (43%)*
1	19 (24%)	14 (27%)	5 (18%)
0	27 (33%)	10 (20%)	16 (57%)
Coronary arteries with >75% ↓ in CSA by plaque			
Left main	4 (5%)	2 (4%)	2 (7%)
Left anterior descending	47 (59%)	38 (73%)*	9 (32%)*
Left circumflex	21 (26%)	14 (27%)	7 (25%)
Right	34 (43%)	27 (52%)*	7 (25%)*
Left ventricular fibrosis	22 (28%)	18 (35%)*	4 (14%)*
Left ventricular necrosis	15 (19%)	10 (19%)	5 (18%)
Mitral annular calcium	21 (26%)	14 (27%)	7 (25%)
Thickness of atrial septum (cm), range (mean)			
Cephalad portion	2–6 (2.5 ± 0.7)	2–5 (2.4 ± 0.5)*	2–6 (2.8 ± 0.9)*
Caudal portion	0.3–2.4 (1.0 ± 0.3)	0.4–1.5 (0.9 ± 0.2)	0.3–2.4 (1.0 ± 0.5)
Thickness of fat in atrioventricular groove, range (mean) (cm)	0.7–2.6 (1.7 ± 0.5)	0.7–2.6 (1.6 ± 0.5)	0.7–2.5 (1.8 ± 0.6)
Thickness of fat over the right ventricle, range (mean) (cm)	0.2–1.5 (0.7 ± 0.2)	0.3–1.5 (0.7 ± 0.2)	0.2–1.3 (0.7 ± 0.3)

*p ≤ 0.05. †Data available in 40 patients. Abbreviations as in Table 1.

showed atrial arrhythmias (9 atrial premature complexes, 7 AF, 3 atrial tachycardia, 1 ectopic atrial rhythm, and 1 junctional rhythm). Thus, massive fatty deposits in the atrial septum are associated with large deposits of fat elsewhere in the body and other parts of the heart. They are frequently associated with atrial arrhythmias and atherosclerotic CAD.

Transesophageal Echocardiography in the Elderly

In an investigation by Stoddard and Longaker,[32] from Louisville, Ky, the safety of transesophageal echocardiography in elderly patients (aged ≥70 years) and younger patients (aged ≤50 years) was compared in a retrospective study of 283 examinations in each group. A greater percentage of studies was performed in an intensive care unit in the elderly group (22%) as compared with the younger group (13%). In studies performed in an intensive care unit, 39% (24/61) of patients in the elderly group and 45% (17/38) in the younger group were on ventilators. Transient systemic hypotension complicating transesophageal echocardiography

Table 10-9. Comparison of the Clinical and Morphologic Findings in 20 Patients with Small (Septal Thickness < 3 cm) and Large (Septal Thickness ≥ 3 cm) Fatty Deposits in the Atrial Septum in Whom 12-Lead Electrocardiogram was Available. Reproduced with permission from Shirani et al.[31]

	Atrial Septal Thickness <3 cm (n = 16)	Atrial Septal Thickness ≥3 cm (n = 12)
Age (yr) (mean)	(69)	(73)
Gender		
Men	7	5
Women	9	7
Systemic hypertension	10 (63%)	9 (75%)
Interval ECG to death (days)	19*	32*
Heart rhythm		
Sinus	13 (82%)*	3 (25%)*
Junctional	1 (6%)	0
Atrial tachycardia	1 (6%)	2 (17%)
Atrial fibrillation	1 (6%)	6 (50)%
Ectopic atrial rhythm	0	1 (8%)
Any atrial rhythm other than sinus	3 (18%)*	9 (75%)*
Conduction abnormality		
QRS voltage		
12-lead	115*	150*
Precordial leads	46	51
Limb leads	69*	99*
Heart weight (g)	515	520
LV fibrosis	3	3
LV necrosis	4	2
Thickness of atrial septum (cm)	2.2*	3.4*
≥1 CA with >75% ↓ in CSA by plaque	12 (75%)	6 (50%)

*p = 0.05. Abbreviations as in Table 1.

was 3.5 times more frequent in the elderly (5%) as compared with the younger group (1.4%). Life-threatening complications associated with transesophageal echocardiography were rare and included third-degree AV block in 1 patient and profound vasovagal reaction in 1 patient in the elderly group and myocardial ischemia in 1 patient in the younger group. Being elderly and on a ventilator were independent predictors of the development of systemic hypotension during transesophageal echocardiography. Overall, transesophageal echocardiography was a low-risk procedure but was associated with a 3.5 times greater risk of systemic hypotension in elderly patients as compared with younger individuals. The benefit and risk should be assessed in all patients before transesophageal echocardiography, particularly in the elderly.

Transesophageal Echocardiography in Cerebral Ischemia

Labovitz and associates,[33] from St. Louis, Mo, studied 270 consecutive patients with "unexplained cerebral ischemia" with transesophageal echocardiography to determine the value of this test in identifying potential cardiac sources of cerebral embolism. The findings of this group were compared with those of 772 consecutive patients undergoing trans-esophageal echocardiographic evaluation for indications other than cere-bral ischemia. This study also examined this group of patients with unexplained cerebral ischemia to determine differences in relation to underlying cardiac rhythm and patient age. Intracardiac thrombus, atrial septal aneurysm, patent foramen ovale, spontaneous LA contrast, and protruding debris in the thoracic aorta were found more often in patients with unexplained cerebral ischemia (Figure 10-2). LV wall-motion ab-normalities, as well as mild to moderate valvular lesions including MVP, were found to be similar in both groups. Spontaneous LA contrast, as well as mild to moderate valvular abnormalities, were found more often in patients with AF (22% of the group with unexplained cerebral isch-emia). The presence of intracardiac thrombus was no more frequent in patients with AF than in those with normal sinus rhythm. Patients aged >50 years were found to have AF and larger LA size more often than their younger cohorts, as well as a greater incidence of valvular abnor-malities and LV wall-motion abnormalities. MVP was seen more fre-quently in the younger cohort of patients.

Transesophageal echocardiography improves the diagnostic accuracy of transthoracic echocardiography in the identification of potential car-diac sources of embolus. However, there are few studies of the impact of transesophageal echocardiography on the medical management of pa-tients with focal cerebral ischemia. Hata and associates,[34] from Iowa City, Iowa, reviewed the records of 52 consecutive, hospitalized patients un-dergoing both transesophageal and transthoracic echocardiography for suspected cardiac source of embolus to determine the influence of trans-esophageal echocardiography on the decision to anticoagulate patients. Of 52 patients, 39 had focal cerebral ischemia (transient ischemic attack, n = 9; acute cerebral infarction, n = 30). In 4 of these 39 patients (10%),

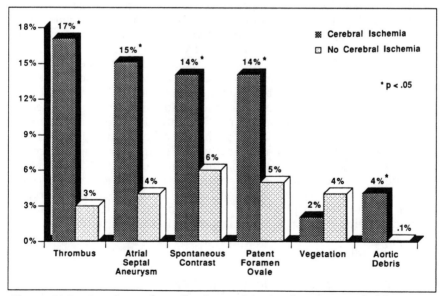

Figure 10-2. Prevalence of specific abnormalities in all patients studied by trans-esophageal echocardiography, including those with (Cerebral Ischemia) and without (No Cerebral Ischemia) stroke or transient ischemic attack. Reproduced with permission from Labovitz et al.[33]

the transesophageal echocardiography results changed the management of anticoagulation. In 19 of 39 patients (49%), the transesophageal echocardiography results helped confirm anticoagulation decisions; and in 16 (41%), the results had no effect on anticoagulation decisions, because of overriding clinical information. Ten of the latter 16 patients had transesophageal echocardiographic evidence for a possible source of an embolus but were not anticoagulated; 5 of these were poor candidates for long-term anticoagulation, and the others had right-to-left shunting across a patent foramen ovale or an interatrial septal aneurysm. Clinical variables (AF, transesophageal echocardiographic findings, and pretransesophageal echocardiographic anticoagulation status) were considered as possible predictors of post-transesophageal echocardiographic anticoagulation status using logistic regression analysis; the strongest predictor of post-transesophageal echocardiographic anticoagulation status was pretransesophageal echocardiographic anticoagulation status. Despite the selection of patients presumed to receive maximal benefit from transesophageal echocardiography, this study suggested that transesophageal echocardiography findings are not predictive of subsequent anticoagulation management. However, transesophageal echocardiography is at least confirmatory of anticoagulation decisions in most cases.

Transesophageal Echocardiography for Determining Cardiac Output

Measurement of cardiac output is a clinically valuable and widely used index of cardiac function. Although transesophageal echocardiography has been used to assess LV function, little data exist on the accuracy of this technique in the measurement of cardiac output. Therefore, cardiac output derived by pulsed Doppler transesophageal echocardiography and thermodilution methods were compared in adult patients being mechanically ventilated in an investigation by Stoddard and associates,[35] from Louisville, Ky. The LV outflow tract diameter was determined from a transgastric long-axis view of the left ventricle by using the transverse scope. The cross-sectional area of the LV outflow tract was calculated from the diameter assuming a circular shape. Pulsed Doppler recordings were obtained at the LV outflow tract. Doppler time-velocity integrals were measured from the leading edge of the velocity curve. Cardiac output derived by transesophageal echocardiography was calculated as time-velocity integral multiplied by LV outflow tract area and heart rate. Cardiac output derived by transesophageal echocardiography from the transverse plane (n = 26) and longitudinal plane (n = 22) were correlated with simultaneous thermodilution measurements. Thermodilution-derived cardiac output demonstrated excellent correlation with cardiac output measured by using transesophageal echocardiography from the transverse plane and longitudinal plane. Transesophageal echocardiography is a promising technique in the measurement of cardiac output and expands the clinical use of this modality in the assessment of cardiac function.

Intracardiac Chamber Echocardiography

The use of ultrasound catheters has advanced our knowledge of lesions inside coronary arteries. Schwartz and associates[36] extended the use of these catheters to intracardiac echocardiography as a potentially useful technique for imaging and monitoring in certain settings. Intracardiac echocardiography with 12.5 MHz catheters was performed in dogs and 92 patients. Right-sided heart imaging was performed in 68 patients and arterial and left heart imaging in 25 patients. No complications occurred, and useful anatomic and physiologic information was obtained. This study outlines the feasibility of using intracardiac echocardiography as an alternative way of visualizing cardiac chambers.

Atherosclerosis and Thrombosis in Systemic Lupus Erythematosus

Serum lipoproteins contain phospholipids, and modified LDL cholesterol may thus act as a target for antiphospholipid antibodies. Vaarala and associates,[37] from Helsinki, Finland, found raised concentrations of IgG antibodies against oxidized LDL cholesterol in 47 of 61 patients (80%) with systemic lupus erythematosus (SLE); 46% of patients also had raised concentrations of IgG anticardiolipin antibodies. Binding of anticardiolipin antibodies to solid-phase cardiolipin was inhibited by oxidized LDL cholesterol but not by native LDL cholesterol in 16 of 21 sera from SLE patients. These observations suggest cross-reactivity between antiphospholipid antibodies, which are closely associated with thrombosis in SLE, and antibodies to oxidized LDL cholesterol, thus providing a possible link between thrombotic and atherosclerotic complications in SLE.

Cardiac Troponin

Adams and associates,[38] from St. Louis, Mo, determined whether measurements of cardiac troponin I, a myocardial regulatory protein with comparable sensitivity to CK-MB, has comparable sensitivity to MBCK in the detection of myocardial injury and sufficient specificity to distinguish patients with acute or chronic skeletal muscle disease or renal failure from those with heart injury. Among 215 patients studied, 37 had acute skeletal muscle injury, 10 had chronic muscle disease, 9 were marathon runners, and 159 were chronic dialysis patients. Patients were evaluated clinically by ECG and by two-dimensional echocardiography. Total creatine kinase was determined spectrophotometrically and troponin I and MBCK were determined with specific monoclonal antibodies. Values above the upper reference limit were considered "elevated." Increases in total creatine kinase were common and elevations of MBCK occurred in 59% of patients with acute muscle injury, 78% of patients with chronic muscle disease and marathon runners, and 4% of patients with chronic renal failure. Five patients were found to have myocardial infarctions, and one had a myocardial contusion; troponin I values were elevated only in these patients. Thus, elevation of serum troponin I concentration are specific for myocardial injury and should allow distinction between myocardial and skeletal muscle injury when both exist.

Platelet Cyclic GMP and Nitroglycerin

Watanabe and associates,[39] from Ibaraki, Japan, investigated the intracellular production of cyclic GMP in platelets in response to nitroglycerin to determine the potential clinical value of platelet cyclic GMP as an indicator of the effects of nitroglycerin and nitrate tolerance. Platelet cyclic GMP and the diameters of the coronary arteries before and two minutes after intracoronary injection of 200 µg of nitroglycerin were measured in 15 patients who had previously received nitrates and in 16 who had not received any nitrates. Platelet cyclic GMP levels increased significantly after nitroglycerin injection in the two groups, but plasma cyclic GMP levels and plasma atrial natriuretic peptide levels did not change. The percent increase in platelet cyclic GMP levels and percent dilatation of the LAD and LC coronary arteries after nitroglycerin injection were higher in the no-nitrate than in the nitrate group. The percent increase in platelet cyclic GMP levels was significantly correlated with the percent dilatation of the coronary arteries in the no-nitrate group, but it did not correlate in the nitrate group. Thus, these results demonstrated that platelet cyclic GMP may be used as an indicator for in vivo evaluation of nitroglycerin's effects and that patients who have received nitrates develop nitrate tolerance, which affects intracellular production of cyclic GMP and vasodilation in response to nitroglycerin.

Effects of Contrast Material on Platelets

Chronos and associates,[40] from London, United Kingdom, studied the effects of commonly used contrast media on platelets in native blood using immunolabeling and flow cytometry to detect platelet activation in vitro. A nonionic angiographic media (Omnipaque) caused profound platelet degranulation in nearly 80% of platelets compared with 2% to 3% of platelets in the control. In contrast, an ionic angiographic medial (Urografin) caused only 25% degranulation and another ionic angiographic (Hexabrix) caused no platelet activation and inhibited the effects of thrombin on platelets. Platelet degranulation quantified by immunolabeling was paralleled by release of β-thromboglobulin and platelet factor 4 from platelet α-granules. Blood from patients anticoagulated with heparin and treated with standard-dose aspirin in preparation for PTCA showed the same patterns of contrast media-induced platelet activation as normal subjects. Thus, these data indicate that the type of contrast media used during invasive imaging of the vasculature may have a significant effect on platelet activation. Platelet degranulation within a PTCA-damaged vessel is increased by nonionic contrast media, which may contribute to the risk of acute thrombosis and growth factor responses leading to fibroproliferative change at the site of mechanically-induced endothelial injury.

Sealing Arterial Puncture Sites

After angiography, 6 to 24 hours of bedrest is indicated to assure that adequate hemostasis of the femoral artery has been achieved. Recently, de Swart and associates,[41] from Maastricht, The Netherlands, developed a new hemostatic puncture closure device, which consists of a resorbable polymer anchor, a resorbable suture, a small collagen plug, and an 8Fr delivery device. The device is delivered into the femoral artery through the introducer sheath, the anchor is secured against the intraluminal artery wall, and the collagen plug is deployed on the arterial wall. The prototype of the device was used in 20 patients administered heparin. After insertion of the device, hemostasis was achieved in 1.2 minutes; in

2 patients, a light pressure dressing was applied for 4 hours to stop ooz-
ing. No late bleeding occurred. In 1 patient, the positioning suture broke,
requiring the application of a pressure bandage. Patients were unevent-
fully mobilized after 6.7 hours. In all patients, serial duplex scanning of
the femoral artery was performed before and after 1, 7, 30, and 90 days
after device placement. In 5 patients, a small subcutaneous hematoma
close to the site of introduction could be detected by ultrasound 1 day
after catheterization. All but 1 patient had normalization of the flow patterns in the femoral artery. These investigators concluded that (1) the
hemostatic puncture closure device is an effective device to achieve immediate hemostasis after arterial catheterization despite antithrombotic
therapy, (2) early mobilization was uneventful, (3) duplex ultrasound
studies demonstrated only transient changes in the punctured femoral
artery, and (4) further investigations are needed to establish the efficacy
and safety of the device.

Location of Thrombus in Deep-Veins

Two different diagnostic strategies are used to perform compression
(real-time) ultrasound for the diagnosis of clinically suspected deep-vein
thrombosis. One is to examine the entire proximal venous system from
common femoral to distal popliteal vein; the other is a limited examination of only the common femoral and the entire popliteal vein. The latter
strategy, which is less time consuming and requires less expensive
equipment, is based on a strong impression from prospective studies
using limited compression ultrasound that proximal vein thrombi always
involve the common femoral and popliteal vein. This impression, which
is supported by the demonstrated safety at long-term follow-up of not
treating patients whose limited compression ultrasound is normal at presentation and then repeated within the next week, has not been tested
in a formal study. Cogo and associates,[42] from Padua, Italy, Amsterdam,
The Netherlands, and Hamilton, Canada, reviewed a large series of
venograms performed in consecutive patients with clinically suspected
venous thrombosis to determine the distribution of venous thrombosis
in symptomatic patients. Venograms were performed using 150 mL of
radiographic contrast material. Before the study, a panel of experts
agreed on the standardized criteria for the assessment of venograms.
Venograms were adjudicated blindly for the presence of deep-vein
thrombosis and isolated calf-vein thrombosis, the size of proximal
thrombi, and whether they were occlusive or nonocclusive. Subsequently, the duration of symptoms was related to the venographic findings. Five hundred sixty-two venograms from consecutive patients with
a first episode of clinically suspected deep-vein thrombosis were adjudicated. Of these, 20 (3.6%) were inadequate for interpretation. In the remaining 542, venous thrombosis was demonstrated in 189 instances
(prevalence, 35%) and were located in the proximal veins in 166 (88%)
venograms. Isolated calf-vein thrombosis was present in the remaining
23 (12%) venograms. Proximal with concurrent calf thrombosis was detected in 164 (99%) of the 166 patients. Proximal thrombi involved only
the popliteal vein in 16 (10%); the popliteal and superficial femoral
veins in 70 (42%); and the popliteal, superficial, and common femoral
vein in 8 (5%); whereas thrombi involving the entire proximal deep venous system were detected in 58 (35%) venograms. Isolated thrombosis

of the superficial femoral, common femoral, and iliac vein was not observed. Proximal venous thrombi were occlusive in 146 patients (88%). No relation between the duration of symptoms and the extent or the occlusiveness of venous thrombi could be demonstrated. Thus, most symptomatic patients have extensive occlusive proximal vein thrombosis at the time of presentation. Thrombi isolated to the superficial femoral or iliac vein were not observed in this large sample of consecutive patients. These data support the use of the relatively simple, inexpensive, and rapid compression ultrasound method that limits the examination of the proximal veins to the common femoral and popliteal veins.

Pulmonary Embolism

Data from a nonrandomized study have hinted that in patients with acute pulmonary embolism, thrombolysis followed by heparin more rapidly reverses RV dysfunction and restores pulmonary tissue perfusion than does heparin alone. Goldhaber and associates,[43] from multiple US medical centers, pursued this idea in a randomized protocol. Forty-six hemodynamically stable patients were randomized to recombinant tissue plasminogen activator (alteplase, rt-PA) 100 mg over two hours followed by intravenous heparin and 55 patients to heparin alone. RV wall motion was assessed qualitatively, and RV end-diastolic area was estimated by planimetry for echocardiograms at baseline and at 3 and 24 hours. Pulmonary perfusion scans were obtained at baseline and 24 hours. In 39% of rt-PA patients but in only 17% of heparin alone patients, RV wall motion at 24 hours had improved from baseline and in 2% and 17%, respectively, it worsened. rt-PA patients also had a significant decrease in RV end-diastolic area during the 24 hours after randomization and a significant absolute improvement in pulmonary perfusion (14.6% v 1.5%). No clinical episodes of recurrent PE were noted among rt-PA patients, but there were two fatal and three nonfatal clinically suspected recurrent PEs within 14 days in patients randomized to heparin alone. rt-PA rapidly improves RV function and pulmonary perfusion among patients with PE and may lead to a lower rate of adverse clinical outcomes.

To test the hypothesis that a low D-dimer level has a high negative predictive value for acute pulmonary embolism (PE) among patients undergoing diagnostic pulmonary angiography, Goldhaber and associates,[44] from four US medical centers, analyzed plasma samples of D-dimer levels, measured using a monoclonal antibody assay from 173 patients with suspected acute PE. All 173 patients underwent diagnostic pulmonary angiography. Of 35 patients with D-dimer values <500 ng/mL, only 3 had abnormal pulmonary angiograms. The negative predictive value of a plasma D-dimer level <500 ng/mL for acute PE was 91.4%. D-dimer levels were >500 ng/mL in 42 of 45 patients with PE and in 96 of 128 patients without PE. Sensitivity, specificity, and positive predictive value of a plasma D-dimer level >500 ng/mL for acute PE were 93.3%, 25.0%, and 30.4%, respectively. The results of our study indicate that quantitative plasma D-dimer levels can be useful in screening patients with suspected PE who require pulmonary angiography. Plasma D-dimer values <500 ng/mL may obviate the need for pulmonary angiography, particularly among medical patients for whom the clinical suspicion of PE is low. The plasma D-dimer value, assayed using a commercially available enzyme-linked immunosorbent assay kit, is a sensitive but nonspecific test for the presence of acute PE.

Adenosine + Nifedipine or Diltiazem for Primary Pulmonary Hypertension

Primary pulmonary hypertension remains a major therapeutic problem. Patients continue to have high morbidity and early mortality despite treatment with vasodilator drugs. Because of this variable and inconsistent response to individual vasodilators, Inbar and associates,[45] from Chicago, Ill, examined the effects of vasodilator combination therapy in 12 patients with primary pulmonary hypertension. They elected to combine calcium antagonists and adenosine. Twelve patients were placed on oral nifedipine (mean dose, 103 mg) and 3 on diltiazem therapy (mean dose, 300 mg) which were titrated to maximal effect. One hour after a maintenance dose of calcium blocker, all patients received an infusion of adenosine (50 µg/kg/min), increasing at two-minute intervals to a maximally tolerated dose (180 ± 60 µg/kg/min). Ten of the 15 patients responded to calcium antagonists, which was defined as a greater than 20% decrease in pulmonary vascular resistance. In the calcium channel blocker responders, the combination of adenosine and calcium blocker reduced pulmonary vascular resistance by 49%, which was greater than the 39% decrease produced by the calcium blocker alone. Stroke volume increased by 33% and mean PA pressure decreased by 14% compared with drug-free baseline values. In nonresponders to calcium blockers, combination therapy was not of benefit in reducing pulmonary vascular resistance. These authors concluded that combination therapy with adenosine on top of calcium blockers has the ability to further decrease PA pressure and pulmonary vascular resistance in those who had responded to the calcium channel blockers. This data raises the possibility that combination therapy may be better than single-drug therapy in selected patients. Although adenosine infusion would be a difficult drug to administer long term, it does appear to be a good pulmonary vasodilator and thus set the stage for oral analogs as possible therapeutic agents. It should be noted that adenosine has the potential to produce negative inotropic effects. Furthermore, this was a short-term study, and it is uncertain whether there would be continued response to combination therapy over the long term. Nevertheless, this study does highlight the potential for considering combination vasodilator therapy in this serious condition.

Ventricular Diastolic Function and Hemodialysis

Gupta and associates,[46] from New Delhi, India, evaluated 21 patients (17 men and 4 women; aged 20 to 40 years) with end-stage renal disease for LV diastolic function by Doppler echocardiography before and after hemodialysis. Fifteen patients were on maintenance hemodialysis (group A), and 6 were studied before and after their first hemodialysis (group B). The following indexes of LV diastolic function were studied: (1) isovolumic relaxation time; and (2) Doppler indexes from mitral inflow signal—peak early velocity, peak late velocity (atrial), deceleration of early filling phase, and deceleration time of early filling phase. LV systolic function in groups A and B (LVEF 68% and 77%, fractional shortening 0.39% and 0.46%, respectively) was normal and did not change after hemodialysis. Group A had a prolonged isovolumic relaxation time of 80 ms, which decreased to 57 ms. Deceleration time decreased from 248 to 184 ms, and the deceleration slope increased from 4.3 to 5.1 m/s^2 after hemodialysis. In group B, isovolumic relaxation time decreased from 87 to 73 ms, deceleration time decreased from 256 to 185 ms, and deceleration slope increased from 3.5 to 4.2 m/s^2. This study indicated that patients with end-stage renal disease have impaired LV diastolic function that improves with hemodialysis.

Best Hospitals in the United States for Heart Disease

Roberts,[47] from Dallas, Tex, reviewed an article that was published in the July 12, 1993, issue of the *US News and World Report* entitled "America's Best Hospitals." The 41 "best hospitals" for patients with heart disease are listed in Table 10-10.

Structure of Academic Divisions of Cardiology

The Task Force from the Association of Professors of Cardiology discussing the structure and function of academic divisions of cardiology was published in the Oct 25, 1993 issue of the *Archives of Internal Medicine*.[48] This document outlines a course for training and for clinical research activities in academic cardiology in the future.

Zaret and associates,[49] from three different US medical centers, wrote a piece entitled "Cardiovascular medicine: Subspecialty or specialty," and it was published in the Oct 15, 1993 issue of *The American Journal of Cardiology*. This article, having to do with whether or not cardiology should be a separate department or whether it should remain as a division of the Department of Medicine, is worth reading.

Good Cardiologic Books Appearing in 1993

MAJOR GENERAL CARDIOLOGIC TEXTBOOKS

1. Schlant RC, Alexander RW, editors; O'Rourke RA, Roberts R, Sonnenblick EH, associate editors. *Hurst's The Heart, Arteries and Veins.* Eighth Edition. New York: McGraw-Hill, Inc., 1994:2586, $125.00.

One hundred and 43 chapters by 203 contributors. Words describing this book might be authoritative, heavy, impressive, overwhelming, practical, useful. The Schlant-Alexander and Braunwald books are essential to a cardiovascular library.

2. Cheitlin MD, Sokolow M, and McIlroy MB. *Clinical Cardiology.* Sixth Edition. Norwalk, Connecticut: Appleton & Lange, 1993:741, $37.95.

Good general text. The cost of the Schlant-Alexander book is actually less in proportion to the information supplied.

CARDIOLOGIC TEXTS FOR THE NON-CARDIOLOGIST

3. Hurst JW. *Cardiovascular Diagnosis. The Initial Examination.* St. Louis: Mosby, 1993:556, $39.95.

4. Timmis AD, Nathan AW. *Essentials of Cardiology.* Second Edition. Oxford: Blackwell Scientific Publications, 1993:351, $36.95.

5. Harvey WP. *Cardiac Pearls.* Newton, New Jersey: Laennec Publishing, 1993:345, $74.00.

6. Carabello BA, Ballard WL, Gazes PC. *Cardiology Pearls.* Philadelphia: Hanley & Belfus, Inc., 1994:223, $35.00.

Table 10-10.   Reproduced with permission from Roberts.[47]

Rank	Hospital	Overall Score	Reputa-tional Score	Mortality Rate	COTH Member	Residents to Beds	Tech-nology Score	R.N.'s to Beds	Board-Certified M.D.'s to Beds	Inpatient Operations to Beds
1	Mayo Clinic, Rochester, MN	100.0	43.4%	0.65	+	NA	16	0.86	1.40	21.9
2	Cleveland Clinic	88.8	36.4%	0.75	+	0.50	14	1.44	0.36	20.4
3	Massachusetts General Hospital, Boston	88.5	36.2%	0.78	+	0.47	19	1.20	1.06	19.3
4	Stanford University Hospital, Stanford	60.8	21.1%	0.94	+	0.72	14	0.85	1.56	15.8
5	Johns Hopkins Hospital, Baltimore	60.4	19.1%	0.76	+	0.44	16	1.28	0.97	14.7
6	Duke University Medical Center, Durham	57.3	18.0%	0.85	+	0.38	19	1.37	0.59	13.6
7	Brigham and Women's Hospital, Boston	56.4	16.4%	0.74	+	0.62	17	0.77	1.20	20.1
8	Texas Heart Institute (St. Luke's Episcopal Hospital), Houston	52.9	19.9%	1.22	+	0.17	10	1.03	0.57	17.2
9	Emory University Hospital, Atlanta	51.0	16.0%	0.88	+	0.29	10	1.12	0.54	14.9
10	University of California, San Francisco Medical Center	42.1	7.0%	0.76	+	0.32	17	1.85	1.59	19.0
11	Cedars-Sinai Medical Center, Los Angeles	41.4	9.1%	0.83	+	0.24	15	0.99	1.13	17.7
12	UCLA Medical Center, Los Angeles	41.2	4.6%	0.78	+	1.29	17	1.61	1.64	16.8
13	University of Michigan Medical Center, Ann Arbor	39.7	7.3%	0.84	+	0.41	17	1.26	0.62	18.5
14	Mount Sinai Medical Center, New York	37.2	4.4%	0.78	+	0.52	16	1.58	1.18	12.8
15	Barnes Hospital, St. Louis	36.8	6.4%	0.74	+	0.41	5	0.79	0.85	11.2
16	New York University Medical Center, New York	36.5	3.8%	0.64	+	0.20	12	1.15	1.15	13.6
17	Hospital of the University of Pennsylvania, Philadelphia	35.2	3.0%	0.83	+	1.06	15	1.18	0.94	15.0
18	Indiana University Medical Center, Indianapolis	34.9	1.0%	0.64	+	0.37	17	1.82	0.90	17.6
19	Thomas Jefferson University Hospital, Philadelphia	34.9	1.2%	0.68	+	0.71	17	1.41	1.11	16.5
20	New York Hospital–Cornell Medical Center, New York	34.4	3.4%	0.72	+	0.36	15	0.88	0.95	11.0
21	University of Alabama Hospital, Birmingham	34.3	7.1%	1.03	+	0.21	15	0.67	0.52	17.1
22	Columbia-Presbyterian Medical Center, New York	34.0	3.6%	0.75	+	0.30	16	1.01	0.63	7.6
23	Methodist Hospital, Houston	34.0	6.1%	1.00	+	0.14	15	1.24	0.58	17.3
24	Baylor University Medical Center, Dallas	33.9	5.8%	0.94	+	0.14	14	1.23	0.49	18.7
25	New England Medical Center, Boston	33.7	1.9%	0.75	+	0.58	13	1.66	1.70	15.9
26	Beth Israel Hospital, Boston	33.3	3.7%	0.75	+	0.01	13	1.36	0.83	14.1
27	University of Chicago Hospitals	32.7	2.3%	0.90	+	0.77	17	1.53	0.74	17.5
28	University of Illinois Hospital and Clinics, Chicago	32.6	0.6%	0.75	+	1.23	12	1.06	0.54	13.7
29	University of Wisconsin Hospital and Clinics, Madison	32.0	0.0%	0.68	+	0.65	16	1.25	0.67	18.2
30	University of Iowa Hospitals and Clinics, Iowa City	31.8	1.7%	0.89	+	0.78	18	1.31	0.49	24.6
31	Presbyterian University Hospital, Pittsburgh	31.7	1.1%	0.83	+	0.66	11	2.12	1.20	17.7
32	University of Washington Medical Center, Seattle	31.7	0.6%	0.74	+	0.31	15	1.88	1.86	15.0
33	Rush-Presbyterian-St.Luke's Medical Center, Chicago	31.5	0.9%	0.75	+	0.61	16	1.18	0.84	13.4
34	Montefiore Medical Center, New York	31.0	2.4%	0.83	+	0.53	14	0.91	0.40	11.2
35	University of Virginia Medical Center, Charlottesville	30.9	0.6%	0.85	+	0.78	17	1.70	0.44	16.4
36	Deaconess Hospital, Boston	30.9	0.4%	0.71	+	0.59	13	1.14	0.78	14.2
37	University of California, San Diego Medical Center	30.7	1.2%	0.89	+	0.27	17	2.66	0.91	18.7
38	University Hospitals of Cleveland	30.6	0.6%	0.87	+	0.61	18	1.72	1.16	14.4
39	Green Hospital of Scripps Clinic, La Jolla	30.3	0.0%	0.61	0	0.00	11	0.82	0.58	23.3
40	University of California, Davis Medical Center, Sacramento	30.1	1.9%	0.94	+	0.63	18	2.59	0.60	16.1
41	University of Minnesota Hospital and Clinic, Minneapolis	30.0	0.6%	0.75	+	NA	15	2.05	0.76	16.2

Reputational Score = the percentage of doctors surveyed who named the hospital; Mortality Rate = ratio of actual to expected deaths (lower is better); COTH Member = member of Council of Teaching Hospitals; Residents to Beds = ratio of interns and residents to beds; Technology Score = index from 0 to 19; R.N.'s to Beds = ratio of registered nurses to beds; Board-Certified M.D.'s to Beds = ratio of doctors certified in a specialty to beds; Inpatient Operations to Beds = ratio of annual inpatient operations to beds; NA = not available. Adapted with permission from *U.S. News & World Report*, July 12, 1993.

7. Gessner IH, Victorica BE, editors. *Pediatric Cardiology*. Philadelphia: W.B. Saunders Company, 1993:283, $45.00.

Each of these five books is good reading. My teachers were Hurst and Harvey, so naturally I am biased. The Harvey book, however, is expensive.

CARDIAC DISEASE IN WOMEN

8. Douglas PS, editor. *Cardiovascular Health and Disease in Women*. Philadelphia: W.B. Saunders Company, 1993:374, $65.00.

9. Wenger NK, Speroff L, Packard B, editors. *Cardiovascular Health and Disease in Women, Proceedings of an N.H.L.B.I. Conference.* Greenwich, Connecticut: LeJacq Communications, Inc., 1993:348, $66.00.

10. Pashkow FJ, Libov C. *The Woman's Heart Book. The Complete Guide to Keeping Your Heart Healthy and What to Do if Things Go Wrong.* New York: Dutton, 1993:358, $22.00.

Both the Douglas and the Wenger books are excellent. Obviously, the subject matter is a hot topic. The Pashkow-Libov book is intended for the nonphysician.

HEART FAILURE

11. Hosenpud JD, Greenberg BH, editors. *Congestive Heart Failure. Pathophysiology, Diagnosis, and Comprehensive Approach to Management.* New York: Springer-Verlag, 1994:769, $180.

12. Gwathmey JK, Briggs GM, Allen PD, editors. *Heart Failure, Basic Science and Clinical Aspects.* New York: Marcel Dekker, Inc., 1993:715, $195.00.

13. Barnett DB, Pouleur H, Francis GS, editors. *Congestive Cardiac Failure. Pathophysiology and Treatment.* New York: Marcel Dekker, Inc., 1993:385, $135.00.

14. Gaasch WH, LeWinter MM, editors. *Left Ventricular Diastolic Dysfunction and Heart Failure.* Philadelphia: Lea & Febiger, 1994:498, $89.50.

It is difficult for me to choose the best of these four books. All appear to be good.

ELECTROCARDIOGRAPHY

15. Mirvis DM. *Electrocardiography. A Physiologic Approach.* St. Louis: Mosby, 1993:532, $34.95.

This interesting book on electrocardiography contains few electrocardiograms. It focuses more on underlying physiologic principles. Thus, this book is a different one on a subject that probably has produced more than 100 books.

16. Gomes JA, editor. *Signal Averaged Electrocardiography. Concepts, Methods, and Applications.* Dordrecht: Kluwer Academic Publications, 1993:583, $172.00.

For the wealthy physician interested in this topic, here it is.

ARRHYTHMIAS, CONDUCTION DEFECTS, PACE-MAKERS, CARDIOVERTER-DEFIBRILLATORS

17. Kastor JA, editor. *Arrhythmias.* Philadelphia: W.B. Saunders Company, 1994:430, $85.00.

This comprehensive book was "specifically written for clinicians who are not now or plan to become clinical electrophysiologists." Good reading.

18. Josephson ME, editor. *Sudden Cardiac Death.* Boston: Blackwell Scientific Publications, 1993:432, $95.00.

You can count on Josephson to produce a good product.

19. Singh BN, Wellens HJJ, Hiraoka M, editors. *Electropharmacological Control of Cardiac Arrhythmias. To Delay Conduction or to Prolong Refractori-*

ness? Mount Kisco, New York: Futura Publishing Company, Inc., 1994:746, $97.00.

A major text.

20. Singer I, Kupersmith J, editors. *Clinical Manual of Electrophysiology.* Baltimore: Williams & Wilkins, 1993:453, $70.00.

As J. Thomas Bigger, Jr. states in the foreword, this book provides "an excellent introduction to electrophysiologic concepts and practice."

21. Shenasa M, Borggrefe M, Breithardt G, editors; Haverkamp W, Hindricks G, assistant editors. *Cardiac Mapping.* Mount Kisco, New York: Futura Publishing Company, Inc., 1993:711, $95.00.

I can only guess if this is a good book. It is the first full book I recall seeing on this subject.

22. Naccarelli GV, Veltri EP, editors. *Implantable Cardioverter-Defibrillators.* Boston: Blackwell Scientific Publications, 1993:443, $65.00.

ECHOCARDIOGRAPHY

23. Feigenbaum H. *Echocardiography.* Fifth Edition. Philadelphia: Lea & Febiger, 1994:695, $95.00.

24. Weyman AE. *Principles and Practice of Echocardiography.* Second Edition. Philadelphia: Lea & Febiger, 1994:1335, $169.00.

Two major texts on the same subject published the same year by the same publisher! The Feigenbaum book is the fifth edition of this classic, written entirely by him. He has met his match, however, in the Weyman book, which contains 41 chapters, 31 of which were written by Weyman. If I could afford the difference, I would go for the Weyman book, which is extremely comprehensive.

25. Roelandt JRTC, Sutherland GR, Iliceto S, Linker DT, editors. *Cardiac Ultrasound.* Edinburgh: Churchill Livingstone, 1993:1013, $275.00.

A major book containing 95 chapters by 149 contributors, virtually all from Europe. This book contains the full gamut of cardiac ultrasound.

26. Wilde P, editor. *Cardiac Ultrasound.* Edinburgh: Churchill Livingstone, 1993:552, $165.00.

27. Oh JK, Seward JB, Tajik AJ. *The Echo Manual From the Mayo Clinic.* Boston: Little, Brown and Company, 1994:252, $75.00.

I do not quite understand the purpose of this book. Twenty bucks more and one has the Feigenbaum book. No question where to go.

28. Goldman ME. *Clinical Atlas of Transesophageal Echocardiography.* Mount Kisco, New York: Futura Publishing Company, Inc., 1993:376, $149.00.

29. Mauer G, editor. *Transesophageal Echocardiography.* New York: McGraw-Hill, Inc., 1994:285, $149.00.

Both are good transesophageal books. The best value is the one by Goldman.

30. Hanrath P, Uebis R, Krebs W. *Cardiovascular Imaging by Ultrasound.* Dordrecht: Kluwer Academic Publishers, 1993:479, $237.50.

31. Hodgson J McB, Sheehan HM, editors. *Atlas of Intravascular Ultrasound.* New York: Raven Press, 1994:333, $115.00.

32. Roelandt J, Bom N, Gussenhoven EJ, editors. *Intravascular Ultrasound.* Dordrecht: Kluwer Academic Publishers, 1993:166, $45.00.

33. Nanda NC, Schlief R, editors. *Advances in Echo Imaging Using Contrast Enhancement.* Dordrecht: Kluwer Academic Publishers, 1993:405, $95.00.

NUCLEAR CARDIOLOGY

34. Zaret BL, Kaufman L, Berson AS, Dunn RA, editors. *Frontiers in Cardiovascular Imaging.* New York: Raven Press, 1993:362, $82.00.

This small book reviews imaging of myocardium using ultrafast computed tomography, positron emission tomography, single-photon emission computed tomography, nuclear magnetic resonance, ultrasound, magnetocardiography, digital subtraction angiography, synchrotran radiation, magnetic resonance angiography, echocardiography, radionuclides, and fluorescence spectroscopy in 362 pages! Four companies supported publication of this book.

35. Zaret BL, Beller GA, editors. *Nuclear Cardiology. State of the Art and Future Directions.* St. Louis: Mosby, 1993:347, $72.00.

This book of 31 chapters by 59 contributors is an outgrowth of the International Nuclear Cardiology Workshop held in Wintergreen, Virginia, in July 1991. The text is a state-of-the-art perspective of the field of nuclear cardiology.

INTERVENTIONAL CARDIOLOGY

36. Topol EJ, editor. *Textbook of Interventional Cardiology,* Volumes 1 and 2. Second Edition. Philadelphia: W.B. Saunders Company, 1994:1–684 (volume 1) and 685–1392 (volume 2), $179.00.

This book unquestionably is the tops in this area.

37. Faxon DP, editor. *Practical Angioplasty.* New York: Raven Press, 1994:273, $95.00.

Good but no comparison to the Topol book.

38. Topol EJ, Serruys PW, editors. *Current Review of Interventional Cardiology.* Philadelphia: Current Medicine, 1994:264, $149.00.

Not needed. Get the other Topol book.

39. Rao PS, editor. *Transcatheter Therapy in Pediatric Cardiology.* New York: Wiley-Liss, 1993:509, $124.95.

40. Kern MJ, editor. *Hemodynamic Rounds. Interpretation of Cardiac Pathophysiology from Pressure Waveform Analysis.* New York: Wiley-Liss, 1993:218, $38.95.

41. Herrmann HC, Hirshfield JW Jr, editors. *Clinical Use of the Palmaz-Schatz Intracoronary Stent.* Mount Kisco, New York: Futura Publishing Company, Inc., 1993:196, $45.00.

If you are interested in this stent, here is the information.

42. Vetrovec GW, Goudreau E. *Coronary Angiography for the Interventionalist.* New York: Chapman & Hall, 1994:129, $99.00.

Beautiful angiograms but much wasted space on many pages.

43. Dyer R, editor. *Handbook of Basic Vascular and Interventional Radiology.* New York: Churchill Livingstone, 1993:275, $62.00.

PHARMACOLOGY AND DRUG THERAPY

44. Hurst JW, editor. *Current Therapy in Cardiovascular Disease.* Fourth Edition. St. Louis: Mosby, 1994:454, $79.00.

45. Singh BN, Dzau VJ, Vanhoutte PM, Woosley RL, editors. *Cardiovascular Pharmacology and Therapeutics.* New York: Churchill Livingstone, 1994:1231, $149.95.

46. Frishman WH, Dollery CT, Cruickshank JM. *Current Cardiovascular Drugs.* Philadelphia: Current Medicine, 1994:297, $39.95.

These three books are all good. The Hurst book contains 97 chapters by 124 contributors, and it appears only 3 years after the previous edition. The Singh book has nearly as many contributors. The best buy is the Singh book.

47. O'Rourke MF, Safar ME, Dzau VJ, editors. *Arterial Vasodilation. Mechanisms and Therapy.* Philadelphia: Lea & Febiger, 1993:231, $89.50.

As the editors indicate, this book seeks to explain how and why vasodilator drugs are successful in treatment of stable, as well as variant, angina, and in treatment of cardiac failure and hypertension, and why some vasodilator agents are more effective than others.

48. Rezakovic DE, Alpert JS, editors. *Nitrate Therapy & Nitrate Tolerance. Current Concepts and Controversies.* Basel: Karger, 1993:547, $232.00.

49. Godfraind T, Govoni S, Paoletti R, Vanhoutte PM, editors. *Calcium Antagonists. Pharmacology and Clinical Research.* Dordrecht: Kluwer Academic Publishers, 1993:380, $132.00.

50. Escande D, Standen N, editors. *K+ Channels in Cardiovascular Medicine.* Paris: Springer-Verlag, 1993:332, $179.95.

GOOD CARDIOLOGIC NUTRITION

51. Piscatella JC, Piscatella B. *The Fat Tooth Fat Gram Counter.* New York: Workman Publishing, 1993:299, $6.25.

52. Piscatella JC, Piscatella B. *The Fat Tooth Restaurant & Fast-Food Fat-Gram Counter.* New York: Workman Publishing, 1993:260, $6.25.

The two little Piscatella books together sell for $12.50. Every physician needs to know what is in these two books, and I highly recommend them. They are each pocket-sized so they can go into the kitchen and restaurant easily.

53. Mogadam M. *Choosing Foods for a Healthy Heart.* Yonkers, New York: Consumer Reports Books, 1993:171, $19.95.

54. Chiavetta JM in collaboration with Barrett C and Chiavetta SV. *Eat, Drink and Be Healthy. A Guide to Healthful Eating and Weight Control.* Raleigh, North Carolina: Piedmont Publishers, 1993:419, $24.95.

This book is popular at the Duke University Medical Center. Every physician needs to own at least one good "healthful-eating" book.

CARDIAC FITNESS AND REHABILITATION

55. Fletcher GF, editor. *Cardiovascular Response to Exercise.* Mount Kisco, New York: Futura Publishing Company, Inc., 1994:446, $75.00.

56. Froelicher VF, Myers J, Follansbee WP, Labovitz AJ. *Exercise and the Heart.* Third Edition. St. Louis: Mosby, 1993:394, $59.00.

57. Franklin B. *Making Healthy Tomorrows. Cardiac Fitness and a Healthier Lifestyle.* Clarkston, Michigan: Glovebox Guidebooks Publishing Company, 1993:207, $12.95.

MISCELLANEOUS

58. Loscalzo J, Schafer AI, editors. *Thrombosis and Hemorrhage.* Boston: Blackwell Scientific Publications, 1994:1337, $225.00.

A major book consisting of 63 chapters by 93 contributors.

59. Kaplan JA, editor. *Cardiac Anesthesia*. Third Edition. Philadelphia: W.B. Saunders Company, 1993:1353, $169.00.

The best on this subject.

60. Stark J, de Leval M, editors. *Surgery for Congenital Heart Defects*. Second Edition. Philadelphia: W.B. Saunders Company, 1994:712, $245.00.

A good book, but a stiff price. The foreword by Dr. John W. Kirklin is one of the best I have read. The emphasis in this book is on surgical techniques.

61. Salmasi A-M, Iskandrian AS, editors. *Cardiac Output and Regional Flow in Health and Disease*. Dordrecht: Kluwer Academic Publishers, 1993:555, $259.00.

62. Gravanis MB, editor. *Cardiovascular Disorders. Pathogenesis and Pathophysiology*. St. Louis: Mosby, 1993:576, $95.00.

63. Pohost GM, editor. *Cardiovascular Applications of Magnetic Resonance*. Mount Kisco, New York: Futura Publishing Company, Inc., 1993:459, $86.00.

64. Draznin B., Eckel RH, editors. *Diabetes and Atherosclerosis. Molecular Basis and Clinical Aspects*. New York: Elsevier, 1993:385, $85.00.

This book is divided into three parts: lipids, atherosclerosis, and systemic hypertension in the diabetic patient. Although I know only 6 of the 41 contributors of the 20 chapters, the book appears to be excellent and is timely.

65. Sobel BE, Collen D, editors. *Coronary Thrombolysis in Perspective. Principles Underlying Conjunctive and Adjunctive Therapy*. New York: Marcel Dekker, Inc., 1993:338, $99.75.

66. Cohn PF. *Silent Myocardial Ischemia and Infarction*. Third Edition. New York: Marcel Dekker, Inc., 1993:268, $79.75.

67. Tresch DD, Aronow WS, editors. *Cardiovascular Disease in the Elderly Patient*. New York: Marcel Dekker, Inc., 1994:663, $125.00.

68. Wenger NK, editor. *Inclusion of Elderly Individuals in Clinical Trials. Cardiovascular Disease and Cardiovascular Therapy as a Model*. Kansas City, Missouri: Marion Merrell Dow, Inc., 1993:294.

69. Waller BF. Harvey WP, editors. *Cardiovascular Evaluation of Athletes. Toward Recognizing Athletes at Risk of Sudden Death*. Newton, New Jersey: Laennec Publishing, 1993:213, $75.00.

70. Nagano M, Takeda N, Dhalla NS, editors. *The Cardiomyopathic Heart*. New York: Raven Press, 1994:464, $95.00.

Forty-four chapters by 183 contributors, 2 of whom are from the United States. Much experimental work is included. Not useful clinically.

71. Alpert JS, Francis GS. *Handbook of Coronary Care*. Fifth Edition. Boston: Little, Brown and Company, 1993:228, $27.00.

This neat little book fits nicely into the coat pocket.

72. Kapoor A, Laks H, editors. *Atlas of Heart-Lung Transplantation*. New York: McGraw-Hill, Inc., 1994:212, $150.

A pictorial description of the operations currently performed for end-stage heart and lung failure. There is much unused space on too many pages in this expensive book.

PERIPHERAL VASCULAR DISEASE

73. Veith FJ, Hobson RW II, Williams RA, Wilson SE, editors. *Vascular Surgery. Principles and Practice*. Second Edition. New York: McGraw-Hill, Inc., 1994:1250, $175.00.

74. Strandness DE Jr, van Breda A, editors. *Vascular Diseases. Surgical and Interventional Therapy*. New York: Churchill Livingstone, 1994:1–634 (volume 1) and 635–1270 (volume 2), $250.00.

Both the Veith and the Strandness-van Breda books are major ones, of similar length. One is priced better than the other.

75. Strandness DE Jr. *Duplex Scanning in Vascular Disorders*. Second Edition. New York: Raven Press, 1993:329, $95.00.

76. Lindsay J Jr. *Diseases of the Aorta*. Philadelphia: Lea & Febiger, 1994:315, $75.00.

ANNUAL REVIEWS

77. Schlant RC, Editor-in-Chief; Collins JJ Jr, Engle MA, Gersh BJ, Kaplan NM, Waldo AL, editors. *1993 The Year Book of CARDIOLOGY®*. St. Louis: Mosby, 1993:502, $59.95.

78. Roberts WC, Willerson JT, Rackley CE, Graham TP Jr, Mason DT. *CARDIOLOGY 1993*. Boston: Butterworth-Heineman, 1993:490, $90.00.

The Schlant book is the 33rd in its series. It contains summaries of 337 articles, most published in 1992 but some in 1991, and an editor provides comments on the publisher-written summaries. Additionally, 11 tables and 97 figures are included. The Roberts book contains summaries of 758 articles all published in 1992 plus 122 figures and 34 tables. I obviously prefer the latter book.

79. Frohlich ED, Kotchen TA, editors. *Advances in Hypertension 1993*. Philadelphia: J.B. Lippincott Company, 1993:438, $65.00.

This book contains 475 abstracts of articles on systemic hypertension. Most of the articles were published in 1991. Each abstract is followed by comments from 1 of the 13 contributors.

CARDIOLOGIC HISTORY

80. Favaloro RG. *The Challenging Dream of Heart Surgery From the Pampas to Cleveland*. Boston: Little, Brown and Company, 1994:167, $24.95.

An autobiography by the surgeon who started the aorto-coronary bypass operation is most appropriate. A wonderful story.

81. Roberts CS. *Life and Writings of Steward R. Roberts, M.C., Georgia's First Heart Specialist*. Spartanburg, South Carolina: The Reprint Company Publishers, 1993:138, $12.95.

This book on my father was written by my son. Obviously, I am proud of both of them.

COMMENTS

This annual book column first appeared in December 1985, and it briefly described 16 books, 4 of which had a 1984 publication date, 7 of which had a 1985 date, and 5 of which had a 1986 date; 9 were edited with multiple contributors, and 7 had only one to three authors. The costs of the books ranged from $37.50 to $150.00 (mean, $77.00), and none were published on acid-free paper. Of the 81 books appearing in 1993, 53 (65%) had a 1993 publication date and 28 (35%) had a 1994 date; of the 73 nonhistoric books intended exclusively for physicians, 56 (77%) were multiauthored (>10 contributors), 9 (12%) had two to five authors, and only 8 (11%) had a single author. The costs of the 72 medical books (the 6 books [numbers 10, 51, 52, 53, 54, and 57] intended for the lay public were excluded, as was 1 book [number 68], which is free of charge, and the 2 historic books [numbers 80 and 81]) ranged from $27.00 to $275.00 (mean, $111.00), and 24 (30%) (numbers 11, 12, 13, 19, 21, 28, 30, 32, 33, 39, 40, 41, 41, 48, 49, 55, 61, 63, 64, 65, 66, 67, 78, and 81) were published on acid-free paper. Of the 71 medical books briefly mentioned in this column 1 year ago, only 9 (13%) were published on acid-free, that is, permanent paper; so progress is being made. It is time for all American book publishers to use permanent paper. I encourage all authors to require in their book contracts that the paper used for their books be acid free.

William Clifford Roberts, MD
Editor in Chief

Reprinted from the January 1 issue of **The American Journal of Cardiology,** A Yorke Medical Journal, Published by Cahners Publishing Company, a Division of Reed Publishing USA, 249 West 17th Street, New York, N.Y., 10011. Copyright 1994. All rights reserved. Printed in the U.S.A.

References

1. Corey GR, Campbell PT, Van Trigt P, et al: Etiology of large pericardial effusions. Am J Med 1993 (Aug);95:209–213.
2. Ziskind AA, Pearce AC, Lemmon CC, et al: Percutaneous balloon pericardiotomy for the treatment of cardiac tamponade and large pericardial effusions: Description of technique and report of the first 50 cases. J Am Coll Cardiol 1993 (Jan);21:1–5.
3. OH JK, Hatle LK, Mulvagh SL, et al: Transient constrictive pericarditis: Diagnosis by two-dimensional Doppler echocardiography. Mayo Clin Proc 1993 (Dec);68:1158–1164.
4. Kubo SH, Ormaza SM, Francis GS, et al: Trends in patient selection for heart transplantation. J Am Coll Cardiol 1993 (March 15);21:975–981.
5. Stoddard MF, Longaker RA: The role of transesophageal echocardiography in cardiac donor screening. Am Heart J 1993 (June);125:1676–1681.
6. Murali S, Kormos RL, Uretsky BF, et al: Preoperative pulmonary hemodynamics and early mortality after orthotopic cardiac transplantation: The Pittsburgh experience. Am Heart J 1993 (Oct);126:896–904.
7. Griffith BP, Hardesty RL, Armitage JM, et al: A decade of lung transplantation. Ann Surg 1993;218:310–320.
8. Pflugfelder PW, Boughner DR, Rudas L, et al: Enhanced detection of cardiac allograft arterial disease with intracoronary ultrasonographic imaging. Am Heart J 1993 (June);125:1583–1591.
9. Ventura HO, White CJ, Jain SP, et al: Assessment of intracoronary morphology in cardiac transplant recipients by angioscopy and intravascular ultrasound. Am J Cardiol 1993 (Oct 1);72:805–809.
10. Schroeder JS, Gao S-Z, Alderman EL, et al: A preliminary study of diltiazem in the prevention of coronary artery disease in heart-transplant recipients. N Engl J Med 1993 (Jan 21);328:164–170.
11. Livi U, Luciani GB, Boffa GM, et al: Clinical results of steroid-free induction immunosuppression after heart transplantation. Ann Thorac Surg 1993;55:1160–1165.

12. Arabia FA, Rosado LJ, Huston CL, et al: Incidence and recurrence of gastrointestinal cytomegalovirus infection in heart transplantation. Ann Thorac Surg 1993;55:8–11.
13. Opelz G, Henderson R, for the Collaborative Transplant Study: incidence of non-Hodgkin lymphoma in kidney and heart transplant recipients. Lancet 1993 (Dec 18/25);342:1514–1516.
14. Shane E, Rivas MDC, Silverberg SJ, et al: Osteoporosis after cardiac transplantation. Am J Med 1993 (March);94:257–264.
15. Erbel R, Oelert H, Meyer J, et al, for the European Cooperative Study Group on Echocardiography: Effect of medical and surgical therapy on aortic dissection evaluated by transesophageal echocardiography: Implications for prognosis and therapy. Circulation 1993 (May);87:1604–1615.
16. Nihoyannopoulos P, Joshi J, Athanasopoulos G, et al: Detection of atherosclerotic lesions in the aorta by transesophageal echocardiography. Am J Cardiol 1993 (May 15);71:1208–1212.
17. Eisenberg MJ, Rice SA, Paraschos A, et al: The clinical spectrum of patients with aneurysms of the ascending aorta. Am Heart J 1993 (May);125:1381–1385.
18. Frame PS, Fryback DG, Patterson C: Cost-effectiveness of screening for abdominal aortic aneurysm in men ages 60–80 years. Ann Intern Med 1993 (Sep 1);1119:411–416.
19. Scott RAP, Wilson NM, Ashton HA, et al: Usefulness of operative resection of abdominal aortic aneurysm less than 6 cm in diameter. Lancet 1993 (Dec 4);342:1395–1396.
20. Regensteiner JG, Wolfel EE, Brass EP, et al: Chronic changes in skeletal muscle histology and function in peripheral arterial disease. Circulation 1993 (Feb);87:413–421.
21. Tunis SR, Bass EB, Klag MJ, et al: Variation in utilization of procedures for treatment of peripheral arterial disease. Arch Intern Med 1993 (April 26);153:991–998.
22. Ernst E, Fialka V: A review of the clinical effectiveness of exercise therapy for intermittent claudication. Arch Intern Med 1993 (Oct 25);153:2357–2360.
23. Siegel RJ, Gaines P, Crew JR, et al: Clinical trial of percutaneous peripheral ultrasound angioplasty. J Am Coll Cardiol 1993 (Aug);22:480–488.
24. Bedarida GV, Kim D, Blaschke TF, et al: Venodilation in Raynaud's disease. Lancet 1993 (Dec 11);342:1451–1454.
25. Ranke C, Hecker H, Creutzig A, et al: Dose-dependent effect of aspirin on carotid atherosclerosis. Circulation 1993 (June);87:1873–1879.
26. Hobson RW, Weiss DG, Fields WS, et al: Efficacy of carotid endarterectomy for asymptomatic carotid stenosis. N Engl J Med 1993 (Jan 28);328:221–227.
27. Kugelmass AD, Oda A, Monahan K, et al: Activation of human platelets by cocaine. Circulation 1993 (Sep);88:876–883.
28. Eisenberg MJ, Mendelson J, Evans GT, et al: Left ventricular function immediately after intravenous cocaine: A quantitative two-dimensional echocardiographic study. J Am Coll Cardiol 1993 (Nov 15);22:1581–1586.
29. Zaret BL, Wackers FJ: Nuclear cardiology. N Engl J Med 1993 (Sep 9); 329:775–783 and 855–863.
30. Roberts WC: Ninety-three hearts ≥90 years of age. Am J Cardiol 1993 (March 1);71:599–602.
31. Shirani J, Roberts WC: Clinical, electrocardiographic and morphologic features of massive fatty deposits ("lipomatous hypertrophy") in the atrial septum. J Am Coll Cardiol 1993 (July);22:226–238.
32. Stoddard MF, Longaker RA: The safety of transesophageal echocardiography in the elderly. Am Heart J 1993 (May);125:1358–1362.
33. Labovitz AJ, Camp A, Castello R, et al: Usefulness of transesophageal

echocardiography in unexplained cerebral ischemia. Am J Cardiol 1993 (Dec 15);72:1448–1452.

34. Hata JS, Ayres RW, Biller J, et al: Impact of transesophageal echocardiography on the anticoagulation management of patients admitted with focal cerebral ischemia. Am J Cardiol 1993 (Sep 15);72:707–710.

35. Stoddard MF, Prince CR, Ammash N, et al: Pulsed Doppler transesophageal echocardiographic determination of cardiac output in human beings: Comparison with thermodilution technique. Am Heart J 1993 (Oct);126:956–962.

36. Schwartz SL, Gillam LD, Weingraub AR, et al: Intracardiac echocardiography in humans using a small-sized (6F), low frequency (12.5 MHz) ultrasound catheter. J Am Coll Cardiol 1993 (Jan);21:189–198.

37. Vaarala O, Alfthan G, Jauhiainen M, et al: Crossreaction between antibodies to oxidized low-density lipoprotein and to cardiolipin in systemic lupus erythematosus. Lancet 1993 (April 10);341:923–925.

38. Adams JE III, Bodor GS, Dávila-Román VG, et al: Cardiac troponin I: A marker with high specificity for cardiac injury. Circulation 1993 (July); 88:101–106.

39. Watanabe H, Kakihana M, Ohtsuka S, et al: Platelet cyclic GMP: A potentially useful indicator to evaluate the effects of nitroglycerin and nitrate tolerance. Circulation 1993 (July);88:29–36.

40. Chronos NAF, Goodall AH, Wilson DJ, et al: Profound platelet degranulation is an important side effect of some types of contrast media used in interventional cardiology. Circulation 1993 (Nov);88[part 1]:2035–2044.

41. de Swart H, Dijkman L, Hofstra L, et al: A new hemostatic puncture closure device for the immediate sealing of arterial puncture sites. Am J Cardiol 1993 (Aug 15);72:445–449.

42. Cogo A, Lensing WA, Prandoni P, et al: Distribution of thrombosis in patients with symptomatic deep vein thrombosis. Arch Intern Med 1993 (Dec 27);153:2777–2780.

43. Goldhaber SZ, Haire WD, Feldstein ML, et al: Alteplase versus heparin in acute pulmonary embolism. Lancet 1993 (Feb 1993);341:507–511.

44. Goldhaber SZ, Simons GR, Elliott CG, et al: Quantitative plasma D-dimer levels among patients undergoing pulmonary angiography for suspected pulmonary embolism. JAMA 1993 (Dec 15);270:2819–2822.

45. Inbar S, Schrader BJ, Kaufmann E, et al: Effects of adenosine in combination with calcium channel blockers in patients with primary pulmonary hypertention. J Am Coll Cardiol 1993 (Feb);21(2):413–418.

46. Gupta S, Dev V, Kumar V, et al: Left ventricular diastolic function in end-stage renal disease and the impact of hemodialysis. Am J Cardiol 1993 (June 15);71:1427–1430.

47. Roberts WC: The best hospitals in the USA for patients with heart disease. Am J Cardiol 1993 (Sep 1);72:626–627.

48. The Task Force from the Association of Professors of Cardiology: Structure and function of academic divisions of cardiology. Arch Intern Med 1993 (Oct 25);153:2305–2316.

49. Zaret BL, Hood WB Jr, O'Rourke RA: Cardiovascular medicine: Subspecialty or specialty. Am J Cardiol 1993 (Oct 15);72:968–970.

Index